Research of Pathogenesis and Novel Therapeutics in Arthritis

Research of Pathogenesis and Novel Therapeutics in Arthritis

Special Issue Editor

Chih-Hsin Tang

MDPI • Basel • Beijing • Wuhan • Barcelona • Belgrade

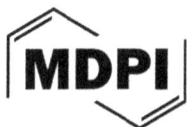

MDPI

Special Issue Editor
Chih-Hsin Tang
China Medical University
Taiwan

Editorial Office
MDPI
St. Alban-Anlage 66
4052 Basel, Switzerland

This is a reprint of articles from the Special Issue published online in the open access journal *International Journal of Molecular Sciences* (ISSN 1422-0067) from 2017 to 2019 (available at: https://www.mdpi.com/journal/ijms/special_issues/arthritis)

For citation purposes, cite each article independently as indicated on the article page online and as indicated below:

LastName, A.A.; LastName, B.B.; LastName, C.C. Article Title. *Journal Name* **Year**, *Article Number*, Page Range.

ISBN 978-3-03897-065-1 (Pbk)
ISBN 978-3-03897-066-8 (PDF)

Contents

Takahiro Makino, Hiroyuki Tsukazaki, Yuichiro Ukon, Daisuke Tateiwa, Hideki Yoshikawa
and Takashi Kaito

The Biological Enhancement of Spinal Fusion for Spinal Degenerative Disease

About the Special Issue Editor

Chih-Hsin Tang, Dr. Chih-Hsin Tang earned his PhD degree at the National Taiwan University, Taiwan, and is Professor and Dean of the Department of Research & Development, China Medical University, Taiwan. His research covers the pharmacology and pathology of arthritis, osteoporosis, bone tumors, and tumor metastasis to bone. He is a member of AACR, ASBMR, and the Pharmacological Society in Taiwan, Editorial Board member in five journals and an ad hoc reviewer for many journals. He has authored 290 articles and 8 reviews.

International Journal of
Molecular Sciences

MDPI

Editorial

Research of Pathogenesis and Novel Therapeutics in Arthritis

Chih-Hsin Tang [1,2,3]

[1] Department of Pharmacology, School of Medicine, China Medical University, Taichung 40402, Taiwan;
chtang@mail.cmu.edu.tw; Tel.: +886-22052121 (ext. 7726); Fax: +886-4-22333641
[2] Chinese Medicine Research Center, China Medical University, Taichung 40402, Taiwan
[3] Department of Biotechnology, College of Health Science, Asia University, Taichung 41354, Taiwan

Received: 29 March 2019; Accepted: 1 April 2019; Published: 2 April 2019

check for updates

Abstract: Arthritis has a high prevalence globally and includes over 100 types, the most common of which are rheumatoid arthritis, osteoarthritis, psoriatic arthritis and inflammatory arthritis. The exact etiology of arthritis remains unclear and no cure exists. Anti-inflammatory drugs are commonly used in the treatment of arthritis, but are associated with significant side effects. Novel modes of therapy and additional prognostic biomarkers are urgently needed for these patients. In this editorial, the twenty articles published in the Special Issue Research of Pathogenesis and Novel Therapeutics in Arthritis 2019 are summarized and discussed as part of the global picture of the current understanding of arthritis.

Keywords: rheumatoid arthritis; osteoarthritis; anti-arthritis; biomarkers

---

Arthritis has a high prevalence globally and includes over 100 types, the most common of which are rheumatoid arthritis (RA), osteoarthritis (OA), psoriatic arthritis and inflammatory arthritis. All types of arthritis share common features of disease, including monocyte infiltration, inflammation, synovial swelling, pannus formation, stiffness in the joints and articular cartilage destruction. The exact etiology of arthritis remains unclear and no cure exists. Anti-inflammatory drugs are commonly used in the treatment of arthritis, but are associated with significant side effects, such as gastric bleeding, an increased risk for heart attacks and other cardiovascular problems. Novel modes of therapy and additional prognostic biomarkers are urgently needed for these patients.

In response to the call for papers, we received many submissions from all over the world. After an initial screening, we selected 20 articles that are appropriate for this Special Issue. All manuscripts underwent a very rigorous peer-review process. The papers included in this issue can be broadly organized into three main categories: (i) the pathogenesis of arthritis, (ii) new biomarkers and (iii) novel strategies in the treatment of arthritis.

(i) Pathogenesis of arthritis. The important role of angiogenesis in arthritis progression has been summarized by MacDonald et al. [1]. The same research team has also summarized the critical role played by adipokines in cartilage and bone homeostasis in the pathogenesis of RA and OA, which has important implications for obesity [2]. The involvement of growth factors, inflammatory cytokines and differential miRNA expression in synovial tissue, articular cartilage and subchondral bone during the onset and progression of OA has been summarized by two research groups [3,4], while another research team has reviewed how the Epstein–Barr virus (EBV) is able to induce the onset of RA in predisposed shared epitope (SE)-positive individuals, by promoting entry of B-cells through direct contact between SE and gp42 in the entry complex [5]. An interesting article from Polish researchers reviews the evidence on the role of mesenchymal stromal cells in the pathogenesis of spondyloarthropathies (SpA) and discusses the potential use of stem cells in regenerative processes and the treatment of inflammatory changes in articular structures [6].

(ii) New biomarkers. Dudics et al. examined the miRNA expression profiles of immune cells from arthritic Lewis rats and arthritic rats treated with celastrol, a natural triterpenoid [7]. Their results indicate that several miRNAs may serve as novel biomarkers of disease activity and therapeutic response in autoimmune arthritis. Another article, by Chen et al., has explored the differential expression of novel miRNAs in RA osteoblasts [8]. The findings suggest that certain candidate genes may help in the evaluation of therapies targeting chemotaxis and neovascularization in an effort to control joint destruction in RA.

(iii) Novel strategies in the treatment of arthritis. Liu et al. describe the synthetization of an analogue, 6-(2,4-difluorophenyl)-3-(3-(trifluoromethyl)phenyl)-2H-benzo[e][1,3]oxazine-2,4(3H)-dione (Cf-02), which shares structural similarity with quercetin, a potent anti-inflammatory flavonoid present in many different fruits and vegetables [9]. Cf-02 was shown to suppress inflammation and cartilage damage. The methodology used by this research team shows considerable promise for the identification of candidate disease-modifying immunomodulatory drugs and lead compounds for arthritis therapies.

Tsai et al. have found that a natural diterpene compound, sclareol, inhibits the release of inflammatory cytokines (TNF-α and IL-6) in synovial fibroblasts and alleviates the severity of arthritis in an experimental model of RA, collagen-induced arthritis (CIA) [10], while the article by Jung et al. indicates that the active component of the herb *Dictamnus dasycarpus*, fraxinellone, alleviates synovial inflammation and osteoclastogenesis in CIA mice [11]. As for OA, Valenti et al. suggest that the bisphosphonate clodronate, already used in the treatment of osteoporosis, may prove to be a good therapeutic tool against OA [12].

Investigations by Wu et al. into the relationship between visfatin (a proinflammatory adipokine) and the expression of IL-6 and TNF-α describe how visfatin promotes their production in human synovial fibroblasts [13]. Another paper provides insight into the mechanism of crosstalk between IL-1β and WNT signaling in primary human chondrocytes, describing the pivotal roles played by inducible nitric oxide synthase (iNOS) and NO in in OA pathogenesis [14]. The evidence from these papers suggests that visfatin and iNOS/NO are novel therapeutic targets in arthritis.

Talotta et al. evaluated changes in percentages of T helper 9 (Th9) cells in response to an in vitro simulation assay that examined the immunogenicity of the infliximab originator (Remicade®) and its biosimilar compound (Remsima®), using peripheral blood mononuclear cells from a cohort of RA patients classified as infliximab responders or inadequate responders [15]. Their findings provide insights into the association between levels of Th9 cells, clinicopathological features of the patient cohort, their use of concomitant methotrexate and steroidal drugs, and the outcome of infliximab therapy.

Chen et al. summarize the current understanding of the immunopathogenic mechanisms underlying RA disease, which has led to the emergence of increasingly novel biologic agents for the treatment of RA [16]. Another article discusses the structural biology of TNF-α antagonists, including etanercept (Enbrel®), infliximab (Remicade®), adalimumab (Humira®), certolizumab-pegol (Cimzia®) and golimumab (Simponi®), all of which are used in the treatment of RA [17]. A review by Nandakumar suggests that it is worthwhile targeting pathogenic IgG molecules in arthritis through the process of glyco-engineering, using bacterial enzymes to specifically cleave IgG/alter N-linked Fc-glycans at Asn 297, or by blocking the downstream effector pathways; these techniques offer new avenues for developing novel therapeutics for arthritis treatment [18]. On this theme, one of the articles in this Special Issue details the potent pharmacodynamic effects, toxicity, and clinical translation of triptolide, a major extract of the herb *Tripterygium wilfordii* Hook F (TWHF), in RA treatment [19]. Makino et al. look to the future with their review of the evidence on novel biological enhancement strategies for spinal degenerative disease [20].

We hope that this collection of research will provide new impetus and directions for all those who are interested in the development of novel prevention and treatment strategies for arthritis.

Conflicts of Interest: The author declares no conflict of interest.

References

1. MacDonald, I.J.; Liu, S.C.; Su, C.M.; Wang, Y.H.; Tsai, C.H.; Tang, C.H. Implications of angiogenesis involvement in arthritis. *Int. J. Mol. Sci.* **2018**, *19*, 2012. [CrossRef] [PubMed]
2. MacDonald, I.J.; Liu, S.C.; Huang, C.C.; Kuo, S.J.; Tsai, C.H.; Tang, C.H. Associations between Adipokines in Arthritic Disease and Implications for Obesity. *Int. J. Mol. Sci.* **2019**, *20*, 1505. [CrossRef] [PubMed]
3. Boehme, K.A.; Rolauffs, B. Onset and progression of human osteoarthritis-can growth factors, inflammatory cytokines, or differential mirna expression concomitantly induce proliferation, ecm degradation, and inflammation in articular cartilage? *Int. J. Mol. Sci.* **2018**, *19*, 2282. [CrossRef] [PubMed]
4. Kim, J.R.; Yoo, J.J.; Kim, H.A. Therapeutics in osteoarthritis based on an understanding of its molecular pathogenesis. *Int. J. Mol. Sci.* **2018**, *19*, 674. [CrossRef] [PubMed]
5. Trier, N.; Izarzugaza, J.; Chailyan, A.; Marcatili, P.; Houen, G. Human mhc-ii with shared epitope motifs are optimal epstein-barr virus glycoprotein 42 ligands-relation to rheumatoid arthritis. *Int. J. Mol. Sci.* **2018**, *19*, 317. [CrossRef] [PubMed]
6. Krajewska-Wlodarczyk, M.; Owczarczyk-Saczonek, A.; Placek, W.; Osowski, A.; Engelgardt, P.; Wojtkiewicz, J. Role of stem cells in pathophysiology and therapy of spondyloarthropathies-new therapeutic possibilities? *Int. J. Mol. Sci.* **2017**, *19*, 80. [CrossRef] [PubMed]
7. Dudics, S.; Venkatesha, S.H.; Moudgil, K.D. The micro-rna expression profiles of autoimmune arthritis reveal novel biomarkers of the disease and therapeutic response. *Int. J. Mol. Sci.* **2018**, *19*, 2293. [CrossRef] [PubMed]
8. Chen, Y.J.; Chang, W.A.; Hsu, Y.L.; Chen, C.H.; Kuo, P.L. Deduction of novel genes potentially involved in osteoblasts of rheumatoid arthritis using next-generation sequencing and bioinformatic approaches. *Int. J. Mol. Sci.* **2017**, *18*, 2396. [CrossRef] [PubMed]
9. Liu, F.C.; Lu, J.W.; Chien, C.Y.; Huang, H.S.; Lee, C.C.; Lien, S.B.; Lin, L.C.; Chen, L.W.; Ho, Y.J.; Shen, M.C.; et al. Arthroprotective effects of cf-02 sharing structural similarity with quercetin. *Int. J. Mol. Sci.* **2018**, *19*, 1453. [CrossRef] [PubMed]
10. Tsai, S.W.; Hsieh, M.C.; Li, S.; Lin, S.C.; Wang, S.P.; Lehman, C.W.; Lien, C.Z.; Lin, C.C. Therapeutic potential of sclareol in experimental models of rheumatoid arthritis. *Int. J. Mol. Sci.* **2018**, *19*, 1351. [CrossRef] [PubMed]
11. Jung, S.M.; Lee, J.; Baek, S.Y.; Lee, J.; Jang, S.G.; Hong, S.M.; Park, J.S.; Cho, M.L.; Park, S.H.; Kwok, S.K. Fraxinellone attenuates rheumatoid inflammation in mice. *Int. J. Mol. Sci.* **2018**, *19*, 829. [CrossRef] [PubMed]
12. Valenti, M.T.; Mottes, M.; Biotti, A.; Perduca, M.; Pisani, A.; Bovi, M.; Deiana, M.; Cheri, S.; Dalle Carbonare, L. Clodronate as a therapeutic strategy against osteoarthritis. *Int. J. Mol. Sci.* **2017**, *18*, 2696. [CrossRef] [PubMed]
13. Wu, M.H.; Tsai, C.H.; Huang, Y.L.; Fong, Y.C.; Tang, C.H. Visfatin promotes il-6 and tnf-alpha production in human synovial fibroblasts by repressing mir-199a-5p through erk, p38 and jnk signaling pathways. *Int. J. Mol. Sci.* **2018**, *19*, 190. [CrossRef] [PubMed]
14. Zhong, L.; Schivo, S.; Huang, X.; Leijten, J.; Karperien, M.; Post, J.N. Nitric oxide mediates crosstalk between interleukin 1beta and wnt signaling in primary human chondrocytes by reducing dkk1 and frzb expression. *Int. J. Mol. Sci.* **2017**, *18*, 2491. [CrossRef] [PubMed]
15. Talotta, R.; Berzi, A.; Doria, A.; Batticciotto, A.; Ditto, M.C.; Atzeni, F.; Sarzi-Puttini, P.; Trabattoni, D. The immunogenicity of branded and biosimilar infliximab in rheumatoid arthritis according to th9-related responses. *Int. J. Mol. Sci.* **2017**, *18*, 2127. [CrossRef] [PubMed]
16. Chen, S.J.; Lin, G.J.; Chen, J.W.; Wang, K.C.; Tien, C.H.; Hu, C.F.; Chang, C.N.; Hsu, W.F.; Fan, H.C.; Sytwu, H.K. Immunopathogenic mechanisms and novel immune-modulated therapies in rheumatoid arthritis. *Int. J. Mol. Sci.* **2019**, *20*, 1332. [CrossRef] [PubMed]
17. Lim, H.; Lee, S.H.; Lee, H.T.; Lee, J.U.; Son, J.Y.; Shin, W.; Heo, Y.S. Structural biology of the tnfalpha antagonists used in the treatment of rheumatoid arthritis. *Int. J. Mol. Sci.* **2018**, *19*, 768. [CrossRef] [PubMed]

18. Nandakumar, K.S. Targeting igg in arthritis: Disease pathways and therapeutic avenues. *Int. J. Mol. Sci.* **2018**, *19*, 677. [CrossRef] [PubMed]

19. Fan, D.; Guo, Q.; Shen, J.; Zheng, K.; Lu, C.; Zhang, G.; Lu, A.; He, X. The effect of triptolide in rheumatoid arthritis: From basic research towards clinical translation. *Int. J. Mol. Sci.* **2018**, *19*, 376. [CrossRef] [PubMed]

20. Makino, T.; Tsukazaki, H.; Ukon, Y.; Tateiwa, D.; Yoshikawa, H.; Kaito, T. The biological enhancement of spinal fusion for spinal degenerative disease. *Int. J. Mol. Sci.* **2018**, *19*, 2430. [CrossRef] [PubMed]

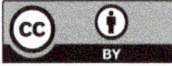

International Journal of
Molecular Sciences

MDPI

Review

Implications of Angiogenesis Involvement in Arthritis

Iona J. MacDonald [1], Shan-Chi Liu [1,2], Chen-Ming Su [3], Yu-Han Wang [4], Chun-Hao Tsai [2,5] and Chih-Hsin Tang [1,5,6,7,*]

[1] Graduate Institute of Basic Medical Science, China Medical University, Taichung 40402, Taiwan; ionamac@gmail.com (I.J.M.); sdsaw.tw@yahoo.com.tw (S.-C.L.)

[2] Department of Orthopedic Surgery, China Medical University Hospital, Taichung 40447, Taiwan; ritsai8615@gmail.com

[3] Department of Biomedical Sciences Laboratory, Wenzhou Medical University, Dongyang 325035, Zhejiang, China; proof814@gmail.com

[4] Graduate Institute of Biomedical Science, China Medical University, Taichung 40402, Taiwan; laecy0313@gmail.com

[5] School of Medicine, China Medical University, Taichung 40402, Taiwan

[6] Chinese Medicine Research Center, China Medical University, Taichung 40402, Taiwan

[7] Department of Biotechnology, College of Health Science, Asia University, Taichung 41354, Taiwan

[*] Correspondence: chtang@mail.cmu.edu.tw; Tel.: +886-04-2205-2121 (ext. 7726)

Received: 31 May 2018; Accepted: 8 July 2018; Published: 10 July 2018

check for
updates

Abstract: Angiogenesis, the growth of new blood vessels, is essential in the pathogenesis of joint inflammatory disorders such as rheumatoid arthritis (RA) and osteoarthritis (OA), facilitating the invasion of inflammatory cells and increase in local pain receptors that contribute to structural damage and pain. The angiogenic process is perpetuated by various mediators such as growth factors, primarily vascular endothelial growth factor (VEGF) and hypoxia-inducible factors (HIFs), as well as proinflammatory cytokines, various chemokines, matrix components, cell adhesion molecules, proteases, and others. Despite the development of potent, well-tolerated nonbiologic (conventional) and biologic disease-modifying agents that have greatly improved outcomes for patients with RA, many remain resistant to these therapies, are only partial responders, or cannot tolerate biologics. The only approved therapies for OA include symptom-modifying agents, such as analgesics, non-steroidal anti-inflammatory drugs (NSAIDs), steroids, and hyaluronic acid. None of the available treatments slow the disease progression, restore the original structure or enable a return to function of the damaged joint. Moreover, a number of safety concerns surround current therapies for RA and OA. New treatments are needed that not only target inflamed joints and control articular inflammation in RA and OA, but also selectively inhibit synovial angiogenesis, while preventing healthy tissue damage. This narrative review of the literature in PubMed focuses on the evidence illustrating the therapeutic benefits of modulating angiogenic activity in experimental RA and OA. This evidence points to new treatment targets in these diseases.

Keywords: rheumatoid arthritis; osteoarthritis; angiogenesis; cytokines; chemokines

1. Introduction

Angiogenesis, the formation of new capillaries from pre-existing vessels, is one of the earliest histopathologic findings in chronic, non-infectious arthritis and is a potential target for therapeutic intervention. The most common forms of chronic, non-infectious arthritis are rheumatoid arthritis (RA) and osteoarthritis (OA). The development of potent, well-tolerated non-biologic (conventional), and biologic disease-modifying agents used alone and in combination to induce and maintain tight control of disease have greatly improved outcomes for patients with RA, but treatment resistance is common or patients achieve only partial responses [1]. Moreover, few treated RA patients achieve sustained remission, so require ongoing pharmacologic therapy [1]. For OA, the only approved therapies include symptom-modifying agents, such as analgesics, non-steroidal anti-inflammatory drugs (NSAIDs), steroids, and hyaluronic acid [2,3]. None of the available treatments slow the disease progression, or restore the original structure and function of the damaged joint [2,3]. Joint replacement surgery is considered to be the definitive treatment for alleviating pain and restoring function [3]. New treatments are needed that not only target inflamed joints and control articular inflammation in RA and OA, but also selectively inhibit angiogenesis, while preventing healthy tissue damage. This article discusses the current therapeutic situation in RA and OA, and focuses on future strategies that look very promising for the management of angiogenesis in these diseases. The literature consulted for this Review is ordered by topics discussed in Table 1 (RA) and Table 2 (OA).

2. Rheumatoid Arthritis

Conventional synthetic disease-modifying anti-rheumatic drugs (csDMARDs) such as methotrexate have long been the mainstay of treatment for RA [4]. However, these treatments fail to slow radiographic progression, with the exception of antimalarials, and safety issues have necessitated additional treatment strategies [4]. An improved understanding of the immunological pathway mediating RA has revealed that pro-inflammatory cytokines such as tumor necrosis factor alpha (TNF-α), interleukin (IL)-1, and IL-6 play a key role in the pathogenesis of RA [4,5]. The development of biologic DMARDs (bDMARDs) that target these cytokine pathways and mediators in the inflammatory cascade has improved outcomes for patients with RA. Compared with the traditional DMARDs, bDMARDs have a more rapid onset of action and are associated with sustained and clinically significant suppression of signs and symptoms, as well as inhibition of joint damage [4,6]. In general, their methods of action are also more directed, defined and targeted, compared with traditional DMARDs.

Together with bDMARD therapies, the introduction of early treatment initiation and the treat-to-target principle have helped to transform the management of RA and many patients achieve clinical remission early in the disease course, although this is not possible for all patients. The level of clinical response and efficacy of bDMARDs differ amongst individual patients [7]. An additional complication with bDMARD therapies is that they are typically given as injectable formulations, which poses a significant burden on health systems worldwide and may severely compromise treatment compliance where patients must travel long distances to access health centers [8]. The majority of patients with RA would prefer oral treatment to an injection or intravenous infusion [9]. Better personalized treatment algorithms are called for that achieve rapid remission in all patients, preventing disability, restoring and maintaining quality of life, without unwanted toxicity [8]. The more that is understood about the disease process in RA, the better.

Angiogenesis is essential for the expansion of synovial tissue in RA: pre-existing vessels facilitate the entry of blood-derived leukocytes into the synovial sublining, to generate and potentiate inflammation. Several steps are involved in angiogenesis, each of which is modulated by specific factors [10]. The process starts with growth factors such as vascular endothelial growth factor (VEGF) and fibroblast growth factor (FGF) binding to their cognate receptors on endothelial cells (ECs) and activation of these cells to produce proteolytic enzymes. Subsequently, the basement membrane is degraded by matrix metalloproteinases (MMPs), leading to migration and further endothelial proliferation to vascular tubules that are in part developed by adhesion molecules such as integrins. Lastly, blood vessels are stabilized by pro-angiogenic factors such as Ang1, followed by incorporation of pericytes into the newly formed basement membrane to facilitate the blood flow process (see Figure 1).

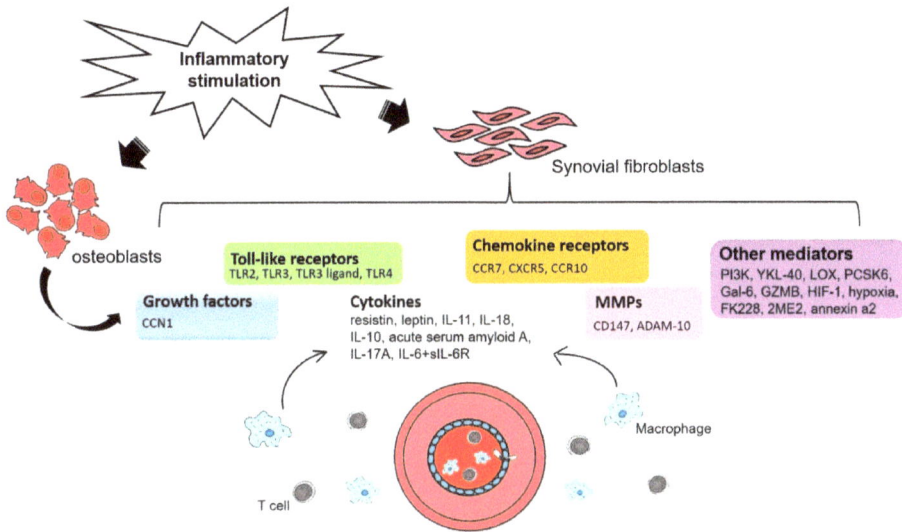

Figure 1. An illustration of the proinflammatory process underlying rheumatoid arthritis (RA) angiogenesis in synovial fluid. Inflammatory stimulation activates RA osteoblasts and synovial fibroblasts that in turn modulate the expression of growth factors, Toll-like receptors, chemokine receptors, cytokines, matrix metalloproteinases (MMPs) and other mediators that are involved at different stages of angiogenesis. Recruitment of macrophages and T cells from the blood into the inflammatory process ensure the maintenance and progression of angiogenesis.

3. The Involvement of Toll-Like Receptors in RA Disease

Toll-like receptors (TLRs), a family of germline-encoded type I trans-membrane proteins, enable the innate immune system to recognize pathogen-associated molecular patterns [11]. High levels of TLR2, TLR3, TLR4, and TLR7 expression have been found in the RA synovium; TLR3 is highly expressed in fibroblast-like synoviocytes (FLS), while TLR2 and TLR4 expression is increased in the perivascular regions of the joint, at the sites of attachment and invasion into cartilage/bone, and on synovial macrophages [11,12]. In vitro and ex vivo studies have investigated the roles of TLR2 and TLR3 in RA pathogenesis.

Evidence indicates that the activation of TLR3 in RA FLS increases VEGF and IL-8 production and upregulates the genes for these proteins at the transcriptional level after stimulation of FLS with the TLR3 ligand, a polyinosinic-polycytidylic acid (poly(I:C)) [11]. Treatment with the nuclear factor-kappa B (NF-κB) inhibitors, pyrrolidine dithiocarbamate and parthenolide, abrogated the stimulatory effect of poly(I:C) on the production of VEGF and IL-8 in RA FLS, which suggests that targeting the NF-κB signaling pathway may prevent the upregulation of pro-angiogenic molecules in RA FLS [11].

Another study used RA whole-tissue synovial membrane explants to demonstrate that TLR2 activation induces angiogenic tube formation and angiopoietin-2 (Ang2) expression, EC invasion and migration, as well as increased MMP-2 and MMP-9 expression by RA synovial explants [12]. These effects were inhibited by Tie2 receptor blockade, suggesting that TLR2-induced angiogenic processes are in part mediated through the Tie2 pathway.

4. Vasohibin-1 mRNA Expression in RA Synovial Fibroblasts

In vitro investigations have shown that expression of vasohibin-1, a novel endothelium-derived VEGF-inducible angiogenesis inhibitor, correlates significantly with histological inflammation score ($r = 0.842$; $p = 0.002$) [13]. Those researchers also found that stimulation with VEGF induced the expression of vasohibin-1 mRNA in RA synovial fibroblasts (RASFs) under normoxic conditions, while stimulation with cytokines TNF-α and IL-1β induced vasohibin-1 mRNA expression under a hypoxic condition (1% O_2).

Japanese researchers have suggested that histone deacetylase (HDAC) inhibitors may help to suppress angiogenesis-related factors in RA synovial tissue [14]. They stimulated RASFs with TNF-α and IL-1β then incubated them under hypoxic conditions (1% O_2) with different concentrations of FK228, a specific HDAC inhibitor. FK228 dose-dependently down-regulated the expression of hypoxia-inducible factor-1 alpha (HIF-1α) and VEGF mRNA. FK228 also reduced the levels of HIF-1α and VEGF protein in the RASFs. Intravenous administration of FK228 (2.5 mg/kg) suppressed VEGF expression and inhibited angiogenesis in synovial tissue analyzed from mice with collagen-induced arthritis (CIA), a frequently used autoimmune animal model in the study of RA, as the signs of disease resemble features of human inflammatory arthritis and thus enable investigators to test hypothetical mechanisms of immune-mediated joint disease and examine the comparative efficacy of pending RA therapies during preclinical development.

The findings from the Japanese researchers are extended by in vivo research demonstrating anti-angiogenic and anti-proliferative activity with 2-methoxyestradiol (2ME2) in the rat CIA model [15]. In preventive protocols, 2ME2 significantly inhibited the onset and reduced the severity of clinical and radiographic CIA. In established CIA, oral 2ME2 reduced disease severity compared with vehicle-treated controls.

5. Cytokines Show Angiogenic Activity

An in vitro investigation has reported angiogenic activity with IL-6 plus soluble IL-6 receptor (sIL-6R) in RA FLS co-cultured with human umbilical vein endothelial cells (HUVECs) [16]. Interestingly, whereas IL-6/sIL-6R complex induced tubule formation and augmented VEGF production in the co-culture system, IL-6 alone had no such effects. IL-6/sIL-6R-induced tubule formation was abolished by the addition of either anti-IL-6R or anti-VEGF antibody. Unlike IL-6/sIL-6R, TNF-α did not induce tubule formation; instead, TNF-α reduced the CD31-positive area compared with RA FLS co-cultured with HUVECs without cytokine augmentation (control).

IL-17A has been found to induce human dermal endothelial cell (HDEC) tube-like structures and extracellular matrix (ECM) invasion, and significantly increase the secretion of chemokines (growth-related oncogene-alpha (GRO-α) and monocyte chemotactic protein-1 (MCP-1)) from RASFs [17]. The same researchers also reported IL-17A induced migration of RASFs, HDECs, and mononuclear cells, which was blocked by anti-GRO-α or anti-MCP-1 antibodies. Interestingly, the studies showed that IL-17A differentially regulated $\alpha v\beta 3$ and $\alpha v\beta 1$ integrin expression, and induced cytoskeletal rearrangement and upregulation of active Rac1, key markers in angiogenic vascular morphology and cell migration.

It may be worthwhile targeting IL-18 or its signaling intermediaries in RA, according to a study confirming IL-18-induced angiogenesis in RA synovial tissue engrafted in severe combined immune-deficient (SCID) mice [18]. In that study, IL-18-induced human microvascular EC (HMVEC) chemotaxis, tube formation, and angiogenesis in Matrigel plugs was blocked by Src and c-Jun N-terminal kinase (JNK) inhibitors, whereas inhibitors of Janus kinase 2 (JAK2), p38, MEK, phosphatidylinositol-3-kinase (PI3K) and neutralizing antibodies to VEGF or stromal-derived factor-1α did not alter IL-18-induced HMVEC migration. The study researchers also report that IL-18 induced Src and JNK phosphorylation in HMVECs.

An in vitro investigation into the mechanism whereby IL-18 contributes to excessive angiogenesis has shown that IL-18 acts synergistically with IL-10 to amplify the production of M2 macrophage (Mφ)-derived mediators like osteopontin (OPN) and thrombin, yielding the thrombin-cleaved form of OPN, which acts through integrins $\alpha 4/\alpha 9$ and augments M2 polarization of Mφ with increasing surface CD163 expression in association with morphological alteration [19]. Furthermore, CD163 appears to mediate the direct cell-cell interaction between Mφs and ECs during angiogenesis.

Other research indicates that IL-11 appears to represent a novel connection between RA joint fibroblasts and ECs, enhancing synovial fibroblast infiltration and further advancing disease severity by increasing the invasion of blood vessels into the RA pannus [20]. Blocking IL-11 impaired RASF capacity to elicit EC transmigration and tube formation.

TLR2 May Amplify the Effects of Serum Amyloid A

Serum amyloid A (A-SAA), an acute-phase protein with cytokine-like properties, promotes cell migrational mechanisms and angiogenesis critical to RA pathogenesis [21]. As that paper observes, the fact that other research has reported localization of TLR2 expression to the RA synovial lining layer and synovial macrophages is consistent with the localized expression of A-SAA, so TLR2 may play a role in the A-SAA-mediated response in RA.

Resistin may be an appropriate target in RA. Resistin promotes endothelial progenitor cell (EPC) homing into the synovium during RA angiogenesis via a signal transduction pathway involving VEGF expression in primary EPCs [22]. Others suggest that it may be useful to inhibit leptin in RA disease, as leptin promotes RA FLS migration by increasing reactive oxygen species (ROS) expression [23]. Leptin is also capable of enhancing HUVEC tube formation in a ROS/HIF-1α-dependent manner, and promoting production of VEGF and IL-6 in RA FLS. It is possible to downregulate leptin-induced ROS production with the use of TNF, IL-6 and IL-1β antagonists, and thus attenuate RA FLS migration and HUVEC tube formation.

IL-1β has been found to play an important role in chondrocyte angiogenesis. IL-1β stimulation of chondrogenic ATDC5 cells increased FGF-2 expression and promoted EPC tube formation and migration [24]. The same research group reports finding that FGF-2-neutralizing antibody abolished ATDC5-conditional medium-mediated angiogenesis in vitro, as well as its angiogenic effects in the chick chorioallantoic membrane (CAM) assay and Matrigel plug nude mice model in vivo.

6. Targeting Stromal Cells and Vascular Responses

Some evidence indicates that targeting stromal cell-derived pro-angiogenic factors and HIF transcriptional responses can reduce the contribution of fibroblasts to the chronic inflammatory response [25,26]. In one study, chronically inflamed synovial tissue from patients with RA or OA significantly enhanced myeloid cell infiltration and angiogenesis in immune-deficient mice, which was associated with increased constitutive and hypoxia-induced VEGF expression in inflammatory fibroblasts compared with healthy fibroblasts [25]. A single intra-peritoneal (IP) injection of a VEGF antagonist (bevacizumab 5 mg/kg) at the time of Matrigel injection significantly inhibited angiogenesis and myeloid cell infiltration. Similar effects were seen in mice treated with daily IP injections of a CXCL12/CXCR4 antagonist (bicyclam AMD3100 at a dose of 300 µg). Targeting HIF-1α expression by lentiviral siRNA transduction of RA fibroblasts reduced both HIF-1α accumulation and significantly reduced angiogenesis in RA fibroblasts.

Hypoxia increases the angiogenic drive of RA cells, by upregulating MMPs responsible for collagen breakdown (MMP-2, MMP-8, and MMP-9), at both mRNA and protein levels [27]. These researchers also describe how hypoxia significantly increases RA fibroblast migration across collagen and is dependent on MMP activity in an in vitro angiogenesis assay. They document increased expression of angiogenic stimuli, such as VEGF, and VEGF/placental growth factor heterodimer.

In rats with adjuvant arthritis, significantly up-regulated levels of VEGF, HIF-1α, and CD34 expression have been observed in synovial tissue [28]. Significant, positive correlations were observed between VEGF mRNA and extent of paw swelling, between HIF-1α protein and the arthritis index, while VEGF mRNA and HIF-1α protein were positively correlated with CD34. Clearly, hypoxia is closely linked to angiogenesis and inflammation in RA; angiogenesis blockade is a worthwhile therapeutic concept.

Possibilities of Stem Cell Therapy and GZMB Gene Silencing

Exogenously administered mesenchymal stromal cells (MSCs) inhibit dendritic cell maturation, promote macrophage polarization towards an anti-inflammatory phenotype and activate regulatory T cells, thereby lowering inflammation and preventing joint damage [26]. Proof-of-concept clinical studies have shown that allogeneic MSC therapy has a satisfactory safety profile and promising efficacy in the management of RA. More data are needed from larger, multicenter studies. Interestingly, when researchers explored the underlying mechanisms of human bone marrow-derived MSCs administered to mice with collagen antibody-induced arthritis (CAIA), they found that the curative effects of MSCs appear to depend on their migration into inflamed tissue, where they directly induce the differentiation of CD4$^+$ T cells into regulatory T cells, and thus suppress inflammation [29]. Such evidence supports the systemic administration of MSCs in the setting of RA.

Investigations suggest that the serine proteinase granzyme B (GZMB) may be a useful prognostic marker in early RA. In CIA rats, silencing of the *GZMB* gene helped to maintain body weight increases, reduce the degree of ankle swelling, as well as relieve RA synovial tissue hyperplasia and articular cartilage tissue injury [30]. *GZMB* gene silencing decreased inflammatory cytokine levels and also Bcl-2, cyclin D1, VEGF and basic fibroblast growth factor (bFGF) expression, while simultaneously increasing mRNA and protein levels of caspase 3.

Recent research indicates a novel role for galectin-9 (Gal-9), a mammalian lectin secreted by ECs that is highly expressed in RASFs and synovial tissues. In a series of in vitro and in vivo investigations, Gal-9 medium significantly increased HMVEC migration and tube formation on Matrigel, as well as in vivo angiogenesis, via the ERK1/2, p38, and JNK pathways [31]. Gal-9 medium also induced monocyte migration and acute inflammation when injected into C57BL/6 mouse knees, indicating a proinflammatory role for Gal-9.

7. Characterizing the Expression and Function of Chemokine Receptors in RA

CCR7 signaling is essential in the pathogenesis of RA [32]; the development of lymphoid neogenesis in RA depends on the homeostatic chemokine receptors CXCR5 and CCR7 [33]. An essential role has also been identified for CCL28, a CCR10 ligand, in RA pathogenesis. The production of CCL28 from joint myeloid and ECs strongly promotes angiogenesis in EPCs and it is now known that both CCL28 and CCR10 are involved in RASF-mediated EPC chemotaxis [34]. The same researchers have also demonstrated that CCL28 can directly mediate neovascularization by attracting CCR10$^+$ ECs. The CCL28/CCR10 cascade is a potential therapeutic target for RA. The CCL19 and CCL21 pathways also play important roles in RA angiogenesis [35].

8. Targeting the MMP Family

Inhibition of CD147 may reduce angiogenesis in RA. CD147, also known as extracellular matrix metalloproteinase inducer (EMMPRIN), is highly expressed in RA synovial tissue and triggers human synoviocytes to produce MMPs. Investigations have shown that CD147 expression is significantly and positively correlated with VEGF and HIF-1α levels, as well as with vascular density, in RA synovium [36]. When those researchers transfected RA FLS with the CD147-specific small interfering RNA (siCD147) or specific antibodies for CD147, VEGF, and HIF-1α expression was significantly decreased. In vivo findings in SCID-HuRAg mice were consistent with the in vitro findings, with both systems showing that CD147 up-regulation on RA FLS induces the up-regulation of VEGF and HIF-1α, which may further augment angiogenesis.

Another research group has suggested that the PI3K/Akt pathway may underlie CD147-induced upregulation of VEGF in U937-derived foam cells [37]. When the cell culture was transfected with CD147 stealth siRNA, the extent to which VEGF production was reduced depended on the inhibition efficiency of CD147 siRNAs. The addition of signaling pathway inhibitors LY294002, SP600125,

SB203580, and U0126 to cultures revealed that LY294002 dose-dependently inhibited the expression of VEGF. Phospho-Akt was also reduced in both the LY294002 and siRNA groups.

An investigation into the role of the cell surface metalloproteinase ADAM-10 (a disintegrin and metalloprotease 10) in RA angiogenesis has reported high levels of ADAM-10 in ECs and lining cells within RA synovial tissue compared with cells from OA and normal synovial tissue [38]. After incubation for 24 h with proinflammatory mediators phorbol myristate acetate (PMA), lipopolysaccharide (LPS), IL-17, IL-1β, or TNF-α, the researchers observed significantly elevated ADAM-10 expression at both the protein and messenger RNA levels in HMVECs and RASFs as compared with unstimulated cells. In addition, EC tube formation and migration was lower in ADAM-10 siRNA-treated HMVECs when compared with control siRNA-treated HMVECs. When untreated HMVECs, ADAM-10 siRNA-treated HMVECs, and control siRNA-treated HMVECs were co-cultured with RASFs, EC tube formation was reduced in ADAM-10 siRNA-treated HMVECs compared with control siRNA-treated HMVECs. As the researchers suggest, ADAM-10 appears to be a potential therapeutic target in RA.

9. Chinese Herbal Preparations

Scopolin isolated from *Erycibe obtusifolia* Benth stems has long been used in traditional Chinese medicine for the treatment of RA. In an adjuvant-induced arthritis (AIA) rat model, animals treated with high doses of scopolin (100 mg/kg) had higher mean body weights, near-normal histology of joint architecture and significantly reduced angiogenesis in synovial tissue compared with untreated controls [39]. The study researchers suggest that scopolin could potentially be used to treat angiogenesis-related disorders and serve as a structural base for screening more potent synthetic analogs.

Another traditional Chinese herbal compound, *Celastrus aculeatus* Merr. (*Celastrus*), has been used in China for centuries to treat rheumatoid disease. Celastraceae plants contain pristimerin, a triterpenoid quinone methide isolated from *Maytenus heterophylla*, a Kenyan medicinal plant. It appears that pristimerin has anti-angiogenic potential in RA. In AIA rats, pristimerin significantly decreased vessel density in synovial membrane tissues of inflamed joints and reduced the expression of pro-angiogenic factors TNF-α, angiopoietin 1 (Ang-1), and MMP-9 in sera [40]. Pristimerin also reduced synovial membrane expression of VEGF and phosphorylated VEGF receptor 2 (pVEGFR2), suppressed capillary sprouting in the rat aortic ring and inhibited migration of VEGF-induced RA-human fibroblast-like synoviocytes (HFLS) in vitro. Furthermore, pristimerin inhibited VEGF-induced proliferation, migration and tube formation by HUVECs, blocked the auto phosphorylation of VEGF-induced VEGFR2 and downregulated VEGFR2-mediated activation of PI3K, Akt, mTOR, ERK1/2, JNK, and p38.

10. Other Potentially Targetable Factors That Participate in RA Angiogenesis

Some evidence suggests that benzophenone analogs could have a role in ameliorating RA. Some researchers have demonstrated that commencing treatment with the synthetic benzophenone analog 2-benzoyl-phenoxy acetamide (BP-1) after the onset of disease in an AIA rat model reduced the arthritic score, paw volume and edema, the degree of inflammation and redness, as well as bone erosion, compared with untreated rats [41]. The researchers report that VEGF expression was clearly down-regulated in hypoxic ECs and AIA rats administered BP-1. Nuclear translocation of HIF-1α was also inhibited in synovium tissue after BP-1 treatment, which subsequently suppressed transcription of the *VEGF* gene.

Evidence suggests that proprotein convertase subtilisin/kexin type 6 (PCSK6) may serve as an important therapeutic target in RA. Stimulation with recombinant human (rh)PCSK6 of cultured RASFs from RA patients significantly increased RASF cell invasion, migration, and proliferation, which was influenced through both reduced cell cycle arrest and reduced apoptosis [42]. rhPCSK6 also stimulated RASFs to secrete IL-1α, IL-1β, and IL-6, and altered gene expression patterns involved in angiogenesis, hypoxia, proliferation, and inflammation. The signaling pathways involved in these cellular effects included the NF-κB, signal transducer and activator of transcription 3 (STAT3) and ERK1/2 pathways.

Other evidence points to the involvement of lysyl oxidase (LOX) in the promotion of synovial hyperplasia and angiogenesis in CIA rats [43]. In this study, the researchers identified higher amounts of rough synovial membranes, higher microvascular density in those membranes and more synovial cell layers in CIA rats compared with saline-treated controls. The CIA rats also exhibited higher LOX enzymatic activity and higher MMP-2 and MMP-9 expression levels compared with controls. Injection of CIA rats with the LOX inhibitor β-aminopropionitrile inhibited paw swelling and decreased the arthritis index, microvascular density in the synovial membranes and MMP-2 and MMP-9 expression levels. Notably, LOX expression levels in the synovial membranes were positively associated with microvascular density, as well as with levels of MMP-2 and MMP-9 expression.

Calreticulin, a multi-functional endoplasmic reticulum protein, has been found to promote RA-related angiogenesis via the activating nitric oxide (NO) signaling pathway [44]. Calreticulin concentrations were significantly higher in serum samples from RA patients than in serum samples from OA patients and healthy controls, and significantly higher in synovial fluid from RA patients than that OA patients. Calreticulin increased NO production and endothelial nitric oxide synthase (eNOS) phosphorylation in HUVECs, and promoted their proliferation, migration and tube formation. The effects of calreticulin on the proliferation, migration and morphological differentiation of HUVECs were significantly inhibited by L-NAME, a specific eNOS inhibitor.

Targeting Proinflammatory YKL-40, Cyr61/CCN1, Axna2, and Axna2R

The proinflammatory protein YKL-40, also known as human cartilage glycoprotein-39 or chitinase-3-like-1, reportedly stimulates IL-18 production in osteoblasts and facilitates EPC angiogenesis [45]. The study researchers found that this process occurs through the suppression of miR-590-3p via the focal adhesion kinase (FAK)/PI3K/Akt signaling pathway. In vivo models of angiogenesis (CAM and Matrigel plug models) confirmed that inhibition of YKL-40 reduced angiogenesis.

Recent observations report that the proinflammatory cytokine cysteine-rich 61 (Cyr61 or CCN1), a secreted protein from the CCN family, induces VEGF expression in osteoblasts and increases EPC angiogenesis in RA [46]. The evidence reveals two major mechanisms through which CCN1 stimulates EPC-dependent angiogenesis. CCN1 inhibits the microRNA miR-126, a potent VEGF inhibitor, inhibitor of angiogenesis, and tumour suppressor, via the protein kinase C-alpha (PKC-α) signaling pathway. Thus, inhibition of miR-126 indirectly stimulates angiogenesis. CCN1 also directly increases VEGF expression in and production by osteoblasts. In vitro and in vivo investigations demonstrated that angiogenesis was inhibited by CCN1 knockdown. In CIA mice injected with lentiviral vectors expressing CCN1 short hairpin RNA (Lenti-CCN1), hind paw swelling was significantly ameliorated compared with that of mice in the control group. Lenti-shCCN1 treatment was also associated with markedly lower numbers of cells positive for CCN1, EPC markers (CD34 and CD133), and vessel markers (CD31, CD144, Endomucin, and VEGF), as well as less cartilage erosion, compared with untreated CIA mice.

Annexin A2 (Axna2) and its receptor (Axna2R) are upregulated in patients with RA compared with patients with OA and healthy controls [47]. Moreover, in CIA mice, exogenous Axna2 promotes the development of arthritis, by aggravating the disease process and joint damage. Suppressing the effects of Axna2 could therefore ameliorate RA pathogenesis.

Table 1. Literature consulted for the RA section of this Review.

Stimulation	Target Factors		Effects in Tissue	Known Pathways	References
Toll-like receptors					
Toll-like receptor 3	VEGF, IL-8	↑	Synovium	NF-κB	[1]
Toll-like receptor 2	Ang2/Tie2	↑	HMVEC	Ang2/Tie2	[2]
Cytokines					
Resistin	VEGF	↑	EPC	PKC AMPK/miR-206	[2]
Leptin	VEGF, IL-8	↑	Synovium	ROS/HIF-1	[2]
IL-11	VEGF, IL-8	↑	Synovium	N/A	[10]
IL-18, IL-10	OPN	↑	M2 macrophage (Mφ)	N/A	[19]
Acute serum amyloid A			Synovium	N/A	[21]
IL-18	IL-18	↑	HMVEC	Src/JNK	[18]
IL-17A	IL-17A	↑	HDECs	N/A	[17]
IL-6/SL-IL-6R	VEGF	↑	Synovium	IL-6/SL-IL-6R	[16]
IL-1β	bFGF	↑	Cartilage	ROS/AMPK/p38/NF-κB	[34]
Chemokine receptors					
CCR7	VEGF	↑	Synovium	N/A	[32]
CCL28	CCR10	↑	Synovium and EPC	ERK1/2	[34]
CXCR5		↑	CIA model	N/A	[3]
MMPs					
CD147	VEGF, HIF-1α	↓	Synovium	PI3K/AKT/HIF-1α	[36]
ADAM-10	ADAM-10	↓	Synovium	N/A	[38]
Chinese Herbs					
Pristimerin	VEGF-A/VEGFR2	↓	Synovium	PI3K/AKT/mTOR and MAPK	[40]
Scopolin	IL-6, VEGF and FGF-2	↓	Synovium	N/A	[39]
Growth factors					
CCN1	VEGF-A	↓	Osteoblast	PKC/miR-126	[44]
VEGF	vasohibin-1	↓	Synovium	N/A	[43]
Other mediators					
YKL-40	IL-18	↑	Osteoblast	FAK/PI3K/AKT	[45]
Lysyl oxidase (LOX)	MMP-2, MMP-9	↑	Synovium	N/A	[43]
PCSK6	IL-1, IL-1, IL-6	↑	Synovium	NF-B	[42]
Galectin-9	Galectin-9	↑	HMVEC	N/A	[31]
GZMB	VEGF and bFGF	↑	CIA model	MEK/ERK	[30]
Annexin A2	VEGF, Ang2, MMP-2	↑	HUVEC	HH signaling	[47]
HIF-1α	HIF-1, VEGF, CD34	↑	Synovium	HIF-1α	[28]
Hypoxia	VEGF and MMP-2, -8, -9	↑	Synovium	N/A	[27]
FK228 (inhibitor)	HIF-1α and VEGF	↓	Synovium	HIF-1α	[14]
2ME2 (inhibitor)	VEGF and bFGF	↓	Synovium	N/A	[5]
BP-1 (inhibitor)	HIF-1α and VEGF	↓	Synovium	HIF-1α	[41]

CCN1, CCN family member 1; VEGF, Vascular endothelial growth factor; VEGF-A, Vascular endothelial growth factor A; IL-11, Interleukin 11; IL-18, Interleukin 18; IL-10, Interleukin 10; OPN, Osteopontin; IL-17A, Interleukin 17A; IL-6, Interleukin 6; SL-IL-6R, Soluble interleukin 6 receptor; CCR7, C-C chemokine receptor type 7; CD147, Basigin; HIF-1α, Hypoxia-inducible factor 1-alpha; ADAM-10, A Disintegrin and metalloproteinase domain-containing protein 10; Ang2, Angiopoietin-2; Tie2, Angiopoietin-1 (Ang1) and Ang2 receptor tyrosine kinase; YKL-40, Chitinase-3-like protein 1; MMP-2, Matrix metalloproteinase 2; MMP-8, Matrix metalloproteinase 8; MMP-9, Matrix metalloproteinase 9; PCSK6, Proprotein convertase subtilisin/kexin type 6; IL-1α, Interleukin 1 alpha; IL-1β, Interleukin 1 beta; GZMB, Granzyme B; bFGF, Basic fibroblast growth factor; CD34, Cluster of differentiation 34; N/A, Not appropriate.

11. Osteoarthritis

Inflammation in OA differs from that in RA. OA pathogenesis is characterized by chronic, low-grade inflammation within the synovial lining [48], whereas patients with RA manifest with persistent, high-grade systemic inflammation [49]. In both diseases, it is essential to halt the inflammatory process, which prevents proper repair by bone, stromal, and/or cartilage cells (see Figure 2). American College of Rheumatology (ACR), American Academy of Orthopaedic Surgeons (AAOS), and Osteoarthritis Research Society International (ORSI) guidelines recommend the use of various symptom-modifying agents for the treatment of OA, which mainly fall into five categories: acetaminophen; opioid analgesics; nonsteroidal anti-inflammatory drugs (NSAIDs); intra-articular injections (corticosteroids and hyaluronic acid); and serotonin-norepinephrine reuptake inhibitors (duloxetine) [2]. Although anti-inflammatory modalities have shown promise in in vitro and preclinical models of OA, there are currently no established United States Food and Drug Administration (US FDA)/European Medicines Agency (EMA)-approved therapies that inhibit the low-grade inflammation in this disease [2,3]. As discussed below, the emerging evidence suggests several promising avenues for pharmacologic therapies that might eventually be used to prevent or slow OA disease progression in patients.

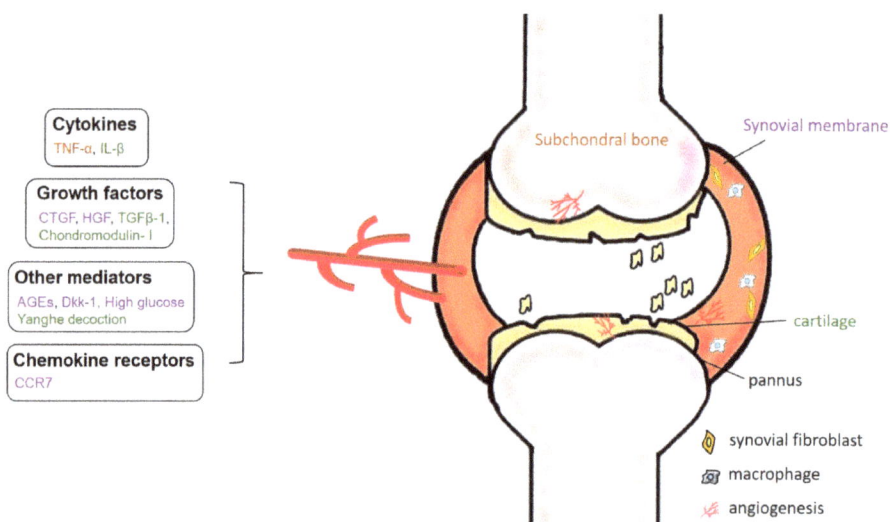

Figure 2. Specific mechanisms underlying angiogenesis in OA. Chronic, low-grade inflammation in OA is driven by increased expression of pro-angiogenic factors including chemokine receptors, cytokines, growth factors, and other mediators such as advanced glycation end-products (AGEs) and Dickkopf-1 (Dkk-1) entering the synovial fluid, enabling them to erode cartilage and subchondral bone.

12. Angiogenesis in the OA Synovium

The role of the inflammatory mediator connective tissue growth factor (CTGF/CCN2) has been investigated in VEGF production and angiogenesis in OA synovial fibroblasts (OASFs) [50]. It appears that CTGF activates the PI3K, Akt, ERK, and NF-κB/ELK1 pathways, leading to the up-regulation of miR-210, contributing to the inhibition of GPD1L expression and prolyl hydroxylase 2 activity, promoting HIF-1α-dependent VEGF expression and angiogenesis in human SFs (see Figure 2).

The discovery that CCR7 is functionally expressed on FLS of patients with RA and OA has revealed that this process enhances VEGF secretion in both diseases [32]. Other researchers have found that hepatocyte growth factor induces concentration- and time-dependent increases in VEGF-A expression in OASFs and that this enhancement involves the activation of the c-Met/PI3K/Akt and mTORC1 pathways [51].

Implantation of inflammatory SFs from patients with chronic arthritis (RA or OA) into immune-deficient mice has been found to enhance myeloid cell recruitment and angiogenesis [25]; these proangiogenic factors correlate with increasing levels of VEGF expression. VEGF and CXCL12 antagonists significantly reduced myeloid cell infiltration and angiogenesis.

13. The Importance of Targeting AGE-Induced Inflammatory Responses

Interference with the activity of the Wnt inhibitor Dickkopf-1 (Dkk-1) has been shown to reduce the expression of angiogenic factors and proteinases, as well as ameliorate synovial vascularity and cartilage injury in an animal model of OA knee joints [52], while insight into the signaling pathway of advanced glycation end-products (AGEs) has led to the understanding that AGEs induce the expression of COX-2 and the production of prostaglandin E2 (PGE2), IL-6 and MMP-13 in human OA synoviocytes [53]. Neutralizing antibody for the receptor for AGEs (RAGE) effectively reversed the AGE-induced inflammatory responses and VEGF production in human synoviocytes, indicating that RAGE plays an important role in the activation of synoviocytes and thereby encourages OA progression. Investigations have highlighted the link between IL-1β and chondrocyte angiogenesis in arthritis. As noted in the RA section above, IL-1β stimulation of chondrogenic ATDC5 cells induces FGF-2 expression and promotes EPC tube formation and migration [24]. FGF-2-neutralizing antibody abolishes ATDC5-conditional medium-mediated angiogenesis in vitro, as well as its angiogenic effects in the chick chorioallantoic membrane (CAM) assay, Matrigel plug nude mice model, and CIA mouse model. In these studies, IL-1β was found to induce FGF-2 expression via IL-1RI, ROS generation, AMP-activated protein kinase (AMPK), the AMPK-dependent p38 pathway, and the NF-κB pathway.

Other researchers have demonstrated that high glucose induces VEGF production in OASFs [54]. They report that high glucose generates increases in ROS production and induces concentration- and time-dependent increases in VEGF expression. This increase in VEGF production is inhibited by pretreating OASFs with NADPH oxidase inhibitors (APO or DPI), a ROS scavenger (NAC), a PI3K inhibitor (Ly294002 or wortmannin), an Akt inhibitor, or AP-1 inhibitor (curcumin or tanshinone IIA). High glucose treatment also increases PI3K and Akt activation and increases the accumulation of phosphorylated c-Jun in the nucleus, AP-1-luciferase activity, and c-Jun binding to the AP-1 element on the VEGF promoter.

14. Targeting OA Cartilage

Targeting the transforming growth factor β1 (TGF-β1) or relevant receptors may help to prevent or lessen angiogenic activity in OA. One group of researchers has reported that TGF-β1 treatment of human chondrocytes cultured in vitro significantly upregulates genes involved in chondrocyte hypertrophy and blood vessel development [55]. Another potential strategy for attenuating angiogenic activity in OA cartilage is to target chondromodulin-I (ChM-I) expression [56]. Investigations have shown that in mildly degenerated human OA cartilage, ChM-I expression is significantly decreased in the extracellular matrix (ECM) of the superficial zone and in the cytoplasm of the superficial and middle zones compared with normal cartilage ($p < 0.05$). In moderately degenerated cartilage, ChM-I protein expression is reduced in the ECM of all zones of articular cartilage, but the immunostaining intensity in the cytoplasm is increased. In severely degenerated cartilage, ChM-I expression is detected primarily in the cytoplasm of the cluster-forming chondrocytes. The density of vascular channels correlates with levels of ChM-I expression in cartilage ECM. The findings suggest that loss of ChM-I may promote angiogenesis in OA cartilage.

15. Subchondral Bone and Articular Cartilage

Some researchers suggest that it may be possible to prevent or reduce joint pathology and pain symptoms in OA by reducing angiogenesis and nerve formation from the subchondral bone into articular cartilage [57]. Their data demonstrated associations between neurovascular growth and expression of proangiogenic factors VEGF, nerve growth factor (NGF) and platelet-derived growth factor (PDGF) at the osteochondral junction. Other researchers suggest that angiogenesis and associated sensory nerve growth in human menisci may be a potential source of pain in knee OA [58]. They found that this increased vascular penetration and nerve growth expression enhanced inflammation and tissue damage, driving OA pathogenesis. OA has also been associated with deficient fluid clearance. Synovia from patients with knee OA is associated with lower lymphatic vessel density (LVD) and lower lymphatic EC fractional areas than synovia from non-arthritic control knees [57]. In the OA cohort, low LVD was associated with clinically detectable lesions. The study researchers hypothesized that impaired SF drainage, due to reduced LVD, may contribute to effusion in OA.

Using lenalidomide to inhibit the activity of TNF-α and leucine-rich-alpha-2-glycoprotein 1 (LRG1) appears to attenuate OA progression [59]. LRG1 expression was upregulated in the subchondral bone and articular cartilage in a mouse OA model (anterior cruciate ligament transection [ACLT] mice) and was associated with angiogenesis. The researchers also found that TNF-α stimulated LRG1 expression in HUVECs and that this effect was inhibited through p38 and NF-κB signaling. The injection of lenalidomide reduced the number of nestin-positive MSCs in the subchondral bone of ACLT mice compared with sham-operated controls. Lenalidomide also reduced the number of osterix-positive osteoprogenitors. Lenalidomide not only attenuated the pathological changes of subchondral bone but also alleviated the degeneration of articular cartilage compared with vehicle-treated mice. Of all surgically-induced OA models, the ACLT model is currently the most commonly used [60]. Other commonly used models include meniscectomy (partial and total), medial meniscal tear, and ovariectomy. Using aseptic techniques to surgically induce OA in animals yields highly reproducible results that progress rapidly. The ACLT model imitates articular cartilage degradation after ACL injury. As the OA lesions in this model develop more slowly than after meniscectomy, ACLT is useful in pharmaceutical investigations.

A Chinese medicinal formulation, Yanghe Decoction, has indicated in preclinical investigations that it may protect articular cartilage in the early stage of OA [61]. The formula contained *Rehmannia glutinosa* (30 g), cinnamon (3 g), ephedra (2 g), antler gum (9 g), white mustard seed (6 g), ginger charcoal (2 g) and licorice (3 g). A rabbit model of OA was established using New Zealand white rabbits randomly allocated to one of three groups: normal healthy controls, untreated OA, or OA treated with Yanghe Decoction for 14 days administered at the end of the study; all animals were sacrificed at 8 weeks. Examination of tibia articular cartilage revealed significant between-group differences for Mankin scores (1.25 vs. 6.25 and 3.22 in the controls, untreated and treated animals, respectively; $p < 0.01$ for both comparisons). Moreover, IHC (immunohistochemistry) staining revealed a significantly higher level of VEGF expression in the untreated OA group compared with controls (1.49 vs. 0.83; $p < 0.01$) and the Yanghe Decoction group (1.05; $p < 0.05$).

Table 2. Literature consulted for the OA section of this Review.

Stimulation	Target Factors		Effect in Tissue	Known Pathways	References
Growth factors					
CTGF	VEGF-A	↑	Synovium	PI3K/AKT/ERK and NF-B/ELK1	[50]
HGF	VEGF-A	↑	Synovium	c-Met/PI3K/Akt and mTORC1	[51]
TGF-β1	VEGF-A	↑	Cartilage	N/A	[55]
Chondromodulin-I	Chondromodulin-I	↑	Cartilage		[56]
Chemokine receptors					
CCR7	VEGF	↑	Synovium	N/A	[32]
Other mediators					
High glucose	VEGF-A	↑	Synovium	ROS, PI3K, Akt, c-Jun and AP-1	[54]
Dkk-1	Dkk-1	↑	Synovium	β-catenin– and ERK-dependent	[52]
AGEs	VEGF-A	↑	Synovium	RAGE-NF-κB pathway	[53]
Cytokines					
TNF-α	LRG1	↑	Subchondral bone	*p*38/ NF-κB	[59]
IL-1β	bFGF	↑	Cartilage	ROS/AMPK/p38/NF-κB	[24]
Chinese Herbs					
Yanghe Decoction	VEGF-A	↓	Cartilage	N/A	[61]

CTGF, Connective tissue growth factor; HGF, Hepatocyte growth factor; TGF-β1, Transforming growth factor beta-1; TNF-α, Tumor necrosis factor alpha; IL-1β, Interleukin 1 beta; Dkk-1, Dickkopf-related protein 1; AGEs, Advanced glycation end-products; N/A, not appropriate.

16. Summary and Future Directions

The evidence discussed in this Review underlines the essential role played by angiogenesis in RA and OA in articular cartilage. Angiogenic activity initiates and perpetuates both arthropathies, contributing to inflammation, joint damage and pain. Notably, the effects of angiogenesis have been confirmed as extending beyond the RA synovium to include RA osteoblasts and also OA subchondral bone and articular cartilage. For example, in preclinical investigations, elevated levels of the pro-inflammatory cytokine TNF-α-induced LRG1 expression during OA progression [32]. Using lenalidomide to inhibit TNF-α successfully reduced TNF-α-induced LRG1 secretion and attenuated degeneration of OA articular cartilage. Interestingly, besides demonstrating angiogenic and anti-inflammatory effects, lenalidomide has also shown antitumor activity in clinical trials for the treatment of multiple myeloma and colorectal cancer, highlighting the importance of angiogenesis as a therapeutic target [62–66]. Other researchers have reported that IL-1β induces FGF-2 expression and promotes EPC angiogenesis in chondrocytes, then subsequently promotes EPC migration and tube formation [24]. Similarly, VEGF production in osteoblasts and EPC angiogenesis is promoted by CCN1, which has been found to inhibit levels of miR-126 expression in RA [46]. Another facet of angiogenesis is the activity of MSCs, which may have potential in RA and OA management [26,67]. Similarly, platelet-rich plasma (PRP) shows potential in arthritis. More high-quality clinical evidence is needed to determine the effectiveness of such therapy in the management of articular cartilage pathology [68] and to confirm its promising data in experimental studies [69]. All in all, the expression of chemokines and cytokines in synovial fluid is the most important element to consider in RA and OA angiogenesis—these molecules control the disease and the more that we learn about the complex process involved in their networks of anti- and pro-inflammatory interactions, the closer we surely edge towards the day when we can arrest these chronic diseases at their earliest stages.

Funding: This work was supported by grants from the Ministry of Science and Technology of Taiwan (MOST 106-2320-B-039-005 and MOST 105-2320-B-039-015-MY3).

Conflicts of Interest: The authors declare no conflict of interest.

References

1. McInnes, I.B.; Schett, G. The pathogenesis of rheumatoid arthritis. *N. Engl. J. Med.* **2011**, *365*, 2205–2219. [CrossRef] [PubMed]
2. Zhang, W.; Ouyang, H.; Dass, C.R.; Xu, J. Current research on pharmacologic and regenerative therapies for osteoarthritis. *Bone Res.* **2016**, *4*, 15040. [CrossRef] [PubMed]
3. Wehling, P.; Evans, C.; Wehling, J.; Maixner, W. Effectiveness of intra-articular therapies in osteoarthritis: A literature review. *Ther. Adv. Musculoskelet. Dis.* **2017**, *9*, 183–196. [CrossRef] [PubMed]
4. Emery, P. Optimizing outcomes in patients with rheumatoid arthritis and an inadequate response to anti-tnf treatment. *Rheumatology* **2012**, *51* (Suppl. 5), v22–v30. [CrossRef] [PubMed]
5. Kihara, M.; Davies, R.; Kearsley-Fleet, L.; Watson, K.D.; Lunt, M.; Symmons, D.P.; Hyrich, K.L. Use and effectiveness of tocilizumab among patients with rheumatoid arthritis: An observational study from the british society for rheumatology biologics register for rheumatoid arthritis. *Clin. Rheumatol.* **2017**, *36*, 241–250. [CrossRef] [PubMed]
6. Jones, G.; Nash, P.; Hall, S. Advances in rheumatoid arthritis. *Med. J. Aust.* **2017**, *206*, 221–224. [CrossRef] [PubMed]
7. Wijbrandts, C.A.; Tak, P.P. Prediction of response to targeted treatment in rheumatoid arthritis. *Mayo Clin. Proc.* **2017**, *92*, 1129–1143. [CrossRef] [PubMed]
8. Castaneda, O.M.; Romero, F.J.; Salinas, A.; Citera, G.; Mysler, E.; Rillo, O.; Radominski, S.C.; Cardiel, M.H.; Jaller, J.J.; Alvarez-Moreno, C.; et al. Safety of tofacitinib in the treatment of rheumatoid arthritis in latin america compared with the rest of the world population. *J. Clin. Rheumatol. Pract. Rep. Rheum. Musculoskelet. Dis.* **2017**, *23*, 193–199. [CrossRef] [PubMed]
9. Barclay, N.; Tarallo, M.; Hendrikx, T.; Marett, S. Patient preference for oral versus injectable and intravenous methods of treatment for rheumatoid arthritis. *Value Health* **2013**, *16*, A568. [CrossRef]

10. Elshabrawy, H.A.; Chen, Z.; Volin, M.V.; Ravella, S.; Virupannavar, S.; Shahrara, S. The pathogenic role of angiogenesis in rheumatoid arthritis. *Angiogenesis* **2015**, *18*, 433–448. [CrossRef] [PubMed]

11. Moon, S.J.; Park, M.K.; Oh, H.J.; Lee, S.Y.; Kwok, S.K.; Cho, M.L.; Ju, J.H.; Park, K.S.; Kim, H.Y.; Park, S.H. Engagement of toll-like receptor 3 induces vascular endothelial growth factor and interleukin-8 in human rheumatoid synovial fibroblasts. *Korean J. Intern. Med.* **2010**, *25*, 429–435. [CrossRef] [PubMed]

12. Saber, T.; Veale, D.J.; Balogh, E.; McCormick, J.; NicAnUltaigh, S.; Connolly, M.; Fearon, U. Toll-like receptor 2 induced angiogenesis and invasion is mediated through the tie2 signalling pathway in rheumatoid arthritis. *PLoS ONE* **2011**, *6*, e23540. [CrossRef] [PubMed]

13. Miyake, K.; Nishida, K.; Kadota, Y.; Yamasaki, H.; Nasu, T.; Saitou, D.; Tanabe, K.; Sonoda, H.; Sato, Y.; Maeshima, Y.; et al. Inflammatory cytokine-induced expression of vasohibin-1 by rheumatoid synovial fibroblasts. *Acta Med. Okayama* **2009**, *63*, 349–358. [PubMed]

14. Manabe, H.; Nasu, Y.; Komiyama, T.; Furumatsu, T.; Kitamura, A.; Miyazawa, S.; Ninomiya, Y.; Ozaki, T.; Asahara, H.; Nishida, K. Inhibition of histone deacetylase down-regulates the expression of hypoxia-induced vascular endothelial growth factor by rheumatoid synovial fibroblasts. *Inflamm. Res. Off. J. Eur. Histamine Res. Soc.* **2008**, *57*, 4–10. [CrossRef] [PubMed]

15. Brahn, E.; Banquerigo, M.L.; Lee, J.K.; Park, E.J.; Fogler, W.E.; Plum, S.M. An angiogenesis inhibitor, 2-methoxyestradiol, involutes rat collagen-induced arthritis and suppresses gene expression of synovial vascular endothelial growth factor and basic fibroblast growth factor. *J. Rheumatol.* **2008**, *35*, 2119–2128. [CrossRef] [PubMed]

16. Hashizume, M.; Hayakawa, N.; Suzuki, M.; Mihara, M. Il-6/sil-6r trans-signalling, but not tnf-alpha induced angiogenesis in a huvec and synovial cell co-culture system. *Rheumatol. Int.* **2009**, *29*, 1449–1454. [CrossRef] [PubMed]

17. Moran, E.M.; Connolly, M.; Gao, W.; McCormick, J.; Fearon, U.; Veale, D.J. Interleukin-17a induction of angiogenesis, cell migration, and cytoskeletal rearrangement. *Arthritis Rheum.* **2011**, *63*, 3263–3273. [CrossRef] [PubMed]

18. Amin, M.A.; Rabquer, B.J.; Mansfield, P.J.; Ruth, J.H.; Marotte, H.; Haas, C.S.; Reamer, E.N.; Koch, A.E. Interleukin 18 induces angiogenesis in vitro and in vivo via src and jnk kinases. *Ann. Rheum. Dis.* **2010**, *69*, 2204–2212. [CrossRef] [PubMed]

19. Kobori, T.; Hamasaki, S.; Kitaura, A.; Yamazaki, Y.; Nishinaka, T.; Niwa, A.; Nakao, S.; Wake, H.; Mori, S.; Yoshino, T.; et al. Interleukin-18 amplifies macrophage polarization and morphological alteration, leading to excessive angiogenesis. *Front. Immunol.* **2018**, *9*, 334. [CrossRef] [PubMed]

20. Elshabrawy, H.A.; Volin, M.V.; Essani, A.B.; Chen, Z.; McInnes, I.B.; Van Raemdonck, K.; Palasiewicz, K.; Arami, S.; Gonzalez, M.; Ashour, H.M.; et al. Il-11 facilitates a novel connection between ra joint fibroblasts and endothelial cells. *Angiogenesis* **2018**, *21*, 215–228. [CrossRef] [PubMed]

21. Connolly, M.; Marrelli, A.; Blades, M.; McCormick, J.; Maderna, P.; Godson, C.; Mullan, R.; FitzGerald, O.; Bresnihan, B.; Pitzalis, C.; et al. Acute serum amyloid a induces migration, angiogenesis, and inflammation in synovial cells in vitro and in a human rheumatoid arthritis/scid mouse chimera model. *J. Immunol.* **2010**, *184*, 6427–6437. [CrossRef] [PubMed]

22. Su, C.M.; Hsu, C.J.; Tsai, C.H.; Huang, C.Y.; Wang, S.W.; Tang, C.H. Resistin promotes angiogenesis in endothelial progenitor cells through inhibition of microrna206: Potential implications for rheumatoid arthritis. *Stem Cells* **2015**, *33*, 2243–2255. [CrossRef] [PubMed]

23. Sun, X.; Wei, J.; Tang, Y.; Wang, B.; Zhang, Y.; Shi, L.; Guo, J.; Hu, F.; Li, X. Leptin-induced migration and angiogenesis in rheumatoid arthritis is mediated by reactive oxygen species. *FEBS Open Bio* **2017**, *7*, 1899–1908. [CrossRef] [PubMed]

24. Chien, S.Y.; Huang, C.Y.; Tsai, C.H.; Wang, S.W.; Lin, Y.M.; Tang, C.H. Interleukin-1beta induces fibroblast growth factor 2 expression and subsequently promotes endothelial progenitor cell angiogenesis in chondrocytes. *Clin. Sci.* **2016**, *130*, 667–681. [CrossRef] [PubMed]

25. del Rey, M.J.; Izquierdo, E.; Caja, S.; Usategui, A.; Santiago, B.; Galindo, M.; Pablos, J.L. Human inflammatory synovial fibroblasts induce enhanced myeloid cell recruitment and angiogenesis through a hypoxia-inducible transcription factor 1alpha/vascular endothelial growth factor-mediated pathway in immunodeficient mice. *Arthritis Rheum.* **2009**, *60*, 2926–2934. [CrossRef] [PubMed]

26. Ansboro, S.; Roelofs, A.J.; De Bari, C. Mesenchymal stem cells for the management of rheumatoid arthritis: Immune modulation, repair or both? *Curr. Opin. Rheumatol.* **2017**, *29*, 201–207. [CrossRef] [PubMed]

27. Akhavani, M.A.; Madden, L.; Buysschaert, I.; Sivakumar, B.; Kang, N.; Paleolog, E.M. Hypoxia upregulates angiogenesis and synovial cell migration in rheumatoid arthritis. *Arthritis Res. Ther.* **2009**, *11*, R64. [CrossRef] [PubMed]

28. Zhang, X.; Liu, J.; Wan, L.; Sun, Y.; Wang, F.; Qi, Y.; Huang, C. Up-regulated expressions of hif-1alpha, vegf and cd34 promote synovial angiogenesis in rats with adjuvant arthritis. *Chin. J. Cell. Mol. Immunol.* **2015**, *31*, 1053–1056.

29. Nam, Y.; Jung, S.M.; Rim, Y.A.; Jung, H.; Lee, K.; Park, N.; Kim, J.; Jang, Y.; Park, Y.B.; Park, S.H.; et al. Intraperitoneal infusion of mesenchymal stem cell attenuates severity of collagen antibody induced arthritis. *PLoS ONE* **2018**, *13*, e0198740. [CrossRef] [PubMed]

30. Bao, C.X.; Chen, H.X.; Mou, X.J.; Zhu, X.K.; Zhao, Q.; Wang, X.G. Gzmb gene silencing confers protection against synovial tissue hyperplasia and articular cartilage tissue injury in rheumatoid arthritis through the mapk signaling pathway. *Biomed. Pharmacother.* **2018**, *103*, 346–354. [CrossRef] [PubMed]

31. O'Brien, M.J.; Shu, Q.; Stinson, W.A.; Tsou, P.S.; Ruth, J.H.; Isozaki, T.; Campbell, P.L.; Ohara, R.A.; Koch, A.E.; Fox, D.A.; et al. A unique role for galectin-9 in angiogenesis and inflammatory arthritis. *Arthritis Res. Ther.* **2018**, *20*, 31. [CrossRef] [PubMed]

32. Bruhl, H.; Mack, M.; Niedermeier, M.; Lochbaum, D.; Scholmerich, J.; Straub, R.H. Functional expression of the chemokine receptor ccr7 on fibroblast-like synoviocytes. *Rheumatology* **2008**, *47*, 1771–1774. [CrossRef] [PubMed]

33. Wengner, A.M.; Hopken, U.E.; Petrow, P.K.; Hartmann, S.; Schurigt, U.; Brauer, R.; Lipp, M. Cxcr5- and ccr7-dependent lymphoid neogenesis in a murine model of chronic antigen-induced arthritis. *Arthritis Rheum.* **2007**, *56*, 3271–3283. [CrossRef] [PubMed]

34. Chen, Z.; Kim, S.J.; Essani, A.B.; Volin, M.V.; Vila, O.M.; Swedler, W.; Arami, S.; Volkov, S.; Sardin, L.V.; Sweiss, N.; et al. Characterising the expression and function of ccl28 and its corresponding receptor, ccr10, in ra pathogenesis. *Ann. Rheum. Dis.* **2015**, *74*, 1898–1906. [CrossRef] [PubMed]

35. Pickens, S.R.; Chamberlain, N.D.; Volin, M.V.; Pope, R.M.; Mandelin, A.M., 2nd; Shahrara, S. Characterization of ccl19 and ccl21 in rheumatoid arthritis. *Arthritis Rheum.* **2011**, *63*, 914–922. [CrossRef] [PubMed]

36. Wang, C.H.; Yao, H.; Chen, L.N.; Jia, J.F.; Wang, L.; Dai, J.Y.; Zheng, Z.H.; Chen, Z.N.; Zhu, P. Cd147 induces angiogenesis through a vascular endothelial growth factor and hypoxia-inducible transcription factor 1alpha-mediated pathway in rheumatoid arthritis. *Arthritis Rheum.* **2012**, *64*, 1818–1827. [CrossRef] [PubMed]

37. Zong, J.; Li, Y.; Du, D.; Liu, Y.; Yin, Y. Cd147 induces up-regulation of vascular endothelial growth factor in u937-derived foam cells through pi3k/akt pathway. *Arch. Biochem. Biophys.* **2016**, *609*, 31–38. [CrossRef] [PubMed]

38. Isozaki, T.; Rabquer, B.J.; Ruth, J.H.; Haines, G.K., 3rd; Koch, A.E. Adam-10 is overexpressed in rheumatoid arthritis synovial tissue and mediates angiogenesis. *Arthritis Rheum.* **2013**, *65*, 98–108. [CrossRef] [PubMed]

39. Pan, R.; Dai, Y.; Gao, X.; Xia, Y. Scopolin isolated from erycibe obtusifolia benth stems suppresses adjuvant-induced rat arthritis by inhibiting inflammation and angiogenesis. *Int. Immunopharmacol.* **2009**, *9*, 859–869. [CrossRef] [PubMed]

40. Deng, Q.; Bai, S.; Gao, W.; Tong, L. Pristimerin inhibits angiogenesis in adjuvant-induced arthritic rats by suppressing vegfr2 signaling pathways. *Int. Immunopharmacol.* **2015**, *29*, 302–313. [CrossRef] [PubMed]

41. Shankar, J.; Thippegowda, P.B.; Kanum, S.A. Inhibition of hif-1alpha activity by bp-1 ameliorates adjuvant induced arthritis in rats. *Biochem. Biophys. Res. Commun.* **2009**, *387*, 223–228. [CrossRef] [PubMed]

42. Jiang, H.; Wang, L.; Wang, F.; Pan, J. Proprotein convertase subtilisin/kexin type 6 promotes in vitro proliferation, migration and inflammatory cytokine secretion of synovial fibroblastlike cells from rheumatoid arthritis via nuclearkappab, signal transducer and activator of transcription 3 and extracellular signal regulated 1/2 pathways. *Mol. Med. Rep.* **2017**, *16*, 8477–8484. [PubMed]

43. Wang, F.; Wan, J.; Li, Q.; Zhang, M.; Wan, Q.; Ji, C.; Li, H.; Liu, R.; Han, M. Lysyl oxidase is involved in synovial hyperplasia and angiogenesis in rats with collageninduced arthritis. *Mol. Med. Rep.* **2017**, *16*, 6736–6742. [CrossRef] [PubMed]

44. Ding, H.; Hong, C.; Wang, Y.; Liu, J.; Zhang, N.; Shen, C.; Wei, W.; Zheng, F. Calreticulin promotes angiogenesis via activating nitric oxide signalling pathway in rheumatoid arthritis. *Clin. Exp. Immunol.* **2014**, *178*, 236–244. [CrossRef] [PubMed]

45. Li, T.M.; Liu, S.C.; Huang, Y.H.; Huang, C.C.; Hsu, C.J.; Tsai, C.H.; Wang, S.W.; Tang, C.H. Ykl-40-induced inhibition of mir-590-3p promotes interleukin-18 expression and angiogenesis of endothelial progenitor cells. *Int. J. Mol. Sci.* **2017**, *18*, 920. [CrossRef] [PubMed]

46. Chen, C.Y.; Su, C.M.; Hsu, C.J.; Huang, C.C.; Wang, S.W.; Liu, S.C.; Chen, W.C.; Fuh, L.J.; Tang, C.H. Ccn1 promotes vegf production in osteoblasts and induces endothelial progenitor cell angiogenesis by inhibiting mir-126 expression in rheumatoid arthritis. *J. Bone Miner. Res. Off. J. Am. Soc. Bone Miner. Res.* **2017**, *32*, 34–45. [CrossRef] [PubMed]

47. Yi, J.; Zhu, Y.; Jia, Y.; Jiang, H.; Zheng, X.; Liu, D.; Gao, S.; Sun, M.; Hu, B.; Jiao, B.; et al. The annexin a2 promotes development in arthritis through neovascularization by amplification hedgehog pathway. *PLoS ONE* **2016**, *11*, e0150363. [CrossRef] [PubMed]

48. Robinson, W.H.; Lepus, C.M.; Wang, Q.; Raghu, H.; Mao, R.; Lindstrom, T.M.; Sokolove, J. Low-grade inflammation as a key mediator of the pathogenesis of osteoarthritis. *Nat. Rev. Rheumatol.* **2016**, *12*, 580–592. [CrossRef] [PubMed]

49. Lazzerini, P.E.; Capecchi, P.L.; Laghi-Pasini, F. Systemic inflammation and arrhythmic risk: Lessons from rheumatoid arthritis. *Eur. Heart J.* **2017**, *38*, 1717–1727. [CrossRef] [PubMed]

50. Liu, S.C.; Chuang, S.M.; Hsu, C.J.; Tsai, C.H.; Wang, S.W.; Tang, C.H. Ctgf increases vascular endothelial growth factor-dependent angiogenesis in human synovial fibroblasts by increasing mir-210 expression. *Cell Death Dis.* **2014**, *5*, e1485. [CrossRef] [PubMed]

51. Lin, Y.M.; Huang, Y.L.; Fong, Y.C.; Tsai, C.H.; Chou, M.C.; Tang, C.H. Hepatocyte growth factor increases vascular endothelial growth factor-a production in human synovial fibroblasts through c-met receptor pathway. *PLoS ONE* **2012**, *7*, e50924. [CrossRef] [PubMed]

52. Weng, L.H.; Ko, J.Y.; Wang, C.J.; Sun, Y.C.; Wang, F.S. Dkk-1 promotes angiogenic responses and cartilage matrix proteinase secretion in synovial fibroblasts from osteoarthritic joints. *Arthritis Rheum.* **2012**, *64*, 3267–3277. [CrossRef] [PubMed]

53. Chen, Y.J.; Chan, D.C.; Chiang, C.K.; Wang, C.C.; Yang, T.H.; Lan, K.C.; Chao, S.C.; Tsai, K.S.; Yang, R.S.; Liu, S.H. Advanced glycation end-products induced vegf production and inflammatory responses in human synoviocytes via rage-nf-kappab pathway activation. *J. Orthop. Res. Off. Publ. Orthop. Res. Soc.* **2016**, *34*, 791–800. [CrossRef] [PubMed]

54. Tsai, C.H.; Chiang, Y.C.; Chen, H.T.; Huang, P.H.; Hsu, H.C.; Tang, C.H. High glucose induces vascular endothelial growth factor production in human synovial fibroblasts through reactive oxygen species generation. *Biochim. Biophys. Acta* **2013**, *1830*, 2649–2658. [CrossRef] [PubMed]

55. Chen, J.L.; Zou, C.; Chen, Y.; Zhu, W.; Liu, W.; Huang, J.; Liu, Q.; Wang, D.; Duan, L.; Xiong, J.; et al. Tgfbeta1 induces hypertrophic change and expression of angiogenic factors in human chondrocytes. *Oncotarget* **2017**, *8*, 91316–91327. [PubMed]

56. Deng, B.; Chen, C.; Gong, X.; Guo, L.; Chen, H.; Yin, L.; Yang, L.; Wang, F. Chondromodulini expression and correlation with angiogenesis in human osteoarthritic cartilage. *Mol. Med. Rep.* **2017**, *16*, 2142–2148. [CrossRef] [PubMed]

57. Walsh, D.A.; McWilliams, D.F.; Turley, M.J.; Dixon, M.R.; Franses, R.E.; Mapp, P.I.; Wilson, D. Angiogenesis and nerve growth factor at the osteochondral junction in rheumatoid arthritis and osteoarthritis. *Rheumatology* **2010**, *49*, 1852–1861. [CrossRef] [PubMed]

58. Ashraf, S.; Wibberley, H.; Mapp, P.I.; Hill, R.; Wilson, D.; Walsh, D.A. Increased vascular penetration and nerve growth in the meniscus: A potential source of pain in osteoarthritis. *Ann. Rheum. Dis.* **2011**, *70*, 523–529. [CrossRef] [PubMed]

59. Wang, Y.; Xu, J.; Zhang, X.; Wang, C.; Huang, Y.; Dai, K. Tnf-alpha-induced lrg1 promotes angiogenesis and mesenchymal stem cell migration in the subchondral bone during osteoarthritis. *Cell Death Dis.* **2017**, *8*, e2715. [CrossRef] [PubMed]

60. Kuyinu, E.L.; Narayanan, G.; Nair, L.S.; Laurencin, C.T. Animal models of osteoarthritis: Classification, update, and measurement of outcomes. *J. Orthop. Surg. Res.* **2016**, *11*, 19. [CrossRef] [PubMed]

61. Chen, Z.W.; Chen, Y.Q. Effects of yanghe decoction on vascular endothelial growth factor in cartilage cells of osteoarthritis rabbits. *J. Chin. Integr. Med.* **2008**, *6*, 372–375. [CrossRef] [PubMed]

62. Richardson, P.G.; Schlossman, R.L.; Weller, E.; Hideshima, T.; Mitsiades, C.; Davies, F.; LeBlanc, R.; Catley, L.P.; Doss, D.; Kelly, K.; et al. Immunomodulatory drug cc-5013 overcomes drug resistance and is well tolerated in patients with relapsed multiple myeloma. *Blood* **2002**, *100*, 3063–3067. [CrossRef] [PubMed]

63. Davies, F.E.; Raje, N.; Hideshima, T.; Lentzsch, S.; Young, G.; Tai, Y.T.; Lin, B.; Podar, K.; Gupta, D.; Chauhan, D.; et al. Thalidomide and immunomodulatory derivatives augment natural killer cell cytotoxicity in multiple myeloma. *Blood* **2001**, *98*, 210–216. [CrossRef] [PubMed]
64. Yang, B.; Yu, R.L.; Chi, X.H.; Lu, X.C. Lenalidomide treatment for multiple myeloma: Systematic review and meta-analysis of randomized controlled trials. *PLoS ONE* **2013**, *8*, e64354. [CrossRef] [PubMed]
65. Bridoux, F.; Chen, N.; Moreau, S.; Arnulf, B.; Moumas, E.; Abraham, J.; Desport, E.; Jaccard, A.; Fermand, J.P. Pharmacokinetics, safety, and efficacy of lenalidomide plus dexamethasone in patients with multiple myeloma and renal impairment. *Cancer Chemother. Pharmacol.* **2016**, *78*, 173–182. [CrossRef] [PubMed]
66. Leuci, V.; Maione, F.; Rotolo, R.; Giraudo, E.; Sassi, F.; Migliardi, G.; Todorovic, M.; Gammaitoni, L.; Mesiano, G.; Giraudo, L.; et al. Lenalidomide normalizes tumor vessels in colorectal cancer improving chemotherapy activity. *J. Transl. Med.* **2016**, *14*, 119. [CrossRef] [PubMed]
67. Luz-Crawford, P.; Ipseiz, N.; Espinosa-Carrasco, G.; Caicedo, A.; Tejedor, G.; Toupet, K.; Loriau, J.; Scholtysek, C.; Stoll, C.; Khoury, M.; et al. Pparbeta/delta directs the therapeutic potential of mesenchymal stem cells in arthritis. *Ann. Rheum. Dis.* **2016**, *75*, 2166–2174. [CrossRef] [PubMed]
68. Dold, A.P.; Zywiel, M.G.; Taylor, D.W.; Dwyer, T.; Theodoropoulos, J. Platelet-rich plasma in the management of articular cartilage pathology: A systematic review. *Clin. J. Sport Med. Off. J. Can. Acad. Sport Med.* **2014**, *24*, 31–43. [CrossRef] [PubMed]
69. Tong, S.; Zhang, C.; Liu, J. Platelet-rich plasma exhibits beneficial effects for rheumatoid arthritis mice by suppressing inflammatory factors. *Mol. Med. Rep.* **2017**, *16*, 4082–4088. [CrossRef] [PubMed]

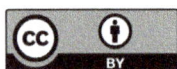

International Journal of
Molecular Sciences

MDPI

Review

Associations between Adipokines in Arthritic Disease and Implications for Obesity

Iona J. MacDonald [1], Shan-Chi Liu [1,2], Chien-Chung Huang [3,4], Shu-Jui Kuo [2,5], Chun-Hao Tsai [2,6] and Chih-Hsin Tang [1,6,7,8,*]

[1]   Graduate Institute of Basic Medical Science, China Medical University, Taichung 40402, Taiwan; ionamac@gmail.com (I.J.M.); sdsaw.tw@yahoo.com.tw (S.-C.L.)
[2]   Department of Orthopedic Surgery, China Medical University Hospital, Taichung 40447, Taiwan; b90401073@gmail.com (S.-J.K.); ritsai8615@gmail.com (C.-H.T.)
[3]   Graduate Institute of Clinical Medical Science, China Medical University, Taichung 40447, Taiwan; u104054003@cmu.edu.tw
[4]   Division of Immunology and Rheumatology, Department of Internal Medicine, China Medical University Hospital, Taichung 40447, Taiwan
[5]   Department of Anatomy, China Medical University, Taichung 40402, Taiwan
[6]   School of Medicine, China Medical University, Taichung 40402, Taiwan
[7]   Chinese Medicine Research Center, China Medical University, Taichung 40447, Taiwan
[8]   Department of Biotechnology, College of Health Science, Asia University, Taichung 41354, Taiwan
[*]   Correspondence: chtang@mail.cmu.edu.tw; Tel.: +886-2205-2121 (ext. 7726)

check for updates

Received: 4 March 2019; Accepted: 21 March 2019; Published: 26 March 2019

Abstract: Secretion from adipose tissue of adipokines or adipocytokines, comprising of bioactive peptides or proteins, immune molecules and inflammatory mediators, exert critical roles in inflammatory arthritis and obesity. This review considers the evidence generated over the last decade regarding the effects of several adipokines including leptin, adiponectin, visfatin, resistin, chemerin and apelin, in cartilage and bone homeostasis in the pathogenesis of rheumatoid arthritis and osteoarthritis, which has important implications for obesity.

Keywords: rheumatoid arthritis; osteoarthritis; adipokines; obesity

1. Introduction

Adipose tissue secretes various bioactive peptides or proteins, immune molecules and inflammatory mediators known as adipokines (only produced by the adipose tissue) or adipocytokines (mainly, but not solely, produced by adipocytes) (Figure 1). In this review, the term "adipokine" refers to these multifunctional molecules. Since the discovery in 1994 of the first adipokine, leptin, profiling studies have identified hundreds of adipokines in the human adipose proteome (adipokinome), all of which can potently modulate inflammation via autocrine/paracrine and endocrine pathways. Some of these multifunctional molecules are critical to the pathogenesis of rheumatoid arthritis (RA) and osteoarthritis (OA), modulating target tissues and cells in cartilage, synovium, bone, and various immune cells [1]. Thus, our review of data details adipose tissue paracrine signaling in RA and OA and discusses correlations identified between adipokines, obesity and the development of RA and OA. These are two of the most important and common arthritic diseases that lead to bone destruction and deformity; we therefore focused on the role of adipokines in these arthritic diseases. Our evidence is drawn from the period of January 2007 through October 2018, because the literature begins to extensively cover the role of adipose tissue and adipokines in obesity, RA and OA from 2007 and our literature search ended in October 2018.

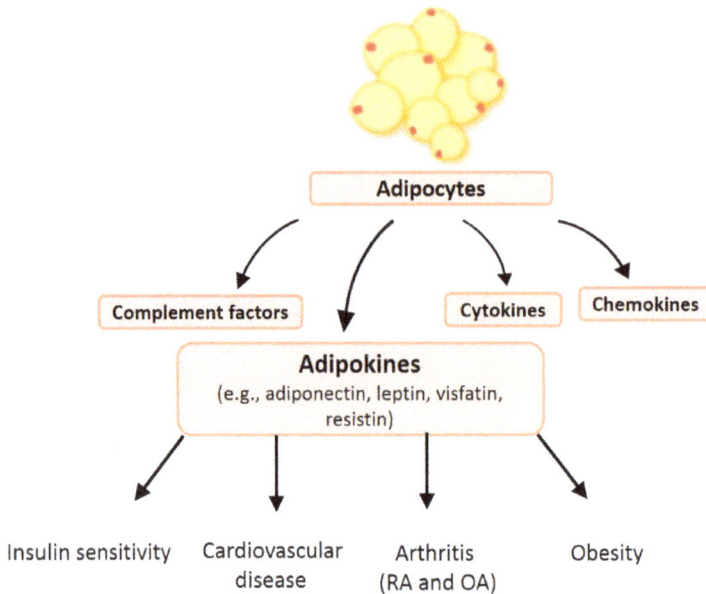

Figure 1. The important role of adipokines. Adipokines are produced mainly by adipocytes and play critical roles in several major disorders including insulin sensitivity, cardiovascular disease, arthritic conditions (i.e., RA and OA), and obesity.

Rheumatoid arthritis, a chronic autoimmune disease marked by persistent synovial and systemic inflammation, damages joints, results in disability and increases cardiovascular burden. The pathogenesis of RA is uncertain, but the underlying pathology appears to commence outside the joints [2]. Obesity is accompanied by low-grade inflammation and is a recognized risk factor for several well-known health problems, including cardiovascular disorders, disorders of metabolic syndrome (MetS), various cancers, and some rheumatic diseases [3]. Evidence demonstrates that obesity independently increases the risk of RA developing in "at-risk", autoantibody-positive people, and that higher birth weight is associated with the future onset of RA [4,5]. Conversely, other evidence suggests that obesity has no influence over the likelihood of developing RA. For instance, researchers have reported that in early RA, higher body mass index (BMI) not only does not influence the progression to clinical RA, but that it may be associated with less radiographic joint damage, with people who are obese developing fewer joint erosions and experiencing slower structural progression [6,7]. Interestingly, an association between lower BMI and progression of radiographic joint damage in early RA has been observed only in seropositive individuals [6,8,9].

In comparison to RA, a more definite link is established between higher BMI and the risk of developing hip and knee OA in men and women [10,11]. Evidence from the Framingham Heart Study reveals a 1.5- to 2-fold higher risk of developing knee OA among people who are obese compared with those who are leaner [1] and, in a US population-based study involving community-dwelling older adults (aged $\geq$70 years), a 5 kg/m^2 increase in BMI increased the likelihood of developing knee OA by 32% [12]. Not only did a 200 pM increase in serum leptin increase the odds of knee OA by 11%, but also, approximately half of the BMI's total effect on knee OA was attributed to leptin. In pooled relative risks (RRs) of a recent meta-analysis, overweight and obesity significantly increased the risk of knee OA by approximately 2.5 and 4.6 times, respectively, compared with normal weight [13]. Other risk factors that predispose to OA include joint trauma, and family history or medical disorders presenting with joint inflammation, such as hemochromatosis, septic arthritis, inflammatory arthritis, avascular necrosis, hemophilia, or gout [12].

As higher BMI fails to totally account for the development or progression of RA, researchers speculate that alterations in the production of inflammatory molecules from adipose tissue may help to activate the immune system and slow the process of damage in the joints [14]. Indeed, the release of adipokines from adipose tissue or joint compartments appears to have critical implications in inflammatory and immune responses of rheumatic diseases [15,16]. For instance, in a cohort of nonarthritic individuals with immunoglobulin M rheumatoid factor (IgM RF) and/or anti-citrullinated protein antibody (ACPA) positivity, serum vaspin levels at study entry related to the clinical manifestation of arthritis after a median 22 months of follow-up [17]. No such association was observed with other adipokines (adiponectin, resistin, leptin, chemerin, or omentin). Moreover, no associations were found between adiponectin, resistin or visfatin synovial expression and the development of arthritis [17]. Some researchers have proposed that lower levels of adiponectin in people with obesity are linked with high adiposity (a surrogate for high BMI) and less joint damage in RA [18].

2. The Involvement of Adiponectin in Arthritis

2.1. Adiponectin in RA

Adiponectin (also known as Acrp30, AdipoQ and GBP28) has attracted much attention for its potential therapeutic use in metabolic disorders, as this adipokine exerts pleiotropic metabolic effects on insulin sensitivity, inflammation and angiogenesis, primarily via the adiponectin receptors 1 and 2 (AdipoR1 and AdipoR2), as well as the non-signaling binding protein T-cadherin, regulating glucose and lipid metabolism [19,20]. Evidence also indicates that adiponectin serves as a possible link between obesity and cancer [19]. Patients with RA have consistently higher serum [21–23] and synovial fluid [24] adiponectin levels than non-RA controls. The data are mixed as to the differential regulation of cytokines by adiponectin: On the one hand, adiponectin is capable of suppressing levels of proinflammatory cytokines tumor necrosis factor alpha (TNF-α) and interleukin 6 (IL-6) that are typically elevated in RA and adiponectin increases levels of the anti-inflammatory cytokine IL-10 in primary human macrophages activated with lipopolysaccharide (LPS) [25]. Conversely, increasing concentrations of adiponectin stimulate cultured synovial fibroblasts from RA and OA patients to produce IL-6 [26]. Adiponectin can also stimulate vascular endothelial growth factor (VEGF) and matrix metalloproteinase (MMP) production in RA fibroblast-like synoviocytes (FLSs), leading to joint inflammation and destruction, respectively [27], and women with erosive OA of the hands have higher serum levels of adiponectin levels compared with those with nonerosive hand OA [28]. Moreover, adiponectin can mediate changes in effector cells in RA disease pathophysiology, inducing gene expression and protein synthesis in human RA synovial fibroblasts (RASFs), lymphocytes, endothelial cells and chondrocytes [29], enhancing prostaglandin E_2 production in RASFs via AdipoR1 [30,31]. In untreated patients with early RA, serum adiponectin levels have been found to predict radiographic disease progression, independently of metabolic status and potentially confounding factors [32]. Other research has failed to find any association between high serum levels of adiponectin and either homeostasis model assessment for insulin resistance (HOMA-IR) index or common carotid artery intima-media thickness (IMT) measurements [23]. Other investigations into the mechanisms underlying adiponectin function have shown that adiponectin induces production of the proinflammatory cytokine, oncostatin M, in human osteoblasts [33].

In severe, infliximab-refractory RA, a negative correlation has been observed between high-grade inflammation (C-reactive protein [CRP]) and low circulating plasma adiponectin levels [34]. That research documented independent, negative correlations between low adiponectin levels with atherogenic dyslipidemia and high plasma glucose levels, findings that are similar to those previously reported in individuals without RA disease, suggesting that low circulating adiponectin levels cluster with features of MetS that are implicated in RA atherogenesis [34]. If higher adiponectin levels are indeed protective against cardiovascular disease and obesity, it may not be wise to modulate those levels.

2.2. Adiponectin in OA

The somewhat puzzling findings as to the inflammatory activity associated with adiponectin is postulated to be because there are several isoforms that have differing, sometimes counteracting functions [35]. Their selective binding to AdipoR1 and AdipoR2 induces specific intracellular signaling cascades; the oligomerization and expression levels of these receptors determine adiponectin bioactivity [36]. For example, high-molecular-weight adiponectin induces IL-6 in human monocytes but has no effect upon LPS-induced IL-6 secretion, while low-molecular-weight adiponectin reduces LPS-induced IL-6 secretion and induces IL-10 in these cells [36]. Intriguingly, positive correlations have been observed between levels of synovial fluid from OA patients and levels of adiponectin and resistin, whereas conversely, the biological active free form of leptin (not the total leptin) appears to be negatively associated with IL-6 [37].

Much higher serum levels of adiponectin, leptin and resistin have been found in patients with severe knee OA compared with controls without radiographic knee OA; that same research also documented weak but positive associations between serum levels of adiponectin, leptin and resistin and synovial inflammation [38]. Another paper, involving female patients with knee OA, identified a significant correlation between synovial adiponectin levels and degradation markers of aggrecan, which suggests that adiponectin regulates the degeneration of cartilage matrix in OA [39]. In an investigation into the effects of adipokines upon the development of OA osteophytes, adiponectin and visfatin stimulated osteoblasts and chondrocytes, respectively, to increase their release of proinflammatory mediators [40]. Adiponectin has been found to enhance nitric oxide, IL-6, MMP-1 and MMP-3 production in OA cartilage and in primary chondrocytes via mitogen-activated protein kinase (MAPK) signaling [29,41]. Similarly, Junker and colleagues found that adiponectin induced p38 MAPK signaling in OA osteoblasts, whereas stimulation with adiponectin, resistin, or visfatin had no effect on Wnt signaling [40]. These findings indicate that adipokines do not directly influence osteophyte development, but that they do influence proinflammatory conditions in OA and that adiponectin possibly mediates cartilage destruction in OA. Other research has reported that monocyte adhesion to the human OA synovial fibroblast (OASF) monolayer is promoted by adiponectin-induced intercellular adhesion molecule 1 (ICAM-1) expression [42]. In contrast, some evidence suggests that serum adiponectin may be protective in OA; a significant, negative association between serum adiponectin and radiographic OA severity in patients with knee OA persisted after adjusting the analyses for age, sex, BMI and duration of disease [43].

3. Leptin Expression in RA and OA

Leptin, a 16 kDa non-glycosylated protein encoded by the *obese* (*ob*) gene, is mainly secreted by adipose tissue and regulates appetite and obesity by inducing anorexigenic factors and suppressing orexigenic neuropeptides [44]. The release of leptin into the circulation enables it to act peripherally and centrally [45]. After entering the brain via a saturable transport mechanism, leptin's central location of action is the hypothalamus [45]. This adipokine also has direct effects on non-neural cells [46], as evidenced by its involvement in immunoregulatory functions, as it is capable of inducing T_H1 immune reactions by increasing the T_H1 phenotype of the effector CD4 T cell and suppressing the T_H2 phenotype; leptin can also induce naïve CD4 T cells to proliferate and inhibit memory CD4 T cells from proliferating [47].

Increased serum leptin levels have been linked to erosion of cartilage and bone in OA [48], synovitis and cartilage defects, bone marrow lesions and osteophytes [49]. Notably, leptin expression correlates with DNA methylation in OA chondrocytes and leptin's downregulation dramatically inhibits MMP-13 gene expression [50]. Single nucleotide polymorphism (SNP) analyses have suggested associations between the leptin gene and its receptor gene with OA in both normal weight and overweight Chinese populations [51,52]. Some research has found a significant correlation between leptin messenger RNA (mRNA) expression in advanced human OA cartilage and BMI, suggesting that leptin could serve as a metabolic link between obesity and OA [53]. That same research also found that leptin expression was significantly increased in synovial fluid, indicating that leptin was locally produced as opposed to diffusing from plasma to synovial fluid via the synovial membrane. The ability of leptin to stimulate IL-1β production and increase MMP-9 and MMP-13 protein expression in OA and normal chondrocytes supports the contention that leptin has proinflammatory and catabolic effects in the metabolism of cartilage [53]. Evidence implicates leptin in obesity and joint damage; a significant association has been found between baseline leptin levels and increased biomarkers of bone formation (osteocalcin and PINP) over a 2-year period; conversely, higher levels of soluble leptin receptor (sOB-Rb), which reduces leptin activity, were associated with lower osteocalcin levels at 2 years of follow-up [54]. Interestingly, serum leptin levels are significantly associated with increased knee OA cartilage volume, whereas serum adiponectin levels are significantly associated with lower levels of disease severity in radiographic OA [43].

Other research has found that adiposity in leptin-impaired mice does not lead to systemic inflammation and knee OA, which suggests that leptin directly influences knee OA pathogenesis rather than via any correlation with obesity and that the loss of leptin signaling pathways may help to prevent the development of OA [55]. Assessing leptin expression could potentially be used to measure RA and OA disease activity. Higher serum leptin levels are found in RA patients with high disease activity compared with those with low disease activity [22,56] and a small but significantly positive correlation exists between leptin levels and RA activity [57,58]; no such correlation exists between serum adiponectin levels and RA disease activity [58]. This lack of association between adiponectin levels and disease activity was seen in another study involving patients with knee OA, in whom synovial fluid leptin levels and plasma levels of adiponectin, soluble leptin receptor and free leptin were not significantly different across categories of OA severity, although the ratio of synovial fluid to plasma leptin level was significantly lower in advanced OA than in early disease [59]. In contrast, other research has revealed a close association between synovial fluid leptin levels and OA radiographic severity, which is highest in stage IV disease [60].

In vitro investigations suggest that leptin increases production of the proinflammatory cytokine IL-8 in RASFs and OASFs by binding to the leptin receptor (OBRl) and activating the Janus kinase 2/signal transducer and activator of transcription 3 (JAK2/STAT3) signaling pathway, which in turn activates the insulin receptor substrate-1/phosphatidylinositol 3 kinase/Akt/nuclear factor-κB (IRS1/PI3K/Akt/NF-κB)-dependent pathway and leads to p300 recruitment [61]. Similarly, leptin induces IL-6 expression in OASFs by activating the OBRl receptor, which in turn activates the IRS-1, PI3K, Akt, and AP-1 signaling pathways and thus upregulates IL-6 expression [62]. Table 1 summarizes the involved receptors, downstream and targeted signaling molecules, and target genes involved in RA and OA. It shows that many leptin receptors exist in individual cells (osteoblasts, FLSs and chondrocytes), but not in the brain. Evidence of brain leptin receptor expression in RA/OA will require much more research. Leptin also increases vascular cell adhesion molecule 1 (VCAM-1) expression in human and murine chondrocytes [63]. Importantly, VCAM-1 functions as a cell adhesion molecule, mediating leukocyte recruitment and extravasation from circulating blood to inflamed joints [63]. Interestingly, leptin appears to induce MAPK signaling in both human chondrocytes [64] and RA FLSs [65]. The presence of leptin stimulates oncostatin M production in osteoblasts from healthy human donors [66].

Table 1. Adipokines implicated in rheumatoid arthritis and osteoarthritis.

Stimulation	Target Factors		Effects in Tissue	Disease	Receptor	Known Pathways	References
			Adiponectin				
	IL-6	↑	FLSs	OA & RA	AdipoR1	AMPK/p38/IKKαβ and NF-κB	[26]
	VEGF, MMPs	↑	FLSs	RA	N/A	N/A	[27]
	IL-6, RANTES, MMP-3	↑	FLSs, lymphocytes, endothelial cells, and chondrocytes	RA	N/A	PKA/NF-κB/p38MAPK/PKC	[29]
	PGE2	↑	FLSs	RA	AdipoR1	NF-κB	[30,31]
	OSM	↑	Osteoblasts	RA	N/A	PI3K/Akt and NF-κB	[33]
	IL-6, IL-8, and CCL2	↑	Osteoblasts and chondrocytes	OA	N/A	p38/MAPK	[40]
	IL-6, MMP-1,-3	↑	Chondrocytes	OA	N/A	p38/ERK1/2/JNK	[41]
	ICAM-1	↑	FLSs	OA	AdipoR1	LKB1, CaMKII, AMPK, and AP-1	[12]
	VCAM-1	↑	Chondrocytes	RA & OA	N/A	JAK2 and PI3K	[63]
			Leptin				
	MMP-13	↑	Chondrocytes	OA	N/A		[50]
	IL-1β, MMP-9 and MMP-13	↑	Chondrocytes	OA	OBRb		[53]
	IL-8	↑	FLSs	RA & OA	OBRI	JAK2/STAT3 and IRS-1/PI3K/Akt/NF-κB	[61]
	IL-6	↑	FLSs	OA	OBRI	IRS-1/PI3K/Akt and AP-1	[62]
	VCAM-1	↑	Chondrocytes	RA & OA	N/A	JAK2 and PI3K	[63]
	ADAMTS-4,-5 and -9	↑	Chondrocytes	OA	N/A	MAPK and NF-κB	[64]
	IL-6	↑	FLSs	RA	OBRb	JAK2/STAT3	[65]
	OSM	↑	Osteoblasts	RA	OBRI	AKT/miR-93	[66]
			Resistin				
	CXCL8, CCL2 and IL-6	↑	FLSs	RA	N/A	CAP1	[67]
	VEGF	↑	EPCs	RA	N/A	PKC-δ/AMPK/miR-206	[68]
			Visfatin				
	IL-6 and IL-8, CCL2 and MMP-3	↑	FLSs	RA	N/A	p38 pathway	[69]
	IGF-1	↓	Chondrocytes	OA	IGF-1R	ERK/MAPK signaling pathway	[70]
	IL-6 and TNF-α	↑	FLSs	OA	N/A	ERK/p38/JNK and miR-199a-5p	[71]
	MMP-3,-12, and -13	↑	Chondrocytes	OA	N/A	HIF-2a	[72]
			Other adipokines				
	MMP-1, -3 and -9, ADAMTS-4 and -5, IL-1β	↑	Chondrocytes	OA	N/A	JNK, ERK and MAPK	[73]

IL-6, interleukin 6; FLSs, fibroblast-like synoviocytes; OA, osteoarthritis; RA, rheumatoid arthritis; AdipoR1, adiponectin receptor 1; AMPK, AMP-activated protein kinase; IKKα/β, IκB kinase alpha/beta; NF-κB, nuclear factor-kappa B; VEGF, vascular endothelial growth factor; MMP, matrix metalloproteinase; RANTES, regulated upon activation, normal T cells expressed and secreted; PKA, protein kinase A; p38MAPK, P38 mitogen-activated protein kinase; PKC, protein kinase C; PGE2, prostaglandin E2; OSM, oncostatin M; PI3K, phosphatidylinositol 3 kinase; IL-8, interleukin-8; CCL2, chemokine (C-C motif) ligand 2; ERK1/2, extracellular signal-regulated protein kinases 1 and 2; JNK, c-Jun N-terminal kinase; ICAM-1, intercellular adhesion molecule 1; LKB1, liver kinase B1; CaMKII, Ca^{2+}/calmodulin-dependent protein kinase II; AP-1, activator protein 1; VCAM-1, vascular cell adhesion molecule 1; JAK2, Janus kinase 2; IL-1β, interleukin-1 beta; OBRb and OBRI, long isoform of leptin receptor; STAT3, signal transducer and activator of transcription 3; IRS1, insulin receptor substrate-1; ADAMTS-4, ADAM metallopeptidase with thrombospondin type 1 motif 4; ADAMTS-5, ADAM metallopeptidase with thrombospondin type 1 motif 5; ADAMTS-9, ADAM metallopeptidase with thrombospondin type 1 motif 9; miR, microRNA; CXCL8, C-X-C motif chemokine ligand 8; CAP1, adenylate cyclase-associated protein 1; EPCs, endothelial progenitor cells; IGF-1, insulin-like growth factor 1; IGF-1R, IGF-1 receptor; TNF-α, tumor necrosis factor alpha; HIF-2α, hypoxia-inducible factor 2 alpha.

4. Resistin in Arthritis

4.1. Resistin in RA

Adipocyte-derived expression and secretion of resistin, a small cysteine-rich adipokine, is linked to inflammation and insulin resistance [68,74]. Some researchers have documented positive correlations between serum resistin levels and inflammatory status (erythrocyte sedimentation rate [ESR], CRP) as well as clinical disease activity (28-joint count Disease Activity Score [DAS28]) in patients with RA [22,75]. Significantly higher resistin levels have been observed in synovial sublining layers from RA patients than from OA patients [75]. Šenolt and colleagues have documented resistin expression within several different cell types within the synovial tissue, including synovial fibroblasts, and in different inflammatory cell types found in RA synovium such as macrophages, B lymphocytes and plasma cells [75]. They proposed that resistin is a secreted signaling molecule that helps to activate these cell types in chronic inflammatory states such as RA. Subsequent investigations support this contention, showing positive associations between serum levels of resistin and leptin with CRP levels in RA, indicating that resistin and leptin act as proinflammatory cytokines in this disease [22]. Indeed, resistin has been found to specifically enhance the concentrations of chemokines CXCL8 and CCL2, as well as IL-6, in RA FLSs; transfecting the FLSs with adenylate cyclase-associated protein 1 (CAP1, a receptor for resistin) significantly reduced CXCL8 expression, which implicates the involvement of the resistin-CAP1 pathway in chemokine production in RA synovial tissue [67]. Plasma resistin levels also correlate with coronary artery calcification, a marker of coronary atherosclerosis [74].

Interestingly, despite finding evidence in support of resistin as a significant mediator of the inflammatory process in RA, Yoshino and colleagues (2011) found that serum resistin levels did not differ between RA patients and healthy controls [22], which is backed by other investigations [76,77]. In contrast, one small study found higher serum and synovial resistin levels in RA patients compared with OA patients, supporting a role for resistin in autoimmune inflammatory rheumatologic disease [78]. The study evidence also suggested that high synovial fluid resistin levels may be a poor prognostic factor for RA in terms of disease progression and radiologic joint damage.

Other researchers have described how resistin directly induces significant increases in VEGF expression in endothelial progenitor cells (EPCs) and promotes EPC homing into the synovium, inducing RA angiogenesis; inhibiting resistin reduces EPC homing into synovial fluid and angiogenesis in mice with collagen-induced arthritis [68]. Those researchers detail the involvement of the protein kinase C delta (PKC-δ) pathway in resistin-induced EPC migration and tube formation; this investigation was the first to show that resistin induces EPC migration and tube formation by downregulating microRNA 206 (miR-206) expression via the PKC-δ/AMPK (AMP-activated protein kinase) signaling pathway, which involves VEGF expression in primary EPCs. This clarification of the mechanisms underlying RA pathogenesis highlights resistin as a therapeutic target in RA and is confirmed by an investigation into resistin gene expression in pathogenetic leukocyte subsets from patients with active RA treated with TNF-α inhibitor therapy (adalimumab) for 3 months [79]. Among those who responded to adalimumab, resistin (*RETN*) gene expression was significantly downregulated in CD14$^+$ and CD4$^+$ monocytes, but was unchanged in CD8$^+$ T cytotoxic lymphocytes and CD19$^+$ B lymphocytes [79]. Conversely, *RETN* gene expression increased in a patient who failed to respond to adalimumab. Some research has explored whether selected gene polymorphisms in Chinese Han patients with RA and healthy controls are associated with RA susceptibility and clinicopathological characteristics [80]. The analysis examined four *RETN* single nucleotide polymorphisms (SNPs rs3745367, rs7408174, rs1862513, and rs3219175). Those carrying the C allele of the *RETN* SNP rs7408174 and those with the AG allele or who had at least one A allele of the SNP rs3219175 were more likely than wild-type carriers to develop RA. In addition, RA patients carrying the AG allele of the *RETN* SNP rs3219175 had higher serum CRP levels compared with controls, and had a high likelihood of being prescribed TNF inhibitors. Besides the risk for RA, genetic variation in *RETN* is linked to a higher likelihood of other diseases, such as MetS and colon cancer, while the *RETN* SNP rs186513 is implicated in a higher risk of type 2 diabetes [74]. Moreover, *RETN* SNPs correlated with lung cancer progression in patients with Chinese Han ethnicity [74].

4.2. Resistin in OA

Resistin may possibly serve as a drug target in OA: Positive correlations have been observed between resistin and inflammatory factors (IL-6, MMP-1 and MMP-3) in human OASFs [81]. Moreover, the researchers found a correlation between release of resistin from cultured OA cartilage and resistin levels in synovial fluid. Similarly, one study has reported that levels of circulating leptin resistin, IL-6 and IL-17, were positively correlated with clinical disease activity in Mexican patients with RA [82].

5. Visfatin in Arthritis

5.1. Visfatin in RA

Visfatin (otherwise known as pre-B-cell colony-enhancing factor [PBEF] or nicotinamide phosphoribosyltransferase [NAMPT]) is actively involved in the synthesis of cellular nicotinamide adenine dinucleotide (NAD$^+$) and helps to regulate cellular growth, angiogenesis and apoptosis in mammalian cells [83]. Visfatin also triggers the release of cytokines, chemokines and proinflammatory enzymes that are characteristically present in RA joints [84] and is overexpressed in plasma and synovial fluid of several inflammatory diseases, including RA and OA [85,86], suggesting that visfatin promotes their development. This is supported by findings showing that visfatin/PBEF contributes to proinflammatory chemokine production in RASFs, matrix-degrading factors and pro-angiogenic molecules in RA synovial tissue [69]. Moreover, other researchers have demonstrated a positive correlation between circulating visfatin levels and RA disease activity as assessed by DAS28 and CRP levels [87]. Interestingly, although the study also reported significantly higher circulating adiponectin levels in RA patients than in controls, there was no apparent link between circulating adiponectin and disease activity.

Insulin-like growth factor-1 (IGF-1) is implicated in the synthesis and repair of cartilage matrix. Visfatin inhibits IGF-1 function in chondrocytes by prolonging the activation of the extracellular signal-regulated kinase (ERK)/MAPK signaling pathway, independently of IGF-1 receptor activation [70]. Visfatin also inhibits IGF-1-stimulated proteoglycan (PG) synthesis, basal and IGF-1-stimulated collagen type II expression and synthesis [70]. These findings help to clarify the local effects of visfatin on joint tissue and its effects upon inflammatory disease.

Substantial epidemiological data characterize cigarette smoking as an important risk factor for RA and attest to the negative impacts of smoking upon all stages of RA disease [88]. Cigarette smoking reduces the clinical response to antirheumatic therapy and to treatment with TNF inhibitors in particular, especially infliximab [88]. In preclinical and early-stage disease, evidence suggests that smoking may interact with HLA-DR shared epitope genes and encourage the development of anticitrulline antibody-positive RA [89]. A strong, positive association has been observed between smoking and radiographic progression in early RA [88]. In established RA disease, cigarette smoking has been associated with progressive joint damage, persistently active RA and the development of rheumatic nodules [89]. Smoking is also associated with high concentrations of inflammatory cytokines [88] and inversely associated with circulating levels of IGF-1 [89]. Intriguingly, researchers have demonstrated lower serum levels of leptin and adiponectin in smokers than in non-smokers, whereas smoking appears to have no such effect upon resistin and visfatin levels, which are similar between smokers and non-smokers [89].

Visfatin is known to increase cardiovascular risk. In untreated patients with early-stage RA, significant positive concentrations have been observed between visfatin and biochemical markers of severe metabolic disturbance (insulin and insulin resistance, total and LDL cholesterol and triglycerides), although other studies have failed to find an association between visfatin concentrations and coronary artery calcification scores in RA, between visfatin concentrations and carotid artery

IMT, or any relationship between NAMPT polymorphisms, disease susceptibility and cardiovascular risk in RA [90]. In patients with established, treated RA, visfatin concentrations have been found to be independently associated with increased diastolic blood pressure and diabetes [90]. Moreover, visfatin concentrations were directly associated with levels of MMP-2 (a plaque stability mediator), even after adjusting for adiposity and Clinical Disease Activity Index (CDAI) scores. It is thought that elevated MMP-2 expression in RA might help to compensate for the visfatin-induced enhancement of cardiovascular risk [90]. Interestingly, several different types of cancers (i.e., colorectal, gastric, breast, prostatic, pancreas and esophageal) exhibit overexpression of visfatin [83].

5.2. Visfatin in OA

Investigations have confirmed an essential role for visfatin in the destruction of OA cartilage mediated by hypoxia-inducible factor 2-alpha (HIF-2α) [72]. Not only does HIF-2α directly target the *Nampt* gene in articular chondrocytes and OA cartilage, but also, visfatin upregulates mRNA levels and activities of MMP-3, MMP-12 and MMP-13 and downregulates aggrecan expression in chondrocytes, all of which are critical for OA pathogenesis. Inhibiting visfatin enzymatic activity blocks the destruction of OA cartilage [72]. In in vitro investigations, visfatin-induced promotion of IL-6 and TNF-α in human synovial fibroblasts occurs through the ERK, p38, and JNK signaling pathways [71].

6. Lipocalin-2 in RA and OA

Lipocalin-2 is upregulated in adipose tissue of obese animals and in vitro evidence suggests that lipocalin-2 homeostatically regulates inflammatory activity and inflammation-mediated adipocyte dysfunction in an autocrine or paracrine fashion [91]. This is supported by findings showing elevated levels of fecal lipocalin-2 in mice with collagen-induced arthritis and concomitant experimental colitis; induction of colitis delayed the onset of arthritis and reduced its severity as compared with the arthritis-only group [92]. Interestingly, the development of arthritis was not affected by colitis severity. Similarly, other researchers have reported that although higher serum lipocalin-2 levels can be used as an indicator of structural damage such as erosions in early-stage RA, they cannot be used to monitor disease activity [93]. A recent investigation into the expression and role of lipocalin-2 in OA osteoblasts and chondrocytes in osteochondral junctions has revealed its importance as a catabolic adipokine and its regulation in osteoblasts by inflammatory, catabolic, and anabolic factors [94]. That investigation also revealed that osteoblasts induced the paracrine expression of lipocalin-2. According to these findings, lipocalin-2 is apparently an active catabolic agent in OA joints and may serve as a link among obesity, aging and OA joint alterations.

7. Apelin in RA and OA

Early in vitro investigations into the role of apelin at any of the following concentrations of 0.5, 1, 10, or 100 nM in cartilage metabolism indicated that this cytokine stimulates chondrocyte proliferation and increases MMP-1, MMP-3 and MMP-9 transcript levels, as well as IL-1β protein expression [73]. These results were supported by in vivo findings: After rats were administered intra-articular injections of apelin (1 nM), MMP-1, MMP-3 and MMP-9 were upregulated, ADAMTS-4 and ADAMTS-5 mRNA levels were markedly increased, as were IL-1β levels, while levels of collagen II gene and protein expression were reduced. Moreover, proteoglycan was depleted in articular cartilage after apelin treatment. In patients with RA, research has reported finding a strong inverse association between apelin concentrations and those of MMP-9 [95]. Patients with early RA exhibit significantly lower serum apelin levels compared with apelin profiles of healthy controls [96]. The published evidence suggests that it could be worth investigating drugs that specifically target apelin and thus inhibit the development of arthritic diseases such as RA and OA.

8. Omentin, Vaspin and Nesfatin in RA, OA, and Other Arthritic Diseases

Similarly, another anti-inflammatory adipokine, omentin, is associated with lower levels of MMP-3 in RA [97], while nesfatin-1 has been found to be inversely associated with carotid IMT (80), suggesting that certain adipokines may protect against cardiovascular disease in RA. Patients with psoriatic arthritis exhibit higher serum levels of omentin and leptin, but lower levels of adiponectin and chemerin, compared with healthy controls [98]. Interestingly, whereas higher serum levels of omentin and leptin are positively correlated with numbers of osteoclast precursors in peripheral blood, lower serum adiponectin levels in psoriatic arthritis are negatively correlated with osteoclast precursors [98]. Those researchers also described finding a positive correlation between leptin and Psoriatic Arthritis Joint Activity Index scores. Serum levels of omentin are also significantly higher in patients with juvenile idiopathic arthritis (JIA) compared with healthy controls; moreover, omentin serum levels are higher in JIA with active joints compared with JIA without active joints, and a positive significant correlation has been observed between omentin serum levels and the presence of active joints in JIA [99]. That same investigation failed to find any such associations between these parameters of disease activity and serum levels of vaspin in JIA [99]. Omentin apparently has no effects upon central effector cells in RA pathophysiology, despite its presence in the synovium and synovial fluid from RA and OA patients [100]. Interestingly, not only do synovial fluid levels of omentin and vaspin appear to differ at the site of local inflammation in patients with RA and OA, but also, patients with RA have demonstrated lower levels of omentin and higher levels of vaspin in synovial fluid compared with patients with OA [101]. Those researchers found that synovial fluid levels of vaspin, but not of omentin, tended to correlated with DAS28 scores, but neither adipokine was correlated with serum CRP or synovial fluid leucocyte counts [101]. Although omentin seems to have anti-inflammatory and antiatherogenic properties in obesity and displays negative associations in inflammatory bowel disease and MetS, these effects may not occur in RA and OA [100]. It may be worth targeting nesfatin-1 in OA; elevated levels in serum and synovial fluid from patients with knee OA have been found to be significantly associated with disease severity as determined by Kellgren–Lawrence grading criteria [102]. Moreover, it is speculated that nesfatin-1 may contribute to pathophysiological changes in OA [103]. Nesfatin-1 has been found in articular cartilage in patients with knee OA, who exhibit significantly higher serum levels of nesfatin-1 compared with serum from healthy controls [103]. Furthermore, serum nesfatin-1 levels are significantly correlated with high-sensitivity CRP levels, while synovial nesfatin-1 is significantly correlated with IL-18 levels in patients with OA [103].

9. Other Adipokines

Importantly, besides those adipokines covered in this review, we cannot discuss other more recently discovered adipokines including adipolin, acylation-stimulating protein, fasting-induced adipose factor, retinol-binding protein-4, and serum amyloid A3, because no available data provide evidence for their roles in RA and OA disease. Interestingly, related research has found that the novel adipokine fatty acid-binding protein 4 (FABP4), closely associated with obesity and metabolic diseases, is significantly higher in the serum and synovial fluid of patients with RA than in those of OA patients [104], while plasma and synovial fluid levels of FABP4 are significantly higher in OA patients than in those of healthy non-OA controls [105]. Furthermore, recent experimental research has indicated that in FABP4 knockout mice (KO) with obesity induced by a high-fat diet, cartilage degradation is significantly alleviated after 6 months of daily oral gavage with a selective FABP4 inhibitor has suggested that FABP4 may be a potential therapeutic target in OA [106]. Further explorations into the pathogenic aspects of novel adipokines involved in obesity may well uncover other such links into RA and OA disease activity; the space limitations of this review prevent us from researching this aspect.

Int. J. Mol. Sci. **2019**, *20*, 1505

10. Summary and Future Directions

Controversially, obesity does not necessarily influence the likelihood of developing RA; the evidential link is more definite for OA, where leptin appears to be a metabolic link between obesity and OA. Other adipokines, such as visfatin and resistin, also play important roles in arthritis pathogenesis (Table 1 and Figure 2). In agreement with previous summaries of evidence on the interaction of adipokines with RA and OA [107,108], the evidence discussed in this review suggests that it could be useful to develop therapeutic molecules that target individual adipokines. We have found no published evidence for any natural product that inhibits adipokines and potentially treats arthritis. To help overcome the lack of treatment opportunities, our laboratory is constructing a full-length adipokine containing luciferase for use as a screening model to identify and test natural products or pharmacochemical structures able to target specific adipokines involved in RA and OA disease. We are also working on the design of anti-adipokine antibodies that we will test for their ability to detect the early development of arthritic diseases, so that in future anti-arthritic therapy can be administered early to prevent disease progression.

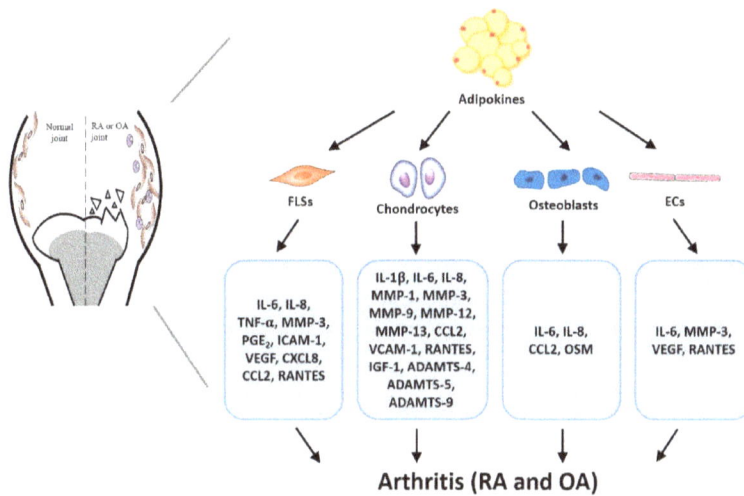

Figure 2. Critical pathways involving adipokines in arthritic diseases. Adipose tissue paracrine signaling in RA and OA demonstrates systemic links between adipokines and arthritic disease.

Author Contributions: All authors except for I.J.M. and C.-C.H. conceptualized the topic for this review; S.-C.L. conceived ideas about the clinical application of anti-adipokine antibodies. S.-J.K. and C.-H.T. (Chun-Hao Tsai) were involved in drafting the article; C.-C.H. and C.-H.T. (Chih-Hsin Tang) critically revised the review for important intellectual content. All authors approved the final version to be published.

Funding: This work was supported by grants from the National Science Council of Taiwan (MOST107-2320-B-039-019-MY3; 105-2320-B-039-015-MY3; 107-2314-B-039-064-) and China Medical University Hospital, Taichung, Taiwan (DMR-108-070).

Conflicts of Interest: The authors declare no conflict of interest.

References

1. Azamar-Llamas, D.; Hernandez-Molina, G.; Ramos-Avalos, B.; Furuzawa-Carballeda, J. Adipokine Contribution to the Pathogenesis of Osteoarthritis. *Mediat. Inflamm.* **2017**, *2017*, 5468023. [CrossRef]
2. Guo, Q.; Wang, Y.; Xu, D.; Nossent, J.; Pavlos, N.J.; Xu, J. Rheumatoid arthritis: Pathological mechanisms and modern pharmacologic therapies. *Bone Res.* **2018**, *6*, 15. [CrossRef]

3. Gremese, E.; Tolusso, B.; Gigante, M.R.; Ferraccioli, G. Obesity as a risk and severity factor in rheumatic diseases (autoimmune chronic inflammatory diseases). *Front. Immunol.* **2014**, *5*, 576. [CrossRef]

4. De Hair, M.J.; Landewe, R.B.; van de Sande, M.G.; van Schaardenburg, D.; van Baarsen, L.G.; Gerlag, D.M.; Tak, P.P. Smoking and overweight determine the likelihood of developing rheumatoid arthritis. *Ann. Rheum. Dis.* **2013**, *72*, 1654–1658. [CrossRef]

5. Mandl, L.A.; Costenbader, K.H.; Simard, J.F.; Karlson, E.W. Is birthweight associated with risk of rheumatoid arthritis? Data from a large cohort study. *Ann. Rheum. Dis.* **2009**, *68*, 514–518. [CrossRef]

6. Van der Helm-van Mil, A.H.; van der Kooij, S.M.; Allaart, C.F.; Toes, R.E.; Huizinga, T.W. A high body mass index has a protective effect on the amount of joint destruction in small joints in early rheumatoid arthritis. *Ann. Rheum. Dis.* **2008**, *67*, 769–774. [CrossRef] [PubMed]

7. Baker, J.F.; George, M.; Baker, D.G.; Toedter, G.; Von Feldt, J.M.; Leonard, M.B. Associations between body mass, radiographic joint damage, adipokines and risk factors for bone loss in rheumatoid arthritis. *Rheumatology* **2011**, *50*, 2100–2107. [CrossRef]

8. Hashimoto, J.; Garnero, P.; van der Heijde, D.; Miyasaka, N.; Yamamoto, K.; Kawai, S.; Takeuchi, T.; Yoshikawa, H.; Nishimoto, N. A combination of biochemical markers of cartilage and bone turnover, radiographic damage and body mass index to predict the progression of joint destruction in patients with rheumatoid arthritis treated with disease-modifying anti-rheumatic drugs. *Mod. Rheumatol.* **2009**, *19*, 273–282. [CrossRef] [PubMed]

9. Westhoff, G.; Rau, R.; Zink, A. Radiographic joint damage in early rheumatoid arthritis is highly dependent on body mass index. *Arthritis Rheum.* **2007**, *56*, 3575–3582. [CrossRef] [PubMed]

10. Lohmander, L.S.; Gerhardsson de Verdier, M.; Rollof, J.; Nilsson, P.M.; Engstrom, G. Incidence of severe knee and hip osteoarthritis in relation to different measures of body mass: A population-based prospective cohort study. *Ann. Rheum. Dis.* **2009**, *68*, 490–496. [CrossRef]

11. Urban, H.; Little, C.B. The role of fat and inflammation in the pathogenesis and management of osteoarthritis. *Rheumatology* **2018**, *57* (Suppl. S4), iv10–iv21. [CrossRef] [PubMed]

12. Fowler-Brown, A.; Kim, D.H.; Shi, L.; Marcantonio, E.; Wee, C.C.; Shmerling, R.H.; Leveille, S. The mediating effect of leptin on the relationship between body weight and knee osteoarthritis in older adults. *Arthritis Rheumatol.* **2015**, *67*, 169–175. [CrossRef] [PubMed]

13. Zheng, H.; Chen, C. Body mass index and risk of knee osteoarthritis: Systematic review and meta-analysis of prospective studies. *BMJ Open* **2015**, *5*, e007568. [CrossRef]

14. Senolt, L. Adipokines: Role in local and systemic inflammation of rheumatic diseases. *Expert Rev. Clin. Immunol.* **2017**, *13*, 1–3. [CrossRef]

15. Gomez, R.; Conde, J.; Scotece, M.; Gomez-Reino, J.J.; Lago, F.; Gualillo, O. What's new in our understanding of the role of adipokines in rheumatic diseases? *Nat. Rev. Rheumatol.* **2011**, *7*, 528–536. [CrossRef] [PubMed]

16. Kontny, E.; Plebanczyk, M.; Lisowska, B.; Olszewska, M.; Maldyk, P.; Maslinski, W. Comparison of rheumatoid articular adipose and synovial tissue reactivity to proinflammatory stimuli: Contribution to adipocytokine network. *Ann. Rheum. Dis.* **2012**, *71*, 262–267. [CrossRef] [PubMed]

17. Maijer, K.I.; Neumann, E.; Muller-Ladner, U.; Drop, D.A.; Ramwadhdoebe, T.H.; Choi, I.Y.; Gerlag, D.M.; de Hair, M.J.; Tak, P.P. Serum Vaspin Levels Are Associated with the Development of Clinically Manifest Arthritis in Autoantibody-Positive Individuals. *PLoS ONE* **2015**, *10*, e0144932. [CrossRef] [PubMed]

18. Giles, J.T.; van der Heijde, D.M.; Bathon, J.M. Association of circulating adiponectin levels with progression of radiographic joint destruction in rheumatoid arthritis. *Ann. Rheum. Dis.* **2011**, *70*, 1562–1568. [CrossRef] [PubMed]

19. Huang, C.Y.; Chang, A.C.; Chen, H.T.; Wang, S.W.; Lo, Y.S.; Tang, C.H. Adiponectin promotes VEGF-C-dependent lymphangiogenesis by inhibiting miR-27b through a CaMKII/AMPK/p38 signaling pathway in human chondrosarcoma cells. *Clin. Sci.* **2016**, *130*, 1523–1533. [CrossRef] [PubMed]

20. Ye, R.; Scherer, P.E. Adiponectin, driver or passenger on the road to insulin sensitivity? *Mol. Metab.* **2013**, *2*, 133–141. [CrossRef]

21. Otero, M.; Lago, R.; Gomez, R.; Lago, F.; Dieguez, C.; Gomez-Reino, J.J.; Gualillo, O. Changes in plasma levels of fat-derived hormones adiponectin, leptin, resistin and visfatin in patients with rheumatoid arthritis. *Ann. Rheum. Dis.* **2006**, *65*, 1198–1201. [CrossRef]

22. Yoshino, T.; Kusunoki, N.; Tanaka, N.; Kaneko, K.; Kusunoki, Y.; Endo, H.; Hasunuma, T.; Kawai, S. Elevated serum levels of resistin, leptin, and adiponectin are associated with C-reactive protein and also other clinical conditions in rheumatoid arthritis. *Intern. Med.* **2011**, *50*, 269–275. [CrossRef]

23. Ozgen, M.; Koca, S.S.; Dagli, N.; Balin, M.; Ustundag, B.; Isik, A. Serum adiponectin and vaspin levels in rheumatoid arthritis. *Arch. Med. Res.* **2010**, *41*, 457–463. [CrossRef]

24. Senolt, L.; Pavelka, K.; Housa, D.; Haluzik, M. Increased adiponectin is negatively linked to the local inflammatory process in patients with rheumatoid arthritis. *Cytokine* **2006**, *35*, 247–252. [CrossRef]

25. Folco, E.J.; Rocha, V.Z.; Lopez-Ilasaca, M.; Libby, P. Adiponectin inhibits pro-inflammatory signaling in human macrophages independent of interleukin-10. *J. Biol. Chem.* **2009**, *284*, 25569–25575. [CrossRef]

26. Tang, C.H.; Chiu, Y.C.; Tan, T.W.; Yang, R.S.; Fu, W.M. Adiponectin enhances IL-6 production in human synovial fibroblast via an AdipoR1 receptor, AMPK, p38, and NF-kappa B pathway. *J. Immunol.* **2007**, *179*, 5483–5492. [CrossRef]

27. Choi, H.M.; Lee, Y.A.; Lee, S.H.; Hong, S.J.; Hahm, D.H.; Choi, S.Y.; Yang, H.I.; Yoo, M.C.; Kim, K.S. Adiponectin may contribute to synovitis and joint destruction in rheumatoid arthritis by stimulating vascular endothelial growth factor, matrix metalloproteinase-1, and matrix metalloproteinase-13 expression in fibroblast-like synoviocytes more than proinflammatory mediators. *Arthritis Res. Ther.* **2009**, *11*, R161.

28. Filkova, M.; Liskova, M.; Hulejova, H.; Haluzik, M.; Gatterova, J.; Pavelkova, A.; Pavelka, K.; Gay, S.; Muller-Ladner, U.; Senolt, L. Increased serum adiponectin levels in female patients with erosive compared with non-erosive osteoarthritis. *Ann. Rheum. Dis.* **2009**, *68*, 295–296. [CrossRef]

29. Frommer, K.W.; Zimmermann, B.; Meier, F.M.; Schroder, D.; Heil, M.; Schaffler, A.; Buchler, C.; Steinmeyer, J.; Brentano, F.; Gay, S.; et al. Adiponectin-mediated changes in effector cells involved in the pathophysiology of rheumatoid arthritis. *Arthritis Rheum.* **2010**, *62*, 2886–2899. [CrossRef]

30. Kusunoki, N.; Kitahara, K.; Kojima, F.; Tanaka, N.; Kaneko, K.; Endo, H.; Suguro, T.; Kawai, S. Adiponectin stimulates prostaglandin E(2) production in rheumatoid arthritis synovial fibroblasts. *Arthritis Rheum.* **2010**, *62*, 1641–1649. [CrossRef]

31. Zuo, W.; Wu, Z.H.; Wu, N.; Duan, Y.H.; Wu, J.T.; Wang, H.; Qiu, G.X. Adiponectin receptor 1 mediates the difference in adiponectin-induced prostaglandin E2 production in rheumatoid arthritis and osteoarthritis synovial fibroblasts. *Chin. Med. J.* **2011**, *124*, 3919–3924.

32. Meyer, M.; Sellam, J.; Fellahi, S.; Kotti, S.; Bastard, J.P.; Meyer, O.; Liote, F.; Simon, T.; Capeau, J.; Berenbaum, F. Serum level of adiponectin is a surrogate independent biomarker of radiographic disease progression in early rheumatoid arthritis: Results from the ESPOIR cohort. *Arthritis Res. Ther.* **2013**, *15*, R210. [CrossRef]

33. Su, C.M.; Lee, W.L.; Hsu, C.J.; Lu, T.T.; Wang, L.H.; Xu, G.H.; Tang, C.H. Adiponectin Induces Oncostatin M Expression in Osteoblasts through the PI3K/Akt Signaling Pathway. *Int. J. Mol. Sci.* **2016**, *17*, 29. [CrossRef]

34. Gonzalez-Gay, M.A.; Llorca, J.; Garcia-Unzueta, M.T.; Gonzalez-Juanatey, C.; De Matias, J.M.; Martin, J.; Redelinghuys, M.; Woodiwiss, A.J.; Norton, G.R.; Dessein, P.H. High-grade inflammation, circulating adiponectin concentrations and cardiovascular risk factors in severe rheumatoid arthritis. *Clin. Exp. Rheumatol.* **2008**, *26*, 596–603.

35. Krysiak, R.; Handzlik-Orlik, G.; Okopien, B. The role of adipokines in connective tissue diseases. *Eur. J. Nutr.* **2012**, *51*, 513–528. [CrossRef]

36. Neumann, E.; Frommer, K.W.; Vasile, M.; Muller-Ladner, U. Adipocytokines as driving forces in rheumatoid arthritis and related inflammatory diseases? *Arthritis Rheum.* **2011**, *63*, 1159–1169. [CrossRef]

37. Gross, J.B.; Guillaume, C.; Gegout-Pottie, P.; Mainard, D.; Presle, N. Synovial fluid levels of adipokines in osteoarthritis: Association with local factors of inflammation and cartilage maintenance. *Bio-med. Mater. Eng.* **2014**, *24* (Suppl. S1), 17–25.

38. De Boer, T.N.; van Spil, W.E.; Huisman, A.M.; Polak, A.A.; Bijlsma, J.W.; Lafeber, F.P.; Mastbergen, S.C. Serum adipokines in osteoarthritis; comparison with controls and relationship with local parameters of synovial inflammation and cartilage damage. *Osteoarthr. Cartil.* **2012**, *20*, 846–853. [CrossRef]

39. Hao, D.; Li, M.; Wu, Z.; Duan, Y.; Li, D.; Qiu, G. Synovial fluid level of adiponectin correlated with levels of aggrecan degradation markers in osteoarthritis. *Rheumatol. Int.* **2011**, *31*, 1433–1437. [CrossRef]

40. Junker, S.; Frommer, K.W.; Krumbholz, G.; Tsiklauri, L.; Gerstberger, R.; Rehart, S.; Steinmeyer, J.; Rickert, M.; Wenisch, S.; Schett, G.; et al. Expression of adipokines in osteoarthritis osteophytes and their effect on osteoblasts. *Matrix Biol.* **2017**, *62*, 75–91. [CrossRef]

41. Koskinen, A.; Juslin, S.; Nieminen, R.; Moilanen, T.; Vuolteenaho, K.; Moilanen, E. Adiponectin associates with markers of cartilage degradation in osteoarthritis and induces production of proinflammatory and catabolic factors through mitogen-activated protein kinase pathways. *Arthritis Res. Ther.* **2011**, *13*, R184. [CrossRef]

42. Chen, H.T.; Tsou, H.K.; Chen, J.C.; Shih, J.M.; Chen, Y.J.; Tang, C.H. Adiponectin enhances intercellular adhesion molecule-1 expression and promotes monocyte adhesion in human synovial fibroblasts. *PLoS ONE* **2014**, *9*, e92741. [CrossRef]

43. Zheng, S.; Xu, J.; Xu, S.; Zhang, M.; Huang, S.; He, F.; Yang, X.; Xiao, H.; Zhang, H.; Ding, C. Association between circulating adipokines, radiographic changes, and knee cartilage volume in patients with knee osteoarthritis. *Scand. J. Rheumatol.* **2016**, *45*, 224–229. [CrossRef]

44. Francisco, V.; Perez, T.; Pino, J.; Lopez, V.; Franco, E.; Alonso, A.; Gonzalez-Gay, M.A.; Mera, A.; Lago, F.; Gomez, R.; et al. Biomechanics, obesity, and osteoarthritis. The role of adipokines: When the levee breaks. *J. Orthop. Res.* **2018**, *36*, 594–604. [CrossRef]

45. Tang, C.H.; Lu, D.Y.; Yang, R.S.; Tsai, H.Y.; Kao, M.C.; Fu, W.M.; Chen, Y.F. Leptin-induced IL-6 production is mediated by leptin receptor, insulin receptor substrate-1, phosphatidylinositol 3-kinase, Akt, NF-kappaB, and p300 pathway in microglia. *J. Immunol.* **2007**, *179*, 1292–1302. [CrossRef]

46. Huang, C.Y.; Yu, H.S.; Lai, T.Y.; Yeh, Y.L.; Su, C.C.; Hsu, H.H.; Tsai, F.J.; Tsai, C.H.; Wu, H.C.; Tang, C.H. Leptin increases motility and integrin up-regulation in human prostate cancer cells. *J. Cell. Physiol.* **2011**, *226*, 1274–1282. [CrossRef]

47. Hasenkrug, K.J. The leptin connection: Regulatory T cells and autoimmunity. *Immunity* **2007**, *26*, 143–145. [CrossRef]

48. Scotece, M.; Conde, J.; Lopez, V.; Lago, F.; Pino, J.; Gomez-Reino, J.J.; Gualillo, O. Adiponectin and leptin: New targets in inflammation. *Basic Clin. Pharmacol. Toxicol.* **2014**, *114*, 97–102. [CrossRef]

49. Karvonen-Gutierrez, C.A.; Harlow, S.D.; Jacobson, J.; Mancuso, P.; Jiang, Y. The relationship between longitudinal serum leptin measures and measures of magnetic resonance imaging-assessed knee joint damage in a population of mid-life women. *Ann. Rheum. Dis.* **2014**, *73*, 883–889. [CrossRef]

50. Iliopoulos, D.; Malizos, K.N.; Tsezou, A. Epigenetic regulation of leptin affects MMP-13 expression in osteoarthritic chondrocytes: Possible molecular target for osteoarthritis therapeutic intervention. *Ann. Rheum. Dis.* **2007**, *66*, 1616–1621. [CrossRef]

51. Qin, J.; Shi, D.; Dai, J.; Zhu, L.; Tsezou, A.; Jiang, Q. Association of the leptin gene with knee osteoarthritis susceptibility in a Han Chinese population: A case-control study. *J. Hum. Genet.* **2010**, *55*, 704–706. [CrossRef]

52. Ma, X.J.; Guo, H.H.; Hao, S.W.; Sun, S.X.; Yang, X.C.; Yu, B.; Jin, Q.H. Association of single nucleotide polymorphisms (SNPs) in leptin receptor gene with knee osteoarthritis in the Ningxia Hui population. *Yi Chuan = Hered.* **2013**, *35*, 359–364. [CrossRef]

53. Simopoulou, T.; Malizos, K.N.; Iliopoulos, D.; Stefanou, N.; Papatheodorou, L.; Ioannou, M.; Tsezou, A. Differential expression of leptin and leptin's receptor isoform (Ob-Rb) mRNA between advanced and minimally affected osteoarthritic cartilage; effect on cartilage metabolism. *Osteoarthr. Cartil.* **2007**, *15*, 872–883. [CrossRef]

54. Berry, P.A.; Jones, S.W.; Cicuttini, F.M.; Wluka, A.E.; Maciewicz, R.A. Temporal relationship between serum adipokines, biomarkers of bone and cartilage turnover, and cartilage volume loss in a population with clinical knee osteoarthritis. *Arthritis Rheum.* **2011**, *63*, 700–707. [CrossRef]

55. Griffin, T.M.; Huebner, J.L.; Kraus, V.B.; Guilak, F. Extreme obesity due to impaired leptin signaling in mice does not cause knee osteoarthritis. *Arthritis Rheum.* **2009**, *60*, 2935–2944. [CrossRef]

56. Lee, S.W.; Park, M.C.; Park, Y.B.; Lee, S.K. Measurement of the serum leptin level could assist disease activity monitoring in rheumatoid arthritis. *Rheumatol. Int.* **2007**, *27*, 537–540. [CrossRef]

57. Lee, Y.H.; Bae, S.C. Circulating leptin level in rheumatoid arthritis and its correlation with disease activity: A meta-analysis. *Z. fur Rheumatol.* **2016**, *75*, 1021–1027. [CrossRef]

58. Cao, H.; Lin, J.; Chen, W.; Xu, G.; Sun, C. Baseline adiponectin and leptin levels in predicting an increased risk of disease activity in rheumatoid arthritis: A meta-analysis and systematic review. *Autoimmunity* **2016**, *49*, 547–553. [CrossRef]

59. Staikos, C.; Ververidis, A.; Drosos, G.; Manolopoulos, V.G.; Verettas, D.A.; Tavridou, A. The association of adipokine levels in plasma and synovial fluid with the severity of knee osteoarthritis. *Rheumatology* **2013**, *52*, 1077–1083. [CrossRef]

60. Ku, J.H.; Lee, C.K.; Joo, B.S.; An, B.M.; Choi, S.H.; Wang, T.H.; Cho, H.L. Correlation of synovial fluid leptin concentrations with the severity of osteoarthritis. *Clin. Rheumatol.* **2009**, *28*, 1431–1435. [CrossRef]
61. Tong, K.M.; Shieh, D.C.; Chen, C.P.; Tzeng, C.Y.; Wang, S.P.; Huang, K.C.; Chiu, Y.C.; Fong, Y.C.; Tang, C.H. Leptin induces IL-8 expression via leptin receptor, IRS-1, PI3K, Akt cascade and promotion of NF-kappaB/p300 binding in human synovial fibroblasts. *Cell. Signal.* **2008**, *20*, 1478–1488. [CrossRef]
62. Yang, W.H.; Liu, S.C.; Tsai, C.H.; Fong, Y.C.; Wang, S.J.; Chang, Y.S.; Tang, C.H. Leptin induces IL-6 expression through OBRl receptor signaling pathway in human synovial fibroblasts. *PLoS ONE* **2013**, *8*, e75551. [CrossRef] [PubMed]
63. Conde, J.; Scotece, M.; Lopez, V.; Gomez, R.; Lago, F.; Pino, J.; Gomez-Reino, J.J.; Gualillo, O. Adiponectin and leptin induce VCAM-1 expression in human and murine chondrocytes. *PLoS ONE* **2012**, *7*, e52533. [CrossRef] [PubMed]
64. Yaykasli, K.O.; Hatipoglu, O.F.; Yaykasli, E.; Yildirim, K.; Kaya, E.; Ozsahin, M.; Uslu, M.; Gunduz, E. Leptin induces ADAMTS-4, ADAMTS-5, and ADAMTS-9 genes expression by mitogen-activated protein kinases and NF-kB signaling pathways in human chondrocytes. *Cell Biol. Int.* **2015**, *39*, 104–112. [CrossRef] [PubMed]
65. Muraoka, S.; Kusunoki, N.; Takahashi, H.; Tsuchiya, K.; Kawai, S. Leptin stimulates interleukin-6 production via janus kinase 2/signal transducer and activator of transcription 3 in rheumatoid synovial fibroblasts. *Clin. Exp. Rheumatol.* **2013**, *31*, 589–595.
66. Yang, W.H.; Tsai, C.H.; Fong, Y.C.; Huang, Y.L.; Wang, S.J.; Chang, Y.S.; Tang, C.H. Leptin induces oncostatin M production in osteoblasts by downregulating miR-93 through the Akt signaling pathway. *Int. J. Mol. Sci.* **2014**, *15*, 15778–15790. [CrossRef] [PubMed]
67. Sato, H.; Muraoka, S.; Kusunoki, N.; Masuoka, S.; Yamada, S.; Ogasawara, H.; Imai, T.; Akasaka, Y.; Tochigi, N.; Takahashi, H.; et al. Resistin upregulates chemokine production by fibroblast-like synoviocytes from patients with rheumatoid arthritis. *Arthritis Res. Ther.* **2017**, *19*, 263. [CrossRef] [PubMed]
68. Su, C.M.; Hsu, C.J.; Tsai, C.H.; Huang, C.Y.; Wang, S.W.; Tang, C.H. Resistin Promotes Angiogenesis in Endothelial Progenitor Cells Through Inhibition of MicroRNA206: Potential Implications for Rheumatoid Arthritis. *Stem Cells* **2015**, *33*, 2243–2255. [CrossRef]
69. Meier, F.M.; Frommer, K.W.; Peters, M.A.; Brentano, F.; Lefevre, S.; Schroder, D.; Kyburz, D.; Steinmeyer, J.; Rehart, S.; Gay, S.; et al. Visfatin/pre-B-cell colony-enhancing factor (PBEF), a proinflammatory and cell motility-changing factor in rheumatoid arthritis. *J. Biol. Chem.* **2012**, *287*, 28378–28385. [CrossRef]
70. Yammani, R.R.; Loeser, R.F. Extracellular nicotinamide phosphoribosyltransferase (NAMPT/visfatin) inhibits insulin-like growth factor-1 signaling and proteoglycan synthesis in human articular chondrocytes. *Arthritis Res. Ther.* **2012**, *14*, R23. [CrossRef]
71. Wu, M.H.; Tsai, C.H.; Huang, Y.L.; Fong, Y.C.; Tang, C.H. Visfatin Promotes IL-6 and TNF-alpha Production in Human Synovial Fibroblasts by Repressing miR-199a-5p through ERK, p38 and JNK Signaling Pathways. *Int. J. Mol. Sci.* **2018**, *19*, 190. [CrossRef]
72. Yang, S.; Ryu, J.H.; Oh, H.; Jeon, J.; Kwak, J.S.; Kim, J.H.; Kim, H.A.; Chun, C.H.; Chun, J.S. NAMPT (visfatin), a direct target of hypoxia-inducible factor-2alpha, is an essential catabolic regulator of osteoarthritis. *Ann. Rheum. Dis.* **2015**, *74*, 595–602. [CrossRef]
73. Hu, P.F.; Chen, W.P.; Tang, J.L.; Bao, J.P.; Wu, L.D. Apelin plays a catabolic role on articular cartilage: In vivo and in vitro studies. *Int. J. Mol. Med.* **2010**, *26*, 357–363.
74. Yang, W.H.; Wang, S.J.; Chang, Y.S.; Su, C.M.; Yang, S.F.; Tang, C.H. Association of Resistin Gene Polymorphisms with Oral Squamous Cell Carcinoma Progression and Development. *BioMed Res. Int.* **2018**, *2018*, 9531315. [CrossRef]
75. Senolt, L.; Housa, D.; Vernerova, Z.; Jirasek, T.; Svobodova, R.; Veigl, D.; Anderlova, K.; Muller-Ladner, U.; Pavelka, K.; Haluzik, M. Resistin in rheumatoid arthritis synovial tissue, synovial fluid and serum. *Ann. Rheum. Dis.* **2007**, *66*, 458–463. [CrossRef]
76. Forsblad d'Elia, H.; Pullerits, R.; Carlsten, H.; Bokarewa, M. Resistin in serum is associated with higher levels of IL-1Ra in post-menopausal women with rheumatoid arthritis. *Rheumatology* **2008**, *47*, 1082–1087. [CrossRef]
77. Alkady, E.A.; Ahmed, H.M.; Tag, L.; Abdou, M.A. Serum and synovial adiponectin, resistin, and visfatin levels in rheumatoid arthritis patients. Relation to disease activity. *Z. fur Rheumatol.* **2011**, *70*, 602–608. [CrossRef]

78. Fadda, S.M.; Gamal, S.M.; Elsaid, N.Y.; Mohy, A.M. Resistin in inflammatory and degenerative rheumatologic diseases. Relationship between resistin and rheumatoid arthritis disease progression. *Z. fur Rheumatol.* **2013**, *72*, 594–600. [CrossRef]

79. Nagaev, I.; Andersen, M.; Olesen, M.K.; Nagaeva, O.; Wikberg, J.; Mincheva-Nilsson, L.; Andersen, G.N. Resistin Gene Expression is Downregulated in CD4(+) T Helper Lymphocytes and CD14(+) Monocytes in Rheumatoid Arthritis Responding to TNF-alpha Inhibition. *Scand. J. Immunol.* **2016**, *84*, 229–236. [CrossRef]

80. Wang, L.; Tang, C.H.; Lu, T.; Sun, Y.; Xu, G.; Huang, C.C.; Yang, S.F.; Su, C.M. Resistin polymorphisms are associated with rheumatoid arthritis susceptibility in Chinese Han subjects. *Medicine* **2018**, *97*, e0177. [CrossRef]

81. Koskinen, A.; Vuolteenaho, K.; Moilanen, T.; Moilanen, E. Resistin as a factor in osteoarthritis: Synovial fluid resistin concentrations correlate positively with interleukin 6 and matrix metalloproteinases MMP-1 and MMP-3. *Scand. J. Rheumatol.* **2014**, *43*, 249–253. [CrossRef] [PubMed]

82. Bustos Rivera-Bahena, C.; Xibille-Friedmann, D.X.; Gonzalez-Christen, J.; Carrillo-Vazquez, S.M.; Montiel-Hernandez, J.L. Peripheral blood leptin and resistin levels as clinical activity biomarkers in Mexican Rheumatoid Arthritis patients. *Reumatol. Clin.* **2016**, *12*, 323–326. [CrossRef] [PubMed]

83. Mohammadi, M.; Mianabadi, F.; Mehrad-Majd, H. Circulating visfatin levels and cancers risk: A systematic review and meta-analysis. *J. Cell. Physiol.* **2019**, *234*, 5011–5022. [CrossRef] [PubMed]

84. Brentano, F.; Schorr, O.; Ospelt, C.; Stanczyk, J.; Gay, R.E.; Gay, S.; Kyburz, D. Pre-B cell colony-enhancing factor/visfatin, a new marker of inflammation in rheumatoid arthritis with proinflammatory and matrix-degrading activities. *Arthritis Rheum.* **2007**, *56*, 2829–2839. [CrossRef] [PubMed]

85. Jacques, C.; Holzenberger, M.; Mladenovic, Z.; Salvat, C.; Pecchi, E.; Berenbaum, F.; Gosset, M. Proinflammatory actions of visfatin/nicotinamide phosphoribosyltransferase (Nampt) involve regulation of insulin signaling pathway and Nampt enzymatic activity. *J. Biol. Chem.* **2012**, *287*, 15100–15108. [CrossRef] [PubMed]

86. Laiguillon, M.C.; Houard, X.; Bougault, C.; Gosset, M.; Nourissat, G.; Sautet, A.; Jacques, C.; Berenbaum, F.; Sellam, J. Expression and function of visfatin (Nampt), an adipokine-enzyme involved in inflammatory pathways of osteoarthritis. *Arthritis Res. Ther.* **2014**, *16*, R38. [CrossRef] [PubMed]

87. Lee, Y.H.; Bae, S.C. Circulating adiponectin and visfatin levels in rheumatoid arthritis and their correlation with disease activity: A meta-analysis. *Int. J. Rheum. Dis.* **2018**, *21*, 664–672. [CrossRef]

88. Chang, K.; Yang, S.M.; Kim, S.H.; Han, K.H.; Park, S.J.; Shin, J.I. Smoking and rheumatoid arthritis. *Int. J. Mol. Sci.* **2014**, *15*, 22279–22295. [CrossRef]

89. Erlandsson, M.C.; Doria Medina, R.; Toyra Silfversward, S.; Bokarewa, M.I. Smoking Functions as a Negative Regulator of IGF1 and Impairs Adipokine Network in Patients with Rheumatoid Arthritis. *Mediat. Inflamm.* **2016**, *2016*, 3082820. [CrossRef] [PubMed]

90. Robinson, C.; Tsang, L.; Solomon, A.; Woodiwiss, A.J.; Gunter, S.; Mer, M.; Hsu, H.C.; Gomes, M.; Norton, G.R.; Millen, A.M.E.; et al. Nesfatin-1 and visfatin expression is associated with reduced atherosclerotic disease risk in patients with rheumatoid arthritis. *Peptides* **2018**, *102*, 31–37. [CrossRef]

91. Zhang, J.; Wu, Y.; Zhang, Y.; Leroith, D.; Bernlohr, D.A.; Chen, X. The role of lipocalin 2 in the regulation of inflammation in adipocytes and macrophages. *Mol. Endocrinol.* **2008**, *22*, 1416–1426. [CrossRef] [PubMed]

92. Hablot, J.; Peyrin-Biroulet, L.; Kokten, T.; El Omar, R.; Netter, P.; Bastien, C.; Jouzeau, J.Y.; Sokol, H.; Moulin, D. Experimental colitis delays and reduces the severity of collagen-induced arthritis in mice. *PLoS ONE* **2017**, *12*, e0184624. [CrossRef] [PubMed]

93. Gulkesen, A.; Akgol, G.; Poyraz, A.K.; Aydin, S.; Denk, A.; Yildirim, T.; Kaya, A. Lipocalin 2 as a clinical significance in rheumatoid arthritis. *Cent. -Eur. J. Immunol.* **2017**, *42*, 269–273. [CrossRef] [PubMed]

94. Villalvilla, A.; Garcia-Martin, A.; Largo, R.; Gualillo, O.; Herrero-Beaumont, G.; Gomez, R. The adipokine lipocalin-2 in the context of the osteoarthritic osteochondral junction. *Sci. Rep.* **2016**, *6*, 29243. [CrossRef] [PubMed]

95. Gunter, S.; Solomon, A.; Tsang, L.; Woodiwiss, A.J.; Robinson, C.; Millen, A.M.; Norton, G.R.; Dessein, P.H. Apelin concentrations are associated with altered atherosclerotic plaque stability mediator levels and atherosclerosis in rheumatoid arthritis. *Atherosclerosis* **2017**, *256*, 75–81. [CrossRef]

96. Di Franco, M.; Spinelli, F.R.; Metere, A.; Gerardi, M.C.; Conti, V.; Boccalini, F.; Iannuccelli, C.; Ciciarello, F.; Agati, L.; Valesini, G. Serum levels of asymmetric dimethylarginine and apelin as potential markers of vascular endothelial dysfunction in early rheumatoid arthritis. *Mediat. Inflamm.* **2012**, *2012*, 347268. [CrossRef] [PubMed]

97. Robinson, C.; Tsang, L.; Solomon, A.; Woodiwiss, A.J.; Gunter, S.; Millen, A.M.; Norton, G.R.; Fernandez-Lopez, M.J.; Hollan, I.; Dessein, P.H. Omentin concentrations are independently associated with those of matrix metalloproteinase-3 in patients with mild but not severe rheumatoid arthritis. *Rheumatol. Int.* **2017**, *37*, 3–11. [CrossRef]

98. Xue, Y.; Jiang, L.; Cheng, Q.; Chen, H.; Yu, Y.; Lin, Y.; Yang, X.; Kong, N.; Zhu, X.; Xu, X.; et al. Adipokines in psoriatic arthritis patients: The correlations with osteoclast precursors and bone erosions. *PLoS ONE* **2012**, *7*, e46740. [CrossRef] [PubMed]

99. Cantarini, L.; Simonini, G.; Fioravanti, A.; Generoso, M.; Bacarelli, M.R.; Dini, E.; Galeazzi, M.; Cimaz, R. Circulating levels of the adipokines vaspin and omentin in patients with juvenile idiopathic arthritis, and relation to disease activity. *Clin. Exp. Rheumatol.* **2011**, *29*, 1044–1048. [PubMed]

100. Frommer, K.W.; Vasile, M.; Muller-Ladner, U.; Neumann, E. The Adipokine Omentin in Late-stage Rheumatoid Arthritis and Endstage Osteoarthritis. *J. Rheumatol.* **2017**, *44*, 539–541. [CrossRef]

101. Senolt, L.; Polanska, M.; Filkova, M.; Cerezo, L.A.; Pavelka, K.; Gay, S.; Haluzik, M.; Vencovsky, J. Vaspin and omentin: New adipokines differentially regulated at the site of inflammation in rheumatoid arthritis. *Ann. Rheum. Dis.* **2010**, *69*, 1410–1411. [CrossRef] [PubMed]

102. Zhang, Y.; Shui, X.; Lian, X.; Wang, G. Serum and synovial fluid nesfatin-1 concentration is associated with radiographic severity of knee osteoarthritis. *Med Sci. Monit.* **2015**, *21*, 1078–1082.

103. Jiang, L.; Bao, J.; Zhou, X.; Xiong, Y.; Wu, L. Increased serum levels and chondrocyte expression of nesfatin-1 in patients with osteoarthritis and its relation with BMI, hsCRP, and IL-18. *Mediat. Inflamm.* **2013**, *2013*, 631251. [CrossRef] [PubMed]

104. Andres Cerezo, L.; Kuklova, M.; Hulejova, H.; Vernerova, Z.; Pesakova, V.; Pecha, O.; Veigl, D.; Haluzik, M.; Pavelka, K.; Vencovsky, J.; et al. The level of fatty acid-binding protein 4, a novel adipokine, is increased in rheumatoid arthritis and correlates with serum cholesterol levels. *Cytokine* **2013**, *64*, 441–447. [CrossRef] [PubMed]

105. Zhang, C.; Li, T.; Chiu, K.Y.; Wen, C.; Xu, A.; Yan, C.H. FABP4 as a biomarker for knee osteoarthritis. *Biomark. Med.* **2018**, *12*, 107–118. [CrossRef] [PubMed]

106. Zhang, C.; Chiu, K.Y.; Chan, B.P.M.; Li, T.; Wen, C.; Xu, A.; Yan, C.H. Knocking out or pharmaceutical inhibition of fatty acid binding protein 4 (FABP4) alleviates osteoarthritis induced by high-fat diet in mice. *Osteoarthr. Cartil.* **2018**, *26*, 824–833. [CrossRef] [PubMed]

107. Conde, J.; Scotece, M.; Lopez, V.; Gomez, R.; Lago, F.; Pino, J.; Gomez-Reino, J.J.; Gualillo, O. Adipokines: Novel players in rheumatic diseases. *Discov. Med.* **2013**, *15*, 73–83.

108. Poonpet, T.; Honsawek, S. Adipokines: Biomarkers for osteoarthritis? *World J. Orthop.* **2014**, *5*, 319–327. [CrossRef]

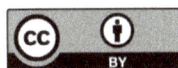

International Journal of
Molecular Sciences

MDPI

Review

Onset and Progression of Human Osteoarthritis—Can Growth Factors, Inflammatory Cytokines, or Differential miRNA Expression Concomitantly Induce Proliferation, ECM Degradation, and Inflammation in Articular Cartilage?

Karen A. Boehme and Bernd Rolauffs *

G.E.R.N. Tissue Replacement, Regeneration & Neogenesis, Department of Orthopedics and Trauma Surgery, Medical Center—Albert-Ludwigs-University of Freiburg, Faculty of Medicine, Albert-Ludwigs-University of Freiburg, 79085 Freiburg im Breisgau, Germany; karen.boehme@web.de
* Correspondence: berndrolauffs@googlemail.com; Tel.: +49-761-270-26101

Received: 3 July 2018; Accepted: 1 August 2018; Published: 3 August 2018

check for
updates

Abstract: Osteoarthritis (OA) is a degenerative whole joint disease, for which no preventative or therapeutic biological interventions are available. This is likely due to the fact that OA pathogenesis includes several signaling pathways, whose interactions remain unclear, especially at disease onset. Early OA is characterized by three key events: a rarely considered early phase of proliferation of cartilage-resident cells, in contrast to well-established increased synthesis, and degradation of extracellular matrix components and inflammation, associated with OA progression. We focused on the question, which of these key events are regulated by growth factors, inflammatory cytokines, and/or miRNA abundance. Collectively, we elucidated a specific sequence of the OA key events that are described best as a very early phase of proliferation of human articular cartilage (AC) cells and concomitant anabolic/catabolic effects that are accompanied by incipient pro-inflammatory effects. Many of the reviewed factors appeared able to induce one or two key events. Only one factor, fibroblast growth factor 2 (FGF2), is capable of concomitantly inducing all key events. Moreover, AC cell proliferation cannot be induced and, in fact, is suppressed by inflammatory signaling, suggesting that inflammatory signaling cannot be the sole inductor of all early OA key events, especially at disease onset.

Keywords: early osteoarthritis; articular cartilage; proliferation; fibroblast growth factor 2; mitogen activated protein kinase; transforming growth factor β; SMA- and MAD-related protein; interleukin; nuclear factor kappa B; miRNA

---

1. Introduction

Osteoarthritis (OA) is a complex degenerative disease of the whole joint leading to progressive articular cartilage (AC) destruction. Even though multiple treatment guidelines have been proposed [1–3], no effective measures exist for the prevention of primary OA. True disease-modifying therapies for OA in the sense of a causal treatment are still missing. However, it is generally accepted that the level of damage occurring in early OA is potentially reversible [4] and that a better insight into the early OA mechanisms is likely the key for developing diagnostic strategies and targeted therapies [5,6].

AC features a specialized architecture consisting of superficial (SZ), middle (MZ), and deep (DZ) zones [7,8], which are formed by modulation of the phenotype of the epiphyseal cartilage cells during skeletal growth and maturation [9]. Of particular interest, it has been shown that, when human

AC samples are fluorescence-tagged and viewed from above, the cells exhibit complex patterns of arrangement in the surface layer of the superficial zone and with an orientation parallel to the joint surface, a feature that has been called superficial cell spatial organization (SCSO) [10,11]. The human SCSO can be highly dynamic, as horizontally orientated cell strings, for example in intact knee AC progress in early OA into double strings, together with an increased SZ cell density suggesting AC cell proliferation, are typical [12]. With OA progression, cell clusters occur, which are ultimately succeeded by a diffuse cell arrangement that is lacking any discernable organization [10,13]. A hallmark of early OA is proliferation of AC-inherent cells [10,13,14], which can be linked to these predictable SCSO changes (see Figure 1) through experimentally inducing AC cell proliferation in early OA AC explants beneath the joint surface. Indeed, proliferation induced via fibroblast growth factor 2 (FGF2) recapitulated SCSO loss and generated a structural AC phenotype that was comparable to advanced OA [13]: human AC explants containing strings and early OA-typical double strings oriented parallel to the surface altered their SCSO through induced proliferation into a diffuse arrangement lacking any discernable organization. Thus, early OA proliferation of SZ cells has a major impact on AC architecture. Moreover, AC cells that transiently proliferate during early OA and form clusters at the margins of extracellular matrix (ECM) fibrillation [14–16] express a large number of proteins that are involved in proliferation, ECM-degradation, and incipient inflammation [14,17], which illustrates the signaling complexity of early OA.

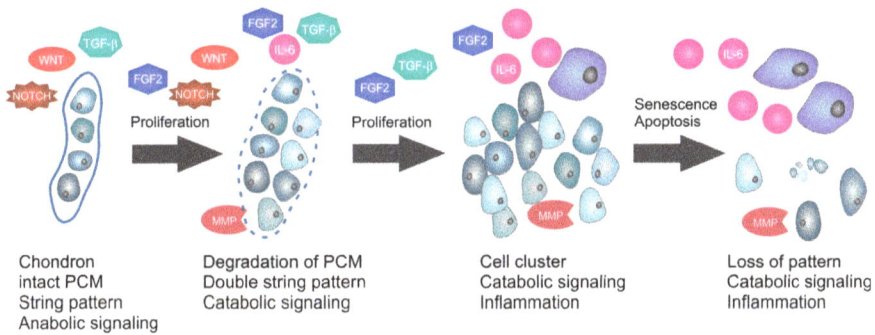

Figure 1. Human osteoarthritis onset and progression. Illustration of the relationship of signaling and superficial cell spatial organization (SCSO). Overview about key proteins in relation to changes in the SCSO of human articular cartilage (AC), which is based on the subsequent chapters that provide a detailed review of the individual pathways. In the superficial zone (SZ) of normal human adult AC differentiated chondrocytes are arranged in string patterns embedded in the pericellular matrix (PCM) and mediate extracellular matrix (ECM) maintenance. The onset of osteoarthritis (OA) is characterized by proliferation. During formation of double string patterns, the PCM is progressively degraded, presumably by MMPs and other catabolic factors. Proliferation in early OA is dependent on fibroblast growth factor 2 (FGF2), transforming growth factor β (TGF-β), wingless-type MMTV integration site family (WNT), and notch homolog (NOTCH) signaling, whereas catabolic matrix metalloproteinase (MMP) expression is mediated by FGF2, a switch in TGF-β signaling and inflammatory cytokines including IL-6. Subsequently, the processes maintaining sustained proliferation and ECM degradation lead to formation of cell clusters that develop from double strings. At the stage of SCSO clusters, pronounced inflammation outweighs attenuated growth factor impact. Late stage OA, accompanied by macroscopic ECM erosion, is characterized by senescence and apoptosis of cartilage-inherent cells and predominance of inflammation.

Indeed, research aimed at establishing a unified theory of the initial OA dysfunction so far has not been successful [18] and this is likely connected to the fact that OA pathogenesis includes several pathways, whose interactions remain unclear, especially at the onset of the disease [19].

The current review focused on the relationship between the signaling pathways that are associated with rarely considered proliferation of human AC cells in early OA and the anabolic, catabolic and pro-inflammatory effects that are well-established and have been associated with OA progression. More specifically, the review focused on the questions, which of the three key events in AC—proliferation, ECM degradation, and inflammation—are inducible by growth factor signaling, inflammatory cytokine signaling, and/or miRNA regulation. Additionally, we aimed to reveal in which sequence(s) these events can and cannot occur, and whether we can identify a single factor that is able to induce all of these key events, according to the currently available knowledge.

The two most examined pro-inflammatory cytokines in early OA are Interleukin-1 beta (IL-1β) and tumor necrosis factor α (TNF-α) [20] but various other pro-inflammatory cytokines and chemokines such as IL-6, IL-8, and IL-17 may also be involved in early OA pathology [20,21]. Proliferation of AC cells is modulated by fibroblast growth factor 2 (FGF2) [22,23] and transforming growth factor β (TGF-β) [24] signaling, in addition to many other effects. Therefore, particularly FGF2, TGF-β, and inflammatory cytokine signaling in combination with their miRNA regulation in human AC have been reviewed.

2. Fibroblast Growth Factor 2 Signaling

FGF2 is participating in several signaling pathways regulating proliferation, migration, inflammation, angiogenesis, differentiation, and senescence [22,23]. FGF2 is produced endogenously in human AC and occurs bound to perlecan, a heparan sulfate proteoglycan (HSPG) in the pericellular matrix (PCM) [25] (see Figure 2). Upon cutting of human AC, FGF2 is released from the PCM, activating mitogen activated protein kinase (MAPK) signaling [26]. Interestingly, FGF2 induces proliferation in both human intact and OA AC [27]. Moreover, FGF2 transduction of human knee AC samples is capable of recapitulating SCSO changes observed in early OA by inducing AC cell proliferation, which cumulates in complete SCSO loss comparable to an advanced OA-like structural phenotype of human AC [13]. In addition, FGF2 expression has been described as a marker of the human AC mesenchymal stem and progenitor cell (MSPC) population and is implicated in MSPC proliferation and chondrogenesis [23]. Besides, FGF2 acts as a chemo-attractant for monocytes and can be released by a variety of immune cells [28]. The FGF2 concentration in plasma and knee synovial fluid (SF) of OA patients is approximately twice of that of patients with normal healthy knee joints. Moreover, the increase of FGF2 abundance in OA plasma and SF correlates positively with radiographic OA severity [29]. Cells in human healthy and OA AC express all four fibroblast growth factor receptors (FGFR), but FGFR1 and FGFR3 dominate by far, compared to FGFR2 and FGFR4 [30,31]. Moreover, in human OA AC cells FGFR1 expression is increased while FGFR3 is concomitantly suppressed, compared to healthy AC cells [30].

In monolayer cell cultures established from human healthy AC, rFGF2 stimulation independently activates both protein kinase C δ (PKC δ) and rat sarcoma viral oncogene homolog (RAS) signaling cascades [32] predominantly via FGFR1 [33]. In parallel, the extracellular signal-regulated kinase (ERK), p38, and JUN N-terminal kinase (JNK) MAPK pathways are activated by PKC δ [32], whereas RAS predominantly activates the ERK signaling cascade [34] (see Figure 2). ERK phosphorylation is enhanced in human OA AC compared to healthy AC [35,36]. Moreover, human OA AC shows higher phosphorylated and therefore activated p38 MAPK level compared with normal AC [36,37]. Also, JNK activation is enhanced in human OA AC, compared to healthy control AC [36]. Notably, the highest phosphorylation of all MAPKs is found in the SZ of both healthy and OA AC [38].

The MAPK signaling cascade appears to be the dominating pathway responsible for matrix metalloproteinase (MMP)-1 and MMP-13 mRNA and protein expression in human healthy and OA AC cells in response to rFGF2 [32,39]. MMP-13 transcription in human (OA) AC cells in response to rFGF2 can be mediated by the transcription factor ETS-domain protein ELK-1 (ELK1) [32,35]. rFGF-2 dependent upregulation and activation of MMP-9 regulated by RAS and PKC δ dependent MAPK activation has been reported utilizing a human breast cancer cell line, whereas MMP-2 is not affected by rFGF2 in these cells [40]. In addition, in rat costal chondrocytes, rFGF2 dependent activation of MMP-9 has been reported [41]. Yet, in human AC, the impact of FGF2 induced MAPK signaling on MMP-2 and MMP-9 expression and activation has not been elucidated so far.

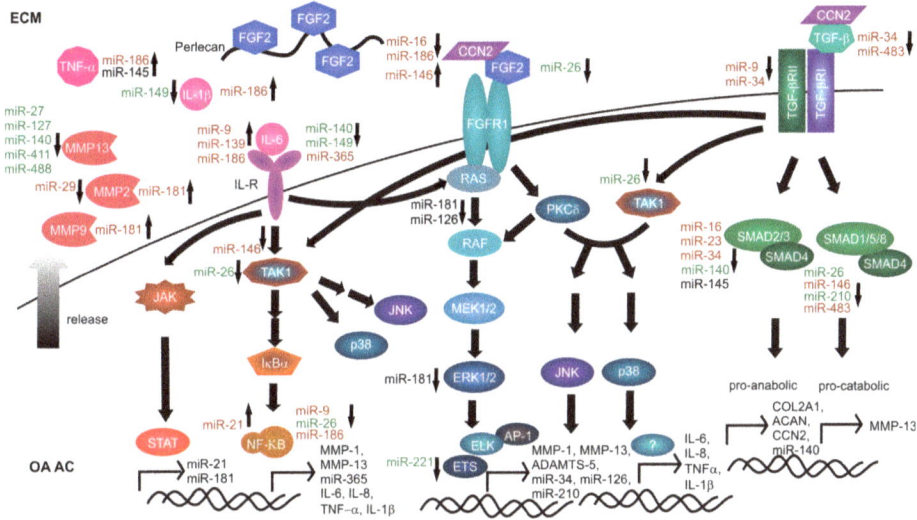

Figure 2. FGF2, TGF-β and inflammatory cytokine induced catabolic and pro-inflammatory signaling in human OA AC. The major components of inflammatory cytokine, FGF2 and TGF-β activated nuclear factor kappa B (NF-κB), mitogen activated protein kinase (MAPK), and SMA- and MAD-related protein (SMAD) signaling as well as their transcriptional targets in human OA AC are depicted. Micro RNAs (miRNAs) upregulated in human OA AC are indicated in red, miRNAs downregulated in human OA AC are indicated in green. For miRNAs with contradictory regulation a black font is chosen. The small arrows beside the miRNAs pointing downwards indicate direct or indirect inhibition of the signaling component by the miRNA, whereas small upward arrows indicate direct or indirect activation of the signaling component by the miRNA. As illustrated, there is an intense crosstalk between the individual pathways. In human OA AC, expression of pro-catabolic target genes is mediated by NF-κB, MAPK and SMAD signaling, whereas pro-inflammatory targets are activated downstream of MAPK and NF-κB signaling. Advanced stages of OA are characterized by activation of inflammatory cytokine signaling. On miRNA level there is primarily a net upregulation of IL-6, whereas both positive and negative regulation of NF-κB signaling is reported. Moreover, in human OA AC upregulation of CCN2 and significantly enhanced activation of extracellular signal-regulated kinase (ERK), JUN N-terminal kinase (JNK) and p38 MAPK pathways has been documented. Yet, evidence for ERK signaling regulation by miRNA is contradictory, whereas JNK and p38 activation is a common downstream event after inflammatory cytokine, FGF2 and TGFβ pathway activation with no direct miRNA regulation reported in OA AC to date. TGF-β signaling is globally downregulated in OA AC with especially negative regulation of the anabolic SMAD3 mediated pathway which is both evident on protein and miRNA level. In addition, in particular at miRNA level, reversal of negative regulation of MMP-13 is obvious in OA AC.

In cells isolated from human macroscopically healthy AC and OA AC, rFGF2 also suppresses expression of aggrecan (ACAN) and collagen type II α 1 chain (COL2A1) [30,39]. Important in the context of this review, rFGF2 promotes the expression of the inflammatory cytokines *TNF-α*, *IL-1β*, *IL-6*, *IL-8*, and *monocyte chemotactic protein 1 (MCP-1)*, also known as *C-C motif chemokine ligand 2 (CCL2)* [32], highlighting an important pro-inflammatory role of FGF2. Moreover, rFGF2 upregulates runt related transcription factor 2 (RUNX2) activity in bovine, murine and human cells of different mesenchymal tissue origin, which, in turn, controls *collagen type X α 1 chain (COL10A1)*, *MMP-13* and *A disintegrin and metalloproteinase with thrombospondin motifs (ADAMTS)-5* at the level of transcription [42–45]. Interestingly, treatment of human AC cells from young and healthy donors (Collins grade 0 or 1, <35-year-old) with rFGF2 shows no significant anti-anabolic or catabolic effect; rFGF2 fails to repress ACAN expression or induce MMP-13 and ADAMTS-5 expression in these cells. By contrast, notable effects on expression of these genes are observed when the same dose of rFGF2 is applied to damaged AC from older donors (grade 2 or higher, >40-year-old) [33]. These findings suggest a contextual property of FGF2 in AC biology, probably mediated by changes in abundance and activity of FGFR and other downstream components of FGF2 signaling. Constitutive rFGF2 expression after recombinant *adeno-associated virus* (rAAV)-hFGF2 transduction of human early OA AC explants induces cell proliferation within the native tissue [13]. Also, in monolayer cultures of human OA AC cells, rFGF2 enhances proliferation and prevents cell death [46].

In contrast to the above discussed human signaling profile showing predominant expression of FGFR1 and FGFR3, in murine healthy and surgically induced OA AC Fgfr2 and Fgfr4 are predominantly expressed, while Fgfr3 is barely detectable [31]. Surgical induction of OA in murine AC slightly reduces the expression of all Fgfr subtypes, but rFgf2 local injection markedly induces Fgfr3 expression, which is opposite to the human OA scenario [30,31], where rFGF2 selectively reduces FGFR3 expression. Indeed, Fgf2 has anabolic functions in murine AC that are mediated by Fgfr3. This is in strong contrast to the rFGF2-mediated anti-anabolic and catabolic in human aged healthy and OA AC [34]. In murine OA models rFgf2 mediates proteoglycan deposition in AC [31,47]. In addition to its species-dependent effects, the AC protective activity of rFGF2 in animal models appears to be age-dependent, too, as seen in rabbit [48] and bovine AC [49], where the anabolic activity is restricted to AC from young animals. Moreover, in calf AC only low doses of 3 ng/mL FGF2 induce proliferation, whereas higher doses of 30–300 ng have no mitotic effect [49]. FGF2 adaptor proteins like CCN2, also known as connective tissue growth factor (CTGF), may fine tune FGF2 signaling in mammalian AC [41]. CCN2 mRNA and protein overexpression has been shown in human OA AC compared to healthy AC [50,51].

Thus, FGF-2 mediates proliferation, anti-anabolism, and catabolism in human AC. However, healthy cells of young donors appear to be resistant against the catabolic effects of FGF2. The important ability of FGF-2 to induce inflammatory cytokine expression in human AC cells isolated from macroscopically healthy, but aged AC may be sufficient to induce or reinforce inflammation, dependent on the context and, thus, trigger OA progression.

3. Transforming Growth Factor β Signaling

TGF-β family ligands are growth factors basically implicated in proliferation, differentiation, and ECM maintenance. Binding to their hetero-tetrameric receptor, consisting of type I and type II subunits (TGF-βR1, TGF-βR2), activates TGF-β signaling [24]. Expression of the three TGF-β isoforms and both receptor subtypes has been examined in human OA AC compared to macroscopically healthy AC. However, the results are contradictory. While an upregulation of TGF-β1, TGF-β3, and TGF-β-R2 proteins with increased severity of OA has been reported in hip AC [52,53], downregulation of TGF-β1 protein in knee OA AC has been observed [54]. In addition, a polymorphism in the *asporin (ASPN)* gene, leading to reinforced TGF-β1 inhibition, has been associated with increased OA susceptibility [55,56]. Also, a single nucleotide polymorphism (SNP) in the *SMA-* and *MAD-related protein 3 (SMAD3)* gene has been linked with an increased risk of hip and knee OA [57].

In healthy adult AC cells all TGF-β isoforms induce proliferation, with an age dependent decline in responsiveness [58]. Moreover, anabolic expression of *COL2A1* and *ACAN* has been reported in response to rTGF-β1 and rTGF-β2 in human healthy AC cells [59] (see Figure 2).

Studies with human OA AC cells show that in OA TGF-β signals predominantly through activin receptor-like kinase 1 (ALK1)/activin A receptor like type 1 (ACVRL1) SMAD1/5/8 pathways, which is linked to the induction of catabolism; e.g., *MMP-13* expression [60,61]. Indeed, it is commonly suggested that ageing or onset of OA switch the receptor in TGF-β signaling from the classical

ALK5/TGF-β-R1 activated Smad2/3 signaling to TGF-β-R1 family member ALK1/ACVRL1 induced SMAD1/5/8 signaling, which converts TGF-β function in AC from an anabolic growth factor into a catabolic cytokine [62].

However, in OA AC both ALK1 and ALK5 expression appears to be largely reduced compared to healthy AC, although with a relative ALK1 excess [63]. rAAV-mediated TGF-β expression induces proliferation and proteoglycan deposition in both human healthy and OA AC cells, while increasing both ALK1 and ALK5 expression, leading to an elevated, balanced receptor expression in OA AC cells resembling healthy AC. Indeed, MMP-13 protein expression is largely reduced in OA AC cells by this approach, while COL2A1 expression increases, indicating simultaneous anabolic and anti-catabolic actions of prolonged TGF-β expression in human OA AC [63].

Although SMAD signaling is dominating in the TGF-β response, additional downstream signaling includes activation of TGF-β-activated kinase-1 (TAK1), also known as mitogen-activated protein kinase kinase kinase 7 (MAP3K7), which acts as upstream activators of MAPK signaling and nuclear factor kappa B (NF-κB) signaling in OA AC, though its role in human AC is not well-investigated [64,65]. Moreover, CCN2 is a transcriptional target of TGF-β and MAPK signaling. Interestingly, in human fibroblast cultures CCN2 is necessary for the TGF-β induced phosphorylation of SMAD1 and ERK1/2, but it is dispensable for activation of the SMAD3 pathway [66]. Yet, in human AC implication of these pathways in CCN2 expression has not been validated so far [67].

Summarized, in human healthy AC TGF-β signaling induces proliferation and anabolic gene expression via ALK5, a function which declines with increasing age. In contrast, in OA AC a pathway switch to ALK1 receptor converts TGF-β from an anabolic cytokine into a catabolic factor promoting AC degradation. In the context of inflammation, TAK1 activation, a downstream event of several signaling pathways including FGF2 or TGF-β signaling (Figure 2) has the potential to induce pro-inflammatory gene expression. Indeed, in a rat OA model, intra-articular injection of Tak1 adenovirus induced the secretion of several pro-inflammatory interleukins in the synovial fluid [68]. However, until today, no pro-inflammatory function of TGF-β signaling has been determined in human AC.

4. Additional Growth Factor Signaling Pathways in Human Adult AC

In addition to FGF2 and TGF-β signaling, several other growth factors and their downstream pathway components appear to be expressed in human adult AC. The differential regulation of these growth factor-induced signaling pathways as well as their impact on proliferation, anabolic/catabolic gene expression, or inflammation in human OA AC is summarized in this chapter.

4.1. WNT Signaling

Evidence for progressive activation of the non-canonical Ca^{2+}/wingless-type MMTV integration site family (WNT) signaling pathway in human OA AC is provided by increased expression of WNT5A mRNA and protein [69–71] as well as *CaMK2 nuclear factor of activated T-cells 5, tonicity-responsive (NFAT5)*, and *nuclear factor of activated T-cells 2 (NFATC2)* mRNA [70]. WNT5A protein expression in healthy human AC is restricted to the SZ, whereas in OA AC also cells of the deeper layers express WNT5A. Indeed, in human normal AC monolayer cultures rWNT5A promotes repression of anabolic genes like *ACAN*, whereas mRNA expression of catabolic genes including *MMP-1, MMP-3, MMP-13* and *ADAMTS-4* is enhanced [69,72]. In addition, rWNT5A induces MMP-1 and MMP-13 protein expression [69].

While *WNT7A* mRNA expression is downregulated in human OA AC compared to normal AC, ectopic lentiviral expression of rWNT7A in human normal AC cell cultures inhibits rIL-1β-induced catabolic gene expression including *MMP-1, MMP-3* and *MMP-13*, which is likely mediated via the non-canonical Ca^{2+}/WNT signaling pathway [73].

Also, *WNT3A* mRNA expression is increasingly downregulated with higher grades of OA severity in human AC [74]. rWNT3A promotes dedifferentiation, indicated by loss of anabolic *COL2A1* and *ACAN* expression in human OA AC monolayer cultures, which is mediated by the

Ca^{2+}/calmodulin-dependent protein kinase 2 (CaMK2) pathway [74]. Indeed, rWNT3A-dependent induction of proliferation, but also *axis inhibition protein 2 (AXIN2)* expression, an inhibitor of canonical WNT signaling, is specifically mediated by the canonical WNT/β-catenin pathway in human OA AC cells [74]. Moreover, in another study using rWNT3A in human OA AC cell monolayer cultures, activation of canonical WNT/β-catenin signaling has turned out to be a potent inhibitor of *MMP-1*, *MMP-3*, and *MMP-13* expression and MMP activity both under basal conditions and also after rIL-1β stimulated NF-κB activation [75]. This indicates the ability of WNT3A to induce proliferation in human adult AC, whereas catabolic gene expression is actively repressed.

Interestingly, in human OA AC mRNA and protein expression of intracellular and extracellular inhibitors of both the canonical and planar cell polarity WNT pathways (e.g., AXIN2), as well as dickkopf WNT signaling pathway inhibitor 1 and 3 (DKK1 and DKK3), are significantly upregulated compared to normal AC [70,76]. AXIN2, DKK1, and DKK3 proteins in normal human AC are predominantly localized to the SZ, whereas their expression is extended to the cells located in the deeper layers of human OA AC [70]. Yet, another study shows reduced *DKK1* mRNA expression in human OA AC with increased OA grading [77]. However, despite obviously enhanced expression of canonical WNT signaling inhibitors upon onset of OA [70], increased nuclear localization of β-catenin protein occurs in human early and late OA AC, compared to normal control AC, indicating sustained activation of canonical WNT signaling in OA AC [78].

Human female hip and knee OA has been associated with a polymorphism in the *frizzled related protein (FRZB)* gene [79–81]. FRZB functions as a soluble WNT decoy receptor and, thus, can inhibit canonical and non-canonical WNT signaling pathways [82]. Interestingly, a FRZB double mutant associated with human AC OA exhibits decreased affinity for WNT molecules, suggesting a compromised ability to suppress WNT signaling [82]. In addition, decreased *FRZB* mRNA expression in human AC has been associated with increased OA grading [77].

Summarized, WNT signaling in human adult AC is complex. Whereas canonical WNT/β-catenin signaling may play a proliferation-inducing and anti-catabolic role in human healthy and early OA AC, the Ca^{2+}/CaMK2 arm of WNT signaling may induce dedifferentiation and catabolic gene expression. Progression of OA apparently depends on the balance of inhibition and activation of different WNT pathways, ultimately leading to cessation of proliferation and increased catabolism. To date, there is no evidence for a pro-inflammatory activity of WNT signaling in human AC.

4.2. Hedgehog Signaling

Indian hedgehog (IHH)-induced hedgehog (Hh) signaling is a key pathway implicated in proliferation and differentiation during vertebrate AC development and longitudinal growth at the growth plate [83–85]. In human OA AC and OA SF, IHH abundance is increased compared to normal controls. Indeed, IHH protein expression is already enhanced in early human OA AC lesions and its expression increases with OA severity. In contrast, in the SF of late stage OA patients, the IHH protein content declines, compared to early OA [86,87]. Interestingly, the IHH protein is predominantly located in the SZ of human OA AC [86]. Additionally, in human knees categorized with the most severe OA, AC expresses the highest levels of Hh downstream target genes *glioma-associated oncogene homolog 1 (GLI1), patched 1 (PTCH1)* and *hedgehog interacting protein (HHIP)* [88]. rIHH activates Hh signaling in human first passage monolayer cultures derived from normal adult AC without inducing catabolic *ADAMTS-5* or *MMP-13* expression. These results show that IHH signaling by itself does not cause catabolic ECM degradation in human normal AC [89]. Indeed, the lack of catabolic response to IHH signaling in healthy AC is in contrast to another study demonstrating in human OA AC explants that recombinant sonic hedgehog (SHH), another Hh ligand, induces catabolic *ADAMTS-5* mRNA expression [88].

In short, the outcome of Hh signaling activation during vertebrate AC development and longitudinal bone growth has been determined in many studies. However, the impact of apparent Hh pathway component overexpression on human adult AC proliferation remains to be elucidated.

In addition, the mechanistic background of Hh signaling-induced catabolic gene expression in human OA AC has to be resolved by additional research. Until today, there is no evidence for any pro-inflammatory activity of Hh signaling in human AC.

4.3. Bone Morphogenetic Protein Signaling

Bone morphogenetic protein (BMP) signaling, like Hh signaling, has a central function in vertebrate cartilage development, stimulating both proliferation and anabolic gene expression [90]. Also, in human adult AC BMP ligand expression can be detected. BMP-2 mRNA and protein expression is up-regulated in OA AC and OA AC derived monolayer cell cultures [91–94]. Indeed, *BMP-2* mRNA expression can be detected in OA AC cell clusters and single cells of the SZ and MZ. Only in severely damaged AC, *BMP-2* mRNA is also located in the DZ [92]. In primary cultures of human OA AC cells BMP-4 is upregulated compared to normal control AC cells [93]. Also, BMP-1, BMP6, and BMP-11 expression is abundant in human adult AC, but without apparent differential regulation upon OA onset [95,96]. In contrast, BMP-3 and BMP-7 are clearly downregulated in human OA AC, although data concerning BMP-7 expression are contradictory. One study found both BMP-3 and BMP-7 predominantly expressed in the SZ of normal AC. Moreover, BMP-7 was detected in early OA AC cell clusters, whereas BMP-3 expression was absent upon OA onset [97]. In another study, both human normal and OA AC lacked BMP-7 protein expression, which was only detected in fetal, developing AC [96]. rBMP-2 induces anabolic gene expression, including *ACAN* and *COL2A1* as well as increased proteoglycan deposition in human normal adult AC (both young and aged) cell cultures as well as OA AC cell cultures [91,98–101]. Expression of catabolic *MMP-2* and *MMP-3* mRNA is not affected by rBMP-2 [99]. Yet, another study in human OA AC monolayer cultures shows rBMP-2 induced catabolic *MMP-9*, *MMP-13* and *ADAMTS-5* mRNA expression, which is at least partially mediated by WNT/β-catenin signaling [93]. Interestingly, the proteoglycan synthesis induced by rBMP-6 in normal adult AC derived monolayer cultures shows an age dependent decrease. Also, OA AC cell cultures exhibit a limited proteoglycan deposition upon rBMP-6 comparable to aged normal AC [95]. rBMP-7 specifically promotes anabolic *ACAN* and *COL2A1* mRNA expression in human adult OA AC cell high density monolayer cultures. Yet, expression of catabolic *MMP-1*, *MMP-3*, *MMP-13* and *ADAMTS-4* genes is not affected by rBMP-7 [102] or in case of human adult AC cell alginate bead cultures even reduced [100]. No positive effect of rBMP-2, rBMP-4, rBMP-6 or rBMP-7 on proliferation of human adult AC cell monolayer or alginate bead cultures was observed [95,100]. In addition, there is no indication that BMP signaling can promote inflammation in human OA AC, whereas rIL-1β and rTNF-α increase BMP-2 mRNA and protein levels in human OA AC explant cultures [91]. Yet, in the context of rheumatoid arthritis, BMP signaling may have anti-inflammatory functions [103].

Summarized, in human adult normal and OA AC, the outcome of BMP signaling is anabolic and potentially also catabolic, via a cross-talk with canonical WNT signaling. However, there is no evidence for a pro-proliferative or inflammation-inducing function.

4.4. NOTCH Signaling

In human macroscopically intact adult AC, notch homolog (NOTCH) receptors and ligands are scarcely expressed. However, in human OA AC mRNA and protein expression of all four NOTCH receptors, jagged 1 (JAG1) and delta-like 1 (DLL1) ligands as well as hairy and enhancer of split 1 (HES1) and HES5 are abundant, especially in cell clusters within the SZ [104–107]. Moreover, proliferation of human OA AC cell cultures in vitro is induced by and depends on active NOTCH signaling [105]. In monolayer cultures of human OA AC cells, NOTCH signaling represses the expression of *BMP-2*, which is implicated in anabolic gene expression. Simultaneously, the expression of pro-inflammatory and catabolic genes, including *IL-8* and *MMP-9*, is repressed by active NOTCH signaling [105].

Taken together, NOTCH signaling appears to be activated specifically in human OA AC and to contribute to increased proliferation, whereas it likely inhibits catabolic and inflammatory gene expression.

4.5. Insulin-Like Growth Factor Signaling

In normal human adult AC insulin like growth factor 1 (IGF-1) is predominantly localized in the SZ. Intriguingly, both in human OA AC and OA SF the IGF-1 protein concentration significantly increases [108,109]. Both in monolayer cultures and explants of human normal adult AC rIGF-1 has pro-proliferative and anabolic effects, indicated by increased proteoglycan synthesis and expression of collagen type II [110,111]. Interestingly, rFGF2 dose dependently antagonizes rIGF-1-mediated proteoglycan deposition in human normal AC alginate cultures, whereas both promote proliferation [112]. For human OA AC no data concerning IGF-1 signaling outcome are available.

Summarized, in human normal adult AC, IGF-1 has mitogenic and anabolic functions. Until today, IGF-1 signaling has neither been implicated in human AC catabolic gene expression nor in inflammation.

4.6. Vascular Endothelial Growth Factor Signaling

Angiogenesis mediated by vascular endothelial growth factor (VEGF) is a contributing factor in OA pathogenesis. Yet, angiogenesis, comprising catabolic ECM degradation and endothelial cell proliferation, remains restricted to tissues such as the synovium and the subchondral bone, whereas AC itself remains avascular during OA progression [113]. Nevertheless, VEGF A is actively expressed in human adult AC. In human normal and OA AC the mRNAs of three VEGF A isoforms (*VEGF121*, *VEGF165*, and *VEGF189*) can be detected and VEGF protein is predominantly localized in the SZ and MZ of OA AC, both intracellularly and in the PCM [114–116]. Intriguingly, an upregulation of VEGF expression in OA AC compared to normal adult AC has been reported [116–118]. Expression of the VEGF receptors VEGFR-1, also known as Fms related tyrosine kinase 1 (FLT-1) and VEGFR-2, also known as kinase insert domain receptor (KDR) is either restricted to OA AC compared to normal AC [115], whereas other studies reported that VEGFR-1 [116] or VEGFR-2 [119] were not detectable at all in human adult AC. Moreover, in human OA AC VEGFR-3, also known as Fms-like tyrosine kinase 4 (FLT4), is expressed in the SZ cells located in cytoplasm and on cell membrane [120]. In primary OA AC monolayer cultures catabolic *MMP-1* and *MMP-3* mRNA expression, but not *MMP-2*, *MMP-9* or *MMP-13* expression, can be induced by rVEGF165, whereas cultured normal AC cells exhibit no catabolic gene expression upon rVEGF165 treatment at all [115]. No proliferation-inducing effect can be attributed to rVEGF in human OA AC cells [115,119].

In summary, active VEGF signaling appears to be restricted to human OA AC, where its outcome is catabolic. Yet, proliferation of human OA AC cells is not affected by VEGF. Until today, no VEGF induced expression of pro-inflammatory genes in human OA AC has been reported. Nevertheless, in other tissues pro-inflammatory VEGF action is renowned [121].

5. Inflammatory Cytokine Signaling

It is well-accepted that inflammation is ubiquitous during OA progression [122]. Yet, it is being debated whether inflammation may also be a primary conductive trigger for the onset of OA [123,124].

IL-1β and TNF-α are the best-studied pro-inflammatory cytokines in human AC experimental OA induction [21]. Apart from that, also IL-6, the IL-6 like cytokine oncostatin M (OSM), IL-17, and IL-8 have been implicated in human OA pathogenesis [20,125]. Yet, IL-1β, which has been discovered as AC destructive factor in porcine tissue, is apparently not substantially upregulated in the human SF of joints with different OA stages [125,126]. Moreover, in SF of OA patients the abundance of IL-1 receptor antagonist (IL-1Ra), competing with IL-1β for IL-1 receptor (IL-1R) binding, was 1800 times higher compared to IL-1β [125], whereas the IL-1R density on human OA AC cells was less than a 2-fold increased [127]. Together, these findings suggest in human OA SF in vivo an inhibition of IL-1β signaling at endogenous IL-1β concentrations [125].

Increased expression of IL-17a, IL-8, monokine induced by interferon-gamma (MIG) and interferon-inducible T-cell alpha chemoattractant (I-TAC) has been found in SF and serum of OA patients [128]. Another study identifies IL-6, but also IL-1β and TNF-α protein, to be specifically upregulated in serum of OA patients [36]. Moreover, *IL-6* mRNA expression is enhanced in human fibrillated OA AC, whereas no *IL-6* signal was evident in histologically normal AC from OA patients or healthy human control AC [129]. Interestingly, this study also revealed that IL-1β expression in human AC did not to correlate with the presence or grading of OA, whereas another study reported decreased IL-1β protein abundance in human OA AC with increased OA grading [130].

rIL-1β stimulates the expression of MMP-1, MMP-3, and MMP-13 mRNA and protein in human healthy and OA AC monolayer cultures [42,131]. In addition, rIL-1 induces IL-8 release from human OA AC cells [132]. Also, *IL-6* and *FGF2* mRNA expression are markedly enhanced by rIL-1β in human healthy AC cell cultures [131]. Indeed, rIL-17 is able to induce IL-8, IL-1β and IL-6 protein release in human healthy and OA AC cells [132,133]. In addition, rIL-8 upregulates secretion of IL-1β, IL-6, TNF-α, MMP-1, MMP-3, and MMP-13 by human OA AC cells [128]. Interestingly, in human OA AC cell cultures depletion of IL-6 prevents rIL-1β-induced MMP-13 expression [134], underlining the possibility that IL-1β may not be the primary cytokine involved in OA AC inflammation. Although human healthy and OA SF contains about 20 pg/mL IL-1β and less than 3 ng/mL TNF-α, many studies using inflammatory cytokines for experimental OA induction apply apparently supra-physiological doses of 1–100 ng/mL rIL-1β and up to 50 ng/mL rTNF-α for activation of downstream signaling [21,125], which may probably not reflect the natural OA pathogenesis in vivo [21].

In human AC, the signaling cascades originating from IL-1β and TNF-α converge on MAPK and NF-κB signaling [135] (see Figure 2). NF-κB in cooperation with ERK, p38 and JNK regulate rIL-1β and rTNF-α-dependent catabolic *MMP-13* production in human OA AC cells via E74-like factor 3 (ELF3) and activator protein 1 (AP-1) [136–138]. Knockdown of NF-κB p65/RelA suppresses the expression of basal and rIL-1β-induced *MMP-1* and *MMP-13* mRNA in human OA AC cells [75].

Notably, IL-17 activates ERK, JNK and p38 as well as NF-κB in normal human AC cells to induce *IL-1β* and *IL-6* expression [133]. Intriguingly, in human OA AC cells, rIL-17 activates FBJ murine osteosarcoma viral oncogene homolog B (FOSB) (AP-1 subunit), whereas IL-1β activates cellular oncogene Fos (cFOS) (AP-1 subunit) to induce MMP-13 release, indicating a different fine tuning of downstream signaling depending on the cytokine [139]. In addition, rIL-8 activates NF-κB and JNK signaling in human OA AC cells to induce IL-1β, IL-6, TNF-α, MMP-1, MMP-3, and MMP-13 secretion [128].

Overall, there is an intense crosstalk of inflammatory cytokine signaling with different growth factor-induced signaling pathways.

Interestingly, in human OA AC, rIL-1β treatment simultaneously down-regulates mRNA expression of the WNT signaling inhibitors *FRZB* and *DKK1*, whereas *WNT5A* mRNA expression is increased by rIL-1β treatment both in human healthy and OA AC. While *FRZB* downregulation and *WNT5A* overexpression have also been observed in OA patients, data for DKK1 expression in OA patients are contentious [70,77]. In human OA AC cells canonical WNT/β-catenin signaling, activated by rWNT3A, counteracts NF-κB-mediated *MMP* expression induced by rIL-1β. Additionally, rWNT3A inhibits rIL-1β induced *IL-6* expression [75], indicating an attenuating role of canonical WNT signaling on human AC inflammation.

Both rTNF-α and rIL-1β significantly repress mRNA expression of several NOTCH pathway components, including *NOTCH1*, *NOTCH3*, *JAG1*, and *HES5* in human healthy and OA AC cells in vitro [105]. Intriguingly, these proteins have been shown to be upregulated in human OA AC in vivo [104,105], revealing the absence of inflammatory cytokine-mediated suppression of NOTCH signaling at least during early OA in vivo.

Hh pathway activation is suppressed by addition of rIL-1β in adult bovine AC explants. Conversely, rIHH weakly suppresses rIL-1β-induced *ADAMTS-5* expression in this model [89], indicating a negative feedback of both pathways. In healthy human AC cell alginate bead cultures rIGF-1 upregulates IL-1RII protein expression, a decoy receptor for IL-1, which may override catabolic IL-1β actions in healthy AC [140].

Remarkably, FGF2 is the only growth factor considered, which directly promotes the mRNA expression of *TNF-α, IL-1β, IL-6, IL-8,* and *MCP-1* in human healthy AC cells, thereby promoting inflammation after 5 days of monolayer culture [32]. On the other hand, in healthy human AC and in the murine teratocarcinoma ATDC5 cell line, rIL-1β increases FGF2 mRNA and protein expression [32,141], indicating a potential feedback loop between FGF2 and Il-1ß.

As discussed, proliferation-induced changes in the SCSO of human AC and formation of cell clusters are early OA marker [10,14]. Increased expression of the proliferation markers *cyclin D1 (CCDN1)* and *cyclin dependent kinase 6 (CDK6)* has been observed in human OA AC compared to healthy control AC [142]. In addition to FGF2, growth factors like IGF-1, NOTCH ligands, and WNT have also been implicated in human adult AC cell proliferation [13,74,105,112]. In contrast, inflammatory cytokines clearly inhibit adult human AC cell proliferation. This is obvious in human OA AC for rIL-1β, which inhibits proliferation and induces apoptosis [36], but also for rIL-8, which even suppresses proliferation [128]. Moreover, in rabbit AC rIL-6 represses proliferation [143]. Interestingly, in healthy human AC cell agarose bead cultures rIL-1β also represses rFGF2-induced proliferation and cluster formation; only IL-17R overexpression has been associated with increased *FGF2* mRNA expression and cluster formation [144].

Summarized, inflammatory cytokines play an important role in human OA AC catabolism and inflammation, but it appears that they cannot be responsible for the observed OA AC proliferation, which is a hallmark of early OA. In contrast, OA AC proliferation can only be attributed to a variety of growth factors. Remarkably, of all growth factors discussed in this chapter, only FGF2 is able to concomitantly upregulate proliferation as well as induce catabolic and inflammatory gene expression, which may represent a so far not considered yet potentially important novel concept for onset of inflammation in human OA.

6. MiRNA Regulation of Fibroblast Growth Factor 2, Transforming Growth Factor β and Inflammatory Cytokine Signaling Pathways

During the last years a myriad of publications addressing the differential regulation and effects of miRNA in human OA AC compared to normal AC have been published, which opened new insights into the intensive regulation and crosstalk of signaling pathways. This chapter focuses on those miRNAs with demonstrated regulatory effects in human OA AC, compared to normal AC, and with established targets in FGF2, inflammatory cytokine or TGF-β signaling pathways (see Figure 2).

Concerning miR-9, most studies report an enhanced abundance in OA AC. Both miR-9 and *IL-6* have been reported to be upregulated in damaged hip OA AC compared to undamaged AC areas of the same patients. Furthermore, rIL-1β and rIL-6 may induce miR-9 expression in monolayer cultures of hip OA AC cells. In the same study, *monocyte chemoattractant protein-induced protein 1 (MCPIP-1)*, a post-transcriptional repressor of IL-6 mRNA, has been established as miR-9 target [145]. In a second study, moderate upregulation of miR-9 in hip OA AC compared to age matched healthy AC has been reported [146]. Also, another group documented upregulation of miR-9 expression in both AC and bone of knee OA patients compared to healthy cartilage and bone from donors of the same age. Interestingly, miR-9 reduces basal and also rIL-1β induced MMP-13 protein expression in primary AC cells [147]. Yet, downregulation of miR-9 expression in human knee OA AC compared to age matched normal AC has been shown [148]. In this study, *NF-κB1* has been established as a direct target of miR-9. In liver fibrosis, TGF-β1 downregulates miR-9 expression by promotor methylation, whereas *TGFBR1* (ALK5) and *TGFBR2* have been established as direct targets of miR-9 [149]. Therefore, miR-9 seems to fine-tune inflammatory cytokine signaling, whereas anabolic TGF-β signaling is attenuated.

MiR-16 levels are upregulated in the plasma of knee OA patients [150]. Also knee and hip AC of OA patients exhibit increased miR-16 expression compared to healthy AC [151,152]. *SMAD3* has been determined as a direct target of miR-16, implicating this miRNA in the switch to catabolic TGF-β signaling [152]. Notably, *FGF2* is a direct transcriptional target of miR-16 in human nasopharyngeal carcinoma cells [153], indicating additional repression of FGF2 signaling by this miRNA.

MiR-21 expression is elevated in human OA AC. Indeed, miR-21 suppresses chondrogenesis by directly targeting *growth differentiation factor 5* (*GDF5*), whereas NF-κB signaling is induced [154]. Another direct target of miR-21 is *tissue inhibitor of metalloproteinases 3* (*TIMP3*). In HUVEC, miR-21 dependent downregulation of *TIMP3* coincided with increased MMP-2 and MMP-9 mRNA, and protein expression [155]. Interestingly, rIL-6-induced signal transducer and activator of transcription 3 (STAT3) activation has been implicated in increased miR-21 and miR-181 expression and malignant transformation of a human mammary epithelial cell line by constitutively activating NF-κB signaling [156]. Moreover, miR-21 has been implicated in several chronic diseases related to an aging-dependent increase of inflammation [157]. Collectively, this indicates a contribution of miR-21 to catabolic NF-κB signaling and MMP activation in response to inflammatory cytokines.

MiR-23a is another miRNA directly suppressing *SMAD3* expression, alleviating anabolic TGF-β signaling. Hypomethylation of the promoter region of miR-23a may contribute to its increased expression, which is observed for both, miR-23a and miR-23b in human hip and knee OA AC compared to healthy AC [151,158]. Yet, another study shows downregulation of miR-23a expression in human knee OA AC explant cultures upon rIL-1β treatment, whereas miR-23 expression and release were enhanced in synovial explants from OA patients [159]. This indicates an opposing scenario in rIL-1β treated ex vivo OA AC cultures compared to the in vivo observed upregulation.

Decreased abundance of miR-26a and miR-26b has been detected in human knee and hip OA AC compared to normal AC [151,160,161]. Notably, increasing body mass index (BMI) and NF-κB pathway activity in OA patients has been related to progressive miR-26a downregulation [162]. Direct targets for miR-26a and miR-26b dependent suppression are *karyopherin subunit alpha 3* (*KPNA3*) that modulates NF-κB p65 translocation [161], *high mobility group protein A1* (*HMGA1*), and *mucosa-associated lymphoid tissue lymphoma translocation protein 1* (*MALT1*), which are also involved in positive regulation of NF-κB signaling and *IL-6* expression [163]. Moreover, *TAK1* and *TGF-β activated kinase 1 and MAP3K7 binding protein 3* (*TAB3*), two additional positive regulators of NF-κB signaling are directly targeted by miR-26b [164]. Besides, *SMAD1* and *SMAD4* are directly repressed by miR-26a [165]. Also, *CCN2* is a target of miR-26a [166]. Therefore, miR-26 family downregulation activates NF-κB signaling, promotes catabolic TGF-β signaling, and probably also interferes with FGF2 signaling.

MiR-27b, which directly targets *MMP-13*, is downregulated in human knee OA AC, compared to AC from young and healthy AC donors [167]. Hydrostatic pressure increases both miR-27a and miR-27b expression specifically in human hip OA AC monolayer cell cultures, but not in cell cultures derived from normal hip AC [168]. Remarkably, though rIL-1β downregulates miR-27a and miR-27b in human late stage knee OA AC explant cultures, in synovial explant cultures of patients with late stage knee OA AC an upregulation and enhanced secretion of miR-27a and miR-27b was detectable upon rIL-1β stimulation [159]. Long non-coding RNA-cartilage injury-related (lncRNA-CIR), which is upregulated in OA AC, acts as a sponge for miR-27, whereas miR-27 directly represses lncRNA-CIR expression [167]. In addition, in human chondrosarcoma cells, expression of miR-27b is negatively regulated by adiponectin (ADPN), an adipokine [169]. This indicates a differential expression of miR-27 family members in OA AC and synovium in response to rIL-1β, whereas enhanced catabolic *MMP-13* expression in may be reinforced by adipokines.

The human miR-29 family consists of three mature members, miR-29a, miR-29b, and miR-29c. Although, their targets are largely overlapping, differential regulation has been reported [170]. Indeed, upregulation of all three miR-29 members in human hip OA AC compared to normal AC has been reported, whereas serial passaging of OA AC cells in monolayer culture leads to miR-29 downregulation [171]. In addition, miR-29c is upregulated in the plasma of human knee OA patients compared to healthy controls [150]. Yet, another study documents miR-29a downregulation in human hip and knee OA AC compared to healthy AC and also shows a negative correlation of miR-29a expression with increasing BMI, whereas IL-1β abundance positively correlates with increasing BMI [151]. Interestingly, rFGF2 can increase miR-29a and miR-29b expression in first passage monolayer cultures of human knee AC [172], whereas both, NF-κB and SMAD3 have been implicated in repression of miR-29 family members [170]. rTGF-β1 reduces miR-29 level in human primary OA AC cell cultures. Yet, while NF-κB inhibits miR-29 expression, rIL-1β increases miR-29a and miR-29b expression in a p38 MAPK dependent manner [171]. Indeed, rTNF-α has been identified as miR-29b suppressor in the human chondrosarcoma cell line SW1353 in another study [173]. Notably, miR-29c directly suppresses *MMP-2* expression in human lung cancer cells [174]. Moreover, several collagen genes are predicted targets of the miR-29 family [175] and especially *COL2A1* is repressed by miR-29b, whereas *COL10A1* is lacking a binding site [176]. Additionally, the miR-29 family has been implicated in alterations of DNA methylation and stem cell exhaustion, which is observed during aging [157]. The fact that miR-29 is upregulated in human OA AC suggests a greater effect of FGF2 and inflammatory cytokine regulated MAPK signaling on miR-29 regulation than of NF-κB, as one would expect a miR-29 upregulation under predominating FGF2 and inflammatory cytokine regulated MAPK signaling and a miR-29 downregulation under predominating NF-κB activation. Especially *SMAD3* is targeted by other upregulated miRNAs in human OA AC, suspending negative regulation by TGF-β signaling. Therefore, miR-29 family members may actively contribute to catabolic ECM remodeling by promoting a collagen II/X imbalance in OA AC.

MiR-30a is upregulated in primary AC cells from knee OA patients compared to young healthy donors [177]. Also, a second family member, miR-30b is overexpressed in human hip and knee OA AC compared to healthy AC [151,178]. Moreover, miR-30b abundance is elevated in the plasma of human knee OA patients compared to healthy controls [150]. *SRY-related HMG box-containing 9 (SOX9)* is a direct target of miR-30a [177], whereas miR-30b targets the *ETS-related gene (ERG)* [178], both reducing anabolic mRNA expression. Yet, also *ADAMTS-5* is a direct target of miR-30a [179]. Notably, rIL-1β represses miR-30a expression in monolayer cell cultures established from normal AC and OA AC by recruiting of AP-1 to the miR-30a promoter [179]. Therefore, in human OA AC the miR-30 family is apparently involved in inhibition of anabolic matrix deposition, whereas it is not pro-catabolic. However, the mechanism of miR-30a upregulation in OA AC remains elusive.

Both miR-33a and its host gene *sterol regulatory element-binding protein 2 (SREBP-2)* are upregulated primary cell cultures of human knee OA AC compared to healthy AC. Treatment of monolayer cultures of human OA AC cells with rTGF-β1 increased expression miR-33a. MiR-33a reduced *ATP-binding cassette transporter A1 (ABCA1)* and *apolipoprotein A1 (APOA1)* mRNA expression levels, which are both involved in cholesterol efflux and elevated *MMP-13* expression levels. While *ABCA1* contains a miR-33 target sequence, the other effects are rather indirect. Indeed, in OA AC reverse cholesterol transport appears to be reduced [180].

Both miR-34a and miR-34b are upregulated in human knee OA AC compared to normal AC [147,181]. Also primary cell cultures of human knee OA AC show increased miR-34a expression compared to healthy controls [182]. In AC, miR-34a targets *sirtuin 1 (SIRT1)*, which is involved in epigenetic gene silencing [182]. Another target is *cysteine-rich angiogenic inducer 61 (CYR61)*, which inhibits ADAMTS-4. Indeed, upregulation of miR-34a by rIL-1β promotes ADAMTS-4 expression in human AC cells [181]. In human primary immortalized fibroblasts the MAPK activated transcription factor ELK1 is involved in miR-34a expression [183]. In prostate cancer cell lines, miR-34b significantly inhibits protein expression of TGF-β, TGF-βR1 and p-SMAD3, but does not affect mRNA level indicating translational repression [184]. Additionally, miR-34 family members have been implicated in altered DNA damage response and telomere shortening associated with cellular senescence [157]. Therefore, this miRNA family promotes catabolic gene expression and contributes to global repression of TGF-β signaling with a focus on the anabolic SMAD3 pathway.

MiR-105 is downregulated by rFGF2 in cell cultures established from human healthy knee AC. Mechanistically, the p65 subunit of NF-kB is implicated in FGF2-mediated miR-105 downregulation. *RUNX2*, involved in the transcription of *ADAMTS-4*, *ADAMTS-5*, *ADAMTS-7* and *ADAMTS-12*, has been identified as direct target of miR-105 [172]. Moreover, *SOX9* is a direct target of miR-105 in human glioma cells [185]. This indicates that miR-105 acts both anti-anabolically and anti-catabolically, whereas its compensatory effect is alleviated by its downregulation in OA.

MiR-125b, which targets *ADAMTS-4*, is downregulated by rFGF2 [172,186]. In human OA AC miR-125b is repressed compared to healthy AC. In addition, an age dependent decrease of miR-125b abundance in human AC has been observed [186]. This indicates an anti-catabolic role of miR-125b in AC, which is attenuated by its downregulation during aging and onset of OA.

MiR-126 has been reported to be upregulated in the plasma of human knee OA patients compared to healthy controls [150]. Yet, downregulation of miR-126 in healthy and OA AC samples from old patients, compared to AC from young, healthy patients has been detected in another study [187]. In HUVEC cells, the MAPK activated transcription factor avian erythroblastosis virus E26 oncogene homolog 1 (ETS1) has been implicated in miR-126 expression [188]. Though, in human glioma cells, *Kirsten rat sarcoma viral oncogene homolog (KRAS)* has been identified as direct miR-126 target, indicating negative regulation of the ERK pathway [189]. Therefore, downregulation of miR-126 may reinforce MAPK signaling, while its upregulation may prevent over-activation depending on the context.

MiR-127 expression is reduced in knee OA AC compared to normal AC [190,191]. Increased *MMP-13* expression upon rIL-1β treatment in monolayer cell cultures of human OA AC correlated with miR-127 suppression, with *MMP-13* as a direct target of miR-127. In addition, miR-127 inhibits also *MMP-1* expression in response to rIL-1β [190]. Collectively, with downregulation of miR-127 in OA AC, another anti-catabolic miRNA in AC is disenabled.

MiR-139 is specifically upregulated in the macroscopically degenerated areas of knee OA AC, compared to macroscopically intact appearing AC from the same patient [192]. rIL-1β and rIL-6 increase miR-139 level OA AC cell cultures, whereas inhibition of miR-139 markedly reduces *IL-6* mRNA and protein expression. *MCPIP1*, a post-transcriptional repressor of *IL-6* mRNA, is a direct target of miR-139. Beyond, *ADAMTS-4* and *MMP-13* mRNA expression is significantly increased by miR-139 mimic. This indicates the involvement of miR-139 in inflammatory cytokine-mediated catabolic gene expression in advanced OA.

Downregulation of miR-140 in human knee and hip OA AC compared to normal AC has been reported [151,161,193]. In cell cultures of knee OA AC and synovial fluid, expression of miR-140 negatively correlates with OA severity [194]. Yet, hydrostatic pressure increases miR-140 expression in human hip OA AC monolayer cell cultures [168]. *MMP-13* [195] and *IL-6* [196] are direct targets of miR-140. In the human rib cartilage cell line C28/I2 rIL-1β reduces miR-140 expression [195]. In contrast, TGF-β signaling can induce miR-140 expression via SMAD3, whereas *SMAD3* is also a target of miR-140 [197]. Summarized, the anti-catabolic miR-140 is repressed in human OA AC and this repression may be mediated by inflammatory cytokines, whereas the TGF-β-dependent miR-140 expression is alleviated by SMAD3 depletion.

MiR-145, upregulated in aged knee OA AC compared to normal AC from younger donors, can be induced by rIL-1β in monolayer cell cultures established from normal and OA AC, with stronger induction of miR-145 observed in OA AC cells [198]. Yet, others documented the downregulation of miR-145 in late stage OA AC, compared to early stage OA AC of the same patients [199] or normal AC [200]. Indeed, in human OA AC increased TNF-α levels correlated with a reduced miR-145 abundance [199]. *SMAD3* is a direct target of miR-145 [198]. Also, human *SOX9* is directly downregulated by miR-145 in cell cultures from human normal knee AC, while the target sequence is not conserved in murine *Sox9*. Notably, in human AC cell cultures miR-145 expression significantly increases from P0 to P2 concomitantly with dedifferentiation [201]. Another miR-145 target in human AC cell lines is *tumor necrosis factor receptor superfamily member 11b (TNFRSF11B)*. TNFRSF11B downregulation originates upregulation of Collagen II, V and X and reduction of MMP-1, MMP-8 and MMP-13 proteins [200]. Moreover, *A disintegrin and metalloproteinase domain-containing protein 17 (ADAM17)* can be directly targeted by miR-145 [202], which initiates a negative feedback loop involving the ADAM17 substrate TNF-α, which is upregulated and subsequently reduces miR-145 expression in renal carcinoma cell lines [203]. In human adipocytes miR-145 increases both glycerol release and TNF-α secretion via activation of NF-κB signaling [202]. Therefore, inflammatory cytokine signaling both positively and negatively interferes with miR-145 abundance, with increasing inflammation probably depleting miR-145 levels. Hence, miR-145 is involved in anti-anabolic and catabolic signaling during OA progression.

In human late stage OA AC cells miR-146a is upregulated, while during chondrogenesis of human bone MSPCs downregulation of miR-146a is observed [204]. Increased expression of miR-146a has been also detected in the plasma of human knee OA patients compared to healthy controls older than 40 years [150]. Moreover, miR-146a expression is elevated in peripheral blood mononuclear cells (PBMC) from late stage OA patients [205]. Mechanical pressure injury increases miR-146a abundance in human healthy AC cells, wherein *SMAD4* has been identified as direct target of miR-146a [206]. In addition, hydrostatic pressure increases miR-146a expression in human hip OA AC monolayer cell cultures, which exhibit reduced basal miR-146a level compared normal hip AC cells [168]. However, transfection of synthetic miR-146a dose-dependently antagonized rIL-1-mediated suppression of both *ACAN* and *COL2A1* expression in cells isolated from human early OA AC. Moreover, rIL-1 induced expression of *MMP-13* and *ADAMTS-5* in human early OA AC cells is significantly suppressed by miR-146a [207]. In THP-1 cells, rIL-1β and rTNF-α induce miR-146a expression mediated by NF-κB. *TNF receptor-associated factor 6* (*TRAF6*) and *IL-1 receptor-associated kinase 1* (*IRAK1*) have been identified as direct miR-146a target genes in these cells [208]. Interestingly, lentiviral overexpression of miR-146a increases FGF2 secretion of HUVECs by upregulation of fibroblast growth factor binding protein 1 (FGFBP1) expression via directly targeting *CAMP responsive element binding protein 3 like 1* (*CREB3L1*) [209]. Moreover, miR-146a has been implicated in several chronic diseases related to aging dependent increase of inflammation [157]. Therefore, miR-146a is apparently fine-tuning inflammatory cytokine, TGF-β and FGF2 signaling to prevent over-activation of inflammatory and catabolic pathways in advanced OA.

MiR-149 is significantly downregulated in human knee OA AC and micropellet cultures from OA AC, compared to normal AC. Yet, in bone it is concurrently upregulated [147,210]. In the chondrosarcoma cell line SW1353 both rIL-1β and rTNF-α reduce miR-149 abundance, whereas *IL-6*, *IL-1β* and *TNF-α* are direct targets of miR-149 [173]. Therefore, inflammatory cytokine mediated downregulation of miR-149 appears to be a self-reinforcing system to promote inflammation in advanced OA.

MiR-181a expression is increased in monolayer cell cultures isolated from aged OA AC compared to cells from aged healthy AC. Yet, specifically in cells derived from OA AC hydrostatic pressure downregulates miR-181 [211]. In human knee AC cell monolayer cultures transfection with miR-181 mimic decreases proliferation and increases apoptosis. Moreover, activity of MMP-2 and MMP-9 is enhanced by miR-181 mimic [212]. In addition, elevated miR-181a expression is associated with successful chondrogenesis of human MSPCs [213]. However, there are also studies showing a decreased expression of miR-181 family members, including miR-181a, in OA AC cell monolayer cultures, compared to healthy AC cells from younger donors [191,214]. Notably, in acute myeloid leukemia (AML) cells *KRAS*, *neuroblastoma RAS viral oncogene homolog* (*NRAS*) and *ERK2* have been identified as direct targets of miR-181a [215]. STAT3, activated by inflammatory cytokine signaling, activates miR-181b in human MCF10A cells [216]. Apparently, the miR-181 family promotes catabolic gene expression, while repressing ERK MAPK signaling.

MiR-186 is upregulated in the plasma of human knee OA patients, compared to healthy controls [150]. In human AC, no direct regulation or transcriptional targets have been identified to date. Remarkably, in human THP-1 macrophages miR-186 enhances secretion of IL-6, IL-1β and TNF-α as well as lipid accumulation via targeting *cystathionine-γ-lyase* (*CSE*) [217]. Moreover, in human glioblastoma cells *FGF2* and the *NF-κB* subunit RelA have been identified as miR-186 targets [218]. Summarized, despite induction of inflammatory cytokine expression by miR-186, the inflammatory response is apparently attenuated via NF-κB depletion.

MiR-210 expression is downregulated in human knee and hip OA AC compared to normal AC [151,219]. Transfection of a miR-210 precursor in human OA AC derived monolayer cell cultures induces *COL2A1* mRNA expression, whereas *COL10A1* and *MMP-13* expression is significantly reduced [219]. In human cervical cancer cells, *SMAD4* has been identified as a direct target of miR-210 [220]. Hypoxia-inducible factor-1α (HIF-1α) can induce miR-210 expression in various human cell lines [221]. Notably, in synovial fibroblasts from OA patients rCCN2 induces VEGF secretion by raising miR-210 expression which involves phosphatidylinositol 3-kinase (PI3K)-AKT, ERK, and NF-κB/ELK1 signaling [222]. This indicates that miR-210-mediated anabolic and anti-catabolic signaling is alleviated in human OA AC, whereas in OA synovium miR-210 acts a pro-angiogenic factor.

In human knee OA AC, miR-221 expression is downregulated with an increasing Mankin score. rIL-1β reduces miR-221 expression in monolayer cultures of human OA AC cells. *Stromal cell derived factor 1 (SDF1)*, also known as *C-X-C Motif Chemokine Ligand 12 (CXCL12)*, has been determined as direct target of miR-221 [223]. Moreover, miR-221 is downregulated in synovial fibroblasts derived from patients with OA of the temporomandibular joint (TMJ), compared to synovial fibroblasts of healthy donors. In addition, treatment with rIL-1β suppresses miR-221 expression in TMJ OA synovial fibroblasts. ETS1, a transcription factor involved in *MMP-1, MMP-2* and *MMP-9* expression, has been identified as direct miR-221 target in TMJ OA synovial fibroblasts [224]. Interestingly, increasing BMI has also been linked to reduced miR-221 abundance [225]. Therefore, reduction of miR-221 abundance by inflammatory cytokines may reinforce their catabolic target gene expression, which, in addition, appears augmented by obesity.

MiR-365 is upregulated in human late stage knee OA AC, compared to macroscopically intact cartilage from the same patients. In cell cultures established from macroscopically normal OA AC, both cyclic loading and rIL-1β increase miR-365 expression by a mechanism involving NF-κB. Yet, hydrostatic pressure reduces miR-365 expression in human hip OA AC monolayer cell cultures [168]. *Histone deacetylase 4 (HDAC4)* is a direct target of miR-365 and its downregulation has been implicated in catabolic *MMP-13* and *COL10A1* expression [226]. Interestingly, also *IL-6* is a direct target of miR-365 [227]. Therefore, miR-365 is involved in catabolic gene expression, but its inflammatory cytokine induced overexpression may also alleviate inflammatory gene expression in a feedback loop.

Expression of miR-411 is reduced in human knee OA AC compared with normal AC. rIL-1β represses miR-411 in the human immortalized juvenile costal chondrocyte cell line C28/I2. Moreover, *MMP-13* has been identified as direct target of miR-411 and overexpression of miR-411 mimic increases both COL2A1 and COL4A2 at mRNA and protein level [228]. This indicates an anabolic and anti-catabolic function of miR-411, which is apparently overridden by inflammatory cytokines.

Upregulation of miR-483 has been observed in human knee and hip OA AC, compared to normal AC [151,229]. Also, OA AC micropellet cultures have higher miR-483 level, compared to normal AC micropellet cultures [210]. TGF-β1 is downregulated by overexpression of miR-483 mimic in monolayer cultures from human normal knee AC, which coincides with *COL2A1* and *ACAN* mRNA depletion and *RUNX2* and *MMP13* upregulation [230]. In human MSPC miR-483 directly targets *SMAD4*, which suppresses chondrogenesis. In mice, *matrilin 3 (Matn3)* and *Timp2* have been identified as direct miR-483 targets [229]. Summarized, miR-483 negatively regulates TGF-β signaling and apparently acts anti-anabolic and pro-catabolic in OA AC.

In monolayer cell cultures derived from human knee OA AC miR-488 expression is reduced, compared to normal AC cell cultures [231]. Exposure to rIL-1β reduces and rTGF-β3 increases miR-488 abundance in normal AC cell cultures. Thereby, miR-488 inhibits MMP-13 activity through targeting the zinc-ion transporter *Zrt- and Irt-like protein 8 (ZIP8)* [231]. Interestingly, ZIP8 expression can be induced through the canonical NF-κB pathway, which is activated in response to several inflammatory cytokines. Increased intracellular zinc level activate metal regulatory transcription factor-1 (Mtf-1), which positively regulates Mmp-3, Mmp-9, Mmp-13, and Adamts-5 mRNA and protein expression in murine AC monolayer cell cultures [232]. In short, miR-488 obviously exerts its anti-catabolic function by reduction of intracellular zinc availability. Yet, its inflammatory cytokine-mediated downregulation permits catabolic gene expression and MMP activity.

This chapter summarizes the current evidence concerning 27 miRNAs, respectively miRNA families, with a significant up- or downregulation in human OA AC, compared to normal AC. As illustrated in Figure 2, differentially regulated miRNAs interfere with inflammatory cytokine, FGF2 and TGF-β downstream signaling, which, additionally, exhibit an intense crosstalk at the protein level. In human OA AC expression of pro-catabolic target genes is mediated by NF-κB, MAPK and SMAD signaling, whereas pro-inflammatory targets are activated downstream of MAPK and NF-κB signaling. Though proliferation prevails during early OA, expression of catabolic ECM degrading proteins is concomitantly induced. Advanced stages of OA are characterized by sustained activation of inflammatory cytokine signaling, whereas proliferation ceases. Regarding the here discussed miRNAs, there is primarily a net upregulation of IL-6, whereas both positive and negative regulation of NF-κB signaling is reported. Moreover, in human OA AC upregulation of CCN2 and significantly enhanced activation of ERK, JNK and p38 MAPK pathways has been documented. Yet, evidence for ERK signaling regulation by miRNAs is contradictory. In contrast, TGF-β signaling is globally downregulated as a consequence of miRNA presence, especially with a negative regulation of the anabolic SMAD3-mediated pathway, both on protein and miRNA level. In addition, at miRNA level, particularly a reversal of negative regulation of MMP-13 is present in OA AC, which might be also due to many studies specifically examining MMP-13, since several other MMPs are upregulated at protein level, whereas no miRNA-dependent regulation has been examined to date.

7. Conclusions

This review focused on the following question: which of the three key events in early OA AC—proliferation, ECM degradation, and inflammation—are inducible by growth factor signaling, inflammatory cytokine signaling, and/or miRNA regulation. Additionally, we aimed to reveal in which sequence(s) these processes can and cannot occur, and whether we can identify a single factor that is able to induce all of these key processes, according to the currently available knowledge. In this context, it is relevant to summarize that differentiated chondrocytes in the SZ of human normal adult AC are predominantly arranged in string patterns embedded in the PCM [12,13] (see Figure 1). Here, growth factors including TGF-β, BMP, and IGF signaling effects mediate AC maintenance-associated anabolic PCM component deposition. However, a hallmark of early OA is proliferation of cartilage-inherent cells [10,13,14], during which the cellular organization changes from single strings to double strings and eventually to small cell clusters [12,233]. During this proliferative phase, the PCM is progressively degraded, apparently by MMPs and other catabolic factors [13]. The proliferating cells may be either dedifferentiated chondrocytes reentering cell cycle or resident or immigrated MSPCs [12,13,23,233]. Whether the proliferation in OA AC is associated with an attempt of cartilage intrinsic anabolic repair or rather a prerequisite for macroscopic cartilage degradation due to a simultaneously lack of extracellular matrix (ECM) maintenance, respectively proliferation-associated degradation, remains elusive. As discussed, proliferation in early OA AC is obviously dependent on FGF2, TGF-β, WNT and NOTCH signaling [13,63,74,105], whereas catabolic gene expression may be induced by FGF2, a switch in TGF-β signaling, and inflammatory cytokines including IL-6 [30,39,60,134]. Importantly, according to what is known, inflammatory cytokines do not induce but in fact suppress human AC cell proliferation [36,128], which in turn means that the proliferative phase during early OA is probably not inducible by inflammatory cytokines and occurs prior to inflammation, whereas catabolic ECM degradation is already apparent during the proliferative phase but steadily increasing with OA severity. Thus, the specific sequence of OA key events is described best by a very early phase of proliferation of human articular cartilage (AC) cells and concomitant anabolic/catabolic effects that are accompanied by incipient pro-inflammatory effects.

Remarkably, it was highly interesting to ask the question whether it was possible to identify any cytokine or growth factor that is potentially able to induce or reinforce all three key events promoting early OA onset and progression. In detail, in human OA AC, proliferation and anabolism, but also catabolism, are associated with TGF-β effects, depending on the receptor utilization. Proliferation and anti-catabolism are associated with canonical WNT/β-catenin signaling effects, whereas non-canonical WNT signaling may contribute to catabolic gene expression. In normal adult AC, proliferation and anabolism are associated with IGF-1 effects. NOTCH signaling contributes to proliferation in human OA AC, whereas it likely inhibits catabolic and inflammatory gene expression. BMP signaling outcome in human AC is anabolic and via a cross-talk with WNT signaling potentially also catabolic. For Hh signaling there are only very few data for human adult AC available. Yet, a potential catabolic role may be assumed. Catabolism is also associated with VEGF signaling in human OA AC. Neither for BMP nor for VEGF experimental evidence reveals a pro-proliferative effect in human AC. In human AC, both catabolism and reinforced pro-inflammatory effects are associated with inflammatory cytokines; yet, proliferation is demonstrably inhibited. Interestingly, based on currently available data, proliferation, catabolism, and pro-inflammatory effects in human AC are solely associated with FGF2. Thus, many factors are able to induce one or two of these three events examined but, importantly, FGF2 was identified as a unique factor capable of concomitantly inducing all three key events. FGF2 is not only involved in proliferative and catabolic gene expression but also in the mRNA expression of the inflammatory cytokines *TNF-α, IL-1β, IL-6, IL-8,* and *MCP-1* [32]. Thus, FGF2-promoted MAPK and NF-κB signaling appears to be uniquely able to induce self-reinforcing inflammation in human adult AC, which is a hallmark of late OA. Therefore, FGF2 is the only cytokine that we can implicate in both the proliferative aspect seen in early OA and also in the degradative and inflammatory progression of later OA. According to the reviewed literature, these properties appear unique to FGF2, as this role cannot be assumed by any other growth factor or inflammatory cytokine.

This review focused on growth factor-, inflammatory cytokine-, or differential miRNA expression-induced signaling effects in the context of human *primary* osteoarthritis. However, it is important to mention that AC degeneration due to acute injury or due to long-standing mechanical problems such as anterior cruciate rupture or laxity, meniscal damage, and/or joint malalignment is known to lead to *post-traumatic* osteoarthritis (PTOA). Many differences between OA and PTOA are known; we refer to the PTOA literature [234,235]. The here discussed data have not been derived from studies that had PTOA in mind; e.g., models of mechanical overload such as those described in [236,237], or studied therapeutic options after AC injury [238–240]. Thus, it remains unclear whether the here derived insights are valid under conditions known to lead to PTOA and designated studies using standardized injury models are needed.

Another important point is that the here discussed signaling effects should not be viewed as isolated events in AC, as several adjacent tissues, including meniscal fibrocartilage, synovium, fat, and bone, with each tissue having its own genetic propensity for anabolic, catabolic, or pro-inflammatory responses, may affect AC by secreted factors. Nevertheless, we focused in this review solely on human AC to produce a systematic foundation for events occurring in human AC, to which the other tissues; e.g., as cytokine and miRNA molecule sources may also contribute.

Collectively, the here presented view represents a novel molecular concept to interpret early OA signaling. However, designated experimental evidence is needed for its confirmation and for judging its potential value in developing novel therapeutic or preventive avenues.

Author Contributions: K.A.B. and B.R. wrote the initial manuscript and edited it until it reached its current form.

Funding: This research was funded by the VolkswagenStiftung, grant number 92701, and by the Deutsche Arthrose-Hilfe, grant number P346-A825-Rolauffs-EP1.

Acknowledgments: The article processing charge was funded by the German Research Foundation (DFG) and the University of Freiburg in the funding programme Open Access Publishing.

Conflicts of Interest: The authors declare no conflict of interest.

Abbreviations

AAV	*adeno-associated virus*
ABCA1	ATP-binding cassette transporter A1
AC	articular cartilage
ACAN	Aggrecan
ACVRL1	activin A receptor like type 1
ADAM17	A disintegrin and metalloproteinase domain-containing protein 17
ADAMTS	A disintegrin and metalloproteinase with thrombospondin motifs
ADPN	adiponectin
ALK	activin receptor-like kinase
AML	acute myeloid leukemia
AP-1	activator protein 1
APOA1	apolipoprotein A1
ASPN	asporin
BMI	body mass index
BMP	bone morphogenetic protein
CaMK2	calmodulin-dependent protein kinase 2
CCL2	C-C motif chemokine ligand 2
CCDN1	cyclin D1
CDK6	cyclin dependent kinase 6
cFOS	cellular oncogene Fos
CIR	cartilage injury-related
COL2A1	collagen type II α 1 chain
COL4A2	collagen type IV α 2 chain
COL10A1	collagen type X α 1 chain
CREB3L1	CAMP Responsive Element Binding Protein 3 Like 1
CSE	cystathionine-γ-lyase
CTGF	connective tissue growth factor
CYR61	cysteine-rich angiogenic inducer 61
CXCL12	C-X-C Motif Chemokine Ligand 12
DKK1	dickkopf WNT signaling pathway inhibitor 1
DKK3	dickkopf WNT signaling pathway inhibitor 3
DLL1	Delta-like 1
DZ	deep zone
ECM	extracellular matrix
ELF3	E74-like factor 3
ELK1	ETS-domain protein ELK1
ERG	ETS-related gene
ERK	extracellular signal-regulated kinase
ETS	avian erythroblastosis virus E26 oncogene homolog
FGF2	fibroblast growth factor 2
FGFBP1	fibroblast growth factor binding protein 1
FGFR	fibroblast growth factor receptor
FLT-1	Fms related tyrosine kinase 1
FLT-4	Fms related tyrosine kinase 4
FOSB	FBJ murine osteosarcoma viral oncogene homolog B
FRZB	frizzled related protein
GDF5	growth differentiation factor 5
GLI1	glioma-associated oncogene homolog 1
HDAC4	histone deacetylase 4
HES	hairy and enhancer of split
HES1	hairy and enhancer of split 1
HES5	hairy and enhancer of split 5

Hh	Hedgehog
HHIP	hedgehog interacting protein
HIF-1α	hypoxia-inducible factor-1α
HMGA1	high mobility group protein A1
HSPG	heparan sulfate proteoglycan
IGF	insulin like growth factor
IHH	indian hedgehog
IL	interleukin
IL-1β	IL-1 beta
IL-1R	IL-1 receptor
IL-1Ra	IL-1 receptor antagonist
IRAK1	IL-1 receptor-associated kinase 1
LncRNA	long non-coding RNA
I-TAC	interferon-inducible T-cell alpha chemoattractant
JAG1	jagged 1
JAK	janus kinase
JNK	JUN N-terminal kinase
KDR	kinase insert domain receptor
KPNA3	karyopherin subunit alpha 3
KRAS	Kirsten rat sarcoma viral oncogene homolog
MALT1	mucosa-associated lymphoid tissue lymphoma translocation protein 1
MAPK	mitogen activated protein kinase
MAP3K7	mitogen-activated protein kinase kinase kinase 7
MCP-1	monocyte chemotactic protein 1
MCPIP-1	monocyte chemoattractant protein-induced protein 1
MIG	monokine induced by interferon-gamma
miRNA	Micro RNA
MMP	matrix metalloproteinase
MSPC	mesenchymal stem and progenitor cells
Matn3	matrilin 3
Mtf-1	metal regulatory transcription factor-1
MZ	middle zone
NFAT5	CaMK2 nuclear factor of activated T-cells 5, tonicity-responsive
NFATC2	nuclear factor of activated T-cells 2
NF-κB	nuclear factor kappa B
NOTCH	notch homolog
NRAS	neuroblastoma RAS viral oncogene homolog
OA	osteoarthritis
OSM	oncostatin M
PBMC	*peripheral blood mononuclear cells*
PCM	pericellular matrix
PI3K	phosphatidylinositol 3-kinase
PKC δ	protein kinase C δ
PTCH1	patched 1
R	recombinant
RAS	rat sarcoma viral oncogene homolog
RUNX2	runt related transcription factor 2
SCSO	superficial cell spatial organization
SDF1	Stromal cell derived factor 1
SF	synovial fluid
SHH	sonic hedgehog
SIRT1	sirtuin 1

SMAD	SMA- and MAD-related protein
SNP	single nucleotide polymorphism
SOX9	SRY-related HMG box-containing
SREBP-2	sterol regulatory element-binding protein 2
HIF-1α	hypoxia-inducible factor-1α
STAT3	signal transducer and activator of transcription 3
SZ	superficial zone
TAB3	TGF-β activated kinase 1 and MAP3K7 binding protein 3
TAK1	TGF-β-activated kinase-1
TGF-β	transforming growth factor β
TGFBR	transforming growth factor β receptor
TIMP	tissue inhibitor of metalloproteinases
TMJ	temporomandibular joint
TNF-α	tumor necrosis factor α
TNFRSF11B	tumor necrosis factor receptor superfamily member 11b
TRAF6	TNF receptor-associated factor 6
VEGF	vascular endothelial growth factor
WNT	wingless-type MMTV integration site family
ZIP8	Zrt- and Irt-like protein 8

References

1. McAlindon, T.E.; Bannuru, R.R.; Sullivan, M.C.; Arden, N.K.; Berenbaum, F.; Bierma-Zeinstra, S.M.; Hawker, G.A.; Henrotin, Y.; Hunter, D.J.; Kawaguchi, H.; et al. Oarsi guidelines for the non-surgical management of knee osteoarthritis. *Osteoarthr. Cartil.* **2014**, *22*, 363–388. [CrossRef] [PubMed]

2. Ondresik, M.; Azevedo Maia, F.R.; da Silva Morais, A.; Gertrudes, A.C.; Dias Bacelar, A.H.; Correia, C.; Goncalves, C.; Radhouani, H.; Amandi Sousa, R.; Oliveira, J.M.; et al. Management of knee osteoarthritis. Current status and future trends. *Biotechnol. Bioeng.* **2017**, *114*, 717–739. [CrossRef] [PubMed]

3. Murphy, N.J.; Eyles, J.P.; Hunter, D.J. Hip osteoarthritis: Etiopathogenesis and implications for management. *Adv. Ther.* **2016**, *33*, 1921–1946. [CrossRef] [PubMed]

4. Chevalier, X.; Eymard, F.; Richette, P. Biologic agents in osteoarthritis: Hopes and disappointments. *Nat. Rev. Rheumatol.* **2013**, *9*, 400–410. [CrossRef] [PubMed]

5. Chu, C.R.; Williams, A.A.; Coyle, C.H.; Bowers, M.E. Early diagnosis to enable early treatment of pre-osteoarthritis. *Arthritis Res. Ther.* **2012**, *14*, 212. [CrossRef] [PubMed]

6. Mobasheri, A. The future of osteoarthritis therapeutics: Targeted pharmacological therapy. *Curr. Rheumatol. Rep.* **2013**, *15*, 364. [CrossRef] [PubMed]

7. Marles, P.J.; Hoyland, J.A.; Parkinson, R.; Freemont, A.J. Demonstration of variation in chondrocyte activity in different zones of articular cartilage: An assessment of the value of in-situ hybridization. *Int. J. Exp. Pathol.* **1991**, *72*, 171–182. [PubMed]

8. Asari, A.; Miyauchi, S.; Kuriyama, S.; Machida, A.; Kohno, K.; Uchiyama, Y. Localization of hyaluronic acid in human articular cartilage. *J. Histochem. Cytochem.* **1994**, *42*, 513–522. [CrossRef] [PubMed]

9. Kuettner, K.E.; Aydelotte, M.B.; Thonar, E.J. Articular cartilage matrix and structure: A minireview. *J. Rheumatol. Suppl.* **1991**, *27*, 46–48. [PubMed]

10. Aicher, W.K.; Rolauffs, B. The spatial organisation of joint surface chondrocytes: Review of its potential roles in tissue functioning, disease and early, preclinical diagnosis of osteoarthritis. *Ann. Rheum. Dis.* **2014**, *73*, 645–653. [CrossRef] [PubMed]

11. Rolauffs, B.; Williams, J.M.; Grodzinsky, A.J.; Kuettner, K.E.; Cole, A.A. Distinct horizontal patterns in the spatial organization of superficial zone chondrocytes of human joints. *J. Struct. Biol.* **2008**, *162*, 335–344. [CrossRef] [PubMed]

12. Rolauffs, B.; Williams, J.M.; Aurich, M.; Grodzinsky, A.J.; Kuettner, K.E.; Cole, A.A. Proliferative remodeling of the spatial organization of human superficial chondrocytes distant from focal early osteoarthritis. *Arthritis Rheumtol.* **2010**, *62*, 489–498.

13. Felka, T.; Rothdiener, M.; Bast, S.; Uynuk-Ool, T.; Zouhair, S.; Ochs, B.G.; De Zwart, P.; Stoeckle, U.; Aicher, W.K.; Hart, M.L.; et al. Loss of spatial organization and destruction of the pericellular matrix in early osteoarthritis in vivo and in a novel in vitro methodology. *Osteoarthr. Cartil.* **2016**, *24*, 1200–1209. [CrossRef] [PubMed]

14. Lotz, M.K.; Otsuki, S.; Grogan, S.P.; Sah, R.; Terkeltaub, R.; D'Lima, D. Cartilage cell clusters. *Arthritis Rheumtol.* **2010**, *62*, 2206–2218. [CrossRef] [PubMed]

15. Goldring, M.B. The role of the chondrocyte in osteoarthritis. *Arthritis Rheumtol.* **2000**, *43*, 1916–1926. [CrossRef]

16. Schumacher, B.L.; Su, J.L.; Lindley, K.M.; Kuettner, K.E.; Cole, A.A. Horizontally oriented clusters of multiple chondrons in the superficial zone of ankle, but not knee articular cartilage. *Anat. Rec.* **2002**, *266*, 241–248. [CrossRef] [PubMed]

17. Tetlow, L.C.; Adlam, D.J.; Woolley, D.E. Matrix metalloproteinase and proinflammatory cytokine production by chondrocytes of human osteoarthritic cartilage: Associations with degenerative changes. *Arthritis Rheumtol.* **2001**, *44*, 585–594. [CrossRef]

18. Bush, J.R.; Beier, F. TGF-beta and osteoarthritis—The good and the bad. *Nat. Med.* **2013**, *19*, 667–669. [CrossRef] [PubMed]

19. Bertrand, J.; Cromme, C.; Umlauf, D.; Frank, S.; Pap, T. Molecular mechanisms of cartilage remodelling in osteoarthritis. *Int. J. Biochem. Cell Biol.* **2010**, *42*, 1594–1601. [CrossRef] [PubMed]

20. Kapoor, M.; Martel-Pelletier, J.; Lajeunesse, D.; Pelletier, J.P.; Fahmi, H. Role of proinflammatory cytokines in the pathophysiology of osteoarthritis. *Nat. Rev. Rheumatol.* **2011**, *7*, 33–42. [CrossRef] [PubMed]

21. Johnson, C.I.; Argyle, D.J.; Clements, D.N. In vitro models for the study of osteoarthritis. *Vet. J.* **2016**, *209*, 40–49. [CrossRef] [PubMed]

22. Yun, Y.R.; Won, J.E.; Jeon, E.; Lee, S.; Kang, W.; Jo, H.; Jang, J.H.; Shin, U.S.; Kim, H.W. Fibroblast growth factors: Biology, function, and application for tissue regeneration. *J. Tissue Eng.* **2010**, *2010*, 218142. [CrossRef] [PubMed]

23. Boehme, K.A.; Schleicher, S.B.; Traub, F.; Rolauffs, B. Chondrosarcoma: A rare misfortune in aging human cartilage? The role of stem and progenitor cells in proliferation, malignant degeneration and therapeutic resistance. *Int. J. Mol. Sci.* **2018**, *19*, 311. [CrossRef] [PubMed]

24. Zhai, G.; Dore, J.; Rahman, P. TGF-beta signal transduction pathways and osteoarthritis. *Rheumatol. Int.* **2015**, *35*, 1283–1292. [CrossRef] [PubMed]

25. Vincent, T.L.; McLean, C.J.; Full, L.E.; Peston, D.; Saklatvala, J. FGF-2 is bound to perlecan in the pericellular matrix of articular cartilage, where it acts as a chondrocyte mechanotransducer. *Osteoarthr. Cartil.* **2007**, *15*, 752–763. [CrossRef] [PubMed]

26. Vincent, T.; Hermansson, M.; Bolton, M.; Wait, R.; Saklatvala, J. Basic fgf mediates an immediate response of articular cartilage to mechanical injury. *Proc. Natl. Acad. Sci. USA* **2002**, *99*, 8259–8264. [CrossRef] [PubMed]

27. Cucchiarini, M.; Terwilliger, E.F.; Kohn, D.; Madry, H. Remodelling of human osteoarthritic cartilage by FGF-2, alone or combined with SOX9 via RAAV gene transfer. *J. Cell. Mol. Med.* **2009**, *13*, 2476–2488. [CrossRef] [PubMed]

28. Presta, M.; Andres, G.; Leali, D.; Dell'Era, P.; Ronca, R. Inflammatory cells and chemokines sustain FGF2-induced angiogenesis. *Eur. Cytokine Netw.* **2009**, *20*, 39–50. [PubMed]

29. Honsawek, S.; Yuktanandana, P.; Tanavalee, A.; Saetan, N.; Anomasiri, W.; Parkpian, V. Correlation between plasma and synovial fluid basic fibroblast growth factor with radiographic severity in primary knee osteoarthritis. *Int. Orthop.* **2012**, *36*, 981–985. [CrossRef] [PubMed]

30. Yan, D.; Chen, D.; Cool, S.M.; van Wijnen, A.J.; Mikecz, K.; Murphy, G.; Im, H.J. Fibroblast growth factor receptor 1 is principally responsible for fibroblast growth factor 2-induced catabolic activities in human articular chondrocytes. *Arthritis Res. Ther.* **2011**, *13*, R130. [CrossRef] [PubMed]

31. Li, X.; Ellman, M.B.; Kroin, J.S.; Chen, D.; Yan, D.; Mikecz, K.; Ranjan, K.C.; Xiao, G.; Stein, G.S.; Kim, S.G.; et al. Species-specific biological effects of FGF-2 in articular cartilage: Implication for distinct roles within the fgf receptor family. *J. Cell. Biochem.* **2012**, *113*, 2532–2542. [CrossRef] [PubMed]

32. Im, H.J.; Muddasani, P.; Natarajan, V.; Schmid, T.M.; Block, J.A.; Davis, F.; van Wijnen, A.J.; Loeser, R.F. Basic fibroblast growth factor stimulates matrix metalloproteinase-13 via the molecular cross-talk between the mitogen-activated protein kinases and protein kinase cdelta pathways in human adult articular chondrocytes. *J. Biol. Chem.* **2007**, *282*, 11110–11121. [CrossRef] [PubMed]

33. Yan, D.; Chen, D.; Im, H.J. Fibroblast growth factor-2 promotes catabolism via FGFR1-Ras-Raf-MEK1/2-ERK1/2 axis that coordinates with the PKCdelta pathway in human articular chondrocytes. *J. Cell. Biochem.* **2012**, *113*, 2856–2865. [CrossRef] [PubMed]

34. Ellman, M.B.; Yan, D.; Ahmadinia, K.; Chen, D.; An, H.S.; Im, H.J. Fibroblast growth factor control of cartilage homeostasis. *J. Cell. Biochem.* **2013**, *114*, 735–742. [CrossRef] [PubMed]

35. Muddasani, P.; Norman, J.C.; Ellman, M.; van Wijnen, A.J.; Im, H.J. Basic fibroblast growth factor activates the MAPK and NFkappaB pathways that converge on Elk-1 to control production of matrix metalloproteinase-13 by human adult articular chondrocytes. *J. Biol. Chem.* **2007**, *282*, 31409–31421. [CrossRef] [PubMed]

36. Sun, H.Y.; Hu, K.Z.; Yin, Z.S. Inhibition of the p38-mapk signaling pathway suppresses the apoptosis and expression of proinflammatory cytokines in human osteoarthritis chondrocytes. *Cytokine* **2016**, *90*, 135–143. [CrossRef] [PubMed]

37. Takebe, K.; Nishiyama, T.; Hayashi, S.; Hashimoto, S.; Fujishiro, T.; Kanzaki, N.; Kawakita, K.; Iwasa, K.; Kuroda, R.; Kurosaka, M. Regulation of p38 MAPK phosphorylation inhibits chondrocyte apoptosis in response to heat stress or mechanical stress. *Int. J. Mol. Med.* **2011**, *27*, 329–335. [PubMed]

38. Fan, Z.; Soder, S.; Oehler, S.; Fundel, K.; Aigner, T. Activation of interleukin-1 signaling cascades in normal and osteoarthritic articular cartilage. *Am. J. Pathol.* **2007**, *171*, 938–946. [CrossRef] [PubMed]

39. Nummenmaa, E.; Hamalainen, M.; Moilanen, T.; Vuolteenaho, K.; Moilanen, E. Effects of FGF-2 and FGF receptor antagonists on mmp enzymes, aggrecan, and type II collagen in primary human OA chondrocytes. *Scand. J. Rheumatol.* **2015**, *44*, 321–330. [CrossRef] [PubMed]

40. Liu, J.F.; Crepin, M.; Liu, J.M.; Barritault, D.; Ledoux, D. FGF-2 and TPA induce matrix metalloproteinase-9 secretion in MCF-7 cells through PKC activation of the RAS/ERK pathway. *Biochem. Biophys. Res. Commun.* **2002**, *293*, 1174–1182. [CrossRef]

41. Nishida, T.; Kubota, S.; Aoyama, E.; Janune, D.; Maeda, A.; Takigawa, M. Effect of CCN2 on FGF2-induced proliferation and MMP9 and MMP13 productions by chondrocytes. *Endocrinology* **2011**, *152*, 4232–4241. [CrossRef] [PubMed]

42. Wang, X.; Manner, P.A.; Horner, A.; Shum, L.; Tuan, R.S.; Nuckolls, G.H. Regulation of MMP-13 expression by RUNX2 and FGF2 in osteoarthritic cartilage. *Osteoarthr. Cartil.* **2004**, *12*, 963–973. [CrossRef] [PubMed]

43. Kamekura, S.; Kawasaki, Y.; Hoshi, K.; Shimoaka, T.; Chikuda, H.; Maruyama, Z.; Komori, T.; Sato, S.; Takeda, S.; Karsenty, G.; et al. Contribution of runt-related transcription factor 2 to the pathogenesis of osteoarthritis in mice after induction of knee joint instability. *Arthritis Rheumtol.* **2006**, *54*, 2462–2470. [CrossRef] [PubMed]

44. Kim, B.G.; Kim, H.J.; Park, H.J.; Kim, Y.J.; Yoon, W.J.; Lee, S.J.; Ryoo, H.M.; Cho, J.Y. RUNX2 phosphorylation induced by fibroblast growth factor-2/protein kinase c pathways. *Proteomics* **2006**, *6*, 1166–1174. [CrossRef] [PubMed]

45. Tetsunaga, T.; Nishida, K.; Furumatsu, T.; Naruse, K.; Hirohata, S.; Yoshida, A.; Saito, T.; Ozaki, T. Regulation of mechanical stress-induced MMP-13 and ADAMTS-5 expression by RUNX-2 transcriptional factor in SW1353 chondrocyte-like cells. *Osteoarthr. Cartil.* **2011**, *19*, 222–232. [CrossRef] [PubMed]

46. Wang, X.; Song, Y.; Jacobi, J.L.; Tuan, R.S. Inhibition of histone deacetylases antagonized FGF2 and IL-1beta effects on MMP expression in human articular chondrocytes. *Growth Factors* **2009**, *27*, 40–49. [CrossRef] [PubMed]

47. Chia, S.L.; Sawaji, Y.; Burleigh, A.; McLean, C.; Inglis, J.; Saklatvala, J.; Vincent, T. Fibroblast growth factor 2 is an intrinsic chondroprotective agent that suppresses ADAMTS-5 and delays cartilage degradation in murine osteoarthritis. *Arthritis Rheumtol.* **2009**, *60*, 2019–2027. [CrossRef] [PubMed]

48. Yamamoto, T.; Wakitani, S.; Imoto, K.; Hattori, T.; Nakaya, H.; Saito, M.; Yonenobu, K. Fibroblast growth factor-2 promotes the repair of partial thickness defects of articular cartilage in immature rabbits but not in mature rabbits. *Osteoarthr. Cartil.* **2004**, *12*, 636–641. [CrossRef] [PubMed]

49. Sah, R.L.; Chen, A.C.; Grodzinsky, A.J.; Trippel, S.B. Differential effects of bFGF and IGF-I on matrix metabolism in calf and adult bovine cartilage explants. *Arch. Biochem. Biophys.* **1994**, *308*, 137–147. [CrossRef] [PubMed]

50. Komatsu, M.; Nakamura, Y.; Maruyama, M.; Abe, K.; Watanapokasin, R.; Kato, H. Expression profiles of human CCN genes in patients with osteoarthritis or rheumatoid arthritis. *J. Orthop. Sci.* **2015**, *20*, 708–716. [CrossRef] [PubMed]

51. Omoto, S.; Nishida, K.; Yamaai, Y.; Shibahara, M.; Nishida, T.; Doi, T.; Asahara, H.; Nakanishi, T.; Inoue, H.; Takigawa, M. Expression and localization of connective tissue growth factor (CTGF/Hcs24/CCN2) in osteoarthritic cartilage. *Osteoarthr. Cartil.* **2004**, *12*, 771–778. [CrossRef] [PubMed]

52. Verdier, M.P.; Seite, S.; Guntzer, K.; Pujol, J.P.; Boumediene, K. Immunohistochemical analysis of transforming growth factor beta isoforms and their receptors in human cartilage from normal and osteoarthritic femoral heads. *Rheumatol. Int.* **2005**, *25*, 118–124. [CrossRef] [PubMed]

53. Pombo-Suarez, M.; Castano-Oreja, M.T.; Calaza, M.; Gomez-Reino, J.; Gonzalez, A. Differential upregulation of the three transforming growth factor beta isoforms in human osteoarthritic cartilage. *Ann. Rheum. Dis.* **2009**, *68*, 568–571. [CrossRef] [PubMed]

54. Wu, J.; Liu, W.; Bemis, A.; Wang, E.; Qiu, Y.; Morris, E.A.; Flannery, C.R.; Yang, Z. Comparative proteomic characterization of articular cartilage tissue from normal donors and patients with osteoarthritis. *Arthritis Rheumtol.* **2007**, *56*, 3675–3684. [CrossRef] [PubMed]

55. Kizawa, H.; Kou, I.; Iida, A.; Sudo, A.; Miyamoto, Y.; Fukuda, A.; Mabuchi, A.; Kotani, A.; Kawakami, A.; Yamamoto, S.; et al. An aspartic acid repeat polymorphism in asporin inhibits chondrogenesis and increases susceptibility to osteoarthritis. *Nat. Genet.* **2005**, *37*, 138–144. [CrossRef] [PubMed]

56. Nakajima, M.; Kizawa, H.; Saitoh, M.; Kou, I.; Miyazono, K.; Ikegawa, S. Mechanisms for asporin function and regulation in articular cartilage. *J. Biol. Chem.* **2007**, *282*, 32185–32192. [CrossRef] [PubMed]

57. Valdes, A.M.; Spector, T.D.; Tamm, A.; Kisand, K.; Doherty, S.A.; Dennison, E.M.; Mangino, M.; Tamm, A.; KeRNA, I.; Hart, D.J.; et al. Genetic variation in the SMAD3 gene is associated with hip and knee osteoarthritis. *Arthritis Rheumtol.* **2010**, *62*, 2347–2352. [CrossRef] [PubMed]

58. Guerne, P.A.; Blanco, F.; Kaelin, A.; Desgeorges, A.; Lotz, M. Growth factor responsiveness of human articular chondrocytes in aging and development. *Arthritis Rheumtol.* **1995**, *38*, 960–968. [CrossRef]

59. Yaeger, P.C.; Masi, T.L.; de Ortiz, J.L.; Binette, F.; Tubo, R.; McPherson, J.M. Synergistic action of transforming growth factor-beta and insulin-like growth factor-I induces expression of type II collagen and aggrecan genes in adult human articular chondrocytes. *Exp. Cell Res.* **1997**, *237*, 318–325. [CrossRef] [PubMed]

60. Blaney Davidson, E.N.; Remst, D.F.; Vitters, E.L.; van Beuningen, H.M.; Blom, A.B.; Goumans, M.J.; van den Berg, W.B.; van der Kraan, P.M. Increase in ALK1/ALK5 ratio as a cause for elevated MMP-13 expression in osteoarthritis in humans and mice. *J. Immunol.* **2009**, *182*, 7937–7945. [CrossRef] [PubMed]

61. Finnson, K.W.; Parker, W.L.; ten Dijke, P.; Thorikay, M.; Philip, A. ALK1 opposes ALK5/SMAD3 signaling and expression of extracellular matrix components in human chondrocytes. *J. Bone Miner. Res.* **2008**, *23*, 896–906. [CrossRef] [PubMed]

62. Van der Kraan, P.M.; Goumans, M.J.; Blaney Davidson, E.; ten Dijke, P. Age-dependent alteration of tgf-beta signalling in osteoarthritis. *Cell Tissue Res.* **2012**, *347*, 257–265. [CrossRef] [PubMed]

63. Venkatesan, J.K.; Rey-Rico, A.; Schmitt, G.; Wezel, A.; Madry, H.; Cucchiarini, M. rAAV-mediated overexpression of TGF-beta stably restructures human osteoarthritic articular cartilage in situ. *J. Transl. Med.* **2013**, *11*, 211. [CrossRef] [PubMed]

64. Blaney Davidson, E.N.; van der Kraan, P.M.; van den Berg, W.B. TGF-beta and osteoarthritis. *Osteoarthr. Cartil.* **2007**, *15*, 597–604. [CrossRef] [PubMed]

65. Finnson, K.W.; Chi, Y.; Bou-Gharios, G.; Leask, A.; Philip, A. TGF-b signaling in cartilage homeostasis and osteoarthritis. *Front. Biosci. (Schol. Ed.)* **2012**, *4*, 251–268. [CrossRef] [PubMed]

66. Nakerakanti, S.S.; Bujor, A.M.; Trojanowska, M. CCN2 is required for the TGF-beta induced activation of SMAD1-ERK1/2 signaling network. *PLoS ONE* **2011**, *6*, e21911. [CrossRef] [PubMed]

67. Tran, C.M.; Markova, D.; Smith, H.E.; Susarla, B.; Ponnappan, R.K.; Anderson, D.G.; Symes, A.; Shapiro, I.M.; Risbud, M.V. Regulation of CCN2/connective tissue growth factor expression in the nucleus pulposus of the intervertebral disc: Role of Smad and activator protein 1 signaling. *Arthritis Rheumtol.* **2010**, *62*, 1983–1992.

68. Cheng, J.; Hu, X.; Dai, L.; Zhang, X.; Ren, B.; Shi, W.; Liu, Z.; Duan, X.; Zhang, J.; Fu, X.; et al. Inhibition of transforming growth factor beta-activated kinase 1 prevents inflammation-related cartilage degradation in osteoarthritis. *Sci. Rep.* **2016**, *6*, 34497. [CrossRef] [PubMed]

69. Huang, G.; Chubinskaya, S.; Liao, W.; Loeser, R.F. Wnt5a induces catabolic signaling and matrix metalloproteinase production in human articular chondrocytes. *Osteoarthr. Cartil.* **2017**, *25*, 1505–1515. [CrossRef] [PubMed]

70. Thorfve, A.; Dehne, T.; Lindahl, A.; Brittberg, M.; Pruss, A.; Ringe, J.; Sittinger, M.; Karlsson, C. Characteristic markers of the wnt signaling pathways are differentially expressed in osteoarthritic cartilage. *Cartilage* **2012**, *3*, 43–57. [CrossRef] [PubMed]

71. Li, Y.; Xiao, W.; Sun, M.; Deng, Z.; Zeng, C.; Li, H.; Yang, T.; Li, L.; Luo, W.; Lei, G. The expression of osteopontin and wnt5a in articular cartilage of patients with knee osteoarthritis and its correlation with disease severity. *Biomed. Res. Int.* **2016**, *2016*, 9561058. [CrossRef] [PubMed]

72. Thirunavukkarasu, K.; Pei, Y.; Moore, T.L.; Wang, H.; Yu, X.P.; Geiser, A.G.; Chandrasekhar, S. Regulation of the human adamts-4 promoter by transcription factors and cytokines. *Biochem. Biophys. Res. Commun.* **2006**, *345*, 197–204. [CrossRef] [PubMed]

73. Gibson, A.L.; Hui Mingalone, C.K.; Foote, A.T.; Uchimura, T.; Zhang, M.; Zeng, L. Wnt7a inhibits il-1beta induced catabolic gene expression and prevents articular cartilage damage in experimental osteoarthritis. *Sci. Rep.* **2017**, *7*, 41823. [CrossRef] [PubMed]

74. Nalesso, G.; Sherwood, J.; Bertrand, J.; Pap, T.; Ramachandran, M.; De Bari, C.; Pitzalis, C.; Dell'accio, F. Wnt-3a modulates articular chondrocyte phenotype by activating both canonical and noncanonical pathways. *J. Cell. Biol.* **2011**, *193*, 551–564. [CrossRef] [PubMed]

75. Ma, B.; van Blitterswijk, C.A.; Karperien, M. A Wnt/beta-catenin negative feedback loop inhibits interleukin-1-induced matrix metalloproteinase expression in human articular chondrocytes. *Arthritis Rheumtol.* **2012**, *64*, 2589–2600. [CrossRef] [PubMed]

76. Snelling, S.J.; Davidson, R.K.; Swingler, T.E.; Le, L.T.; Barter, M.J.; Culley, K.L.; Price, A.; Carr, A.J.; Clark, I.M. Dickkopf-3 is upregulated in osteoarthritis and has a chondroprotective role. *Osteoarthr. Cartil.* **2016**, *24*, 883–891. [CrossRef] [PubMed]

77. Leijten, J.C.; Bos, S.D.; Landman, E.B.; Georgi, N.; Jahr, H.; Meulenbelt, I.; Post, J.N.; van Blitterswijk, C.A.; Karperien, M. GREM1, FRZB and DKK1 mRNA levels correlate with osteoarthritis and are regulated by osteoarthritis-associated factors. *Arthritis Res. Ther.* **2013**, *15*, R126. [CrossRef] [PubMed]

78. Zhu, M.; Tang, D.; Wu, Q.; Hao, S.; Chen, M.; Xie, C.; Rosier, R.N.; O'Keefe, R.J.; Zuscik, M.; Chen, D. Activation of beta-catenin signaling in articular chondrocytes leads to osteoarthritis-like phenotype in adult beta-catenin conditional activation mice. *J. Bone Miner. Res.* **2009**, *24*, 12–21. [CrossRef] [PubMed]

79. Min, J.L.; Meulenbelt, I.; Riyazi, N.; Kloppenburg, M.; Houwing-Duistermaat, J.J.; Seymour, A.B.; Pols, H.A.; van Duijn, C.M.; Slagboom, P.E. Association of the frizzled-related protein gene with symptomatic osteoarthritis at multiple sites. *Arthritis Rheumtol.* **2005**, *52*, 1077–1080. [CrossRef] [PubMed]

80. Loughlin, J.; Dowling, B.; Chapman, K.; Marcelline, L.; Mustafa, Z.; Southam, L.; Ferreira, A.; Ciesielski, C.; Carson, D.A.; Corr, M. Functional variants within the secreted frizzled-related protein 3 gene are associated with hip osteoarthritis in females. *Proc. Natl. Acad. Sci. USA* **2004**, *101*, 9757–9762. [CrossRef] [PubMed]

81. Valdes, A.M.; Loughlin, J.; Oene, M.V.; Chapman, K.; Surdulescu, G.L.; Doherty, M.; Spector, T.D. Sex and ethnic differences in the association of ASPN, CALM1, COL2A1, COMP, and FRZB with genetic susceptibility to osteoarthritis of the knee. *Arthritis Rheumtol.* **2007**, *56*, 137–146. [CrossRef] [PubMed]

82. Oldefest, M.; Dusterhoft, S.; Desel, C.; Thysen, S.; Fink, C.; Rabe, B.; Lories, R.; Grotzinger, J.; Lorenzen, I. Secreted frizzled-related protein 3 (sFRP3)-mediated suppression of interleukin-6 receptor release by a disintegrin and metalloprotease 17 (ADAM17) is abrogated in the osteoarthritis-associated rare double variant of sFRP3. *Biochem. J.* **2015**, *468*, 507–518. [CrossRef] [PubMed]

83. Minina, E.; Wenzel, H.M.; Kreschel, C.; Karp, S.; Gaffield, W.; McMahon, A.P.; Vortkamp, A. BMP and Ihh/PTHrP signaling interact to coordinate chondrocyte proliferation and differentiation. *Development* **2001**, *128*, 4523–4534. [PubMed]

84. Ohba, S. Hedgehog signaling in endochondral ossification. *J. Dev. Biol.* **2016**, *4*, 20. [CrossRef] [PubMed]

85. Kronenberg, H.M. PTHrP and skeletal development. *Ann. N. Y. Acad. Sci.* **2006**, *1068*, 1–13. [CrossRef] [PubMed]

86. Wei, F.; Zhou, J.; Wei, X.; Zhang, J.; Fleming, B.C.; Terek, R.; Pei, M.; Chen, Q.; Liu, T.; Wei, L. Activation of Indian hedgehog promotes chondrocyte hypertrophy and upregulation of mmp-13 in human osteoarthritic cartilage. *Osteoarthr. Cartil.* **2012**, *20*, 755–763. [CrossRef] [PubMed]

87. Zhang, C.; Wei, X.; Chen, C.; Cao, K.; Li, Y.; Jiao, Q.; Ding, J.; Zhou, J.; Fleming, B.C.; Chen, Q.; et al. Indian hedgehog in synovial fluid is a novel marker for early cartilage lesions in human knee joint. *Int. J. Mol. Sci.* **2014**, *15*, 7250–7265. [CrossRef] [PubMed]

88. Lin, A.C.; Seeto, B.L.; Bartoszko, J.M.; Khoury, M.A.; Whetstone, H.; Ho, L.; Hsu, C.; Ali, S.A.; Alman, B.A. Modulating hedgehog signaling can attenuate the severity of osteoarthritis. *Nat. Med.* **2009**, *15*, 1421–1425. [CrossRef] [PubMed]

89. Thompson, C.L.; Patel, R.; Kelly, T.A.; Wann, A.K.; Hung, C.T.; Chapple, J.P.; Knight, M.M. Hedgehog signalling does not stimulate cartilage catabolism and is inhibited by interleukin-1beta. *Arthritis Res. Ther.* **2015**, *17*, 373. [CrossRef] [PubMed]

90. Van der Kraan, P.M.; Blaney Davidson, E.N.; van den Berg, W.B. Bone morphogenetic proteins and articular cartilage: To serve and protect or a wolf in sheep clothing's? *Osteoarthr. Cartil.* **2010**, *18*, 735–741. [CrossRef] [PubMed]

91. Fukui, N.; Zhu, Y.; Maloney, W.J.; Clohisy, J.; Sandell, L.J. Stimulation of BMP-2 expression by pro-inflammatory cytokines IL-1 and TNF-alpha in normal and osteoarthritic chondrocytes. *J. Bone Jt. Surg. Am.* **2003**, *85-A* (Suppl. 3), 59–66. [CrossRef]

92. Nakase, T.; Miyaji, T.; Tomita, T.; Kaneko, M.; Kuriyama, K.; Myoui, A.; Sugamoto, K.; Ochi, T.; Yoshikawa, H. Localization of bone morphogenetic protein-2 in human osteoarthritic cartilage and osteophyte. *Osteoarthr. Cartil.* **2003**, *11*, 278–284. [CrossRef]

93. Papathanasiou, I.; Malizos, K.N.; Tsezou, A. Bone morphogenetic protein-2-induced Wnt/beta-catenin signaling pathway activation through enhanced low-density-lipoprotein receptor-related protein 5 catabolic activity contributes to hypertrophy in osteoarthritic chondrocytes. *Arthritis Res. Ther.* **2012**, *14*, R82. [CrossRef] [PubMed]

94. Schmal, H.; Pilz, I.H.; Mehlhorn, A.T.; Dovi-Akue, D.; Kirchhoff, C.; Sudkamp, N.P.; Gerlach, U.; Niemeyer, P. Expression of BMP-receptor type 1A correlates with progress of osteoarthritis in human knee joints with focal cartilage lesions. *Cytotherapy* **2012**, *14*, 868–876. [CrossRef] [PubMed]

95. Bobacz, K.; Gruber, R.; Soleiman, A.; Erlacher, L.; Smolen, J.S.; Graninger, W.B. Expression of bone morphogenetic protein 6 in healthy and osteoarthritic human articular chondrocytes and stimulation of matrix synthesis in vitro. *Arthritis Rheumtol.* **2003**, *48*, 2501–2508. [CrossRef] [PubMed]

96. Chen, A.L.; Fang, C.; Liu, C.; Leslie, M.P.; Chang, E.; Di Cesare, P.E. Expression of bone morphogenetic proteins, receptors, and tissue inhibitors in human fetal, adult, and osteoarthritic articular cartilage. *J. Orthop. Res.* **2004**, *22*, 1188–1192. [CrossRef] [PubMed]

97. Bobinac, D.; Spanjol, J.; Marinovic, M.; Zoricic Cvek, S.; Maric, I.; Cicvaric, T.; Fuckar, D.; Markic, D.; Vojnikovic, B. Expression of bone morphogenetic proteins, cartilage-derived morphogenetic proteins and related receptors in normal and osteoarthritic human articular cartilage. *Coll. Antropol.* **2008**, *32* (Suppl. 2), 83–87.

98. Lafont, J.E.; Poujade, F.A.; Pasdeloup, M.; Neyret, P.; Mallein-Gerin, F. Hypoxia potentiates the bmp-2 driven COL2A1 stimulation in human articular chondrocytes via p38 MAPK. *Osteoarthr. Cartil.* **2016**, *24*, 856–867. [CrossRef] [PubMed]

99. Smith, R.L.; Lindsey, D.P.; Dhulipala, L.; Harris, A.H.; Goodman, S.B.; Maloney, W.J. Effects of intermittent hydrostatic pressure and BMP-2 on osteoarthritic human chondrocyte metabolism in vitro. *J. Orthop. Res.* **2011**, *29*, 361–368. [CrossRef] [PubMed]

100. Chubinskaya, S.; Segalite, D.; Pikovsky, D.; Hakimiyan, A.A.; Rueger, D.C. Effects induced by BMPs in cultures of human articular chondrocytes: Comparative studies. *Growth Factors* **2008**, *26*, 275–283. [CrossRef] [PubMed]

101. Murphy, M.K.; Huey, D.J.; Hu, J.C.; Athanasiou, K.A. TGF-beta1, GDF-5, and BMP-2 stimulation induces chondrogenesis in expanded human articular chondrocytes and marrow-derived stromal cells. *Stem Cells* **2015**, *33*, 762–773. [CrossRef] [PubMed]

102. Fan, Z.; Chubinskaya, S.; Rueger, D.C.; Bau, B.; Haag, J.; Aigner, T. Regulation of anabolic and catabolic gene expression in normal and osteoarthritic adult human articular chondrocytes by osteogenic protein-1. *Clin. Exp. Rheumatol.* **2004**, *22*, 103–106. [PubMed]

103. Varas, A.; Valencia, J.; Lavocat, F.; Martinez, V.G.; Thiam, N.N.; Hidalgo, L.; FeRNAndez-Sevilla, L.M.; Sacedon, R.; Vicente, A.; Miossec, P. Blockade of bone morphogenetic protein signaling potentiates the pro-inflammatory phenotype induced by interleukin-17 and tumor necrosis factor-alpha combination in rheumatoid synoviocytes. *Arthritis Res. Ther.* **2015**, *17*, 192. [CrossRef] [PubMed]

104. Mahjoub, M.; Sassi, N.; Driss, M.; Laadhar, L.; Allouche, M.; Hamdoun, M.; Romdhane, K.B.; Sellami, S.; Makni, S. Expression patterns of notch receptors and their ligands in human osteoarthritic and healthy articular cartilage. *Tissue Cell* **2012**, *44*, 182–194. [CrossRef] [PubMed]

105. Karlsson, C.; Brantsing, C.; Egell, S.; Lindahl, A. Notch1, Jagged1, and HES5 are abundantly expressed in osteoarthritis. *Cells Tissues Organs* **2008**, *188*, 287–298. [CrossRef] [PubMed]

106. Grogan, S.P.; Miyaki, S.; Asahara, H.; D'Lima, D.D.; Lotz, M.K. Mesenchymal progenitor cell markers in human articular cartilage: Normal distribution and changes in osteoarthritis. *Arthritis Res. Ther.* **2009**, *11*, R85. [CrossRef] [PubMed]

107. Lin, N.Y.; Distler, A.; Beyer, C.; Philipi-Schobinger, A.; Breda, S.; Dees, C.; Stock, M.; Tomcik, M.; Niemeier, A.; Dell'Accio, F.; et al. Inhibition of notch1 promotes hedgehog signalling in a HES1-dependent manner in chondrocytes and exacerbates experimental osteoarthritis. *Ann. Rheum. Dis.* **2016**, *75*, 2037–2044. [CrossRef] [PubMed]

108. Schneiderman, R.; Rosenberg, N.; Hiss, J.; Lee, P.; Liu, F.; Hintz, R.L.; Maroudas, A. Concentration and size distribution of insulin-like growth factor-I in human normal and osteoarthritic synovial fluid and cartilage. *Arch. Biochem. Biophys.* **1995**, *324*, 173–188. [CrossRef] [PubMed]

109. Tavera, C.; Abribat, T.; Reboul, P.; Dore, S.; Brazeau, P.; Pelletier, J.P.; Martel-Pelletier, J. IGF and IGF-binding protein system in the synovial fluid of osteoarthritic and rheumatoid arthritic patients. *Osteoarthr. Cartil.* **1996**, *4*, 263–274. [CrossRef]

110. Starkman, B.G.; Cravero, J.D.; Delcarlo, M.; Loeser, R.F. IGF-I stimulation of proteoglycan synthesis by chondrocytes requires activation of the PI 3-kinase pathway but not ERK MAPK. *Biochem. J.* **2005**, *389*, 723–729. [CrossRef] [PubMed]

111. Weimer, A.; Madry, H.; Venkatesan, J.K.; Schmitt, G.; Frisch, J.; Wezel, A.; Jung, J.; Kohn, D.; Terwilliger, E.F.; Trippel, S.B.; et al. Benefits of recombinant adeno-associated virus (rAAV)-mediated insulinlike growth factor I (IGF-I) overexpression for the long-term reconstruction of human osteoarthritic cartilage by modulation of the IGF-I axis. *Mol. Med.* **2012**, *18*, 346–358. [CrossRef] [PubMed]

112. Loeser, R.F.; Chubinskaya, S.; Pacione, C.; Im, H.J. Basic fibroblast growth factor inhibits the anabolic activity of insulin-like growth factor 1 and osteogenic protein 1 in adult human articular chondrocytes. *Arthritis Rheumtol.* **2005**, *52*, 3910–3917. [CrossRef] [PubMed]

113. Murata, M.; Yudoh, K.; Masuko, K. The potential role of vascular endothelial growth factor (VEGF) in cartilage: How the angiogenic factor could be involved in the pathogenesis of osteoarthritis? *Osteoarthr. Cartil.* **2008**, *16*, 279–286. [CrossRef] [PubMed]

114. Fay, J.; Varoga, D.; Wruck, C.J.; Kurz, B.; Goldring, M.B.; Pufe, T. Reactive oxygen species induce expression of vascular endothelial growth factor in chondrocytes and human articular cartilage explants. *Arthritis Res. Ther.* **2006**, *8*, R189. [CrossRef] [PubMed]

115. Enomoto, H.; Inoki, I.; Komiya, K.; Shiomi, T.; Ikeda, E.; Obata, K.; Matsumoto, H.; Toyama, Y.; Okada, Y. Vascular endothelial growth factor isoforms and their receptors are expressed in human osteoarthritic cartilage. *Am. J. Pathol.* **2003**, *162*, 171–181. [CrossRef]

116. Pufe, T.; Petersen, W.; Tillmann, B.; Mentlein, R. The splice variants VEGF121 and VEGF189 of the angiogenic peptide vascular endothelial growth factor are expressed in osteoarthritic cartilage. *Arthritis Rheumtol.* **2001**, *44*, 1082–1088. [CrossRef]

117. Pfander, D.; Kortje, D.; Zimmermann, R.; Weseloh, G.; Kirsch, T.; Gesslein, M.; Cramer, T.; Swoboda, B. Vascular endothelial growth factor in articular cartilage of healthy and osteoarthritic human knee joints. *Ann. Rheum. Dis.* **2001**, *60*, 1070–1073. [CrossRef] [PubMed]

118. Su, W.; Xie, W.; Shang, Q.; Su, B. The long noncoding RNA MEG3 is downregulated and inversely associated with VEGF levels in osteoarthritis. *Biomed. Res. Int.* **2015**, *2015*, 356893. [CrossRef] [PubMed]

119. Pulsatelli, L.; Dolzani, P.; Silvestri, T.; Frizziero, L.; Facchini, A.; Meliconi, R. Vascular endothelial growth factor activities on osteoarthritic chondrocytes. *Clin. Exp. Rheumatol.* **2005**, *23*, 487–493. [PubMed]

120. Shakibaei, M.; Schulze-Tanzil, G.; Mobasheri, A.; Beichler, T.; Dressler, J.; Schwab, W. Expression of the VEGF receptor-3 in osteoarthritic chondrocytes: Stimulation by interleukin-1 beta and association with beta 1-integrins. *Histochem. Cell Biol.* **2003**, *120*, 235–241. [CrossRef] [PubMed]

121. Takahashi, H.; Shibuya, M. The vascular endothelial growth factor (VEGF)/VEGF receptor system and its role under physiological and pathological conditions. *Clin. Sci. (Lond.)* **2005**, *109*, 227–241. [CrossRef] [PubMed]

122. Loeser, R.F.; Collins, J.A.; Diekman, B.O. Ageing and the pathogenesis of osteoarthritis. *Nat. Rev. Rheumatol.* **2016**, *12*, 412–420. [CrossRef] [PubMed]

123. Berenbaum, F. Osteoarthritis as an inflammatory disease (osteoarthritis is not osteoarthrosis!). *Osteoarthr. Cartil.* **2013**, *21*, 16–21. [CrossRef] [PubMed]

124. Sokolove, J.; Lepus, C.M. Role of inflammation in the pathogenesis of osteoarthritis: Latest findings and interpretations. *Ther. Adv. Musculoskelet. Dis.* **2013**, *5*, 77–94. [CrossRef] [PubMed]

125. Sandy, J.D.; Chan, D.D.; Trevino, R.L.; Wimmer, M.A.; Plaas, A. Human genome-wide expression analysis reorients the study of inflammatory mediators and biomechanics in osteoarthritis. *Osteoarthr. Cartil.* **2015**, *23*, 1939–1945. [CrossRef] [PubMed]

126. Kahle, P.; Saal, J.G.; Schaudt, K.; Zacher, J.; Fritz, P.; Pawelec, G. Determination of cytokines in synovial fluids: Correlation with diagnosis and histomorphological characteristics of synovial tissue. *Ann. Rheum. Dis.* **1992**, *51*, 731–734. [CrossRef] [PubMed]

127. Martel-Pelletier, J.; McCollum, R.; DiBattista, J.; Faure, M.P.; Chin, J.A.; Fournier, S.; Sarfati, M.; Pelletier, J.P. The interleukin-1 receptor in normal and osteoarthritic human articular chondrocytes. Identification as the type I receptor and analysis of binding kinetics and biologic function. *Arthritis Rheumtol.* **1992**, *35*, 530–540. [CrossRef]

128. Yang, P.; Tan, J.; Yuan, Z.; Meng, G.; Bi, L.; Liu, J. Expression profile of cytokines and chemokines in osteoarthritis patients: Proinflammatory roles for CXCL8 and CXCL11 to chondrocytes. *Int. Immunopharmacol.* **2016**, *40*, 16–23. [CrossRef] [PubMed]

129. Middleton, J.; Manthey, A.; Tyler, J. Insulin-like growth factor (IGF) receptor, IGF-i, interleukin-1 beta (IL-1 beta), and IL-6 mRNA expression in osteoarthritic and normal human cartilage. *J. Histochem. Cytochem.* **1996**, *44*, 133–141. [CrossRef] [PubMed]

130. Towle, C.A.; Hung, H.H.; Bonassar, L.J.; Treadwell, B.V.; Mangham, D.C. Detection of interleukin-1 in the cartilage of patients with osteoarthritis: A possible autocrine/paracrine role in pathogenesis. *Osteoarthr. Cartil.* **1997**, *5*, 293–300. [CrossRef]

131. Aigner, T.; McKenna, L.; Zien, A.; Fan, Z.; Gebhard, P.M.; Zimmer, R. Gene expression profiling of serum- and interleukin-1 beta-stimulated primary human adult articular chondrocytes—A molecular analysis based on chondrocytes isolated from one donor. *Cytokine* **2005**, *31*, 227–240. [CrossRef] [PubMed]

132. Honorati, M.C.; Bovara, M.; Cattini, L.; Piacentini, A.; Facchini, A. Contribution of interleukin 17 to human cartilage degradation and synovial inflammation in osteoarthritis. *Osteoarthr. Cartil.* **2002**, *10*, 799–807. [CrossRef] [PubMed]

133. Shalom-Barak, T.; Quach, J.; Lotz, M. Interleukin-17-induced gene expression in articular chondrocytes is associated with activation of mitogen-activated protein kinases and NF-kappaB. *J. Biol. Chem.* **1998**, *273*, 27467–27473. [CrossRef] [PubMed]

134. Haseeb, A.; Ansari, M.Y.; Haqqi, T.M. Harpagoside suppresses IL-6 expression in primary human osteoarthritis chondrocytes. *J. Orthop. Res.* **2017**, *35*, 311–320. [CrossRef] [PubMed]

135. Goldring, M.B.; Otero, M.; Plumb, D.A.; Dragomir, C.; Favero, M.; El Hachem, K.; Hashimoto, K.; Roach, H.I.; Olivotto, E.; Borzi, R.M.; et al. Roles of inflammatory and anabolic cytokines in cartilage metabolism: Signals and multiple effectors converge upon MMP-13 regulation in osteoarthritis. *Eur. Cells Mater.* **2011**, *21*, 202–220. [CrossRef]

136. Otero, M.; Plumb, D.A.; Tsuchimochi, K.; Dragomir, C.L.; Hashimoto, K.; Peng, H.; Olivotto, E.; Bevilacqua, M.; Tan, L.; Yang, Z.; et al. E74-like factor 3 (ELF3) impacts on matrix metalloproteinase 13 (mmp13) transcriptional control in articular chondrocytes under proinflammatory stress. *J. Biol. Chem.* **2012**, *287*, 3559–3572. [CrossRef] [PubMed]

137. Liacini, A.; Sylvester, J.; Li, W.Q.; Zafarullah, M. Inhibition of interleukin-1-stimulated MAP kinases, activating protein-1 (AP-1) and nuclear factor kappa b (NF-kappa b) transcription factors down-regulates matrix metalloproteinase gene expression in articular chondrocytes. *Matrix Biol.* **2002**, *21*, 251–262. [CrossRef]

138. Liacini, A.; Sylvester, J.; Li, W.Q.; Huang, W.; Dehnade, F.; Ahmad, M.; Zafarullah, M. Induction of matrix metalloproteinase-13 gene expression by TNF-alpha is mediated by map kinases, AP-1, and NF-kappab transcription factors in articular chondrocytes. *Exp. Cell Res.* **2003**, *288*, 208–217. [CrossRef]

139. Benderdour, M.; Tardif, G.; Pelletier, J.P.; Di Battista, J.A.; Reboul, P.; Ranger, P.; Martel-Pelletier, J. Interleukin 17 (IL-17) induces collagenase-3 production in human osteoarthritic chondrocytes via AP-1 dependent activation: Differential activation of AP-1 members by IL-17 and IL-1beta. *J. Rheumatol.* **2002**, *29*, 1262–1272. [PubMed]

140. Wang, J.; Elewaut, D.; Veys, E.M.; Verbruggen, G. Insulin-like growth factor 1-induced interleukin-1 receptor ii overrides the activity of interleukin-1 and controls the homeostasis of the extracellular matrix of cartilage. *Arthritis Rheumtol.* **2003**, *48*, 1281–1291. [CrossRef] [PubMed]

141. Chien, S.Y.; Huang, C.Y.; Tsai, C.H.; Wang, S.W.; Lin, Y.M.; Tang, C.H. Interleukin-1beta induces fibroblast growth factor 2 expression and subsequently promotes endothelial progenitor cell angiogenesis in chondrocytes. *Clin. Sci. (Lond.)* **2016**, *130*, 667–681. [CrossRef] [PubMed]

142. De Andres, M.C.; Takahashi, A.; Oreffo, R.O. Demethylation of an NF-kappaB enhancer element orchestrates inos induction in osteoarthritis and is associated with altered chondrocyte cell cycle. *Osteoarthr. Cartil.* **2016**, *24*, 1951–1960. [CrossRef] [PubMed]

143. Jikko, A.; Wakisaka, T.; Iwamoto, M.; Hiranuma, H.; Kato, Y.; Maeda, T.; Fujishita, M.; Fuchihata, H. Effects of interleukin-6 on proliferation and proteoglycan metabolism in articular chondrocyte cultures. *Cell Biol. Int.* **1998**, *22*, 615–621. [CrossRef] [PubMed]

144. Quintavalla, J.; Kumar, C.; Daouti, S.; Slosberg, E.; Uziel-Fusi, S. Chondrocyte cluster formation in agarose cultures as a functional assay to identify genes expressed in osteoarthritis. *J. Cell. Physiol.* **2005**, *204*, 560–566. [CrossRef] [PubMed]

145. Makki, M.S.; Haseeb, A.; Haqqi, T.M. MicroRNA-9 promotion of interleukin-6 expression by inhibiting monocyte chemoattractant protein-induced protein 1 expression in interleukin-1beta-stimulated human chondrocytes. *Arthritis Rheumatol.* **2015**, *67*, 2117–2128. [CrossRef] [PubMed]

146. Kopanska, M.; Szala, D.; Czech, J.; Gablo, N.; Gargasz, K.; Trzeciak, M.; Zawlik, I.; Snela, S. MiRNA expression in the cartilage of patients with osteoarthritis. *J. Orthop. Surg. Res.* **2017**, *12*, 51. [CrossRef] [PubMed]

147. Jones, S.W.; Watkins, G.; Le Good, N.; Roberts, S.; Murphy, C.L.; Brockbank, S.M.; Needham, M.R.; Read, S.J.; Newham, P. The identification of differentially expressed microRNA in osteoarthritic tissue that modulate the production of TNF-alpha and MMP13. *Osteoarthr. Cartil.* **2009**, *17*, 464–472. [CrossRef] [PubMed]

148. Gu, R.; Liu, N.; Luo, S.; Huang, W.; Zha, Z.; Yang, J. MicroRNA-9 regulates the development of knee osteoarthritis through the NF-kappaB1 pathway in chondrocytes. *Medicine (Baltimore)* **2016**, *95*, e4315. [CrossRef] [PubMed]

149. Yu, F.; Chen, B.; Fan, X.; Li, G.; Dong, P.; Zheng, J. Epigenetically-regulated microRNA-9-5p suppresses the activation of hepatic stellate cells via TGFBR1 and TGFBR2. *Cell. Physiol. Biochem.* **2017**, *43*, 2242–2252. [CrossRef] [PubMed]

150. Borgonio Cuadra, V.M.; Gonzalez-Huerta, N.C.; Romero-Cordoba, S.; Hidalgo-Miranda, A.; Miranda-Duarte, A. Altered expression of circulating microRNA in plasma of patients with primary osteoarthritis and in silico analysis of their pathways. *PLoS ONE* **2014**, *9*, e97690. [CrossRef] [PubMed]

151. Iliopoulos, D.; Malizos, K.N.; Oikonomou, P.; Tsezou, A. Integrative microRNA and proteomic approaches identify novel osteoarthritis genes and their collaborative metabolic and inflammatory networks. *PLoS ONE* **2008**, *3*, e3740. [CrossRef] [PubMed]

152. Li, L.; Jia, J.; Liu, X.; Yang, S.; Ye, S.; Yang, W.; Zhang, Y. MicroRNA-16-5p controls development of osteoarthritis by targeting SMAD3 in chondrocytes. *Curr. Pharm. Des.* **2015**, *21*, 5160–5167. [CrossRef] [PubMed]

153. He, Q.; Ren, X.; Chen, J.; Li, Y.; Tang, X.; Wen, X.; Yang, X.; Zhang, J.; Wang, Y.; Ma, J.; et al. miR-16 targets fibroblast growth factor 2 to inhibit NPC cell proliferation and invasion via PI3K/AKT and MAPK signaling pathways. *Oncotarget* **2016**, *7*, 3047–3058. [CrossRef] [PubMed]

154. Zhang, Y.; Jia, J.; Yang, S.; Liu, X.; Ye, S.; Tian, H. MicroRNA-21 controls the development of osteoarthritis by targeting GDF-5 in chondrocytes. *Exp. Mol. Med.* **2014**, *46*, e79. [CrossRef] [PubMed]

155. Hu, J.; Ni, S.; Cao, Y.; Zhang, T.; Wu, T.; Yin, X.; Lang, Y.; Lu, H. The angiogenic effect of microRNA-21 targeting TIMP3 through the regulation of MMP2 and MMP9. *PLoS ONE* **2016**, *11*, e0149537. [CrossRef] [PubMed]

156. Iliopoulos, D.; Hirsch, H.A.; Struhl, K. An epigenetic switch involving NF-kappaB, Lin28, Let-7 microRNA, and IL6 links inflammation to cell transformation. *Cell* **2009**, *139*, 693–706. [CrossRef] [PubMed]

157. Harries, L.W. MicroRNAs as mediators of the ageing process. *Genes (Basel)* **2014**, *5*, 656–670. [CrossRef] [PubMed]

158. Kang, L.; Yang, C.; Song, Y.; Liu, W.; Wang, K.; Li, S.; Zhang, Y. MicroRNA-23a-3p promotes the development of osteoarthritis by directly targeting smad3 in chondrocytes. *Biochem. Biophys. Res. Commun.* **2016**, *478*, 467–473. [CrossRef] [PubMed]

159. Li, Y.H.; Tavallaee, G.; Tokar, T.; Nakamura, A.; Sundararajan, K.; Weston, A.; Sharma, A.; Mahomed, N.N.; Gandhi, R.; Jurisica, I.; et al. Identification of synovial fluid microRNA signature in knee osteoarthritis: Differentiating early- and late-stage knee osteoarthritis. *Osteoarthr. Cartil.* **2016**, *24*, 1577–1586. [CrossRef] [PubMed]

160. Hu, J.; Wang, Z.; Pan, Y.; Ma, J.; Miao, X.; Qi, X.; Zhou, H.; Jia, L. miR-26a and mir-26b mediate osteoarthritis progression by targeting FUT4 via NF-kappaB signaling pathway. *Int. J. Biochem. Cell Biol.* **2018**, *94*, 79–88. [CrossRef] [PubMed]

161. Yin, X.; Wang, J.Q.; Yan, S.Y. Reduced miR26a and miR26b expression contributes to the pathogenesis of osteoarthritis via the promotion of p65 translocation. *Mol. Med. Rep.* **2017**, *15*, 551–558. [CrossRef] [PubMed]

162. Xie, Q.; Wei, M.; Kang, X.; Liu, D.; Quan, Y.; Pan, X.; Liu, X.; Liao, D.; Liu, J.; Zhang, B. Reciprocal inhibition between miR-26a and NF-kappaB regulates obesity-related chronic inflammation in chondrocytes. *Biosci. Rep.* **2015**, *35*, e00204. [CrossRef] [PubMed]

163. Chen, C.Y.; Chang, J.T.; Ho, Y.F.; Shyu, A.B. miR-26 down-regulates TNF-alpha/NF-kappaB signalling and IL-6 expression by silencing HMGA1 and MALT1. *Nucleic Acids Res.* **2016**, *44*, 3772–3787. [CrossRef] [PubMed]

164. Zhao, N.; Wang, R.; Zhou, L.; Zhu, Y.; Gong, J.; Zhuang, S.M. MicroRNA-26b suppresses the nf-kappab signaling and enhances the chemosensitivity of hepatocellular carcinoma cells by targeting TAK1 and TAB3. *Mol. Cancer* **2014**, *13*, 35. [CrossRef] [PubMed]

165. Leeper, N.J.; Raiesdana, A.; Kojima, Y.; Chun, H.J.; Azuma, J.; Maegdefessel, L.; Kundu, R.K.; Quertermous, T.; Tsao, P.S.; Spin, J.M. MicroRNA-26a is a novel regulator of vascular smooth muscle cell function. *J. Cell. Physiol.* **2011**, *226*, 1035–1043. [CrossRef] [PubMed]

166. Wei, C.; Kim, I.K.; Kumar, S.; Jayasinghe, S.; Hong, N.; Castoldi, G.; Catalucci, D.; Jones, W.K.; Gupta, S. NF-kappaB mediated mir-26a regulation in cardiac fibrosis. *J. Cell. Physiol.* **2013**, *228*, 1433–1442. [CrossRef] [PubMed]

167. Li, Y.F.; Li, S.H.; Liu, Y.; Luo, Y.T. Long noncoding RNA CIR promotes chondrocyte extracellular matrix degradation in osteoarthritis by acting as a sponge for mir-27b. *Cell. Physiol. Biochem.* **2017**, *43*, 602–610. [CrossRef] [PubMed]

168. Cheleschi, S.; De Palma, A.; Pecorelli, A.; Pascarelli, N.A.; Valacchi, G.; Belmonte, G.; Carta, S.; Galeazzi, M.; Fioravanti, A. Hydrostatic pressure regulates microRNA expression levels in osteoarthritic chondrocyte cultures via the wnt/beta-catenin pathway. *Int. J. Mol. Sci.* **2017**, *18*, 133. [CrossRef] [PubMed]

169. Huang, C.Y.; Chang, A.C.; Chen, H.T.; Wang, S.W.; Lo, Y.S.; Tang, C.H. Adiponectin promotes VEGF-C-dependent lymphangiogenesis by inhibiting mir-27b through a caMKII/AMPK/p38 signaling pathway in human chondrosarcoma cells. *Clin. Sci. (Lond.)* **2016**, *130*, 1523–1533. [CrossRef] [PubMed]

170. Kriegel, A.J.; Liu, Y.; Fang, Y.; Ding, X.; Liang, M. The mir-29 family: Genomics, cell biology, and relevance to renal and cardiovascular injury. *Physiol. Genom.* **2012**, *44*, 237–244. [CrossRef] [PubMed]

171. Le, L.T.; Swingler, T.E.; Crowe, N.; Vincent, T.L.; Barter, M.J.; Donell, S.T.; Delany, A.M.; Dalmay, T.; Young, D.A.; Clark, I.M. The microRNA-29 family in cartilage homeostasis and osteoarthritis. *J. Mol. Med. (Berl.)* **2016**, *94*, 583–596. [CrossRef] [PubMed]

172. Ji, Q.; Xu, X.; Xu, Y.; Fan, Z.; Kang, L.; Li, L.; Liang, Y.; Guo, J.; Hong, T.; Li, Z.; et al. miR-105/Runx2 axis mediates FGF2-induced ADAMTS expression in osteoarthritis cartilage. *J. Mol. Med. (Berl.)* **2016**, *94*, 681–694. [CrossRef] [PubMed]

173. Santini, P.; Politi, L.; Vedova, P.D.; Scandurra, R.; Scotto d'Abusco, A. The inflammatory circuitry of mir-149 as a pathological mechanism in osteoarthritis. *Rheumatol. Int.* **2014**, *34*, 711–716. [CrossRef] [PubMed]

174. Wang, H.; Zhu, Y.; Zhao, M.; Wu, C.; Zhang, P.; Tang, L.; Zhang, H.; Chen, X.; Yang, Y.; Liu, G. miRNA-29c suppresses lung cancer cell adhesion to extracellular matrix and metastasis by targeting integrin beta1 and matrix metalloproteinase2 (MMP2). *PLoS ONE* **2013**, *8*, e70192.

175. Liu, Y.; Taylor, N.E.; Lu, L.; Usa, K.; Cowley, A.W., Jr.; Ferreri, N.R.; Yeo, N.C.; Liang, M. Renal medullary microRNAs in dahl salt-sensitive rats: Mir-29b regulates several collagens and related genes. *Hypertension* **2010**, *55*, 974–982. [CrossRef] [PubMed]

176. Moulin, D.; Salone, V.; Koufany, M.; Clement, T.; Behm-Ansmant, I.; Branlant, C.; Charpentier, B.; Jouzeau, J.Y. MicroRNA-29b contributes to collagens imbalance in human osteoarthritic and dedifferentiated articular chondrocytes. *BioMed Res. Int.* **2017**, *2017*, 9792512. [CrossRef] [PubMed]

177. Chang, T.; Xie, J.; Li, H.; Li, D.; Liu, P.; Hu, Y. MicroRNA-30a promotes extracellular matrix degradation in articular cartilage via downregulation of Sox9. *Cell Prolif.* **2016**, *49*, 207–218. [CrossRef] [PubMed]

178. Li, L.; Yang, C.; Liu, X.; Yang, S.; Ye, S.; Jia, J.; Liu, W.; Zhang, Y. Elevated expression of microRNA-30b in osteoarthritis and its role in erg regulation of chondrocyte. *Biomed. Pharmacother.* **2015**, *76*, 94–99. [CrossRef] [PubMed]

179. Ji, Q.; Xu, X.; Zhang, Q.; Kang, L.; Xu, Y.; Zhang, K.; Li, L.; Liang, Y.; Hong, T.; Ye, Q.; et al. The IL-1beta/AP-1/miR-30a/ADAMTS-5 axis regulates cartilage matrix degradation in human osteoarthritis. *J. Mol. Med. (Berl.)* **2016**, *94*, 771–785. [CrossRef] [PubMed]

180. Kostopoulou, F.; Malizos, K.N.; Papathanasiou, I.; Tsezou, A. MicroRNA-33a regulates cholesterol synthesis and cholesterol efflux-related genes in osteoarthritic chondrocytes. *Arthritis Res. Ther.* **2015**, *17*, 42. [CrossRef] [PubMed]

181. Yang, B.; Ni, J.; Long, H.; Huang, J.; Yang, C.; Huang, X. IL-1beta-induced miR-34a up-regulation inhibits cyr61 to modulate osteoarthritis chondrocyte proliferation through ADAMTS-4. *J. Cell. Biochem.* **2017**. [CrossRef]

182. Yan, S.; Wang, M.; Zhao, J.; Zhang, H.; Zhou, C.; Jin, L.; Zhang, Y.; Qiu, X.; Ma, B.; Fan, Q. MicroRNA-34a affects chondrocyte apoptosis and proliferation by targeting the sirt1/p53 signaling pathway during the pathogenesis of osteoarthritis. *Int. J. Mol. Med.* **2016**, *38*, 201–209. [CrossRef] [PubMed]

183. Christoffersen, N.R.; Shalgi, R.; Frankel, L.B.; Leucci, E.; Lees, M.; Klausen, M.; Pilpel, Y.; Nielsen, F.C.; Oren, M.; Lund, A.H. P53-independent upregulation of mir-34a during oncogene-induced senescence represses myc. *Cell Death Differ.* **2010**, *17*, 236–245. [CrossRef] [PubMed]

184. Fang, L.L.; Sun, B.F.; Huang, L.R.; Yuan, H.B.; Zhang, S.; Chen, J.; Yu, Z.J.; Luo, H. Potent inhibition of mir-34b on migration and invasion in metastatic prostate cancer cells by regulating the TGF-beta pathway. *Int. J. Mol. Sci.* **2017**, *18*, 2762. [CrossRef] [PubMed]

185. Liu, X.; Wang, H.; Zhu, Z.; Ye, Y.; Mao, H.; Zhang, S. MicroRNA-105 targets SOX9 and inhibits human glioma cell progression. *FEBS Lett.* **2016**, *590*, 4329–4342. [CrossRef] [PubMed]

186. Matsukawa, T.; Sakai, T.; Yonezawa, T.; Hiraiwa, H.; Hamada, T.; Nakashima, M.; Ono, Y.; Ishizuka, S.; Nakahara, H.; Lotz, M.K.; et al. MicroRNA-125b regulates the expression of aggrecanase-1 (ADAMTS-4) in human osteoarthritic chondrocytes. *Arthritis Res. Ther.* **2013**, *15*, R28. [CrossRef] [PubMed]

187. Balaskas, P.; Goljanek-Whysall, K.; Clegg, P.; Fang, Y.; Cremers, A.; Emans, P.; Welting, T.; Peffers, M. MicroRNA profiling in cartilage ageing. *Int. J. Genom.* **2017**, *2017*, 2713725. [CrossRef] [PubMed]

188. Li, P.; Wei, J.; Li, X.; Cheng, Y.; Chen, W.; Cui, Y.; Simoncini, T.; Gu, Z.; Yang, J.; Fu, X. 17beta-estradiol enhances vascular endothelial Ets-1/miR-126-3p expression: The possible mechanism for attenuation of atherosclerosis. *J. Clin. Endocrinol. Metab.* **2017**, *102*, 594–603. [PubMed]

189. Li, Y.; Li, Y.; Ge, P.; Ma, C. Mir-126 regulates the ERK pathway via targeting KRAS to inhibit the glioma cell proliferation and invasion. *Mol. Neurobiol.* **2017**, *54*, 137–145. [CrossRef] [PubMed]

190. Park, S.J.; Cheon, E.J.; Lee, M.H.; Kim, H.A. MicroRNA-127-5p regulates matrix metalloproteinase 13 expression and interleukin-1beta-induced catabolic effects in human chondrocytes. *Arthritis Rheumtol.* **2013**, *65*, 3141–3152. [CrossRef] [PubMed]

191. Tu, M.; Li, Y.; Zeng, C.; Deng, Z.; Gao, S.; Xiao, W.; Luo, W.; Jiang, W.; Li, L.; Lei, G. MicroRNA-127-5p regulates osteopontin expression and osteopontin-mediated proliferation of human chondrocytes. *Sci. Rep.* **2016**, *6*, 25032. [CrossRef] [PubMed]

192. Makki, M.S.; Haqqi, T.M. Mir-139 modulates mcpip1/IL-6 expression and induces apoptosis in human OA chondrocytes. *Exp. Mol. Med.* **2015**, *47*, e189. [CrossRef] [PubMed]

193. Miyaki, S.; Nakasa, T.; Otsuki, S.; Grogan, S.P.; Higashiyama, R.; Inoue, A.; Kato, Y.; Sato, T.; Lotz, M.K.; Asahara, H. MicroRNA-140 is expressed in differentiated human articular chondrocytes and modulates interleukin-1 responses. *Arthritis Rheumtol.* **2009**, *60*, 2723–2730. [CrossRef] [PubMed]

194. Si, H.; Zeng, Y.; Zhou, Z.; Pei, F.; Lu, Y.; Cheng, J.; Shen, B. Expression of miRNA-140 in chondrocytes and synovial fluid of knee joints in patients with osteoarthritis. *Chin. Med. Sci. J.* **2016**, *31*, 207–212. [CrossRef]

195. Liang, Z.J.; Zhuang, H.; Wang, G.X.; Li, Z.; Zhang, H.T.; Yu, T.Q.; Zhang, B.D. MiRNA-140 is a negative feedback regulator of MMP-13 in IL-1beta-stimulated human articular chondrocyte c28/i2 cells. *Inflamm. Res.* **2012**, *61*, 503–509. [CrossRef] [PubMed]

196. Yoshida, A.; Kitajima, S.; Li, F.; Cheng, C.; Takegami, Y.; Kohno, S.; Wan, Y.S.; Hayashi, N.; Muranaka, H.; Nishimoto, Y.; et al. MicroRNA-140 mediates RB tumor suppressor function to control stem cell-like activity through interleukin-6. *Oncotarget* **2017**, *8*, 13872–13885. [CrossRef] [PubMed]

197. Tardif, G.; Pelletier, J.P.; Fahmi, H.; Hum, D.; Zhang, Y.; Kapoor, M.; Martel-Pelletier, J. Nfat3 and TGF-beta/smad3 regulate the expression of mir-140 in osteoarthritis. *Arthritis Res. Ther.* **2013**, *15*, R197. [CrossRef] [PubMed]

198. Yang, B.; Kang, X.; Xing, Y.; Dou, C.; Kang, F.; Li, J.; Quan, Y.; Dong, S. Effect of microRNA-145 on il-1beta-induced cartilage degradation in human chondrocytes. *FEBS Lett.* **2014**, *588*, 2344–2352. [CrossRef] [PubMed]

199. Hu, G.; Zhao, X.; Wang, C.; Geng, Y.; Zhao, J.; Xu, J.; Zuo, B.; Zhao, C.; Wang, C.; Zhang, X. MicroRNA-145 attenuates TNF-alpha-driven cartilage matrix degradation in osteoarthritis via direct suppression of mkk4. *Cell Death Dis.* **2017**, *8*, e3140. [CrossRef] [PubMed]

200. Wang, G.D.; Zhao, X.W.; Zhang, Y.G.; Kong, Y.; Niu, S.S.; Ma, L.F.; Zhang, Y.M. Effects of mir-145 on the inhibition of chondrocyte proliferation and fibrosis by targeting tnfrsf11b in human osteoarthritis. *Mol. Med. Rep.* **2017**, *15*, 75–80. [CrossRef] [PubMed]

201. Martinez-Sanchez, A.; Dudek, K.A.; Murphy, C.L. Regulation of human chondrocyte function through direct inhibition of cartilage master regulator SOX9 by microRNA-145 (miRNA-145). *J. Biol. Chem.* **2012**, *287*, 916–924. [CrossRef] [PubMed]

202. Lorente-Cebrian, S.; Mejhert, N.; Kulyte, A.; Laurencikiene, J.; Astrom, G.; Heden, P.; Ryden, M.; Arner, P. MicroRNAs regulate human adipocyte lipolysis: Effects of mir-145 are linked to TNF-alpha. *PLoS ONE* **2014**, *9*, e86800. [CrossRef] [PubMed]

203. Doberstein, K.; Steinmeyer, N.; Hartmetz, A.K.; Eberhardt, W.; Mittelbronn, M.; Harter, P.N.; Juengel, E.; Blaheta, R.; Pfeilschifter, J.; Gutwein, P. MicroRNA-145 targets the metalloprotease ADAM17 and is suppressed in renal cell carcinoma patients. *Neoplasia* **2013**, *15*, 218–230. [CrossRef] [PubMed]

204. Budd, E.; de Andres, M.C.; Sanchez-Elsner, T.; Oreffo, R.O.C. Mir-146b is down-regulated during the chondrogenic differentiation of human bone marrow derived skeletal stem cells and up-regulated in osteoarthritis. *Sci. Rep.* **2017**, *7*, 46704. [CrossRef] [PubMed]

205. Soyocak, A.; Kurt, H.; Ozgen, M.; Turgut Cosan, D.; Colak, E.; Gunes, H.V. MiRNA-146a, miRNA-155 and jnk expression levels in peripheral blood mononuclear cells according to grade of knee osteoarthritis. *Gene* **2017**, *627*, 207–211. [CrossRef] [PubMed]

206. Jin, L.; Zhao, J.; Jing, W.; Yan, S.; Wang, X.; Xiao, C.; Ma, B. Role of miR-146a in human chondrocyte apoptosis in response to mechanical pressure injury in vitro. *Int. J. Mol. Med.* **2014**, *34*, 451–463. [CrossRef] [PubMed]

207. Li, X.; Gibson, G.; Kim, J.S.; Kroin, J.; Xu, S.; van Wijnen, A.J.; Im, H.J. MicroRNA-146a is linked to pain-related pathophysiology of osteoarthritis. *Gene* **2011**, *480*, 34–41. [CrossRef] [PubMed]

208. Taganov, K.D.; Boldin, M.P.; Chang, K.J.; Baltimore, D. NF-kappaB-dependent induction of microRNA miR-146, an inhibitor targeted to signaling proteins of innate immune responses. *Proc. Natl. Acad. Sci. USA* **2006**, *103*, 12481–12486. [CrossRef] [PubMed]

209. Zhu, H.Y.; Bai, W.D.; Liu, J.Q.; Zheng, Z.; Guan, H.; Zhou, Q.; Su, L.L.; Xie, S.T.; Wang, Y.C.; Li, J.; et al. Up-regulation of FGFBP1 signaling contributes to mir-146a-induced angiogenesis in human umbilical vein endothelial cells. *Sci. Rep.* **2016**, *6*, 25272. [CrossRef] [PubMed]

210. Diaz-Prado, S.; Cicione, C.; Muinos-Lopez, E.; Hermida-Gomez, T.; Oreiro, N.; FeRNAndez-Lopez, C.; Blanco, F.J. Characterization of microRNA expression profiles in normal and osteoarthritic human chondrocytes. *BMC Musculoskelet. Disord.* **2012**, *13*, 144. [CrossRef] [PubMed]

211. De Palma, A.; Cheleschi, S.; Pascarelli, N.A.; Giannotti, S.; Galeazzi, M.; Fioravanti, A. Hydrostatic pressure as epigenetic modulator in chondrocyte cultures: A study on miRNA-155, miRNA-181a and miRNA-223 expression levels. *J. Biomech.* **2018**, *66*, 165–169. [CrossRef] [PubMed]

212. Wu, X.F.; Zhou, Z.H.; Zou, J. MicroRNA-181 inhibits proliferation and promotes apoptosis of chondrocytes in osteoarthritis by targeting PTEN. *Biochem. Cell Biol.* **2017**, *95*, 437–444. [CrossRef] [PubMed]

213. Gabler, J.; Ruetze, M.; Kynast, K.L.; Grossner, T.; Diederichs, S.; Richter, W. Stage-specific mirs in chondrocyte maturation: Differentiation-dependent and hypertrophy-related miR clusters and the miR-181 family. *Tissue Eng. Part A* **2015**, *21*, 2840–2851. [CrossRef] [PubMed]

214. Zhai, X.; Meng, R.; Li, H.; Li, J.; Jing, L.; Qin, L.; Gao, Y. Mir-181a modulates chondrocyte apoptosis by targeting glycerol-3-phosphate dehydrogenase 1-like protein (GPD1L) in osteoarthritis. *Med. Sci. Monit.* **2017**, *23*, 1224–1231. [CrossRef] [PubMed]

215. Huang, X.; Schwind, S.; Santhanam, R.; Eisfeld, A.K.; Chiang, C.L.; Lankenau, M.; Yu, B.; Hoellerbauer, P.; Jin, Y.; Tarighat, S.S.; et al. Targeting the ras/mapk pathway with mir-181a in acute myeloid leukemia. *Oncotarget* **2016**, *7*, 59273–59286. [CrossRef] [PubMed]

216. Iliopoulos, D.; Jaeger, S.A.; Hirsch, H.A.; Bulyk, M.L.; Struhl, K. STAT3 activation of miR-21 and mir-181b-1 via PTEN and CYLD are part of the epigenetic switch linking inflammation to cancer. *Mol. Cell* **2010**, *39*, 493–506. [CrossRef] [PubMed]

217. Yao, Y.; Zhang, X.; Chen, H.P.; Li, L.; Xie, W.; Lan, G.; Zhao, Z.W.; Zheng, X.L.; Wang, Z.B.; Tang, C.K. MicroRNA-186 promotes macrophage lipid accumulation and secretion of pro-inflammatory cytokines by targeting cystathionine gamma-lyase in thp-1 macrophages. *Atherosclerosis* **2016**, *250*, 122–132. [CrossRef] [PubMed]

218. Wang, F.; Jiang, H.; Wang, S.; Chen, B. Dual functional microRNA-186-5p targets both FGF2 and RelA to suppress tumorigenesis of glioblastoma multiforme. *Cell. Mol. Neurobiol.* **2017**, *37*, 1433–1442. [CrossRef] [PubMed]

219. Li, Z.; Meng, D.; Li, G.; Xu, J.; Tian, K.; Li, Y. Overexpression of microRNA-210 promotes chondrocyte proliferation and extracellular matrix deposition by targeting hif-3alpha in osteoarthritis. *Mol. Med. Rep.* **2016**, *13*, 2769–2776. [CrossRef] [PubMed]

220. Phuah, N.H.; Azmi, M.N.; Awang, K.; Nagoor, N.H. Down-regulation of microRNA-210 confers sensitivity towards 1′s-1′-acetoxychavicol acetate (ACA) in cervical cancer cells by targeting SMAD4. *Mol. Cells* **2017**, *40*, 291–298. [CrossRef] [PubMed]

221. Bavelloni, A.; Ramazzotti, G.; Poli, A.; Piazzi, M.; Focaccia, E.; Blalock, W.; Faenza, I. MiRNA-210: A current overview. *Anticancer Res.* **2017**, *37*, 6511–6521. [PubMed]

222. Liu, S.C.; Chuang, S.M.; Hsu, C.J.; Tsai, C.H.; Wang, S.W.; Tang, C.H. CTGF increases vascular endothelial growth factor-dependent angiogenesis in human synovial fibroblasts by increasing miR-210 expression. *Cell Death Dis.* **2014**, *5*, e1485. [CrossRef] [PubMed]

223. Zheng, X.; Zhao, F.C.; Pang, Y.; Li, D.Y.; Yao, S.C.; Sun, S.S.; Guo, K.J. Downregulation of miR-221-3p contributes to IL-1beta-induced cartilage degradation by directly targeting the SDF1/CXCR4 signaling pathway. *J. Mol. Med. (Berl.)* **2017**, *95*, 615–627. [CrossRef] [PubMed]

224. Xu, J.; Liu, Y.; Deng, M.; Li, J.; Cai, H.; Meng, Q.; Fang, W.; Long, X.; Ke, J. MicroRNA221-3p modulates Ets-1 expression in synovial fibroblasts from patients with osteoarthritis of temporomandibular joint. *Osteoarthr. Cartil.* **2016**, *24*, 2003–2011. [CrossRef] [PubMed]

225. Chou, W.W.; Wang, Y.T.; Liao, Y.C.; Chuang, S.C.; Wang, S.N.; Juo, S.H. Decreased microRNA-221 is associated with high levels of TNF-alpha in human adipose tissue-derived mesenchymal stem cells from obese woman. *Cell. Physiol. Biochem.* **2013**, *32*, 127–137. [CrossRef] [PubMed]

226. Yang, X.; Guan, Y.; Tian, S.; Wang, Y.; Sun, K.; Chen, Q. Mechanical and il-1beta responsive mir-365 contributes to osteoarthritis development by targeting histone deacetylase 4. *Int. J. Mol. Sci.* **2016**, *17*, 436. [CrossRef] [PubMed]

227. Xu, Z.; Xiao, S.B.; Xu, P.; Xie, Q.; Cao, L.; Wang, D.; Luo, R.; Zhong, Y.; Chen, H.C.; Fang, L.R. miR-365, a novel negative regulator of interleukin-6 gene expression, is cooperatively regulated by Sp1 and NF-kappaB. *J. Biol. Chem.* **2011**, *286*, 21401–21412. [CrossRef] [PubMed]

228. Wang, G.; Zhang, Y.; Zhao, X.; Meng, C.; Ma, L.; Kong, Y. MicroRNA-411 inhibited matrix metalloproteinase 13 expression in human chondrocytes. *Am. J. Transl. Res.* **2015**, *7*, 2000–2006. [PubMed]

229. Wang, H.; Zhang, H.; Sun, Q.; Wang, Y.; Yang, J.; Yang, J.; Zhang, T.; Luo, S.; Wang, L.; Jiang, Y.; et al. Intra-articular delivery of antago-mir-483-5p inhibits osteoarthritis by modulating matrilin 3 and tissue inhibitor of metalloproteinase 2. *Mol. Ther.* **2017**, *25*, 715–727. [CrossRef] [PubMed]

230. Xu, R.; Li, J.; Wei, B.; Huo, W.; Wang, L. MicroRNA-483-5p modulates the expression of cartilage-related genes in human chondrocytes through down-regulating tgf-beta1 expression. *Tohoku J. Exp. Med.* **2017**, *243*, 41–48. [CrossRef] [PubMed]

231. Song, J.; Kim, D.; Lee, C.H.; Lee, M.S.; Chun, C.H.; Jin, E.J. MicroRNA-488 regulates zinc transporter SLC39A8/ZIP8 during pathogenesis of osteoarthritis. *J. Biomed. Sci.* **2013**, *20*, 31. [CrossRef] [PubMed]

232. Kim, J.H.; Jeon, J.; Shin, M.; Won, Y.; Lee, M.; Kwak, J.S.; Lee, G.; Rhee, J.; Ryu, J.H.; Chun, C.H.; et al. Regulation of the catabolic cascade in osteoarthritis by the zinc-ZIP8-MTF1 axis. *Cell* **2014**, *156*, 730–743. [CrossRef] [PubMed]

233. Rolauffs, B.; Rothdiener, M.; Bahrs, C.; Badke, A.; Weise, K.; Kuettner, K.E.; Kurz, B.; Aurich, M.; Grodzinsky, A.J.; Aicher, W.K. Onset of preclinical osteoarthritis: The angular spatial organization permits early diagnosis. *Arthritis Rheumtol.* **2011**, *63*, 1637–1647. [CrossRef] [PubMed]

234. Anderson, D.D.; Chubinskaya, S.; Guilak, F.; Martin, J.A.; Oegema, T.R.; Olson, S.A.; Buckwalter, J.A. Post-traumatic osteoarthritis: Improved understanding and opportunities for early intervention. *J. Orthop. Res.* **2011**, *29*, 802–809. [CrossRef] [PubMed]

235. Lieberthal, J.; Sambamurthy, N.; Scanzello, C.R. Inflammation in joint injury and post-traumatic osteoarthritis. *Osteoarthr. Cartil.* **2015**, *23*, 1825–1834. [CrossRef] [PubMed]

236. Rolauffs, B.; Kurz, B.; Felka, T.; Rothdiener, M.; Uynuk-Ool, T.; Aurich, M.; Frank, E.; Bahrs, C.; Badke, A.; Stockle, U.; et al. Stress-vs-time signals allow the prediction of structurally catastrophic events during fracturing of immature cartilage and predetermine the biomechanical, biochemical, and structural impairment. *J. Struct. Biol.* **2013**, *183*, 501–511. [CrossRef] [PubMed]

237. Rolauffs, B.; Muehleman, C.; Li, J.; Kurz, B.; Kuettner, K.E.; Frank, E.; Grodzinsky, A.J. Vulnerability of the superficial zone of immature articular cartilage to compressive injury. *Arthritis Rheumtol.* **2010**, *62*, 3016–3027. [CrossRef] [PubMed]

238. Behrendt, P.; Feldheim, M.; Preusse-Prange, A.; Weitkamp, J.T.; Haake, M.; Eglin, D.; Rolauffs, B.; Fay, J.; Seekamp, A.; Grodzinsky, A.J.; et al. Chondrogenic potential of IL-10 in mechanically injured cartilage and cellularized collagen aci grafts. *Osteoarthr. Cartil.* **2018**, *26*, 264–275. [CrossRef] [PubMed]

239. Behrendt, P.; Preusse-Prange, A.; Kluter, T.; Haake, M.; Rolauffs, B.; Grodzinsky, A.J.; Lipbross, S.; Kurz, B. IL-10 reduces apoptosis and extracellular matrix degradation after injurious compression of mature articular cartilage. *Osteoarthr. Cartil.* **2016**, *24*, 1981–1988. [CrossRef] [PubMed]

240. Imgenberg, J.; Rolauffs, B.; Grodzinsky, A.J.; Schunke, M.; Kurz, B. Estrogen reduces mechanical injury-related cell death and proteoglycan degradation in mature articular cartilage independent of the presence of the superficial zone tissue. *Osteoarthr. Cartil.* **2013**, *21*, 1738–1745. [CrossRef] [PubMed]

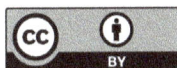

International Journal of
Molecular Sciences

MDPI

Review

Therapeutics in Osteoarthritis Based on an Understanding of Its Molecular Pathogenesis

Ju-Ryoung Kim [1,†], Jong Jin Yoo [2,†] and Hyun Ah Kim [1,*]

1   Rheumatology Division, Department of Internal Medicine, Hallym University Sacred Heart Hospital, 896, Pyongchondong, Dongan-gu, Anyang, Kyunggi-do 431-070, Korea; jurykim75@gmail.com
2   Department of Internal Medicine, Kangdong Sacred Heart Hospital, Seoul 05355, Korea; 99jjyoo@hanmail.net
*   Correspondence: kimha@hallym.ac.kr; Tel.: +82-31-380-1826; Fax: +82-31-381-8812
†   These authors contributed equally to work.

Received: 11 January 2018; Accepted: 21 February 2018; Published: 27 February 2018

Abstract: Osteoarthritis (OA) is the most prevalent joint disease in older people and is characterized by the progressive destruction of articular cartilage, synovial inflammation, changes in subchondral bone and peri-articular muscle, and pain. Because our understanding of the aetiopathogenesis of OA remains incomplete, we haven't discovered a cure for OA yet. This review appraises novel therapeutics based on recent progress in our understanding of the molecular pathogenesis of OA, including pro-inflammatory and pro-catabolic mediators and the relevant signalling mechanisms. The changes in subchondral bone and peri-articular muscle accompanying cartilage damage are also reviewed.

Keywords: osteoarthritis (OA); articular cartilage; molecular pathology; therapeutics

1. Introduction

Osteoarthritis (OA) is the most prevalent joint disease in older people and is characterized by the progressive destruction of articular cartilage, synovial inflammation, changes in subchondral bone and peri-articular muscle, and pain. The progression of OA is usually slow. Nevertheless, it ultimately leads to joint disability because of the poor repair capacity of cartilage [1,2]. Although various risk factors associated with OA are known, including genetic predisposition, aging, obesity, mechanical stress, and traumatic joint injury, the exact aetiology of OA remains largely unknown [3,4] and we have not discovered a cure for it. Therefore, it is important to appreciate the multi-factorial pathology of OA.

This review appraises novel therapeutics based on recent progress in our understanding of the molecular pathogenesis of OA.

2. Molecular Pathology of Cartilage Destruction

In healthy cartilage, chondrocytes respond to their microenvironment to maintain a delicate balance between synthesis and degradation of the extracellular matrix (ECM), the major components of which are type II collagen and aggrecan [5]. When the normal physiological mechanism that maintains the matrix equilibrium fails, ECM components are lost, expanded chondrocytes cluster in the depleted regions, an oxidative state is induced in the stressed cellular environment, and ultimately chondrocyte apoptosis occurs [6,7]. Failure of matrix equilibrium is due to the increased expression of matrix-degrading enzymes [8], inhibition of matrix synthesis [9], and excessive production of pro-inflammatory mediators, including cytokines, chemokines, and matrix degradation products [9]. Subchondral bone changes lead to osteophyte formation and sclerosis; loosening and weakness of the peri-articular muscles accompanies the articular cartilage destruction [10,11].

2.1. Pro-Inflammatory Cytokines

Osteoarthritis was once considered the prototypical non-inflammatory arthropathy distinct from rheumatoid arthritis (RA), a systemic autoimmune disease characterized by chronic inflammation. However, current research has demonstrated that inflammation is one of the key factors leading to the destruction of cartilage in OA. In the OA synovium, inflammatory cell infiltration is frequently observed, sometimes to a similar degree to that seen in RA. However, it is unclear whether this inflammation is the cause or consequence of cartilage destruction. Among inflammatory mediators, the role of cytokines has been studied the most, and many cytokines have been found in OA joints, in correlation with the severity of inflammation, and these play various roles in disrupting the balance of catabolic and anabolic activity in joint tissues [12]. IL-1β, IL-6, and TNF-α cytokines play the most important roles in pathogenesis and disease severity of OA [13], while IL-15, IL-17, IL-18, IL-21 [14], and chemokines and their receptors, such as MCP-1/CCL2, IL-8/CXCL8, and GRO-α/CXCL1, have also been implicated [15]. IL-1β is produced by several cell types in joints, including chondrocytes, immune cells infiltrating the synovium, osteoblasts, adipocytes, and synoviocytes; IL-1β expression is elevated in OA synovial fluid and membranes during the development of OA [16]. IL-1β strongly induces the expression and release of proteolytic enzymes, such as matrix metalloproteinases (MMPs) and aggrecanases, and suppresses the expression of ECM components, including type II collagen and aggrecan [17,18]. It also acts synergistically with other cytokines, IL-6 and chemokines including IL-8, MCP-1, and CCL5, to further increase inflammation [14]. Nevertheless, the elimination of IL-1β in a mouse model of traumatic joint injury aggravated OA, indicating a more complex role for this cytokine in maintaining cartilage metabolism [19]. TNF-α is also elevated in OA joint tissues and synovial fluid compared with healthy individuals [12]. Expression of the p55 TNF-α receptor has been localized in cells at sites of focal loss of cartilage proteoglycans in human OA [20]. TNF-α suppresses the synthesis of proteoglycan and type II collagen in chondrocytes [21] and stimulates pro-inflammatory and pro-catabolic mediators such as MMP-1, -3, and -13, IL-6, IL-8, and chemokines such as MCP-1 and CCL5 [22]. Furthermore, TNF-α promotes the production of nitric oxide (NO), a potent catabolic and pro-apoptotic mediator, in the synovial tissue, while blockade of the TNF-α receptor results in the inhibition of NO production in human cartilage tissue [23].

2.2. Pro-Catabolic Factors

Biomechanical stress, genetic factors, and inflammation contribute to the development of OA by interfering with metabolic responses in chondrocytes that maintain matrix integrity [24]. A series of pro-catabolic and anti-anabolic factors have been identified in the destruction of articular cartilage in OA. In the early phase, anabolic activity is increased, but this response fails to repair the cartilage due to both quantitative and qualitative insufficiency [25], as well as the intrinsic limitation of cartilage repair. During the development of OA, catabolic activity is triggered by pro-inflammatory cytokines, including IL-1β, IL-6, IL-17, and TNF-α. Elevated inducible nitric oxide synthase (iNOS) levels in OA chondrocytes result in an excess of NO, which suppresses proteoglycan and collagen synthesis in chondrocytes [26] and mediates the induction of matrix-degrading MMPs by accelerating the catabolic cascade induced by IL-1β or TNF-α. Chondrocyte-derived MMPs are the main enzymes involved in the breakdown of cartilage collagens and proteoglycans, while pro-inflammatory cytokines up-regulate the expression of MMPs via sequential activation of the catabolic cascade. MMP-13 effectively degrades type II collagen and MMP-13 knockout (KO) mice are protected from cartilage destruction in a surgical OA model [27], while constitutive expression of MMP-13 in transgenic mice induced spontaneous cartilage degradation [28]. MMP activity is partially inhibited by the tissue inhibitors of MMPs (TIMPs), whose synthesis is low compared with MMP production in OA cartilage. The importance of TIMPs in the development of cartilage degradation was demonstrated by elevated serum levels of type II collagen cleavage products in TIMP-3 KO mice [29]. Aggrecan is a large proteoglycan and a critical component of the ECM, along with type II collagen. It is degraded by aggrecanases, particularly ADAMTS-4 and ADAMTS-5, both of which are expressed in human OA cartilage. IL-1 and

TNF-α up-regulate ADAMTS-4, but not ADAMTS-5, in human synovial cells [30]. In contrast to humans, in mice, IL-1 elevates ADAMTS-5 expression [31] and ADAMTS-5 KO mice are resistant to cartilage erosion in a surgical OA model, suggesting that ADAMTS-5 is the predominant aggrecanase responsible for the development of OA in mice [32].

2.3. Transcription Factors

The role of signalling pathways, including the Notch, HIF-2 α, and NF-κB pathways, has been studied in the pathogenesis of OA. The increased expression and activation of Notch signalling components, such as Notch-1 and 2 receptors, Notch ligand, Jag1 and the downstream effector Hes1, have been identified in human OA and a mouse surgical OA model [33,34]. Although several downstream effectors mediate the effect of Notch signalling, including Hes1, 5, 7, Hey 1, 2, and HeyL, only Hes1 expression has been demonstrated in articular chondrocytes and its overexpression induced MMP 13 expression [34]. Furthermore, Hes1 KO mice were resistant to cartilage destruction and showed decreased MMP13 expression in a mouse surgical OA model [34], suggesting that Hes1 mediates the catabolic effect of Notch signalling. However, the role of the Notch signalling pathway in the homeostasis of articular cartilage and OA remains controversial, since transient Notch activation promotes ECM synthesis and helps to maintain articular cartilage under physiological conditions [35]. Articular cartilage is avascular and maintained in a low-oxygen environment with an oxygen gradient in cartilage that ranges from around 6% at the joint surface to 1% in the deep layers [36]. The hypoxia-inducible factor (HIF) protein family permits chondrocytes to adapt to hypoxic conditions. In mice, cartilage-specific HIF-1α deletion leads to articular chondrocyte death, whereas inhibition of HIF-1α degradation increases accumulation of the ECM [37,38]. Mice heterozygous for HIF-2α (or endothelial PAS domain-containing protein 1, EPAS-1) are resistant to developing OA [39]. HIF-2α induces numerous catabolic mediators, including MMPs (MMP1, MMP3, MMP9, MMP12 and MMP13), ADAMTS4, nitric oxide synthase-2 (NOS2), and prostaglandin-endoperoxide synthase-2 (PTGS2) [40]. Therefore, HIF-2 α is believed to be a central transactivator that causes cartilage destruction by regulating key catabolic genes. NF-κB is activated by inflammatory cytokines, elicits the secretion of many degradative enzymes, including MMPs and ADAMTSs, and suppresses ECM synthesis molecules such as Sox9, thereby down-regulating the ECM components type II collagen and aggrecan [30]. NF-κB also acts in a positive feedback loop to augment the catabolic process by stimulating NF-κB-mediated inflammatory cytokines, such as TNF-α, IL-1β, and IL-6, and the chemokine IL-8, and receptor activator of NF-κB (RANK) ligand (RANKL), leading to ECM breakdown and subsequent cartilage destruction [41]. In support of this, knockdown of NF-κB signalling by siRNA has been shown to inhibit cartilage degradation in a mouse model of OA [42]. Adenoviral gene delivery of the NF-κB inhibitor IκBa protects against cartilage loss by suppressing the expression of several MMPs and aggrecanases [43,44], which indicates that the NF-κB signalling plays a central role in degenerative cartilage disease. A recent study showed that the Zn^{2+} transporter ZIP8 was upregulated in OA cartilage of humans and mice, and the ZIP8-mediated Zn^{2+} influx upregulated the expression of matrix-degrading enzymes in chondrocytes [45]. Metal-regulatory transcription factor-1 (MTF1) was identified as an essential transcription factor in the mediation of Zn^{2+}/ZIP8-induced catabolic factor expression, and Ad-Mtf1 injection in mice caused osteophyte formation and subchondral bone sclerosis with more severe cartilage destruction, suggesting that the zinc-ZIP8-MTF1 axis is a major catabolic regulator of the pathogenesis of OA.

2.4. Inherent Changes in Chondrocytes: Senescence, Apoptosis, Autophagy

OA is a disease prevalent in advanced age, characterized by reduction of repair mechanism of cell damage. Cellular senescence is considered a signal transduction process that results in cells entering a stable state of growth arrest, and ultimately results in the loss of cellular replication [46]. Senescent cells are identified by a constellation of characteristics, such as absence of proliferation markers, increase in cell volume, an activated DNA damage response and expression of senescence-associated β-galactosidase (SA-Bgal) [47]. In addition to reduction of tissue regenerative potential, senescent cells chronically secrete proteases and pro-inflammatory mediators, (senescence-associated secretory phenotype (SASP)), which may perturb tissue structure and create a tissue microenvironment promoting proliferation of neoplastic cells [48]. Aged chondrocytes display a number of characteristics detrimental to cartilage integrity: they are more susceptible to cell death induced by an NO donor and less responsive to growth factors, such as insulin-like growth factor(IGF)-1 and osteogenic protein-1 [49]. When compared to cells isolated from young donors, chondrocytes from older adults secrete more MMP-13, IL-1 and IL-7, which are characteristics of SASP [50,51]. Application of cell senescence regulation in the treatment of OA is at its early phase. A recent study using p16-3MR transgenic mouse, which allows selective removal of senescent cells, showed that selective elimination of these cells attenuated the development of cartilage destruction after anterior cruciate ligament transection (ACLT), reduced pain and increased cartilage development [52]. Intra-articular injection of a senolytic molecule that selectively kills senescent chondrocytes led to attenuation of articular cartilage degeneration and amelioration of pain in ACLT-induced OA in C57BL mice as well, suggesting that regulation of senescence may serve as a therapeutic target for OA.

Apoptosis is a highly regulated process of cell death involving specific sets of intracellular signalling pathway. During the late phase of OA, cartilage becomes hypocellular with numerous empty lacunae, and the rate of apoptotic chondrocytes has been reported as high as 20% [53]. While it is intuitive that the death of chondrocytes, the only cell residing in cartilage, would result in the failure to appropriately maintain the structure of articular cartilage, a high rate of apoptosis in cartilage would result in matrix degradation within a short period of time, which is not compatible with the chronic course of OA [54]. Chondrocyte apoptosis may lead to reduction of ECM, and decrease of ECM may in turn result in further chondrocyte apoptosis because of the loss of matrix–cell interaction and anchorage dependence, eventually causing a viscous cycle [55]. Attempts at employing apoptosis modulators for treatment of OA has been hampered by potential harmful effects such as cancer, and inhibitors of apoptosis have been tested mostly in pre-clinical studies. For example, caspase inhibitor, the key regulator of apoptosis, was used in canine and rabbit model of OA, and found to suppress chondrocyte apoptosis as well as cartilage degradation [56–58]. Recently, autophagy, an adaptive response to protect cells from stresses, has been gaining interest as a regulatory mechanism of chondrocyte apoptosis [59]. Autophagy is induced by a variety of stimuli, including metabolic stress and hypoxia, and regulates catabolic processes of energy recycling in eukaryotic cells [60]. Autophagy has been shown to have a complex cross-talk with apoptosis and is induced by common upstream signals. Previous reports have shown that autophagy is decreased in OA cartilage and in an animal OA model, and autophagy activation protected chondrocytes from death, suggesting that autophagy is protective in cartilage degradation [61]. Chondrocyte autophagy is activated by hypoxia inducible factor-1 (HIF-1)-dependent AMP activated protein kinase (AMPK) and mammalian target of rapamycin (mTOR), while HIF-2α inhibits HIF-1α-induced autophagy [62] [63]. Resveratrol (3,4′,5-trihydroxystilbene) is an active food ingredient from grapes and peanuts, which was found to extend life span in nematodes, and ameliorate the fitness of human cells undergoing metabolic stress. Resveratrol was found to prevent cartilage destruction in a mouse model of OA by activating Sirtuin 1 and suppressing the expression of HIF-2α and catabolic mediators such as MMP 13 and ADAMTS5 [64]. Interestingly, a recent study showed that intra-articular injection of resveratrol led to an increase in autophagy markers such as Unc-51-like kinase1, Beclin1, and microtubule-associated protein light chain 3, and delayed articular cartilage degradation in DMM-induced OA. These results indicate that autophagy regulators such as resveratrol may be therapeutic targets for OA.

3. Molecular Pathology of Bone and Peri-Articular Muscle

Bone remodelling is thought to play an important role in the pathophysiology of OA and numerous studies have revealed that changes in cartilage and bone are tightly coupled to the progression of OA. The subchondral bone underneath the articular cartilage is organized into the subchondral cortical plate and a layer of cancellous bone [65]. In the early stage of OA, subchondral bone remodelling increases. Cellular signalling for microdamage repair, stimulation of vascular invasion by angiogenic factors, and the disruption of cartilage crosstalk via pathological microcracks are responsible for this increased subchondral bone remodelling [66]. In the late stage of OA, bone remodelling decreases and subchondral bone sclerosis increases, along with thickening of the cortical plate. Despite this thickening, the stiffness of the subchondral bone decreases due to decreased mineralization [67]. In addition, new bone formation characterized by osteophytes [68] and increased osteoblastic activity, dominate the late phase of OA [69], and subchondral bone cysts and bone marrow lesions are present [70].

In addition to cartilage, subchondral bone is also exposed to catabolic factors, such as MMPs and ADAMTSs, chemokines, and inflammatory cytokines secreted by hypertrophic chondrocytes, and these factors have been implicated in the altered biochemical and functional abilities of osteoblasts [71]. For instance, osteoblasts switch from the normal phenotype to a sclerotic phenotype on exposure to IL-6 in combination with other cytokines, such as IL-1β [71]. The penetration of vessels into articular cartilage exposes chondrocytes to cytokines and growth factors from subchondral bone, such as vascular endothelial growth factor (VEGF), nerve growth factor (NGF), IL-1, IL-6, hepatocyte growth factor (HGF), and insulin-like growth factor (IGF)-1 [69].

Several signalling pathways have been implicated in the changes in subchondral bone that contribute to the progression of OA, including Wnt, TGF-β/BMP, and MAPK signalling. Of these, the Wnt/β-catenin signalling pathway has emerged as a key regulator of bone remodelling. For example, activation of Wnt signalling was observed in osteocytes in subchondral bone, and altered Wnt activation, either by knockdown of Wnt antagonists or overexpression of β-catenin, resulted in increased bone formation in an animal model, leading to thicker and stiffer bones [72–74]. More recently, Zhong et al. [75] provided a possible cross-talk between IL-1b and Wnt signalling in OA. Their findings revealed that IL-1b decreased the expression of Wnt antagonist, Dickkopf-1 (DKK1) and Frizzled related protein (FRZB), through upregulation of iNOS/NO, thereby activating the transcription of WNT target genes in human chondrocyte [75].

In addition to cartilage degradation and abnormal subchondral bone remodelling, pathological peri-articular muscle weakness appears in OA. There is increasing evidence that the consequences of OA, such as pain, joint instability, maladaptive postures, and defective neuromuscular communication, are associated with decreased lower limb muscle strength or function [76]. However, it remains unclear whether this change in peri-articular muscle is responsible for the diseased onset and progression, or is a consequence of the degenerative joint. Although OA is defined as a loss of articular cartilage within the joint, muscle impairment associated with the OA may be the primary underlying cause of the functional limitations [77], and muscle dysfunction may actually lead to a further increase in cartilage deterioration. The quadriceps, hamstrings, and hip muscles are all significantly impaired in patients with knee OA, and the quadriceps, which is involved in functional tasks such as standing up from a chair, going up and down stairs, and level surface walking, is a central determinant of physical function in patients with knee OA [78,79]. Greater quadriceps strength is associated with protection from cartilage loss in the lateral compartment of the patellofemoral joint [80]. The muscle mass loss induced by botulinum type-A toxin injections in rabbits led to cartilage degradation four weeks after injury, suggesting that muscle weakness can cause degenerative joint disease [81]. Proteoglycan loss occurs in the cartilage of mdx/utrophin$^{-/-}$ mice, which lack both dystrophin and utrophin, two important skeletal muscle structural proteins, demonstrating that skeletal muscle plays a crucial role in maintaining cartilage integrity [82]. A surgically induced OA mouse model exhibited impaired muscle function, with changes in twitch and tetanic force in the tibialis anterior muscle [83]. Although the link between the molecular regulation of peri-articular muscle function and knee OA is still under investigation, inflammation in muscles surrounding the knee may cause muscle weakness in knee OA. Inflammatory mediators, such as monocyte chemotactic protein 1 (MCP-1), p65 NF-κB, and JNK-1, are increased in the muscles of patients with knee OA, and were found to correlate with altered knee function, slower gait velocity, and greater physical disability [84,85]. These markers also upregulate pro-inflammatory cytokines, including TNF-α, IL-1β, Il-6, and IL-8, and atrogin-1, a muscle-specific atrophy-related E3 ubiquitin ligase [86,87]. Most studies have focused on the inflammatory responses within the synovium and articular chondrocytes; however, these findings suggest that the inflammatory response in patients with knee OA affects peri-articular tissues, such as subchondral bone and skeletal muscle.

4. Novel Therapeutics Based on the Molecular Pathogenesis of OA

4.1. Anti-Inflammatory and Cytokine Blocker

4.1.1. Anti TNF-α Therapies

TNF-α blockers are very effective in inflammatory joint diseases such as RA, and TNF-α plays a considerable role in the pathogenesis of OA. However, their effects on OA disease modification have not been proven clinically. Adalimumab is a human monoclonal antibody bioengineered to bind to TNF-α and prevent receptor binding [88]. A 12-month randomised, double-blind, placebo-controlled trial evaluated the efficacy of adalimumab (subcutaneously 40 mg every two weeks) in 60 patients with erosive hand OA [89]. Progression from palpable soft tissue swelling to joint damage decreased ten-fold in the adalimumab group compared with the placebo group. Although fewer adalimumab-treated patients developed erosive OA in their interphalangeal joints than the placebo arm (26.7% vs. 40%), the difference was not significant. In a randomised, double-blind, placebo-controlled, multicentre study, 85 patients with hand OA who were non-responders to analgesics and non-steroidal anti-inflammatory drugs (NSAIDs) received adalimumab (40 mg) or placebo subcutaneously every 15 days, and adalimumab was not superior to placebo for alleviating pain [90]. Infliximab has been suggested to reduce the secondary hand OA in patients with RA [91].

An open-label randomized controlled study involving 56 patients with moderate to severe knee OA received an intraarticular injection either 10 mg adalimumab, or 25 mg hyaluronic acid [92]. The decrease in the pain visual analog scale (VAS) score, Western Ontario and McMaster Universities Arthritis Index (WOMAC) score, Patient Global Assessment score, and Physician Global Assessment score from baseline to week 4 were greater in the adalimumab than hyaluronic acid group. There was no difference in adverse events between two groups except one patient who developed a pulmonary infection in the adalimumab group. The pathology of OA is very heterogeneous, with the degree of synovitis varying among patients. In one study, synovitis was not present in half of the patients with early OA [93]. A study examining the benefits of TNF-α blockers in specific subgroups of patients with higher levels of inflammation is needed.

A randomized, double-blind, placebo-controlled, multicenter study [NCT02471118], subcutaneous injection of adalimumab for knee OA with inflammation is recruiting status in a Canadian [94]. Study designed to evaluate the clinical efficacy and safety of adalimumab versus placebo when used to treat subjects with a diagnosis of knee OA, and with clinical features of inflammation, whose pain persists despite receiving maximum tolerated doses of conventional therapy. A total of 130 subjects will be entered into the study.

4.1.2. IL-1β Signalling Inhibitors

IL-1β is a key pathogenic factor in OA. Diacerein, a small-molecule IL-1β inhibitor, reduces the number of IL-1 receptors, resulting in a reduction in functional IL-1 heterodimer receptor complexes [95]. In a three-year randomised, double-blind, placebo-controlled trial, 507 hip OA patients received either diacerein or placebo daily. Although the pain and functional impairment associated with OA remained unchanged, diacerein significantly reduced joint space narrowing compared with placebo [96]. A Cochrane review of the effect of diacerein in OA concluded that the small benefit derived in terms of joint space narrowing was of questionable clinical relevance and has been observed only in hip OA [97]. In vitro and experimental models showed a reduction in cartilage destruction with IL-1 inhibition by IL-1 receptor antagonists (IL-1Ra) [98]. Three patients with aggressive erosive hand OA with major disability who had failed conventional treatment were treated with 100 mg anakinra (an IL-1β receptor antagonist) daily subcutaneously; at the third month, an improvement in pain was observed, and the NSAIDs were withdrawn [99]. A randomised, double-blind, placebo-controlled trial involving 170 patients with painful knee OA, whose joints were injected with either 50 or 150 mg of anakinra or placebo control, showed no improvement in the WOMAC score or cartilage turnover after 4 weeks [100].

4.1.3. NO Inhibitors

Preclinical studies have shown that iNOS KO mice are resistant to developing OA [101], and pharmacological inhibition of iNOS reduced OA progression and pain in a monosodium iodoacetate (MIA) rodent model of OA [102]. A recent clinical trial investigated the safety and efficacy of a novel irreversible iNOS inhibitor on slowing OA progression in a cohort of overweight and obese patients with knee OA [103]. The drug failed to slow the rate of joint space narrowing over the course of 96 weeks. Withdrawn: The study stopped early, before enrolling its first participant.

4.2. Bone Modulators

4.2.1. Bisphosphonates

It has been suggested that the administration of antiresorptive drugs such as bisphosphonates, which are traditionally used to treat osteoporosis, slows the bone remodelling process and could lead to chondroprotection [104]. Zhu et al. showed that early treatment of ovariectomised rats with alendronate significantly attenuated cartilage erosion by inhibiting subchondral bone loss [105]. Strassle et al. demonstrated that when the bisphosphonate zoledronate was administered in a monoiodoacetate model of painful arthritis in rats, it protected against subchondral bone loss, cartilage degradation and, importantly, pain [106]. In a clinical setting, bisphosphonate treatment inhibits bone and cartilage degradation based on an assessment of biochemical markers, although the joint space narrowing observed on X-rays indicated its failure to attenuate the structural deterioration [107]. In a one-year, placebo-controlled trial that included 59 patients with knee OA treated with zoledronic acid 5 mg intravenously as a single infusion, a significant reduction in visual analogue pain scores versus placebo was seen after six months, but not after 12 months; interestingly, a significant reduction in bone marrow lesions was detected with magnetic resonance imaging (MRI) [108]. In a recent meta-analysis of randomised controlled trials that compared bisphosphonate therapy with placebo or conventional medication, Xing et al. assessed the efficacy of bisphosphonates in OA; 15 studies were eligible for analysis and they included 3566 participants (1517 on bisphosphonates) [109]. It was shown that bisphosphonate therapy leads to significant improvements in pain, stiffness and function in OA patients assessed using the WOMAC score. Clodronate is a first-generation, non-amino bisphosphonate, registered in Europe for the treatment of postmenopausal osteoporosis. In a recent study, effects of clodronate in OA patients were investigated [110]. Clodronate increased SOX9 expression, the transcription factor responsible for progenitor stem cells chondrogenic commitment. This study showed that intramuscular 200 mg clodronate weekly injection increased mesenchymal stem cells maturation toward the chondrogenic differentiation. Clodronate also reduced pain VAS score and improved mental and physical performance in patients. In a randomised, double-blind, placebo-controlled trial, 80 symptomatic knee OA patients received either once weekly intraarticular injection of 2 mg clodronate or saline placebo for 4 weeks with 12 weeks of follow-up [111]. The injection of clodronate is associated with significantly greater benefits than placebo in pain VAS, Lequesne index (looking at pain, maximum distance walked and activities of daily living), patient and physician Global Assessment score, WOMAC pain subscale, and acetaminophen requirement. A 6-month randomised pilot trial of 40 patients with active erosive hand OA showed that intramuscular clodronate is effective on pain with a significant reduction in the consumption of anti-inflammatory or analgesic drugs, and improvement of hands function [112]. Reduction of serum Cartilage Oligomeric Matrix Protein (COMP), which bind type I and type II collagen fibers and catalyse fibrillar collagen assembly, was observed after clodronate treatment.

4.2.2. Strontium Ranelate

Strontium ranelate (SR) is an antiosteoporotic drug capable of changing the balance between bone resorption and bone formation, protecting postmenopausal women from spinal and peripheral fractures [113,114]. It has been hypothesised to act on both subchondral bone and cartilage based on the results of in vitro studies [115]. At a dose of 1800 mg/kg/day, SR significantly attenuated cartilage matrix and chondrocyte loss, and decreased chondrocyte apoptosis, in a medial meniscal tear model using Sprague–Dawley rats [116]. Subchondral bone remodelling was also significantly attenuated in the SR-treated group, as shown by the improved microarchitecture and intrinsic mechanical properties. Reginster et al. presented data from a large randomised clinical trial of patients with radiographic and clinical knee OA [115] and showed that SR had a beneficial effect on the radiographic progression of disease based on joint space narrowing after three years of treatment compared with placebo. The effects on pain appeared to be more modest and were only significant for the 2 g group, as assessed using the total WOMAC score and pain subscore. Serial quantitative MRI was analysed in 330 patients to evaluate the effect of SR on cartilage volume loss and bone marrow lesions [117]. The higher-dose of SR (2 g daily) resulted in reduced cartilage volume loss at the tibial plateau versus placebo, assessed after one and three years. In patients with bone marrow lesions in the medial compartment at baseline, a significant decrease in the bone marrow lesion score was detected at 36 months in both treatment groups. These results suggest a beneficial effect of SR on structural progression of primary knee OA.

4.2.3. NGF Inhibitors

Biologic agents that inhibit NGF (fasinumab, tanezumab, and fulranumab) have been tried in OA and have shown promising results in terms of pain relief and improved functional capacity [118,119]. Individuals with knee or hip OA, according to the American College of Rheumatology criteria with radiographic confirmation and who were receiving partial symptom relief with NSAIDs, may benefit more from tanezumab monotherapy; adverse events were more frequent with tanezumab than with NSAIDS, however, and were highest with both in combination [118]. Unfortunately, the rapid progression of OA in NGF inhibitor treated group led the US Food and Drug Administration to impose a partial clinical hold for OA [119]. Three clinical trials are currently being conducted to evaluate the efficacy and long term safety of fasinumab in patients with pain due to osteoarthritis of the knee or hip [NCT03161093] [120] [NCT02683239] [121], and [NCT03304379] [122].

5. Conclusions

Until recently, studies of OA have focused mostly on the inflammatory response within the synovium and articular chondrocytes. Currently, the role of periarticular tissues such as subchondral bone and skeletal muscle is gaining recognition and the mechanism of pain generation independent of cartilage degradation is being increasingly pursued. Experiments using more relevant animal OA models and large-scale clinical trials are needed to evaluate the efficacy of various therapeutic targets.

Acknowledgments: This work was supported by the Basic Science Research Program through the National Research Foundation of Korea (NRF) of Korea funded by the Ministry of Education (2017R1A2B200188) and by the Hallym University Research Fund.

Author Contributions: Conceived and wrote the paper: Ju-Ryoung Kim, Jong Jin Yoo, and Hyun Ah Kim.

Conflicts of Interest: The authors declare no conflict of interest.

References

1. Iannone, F.; Lapadula, G. The pathophysiology of osteoarthritis. *Aging Clin. Exp. Res.* **2003**, *15*, 364–372. [CrossRef] [PubMed]
2. Mortellaro, C.M. Pathophysiology of osteoarthritis. *Vet. Res. Commun.* **2003**, *27* (Suppl. S1), 75–78. [CrossRef] [PubMed]
3. Felson, D.T. Clinical practice. Osteoarthritis of the knee. *N. Engl. J. Med.* **2006**, *354*, 841–848. [CrossRef] [PubMed]
4. Krasnokutsky, S.; Samuels, J.; Abramson, S.B. Osteoarthritis in 2007. *Bull. NYU Hosp. Jt. Dis.* **2007**, *65*, 222–228. [PubMed]
5. Musumeci, G.; Loreto, C.; Carnazza, M.L.; Martinez, G. Characterization of apoptosis in articular cartilage derived from the knee joints of patients with osteoarthritis. *Knee Surg. Sports Traumatol. Arthrosc.* **2011**, *19*, 307–313. [CrossRef] [PubMed]
6. Lane, N.E.; Brandt, K.; Hawker, G.; Peeva, E.; Schreyer, E.; Tsuji, W.; Hochberg, M.C. OARSI-FDA initiative: Defining the disease state of osteoarthritis. *Osteoarthr. Cartil.* **2011**, *19*, 478–482. [CrossRef] [PubMed]
7. Lee, A.S.; Ellman, M.B.; Yan, D.; Kroin, J.S.; Cole, B.J.; van Wijnen, A.J.; Im, H.J. A current review of molecular mechanisms regarding osteoarthritis and pain. *Gene* **2013**, *527*, 440–447. [CrossRef] [PubMed]
8. Im, H.J.; Muddasani, P.; Natarajan, V.; Schmid, T.M.; Block, J.A.; Davis, F.; van Wijnen, A.J.; Loeser, R.F. Basic fibroblast growth factor stimulates matrix metalloproteinase-13 via the molecular cross-talk between the mitogen-activated protein kinases and protein kinase Cδ pathways in human adult articular chondrocytes. *J. Biol. Chem.* **2007**, *282*, 11110–11121. [CrossRef] [PubMed]
9. Maldonado, M.; Nam, J. The role of changes in extracellular matrix of cartilage in the presence of inflammation on the pathology of osteoarthritis. *BioMed Res. Int.* **2013**, *2013*, 284873. [CrossRef] [PubMed]
10. Glyn-Jones, S.; Palmer, A.J.; Agricola, R.; Price, A.J.; Vincent, T.L.; Weinans, H.; Carr, A.J. Osteoarthritis. *Lancet* **2015**, *386*, 376–387. [CrossRef]
11. Van der Kraan, P.M.; van den Berg, W.B. Osteophytes: Relevance and biology. *Osteoarthr. Cartil.* **2007**, *15*, 237–244. [CrossRef] [PubMed]
12. Wojdasiewicz, P.; Poniatowski, L.A.; Szukiewicz, D. The role of inflammatory and anti-inflammatory cytokines in the pathogenesis of osteoarthritis. *Mediat. Inflamm.* **2014**, *2014*, 561459. [CrossRef] [PubMed]
13. Larsson, S.; Englund, M.; Struglics, A.; Lohmander, L.S. Interleukin-6 and tumor necrosis factor alpha in synovial fluid are associated with progression of radiographic knee osteoarthritis in subjects with previous meniscectomy. *Osteoarthr. Cartil.* **2015**, *23*, 1906–1914. [CrossRef] [PubMed]
14. Kapoor, M.; Martel-Pelletier, J.; Lajeunesse, D.; Pelletier, J.P.; Fahmi, H. Role of proinflammatory cytokines in the pathophysiology of osteoarthritis. *Nat. Rev. Rheumatol.* **2011**, *7*, 33–42. [CrossRef] [PubMed]
15. Vergunst, C.E.; van de Sande, M.G.; Lebre, M.C.; Tak, P.P. The role of chemokines in rheumatoid arthritis and osteoarthritis. *Scand. J. Rheumatol.* **2005**, *34*, 415–425. [CrossRef] [PubMed]
16. Sohn, D.H.; Sokolove, J.; Sharpe, O.; Erhart, J.C.; Chandra, P.E.; Lahey, L.J.; Lindstrom, T.M.; Hwang, I.; Boyer, K.A.; Andriacchi, T.P.; et al. Plasma proteins present in osteoarthritic synovial fluid can stimulate cytokine production via Toll-like receptor 4. *Arthritis Res. Ther.* **2012**, *14*, R7. [CrossRef] [PubMed]
17. Dayer, J.M. The process of identifying and understanding cytokines: From basic studies to treating rheumatic diseases. *Best Pract. Res. Clin. Rheumatol.* **2004**, *18*, 31–45. [CrossRef] [PubMed]
18. Chockalingam, P.S.; Varadarajan, U.; Sheldon, R.; Fortier, E.; LaVallie, E.R.; Morris, E.A.; Yaworsky, P.J.; Majumdar, M.K. Involvement of protein kinase Czeta in interleukin-1beta induction of ADAMTS-4 and type 2 nitric oxide synthase via NF-kappaB signaling in primary human osteoarthritic chondrocytes. *Arthritis Rheum.* **2007**, *56*, 4074–4083. [CrossRef] [PubMed]
19. Clements, K.M.; Price, J.S.; Chambers, M.G.; Visco, D.M.; Poole, A.R.; Mason, R.M. Gene deletion of either interleukin-1beta, interleukin-1beta-converting enzyme, inducible nitric oxide synthase, or stromelysin 1 accelerates the development of knee osteoarthritis in mice after surgical transection of the medial collateral ligament and partial medial meniscectomy. *Arthritis Rheum.* **2003**, *48*, 3452–3463. [PubMed]
20. Kobayashi, M.; Squires, G.R.; Mousa, A.; Tanzer, M.; Zukor, D.J.; Antoniou, J.; Feige, U.; Poole, A.R. Role of interleukin-1 and tumor necrosis factor alpha in matrix degradation of human osteoarthritic cartilage. *Arthritis Rheum.* **2005**, *52*, 128–135. [CrossRef] [PubMed]

21. Saklatvala, J. Tumour necrosis factor alpha stimulates resorption and inhibits synthesis of proteoglycan in cartilage. *Nature* **1986**, *322*, 547–549. [CrossRef] [PubMed]
22. Lefebvre, V.; Peeters-Joris, C.; Vaes, G. Modulation by interleukin 1 and tumor necrosis factor alpha of production of collagenase, tissue inhibitor of metalloproteinases and collagen types in differentiated and dedifferentiated articular chondrocytes. *Biochim. Biophys. Acta* **1990**, *1052*, 366–378. [CrossRef]
23. Vuolteenaho, K.; Moilanen, T.; Hamalainen, M.; Moilanen, E. Effects of TNFalpha-antagonists on nitric oxide production in human cartilage. *Osteoarthr. Cartil.* **2002**, *10*, 327–332. [CrossRef] [PubMed]
24. Goldring, M.B. The role of the chondrocyte in osteoarthritis. *Arthritis Rheum.* **2000**, *43*, 1916–1926. [CrossRef]
25. Mueller, M.B.; Tuan, R.S. Anabolic/Catabolic balance in pathogenesis of osteoarthritis: Identifying molecular targets. *PM R* **2011**, *3* (Suppl. S1), S3–S11. [CrossRef] [PubMed]
26. Taskiran, D.; Stefanovic-Racic, M.; Georgescu, H.; Evans, C. Nitric oxide mediates suppression of cartilage proteoglycan synthesis by interleukin-1. *Biochem. Biophys. Res. Commun.* **1994**, *200*, 142–148. [CrossRef] [PubMed]
27. Little, C.B.; Barai, A.; Burkhardt, D.; Smith, S.M.; Fosang, A.J.; Werb, Z.; Shah, M.; Thompson, E.W. Matrix metalloproteinase 13-deficient mice are resistant to osteoarthritic cartilage erosion but not chondrocyte hypertrophy or osteophyte development. *Arthritis Rheum.* **2009**, *60*, 3723–3733. [CrossRef] [PubMed]
28. Neuhold, L.A.; Killar, L.; Zhao, W.; Sung, M.L.; Warner, L.; Kulik, J.; Turner, J.; Wu, W.; Billinghurst, C.; Meijers, T.; et al. Postnatal expression in hyaline cartilage of constitutively active human collagenase-3 (MMP-13) induces osteoarthritis in mice. *J. Clin. Investig.* **2001**, *107*, 35–44. [CrossRef] [PubMed]
29. Sahebjam, S.; Khokha, R.; Mort, J.S. Increased collagen and aggrecan degradation with age in the joints of Timp3(−/−) mice. *Arthritis Rheum.* **2007**, *56*, 905–909. [CrossRef] [PubMed]
30. Ahmad, R.; Sylvester, J.; Ahmad, M.; Zafarullah, M. Adaptor proteins and Ras synergistically regulate IL-1-induced ADAMTS-4 expression in human chondrocytes. *J. Immunol.* **2009**, *182*, 5081–5087. [CrossRef] [PubMed]
31. East, C.J.; Stanton, H.; Golub, S.B.; Rogerson, F.M.; Fosang, A.J. ADAMTS-5 deficiency does not block aggrecanolysis at preferred cleavage sites in the chondroitin sulfate-rich region of aggrecan. *J. Biol. Chem.* **2007**, *282*, 8632–8640. [CrossRef] [PubMed]
32. Stanton, H.; Rogerson, F.M.; East, C.J.; Golub, S.B.; Lawlor, K.E.; Meeker, C.T.; Little, C.B.; Last, K.; Farmer, P.J.; Campbell, I.K.; et al. ADAMTS5 is the major aggrecanase in mouse cartilage in vivo and in vitro. *Nature* **2005**, *434*, 648–652. [CrossRef] [PubMed]
33. Hosaka, Y.; Saito, T.; Sugita, S.; Hikata, T.; Kobayashi, H.; Fukai, A.; Taniguchi, Y.; Hirata, M.; Akiyama, H.; Chung, U.I.; et al. Notch signaling in chondrocytes modulates endochondral ossification and osteoarthritis development. *Proc. Natl. Acad. Sci. USA* **2013**, *110*, 1875–1880. [CrossRef] [PubMed]
34. Sugita, S.; Hosaka, Y.; Okada, K.; Mori, D.; Yano, F.; Kobayashi, H.; Taniguchi, Y.; Mori, Y.; Okuma, T.; Chang, S.H.; et al. Transcription factor Hes1 modulates osteoarthritis development in cooperation with calcium/calmodulin-dependent protein kinase 2. *Proc. Natl. Acad. Sci. USA* **2015**, *112*, 3080–3085. [CrossRef] [PubMed]
35. Liu, Z.; Chen, J.; Mirando, A.J.; Wang, C.; Zuscik, M.J.; O'Keefe, R.J.; Hilton, M.J. A dual role for NOTCH signaling in joint cartilage maintenance and osteoarthritis. *Sci. Signal.* **2015**, *8*, ra71. [CrossRef] [PubMed]
36. Zhang, F.J.; Luo, W.; Lei, G.H. Role of HIF-1alpha and HIF-2alpha in osteoarthritis. *Jt. Bone Spine* **2015**, *82*, 144–147. [CrossRef] [PubMed]
37. Pfander, D.; Kobayashi, T.; Knight, M.C.; Zelzer, E.; Chan, D.A.; Olsen, B.R.; Giaccia, A.J.; Johnson, R.S.; Haase, V.H.; Schipani, E. Deletion of Vhlh in chondrocytes reduces cell proliferation and increases matrix deposition during growth plate development. *Development* **2004**, *131*, 2497–2508. [CrossRef] [PubMed]
38. Schipani, E.; Ryan, H.E.; Didrickson, S.; Kobayashi, T.; Knight, M.; Johnson, R.S. Hypoxia in cartilage: HIF-1alpha is essential for chondrocyte growth arrest and survival. *Genes Dev.* **2001**, *15*, 2865–2876. [PubMed]
39. Saito, T.; Fukai, A.; Mabuchi, A.; Ikeda, T.; Yano, F.; Ohba, S.; Nishida, N.; Akune, T.; Yoshimura, N.; Nakagawa, T.; et al. Transcriptional regulation of endochondral ossification by HIF-2alpha during skeletal growth and osteoarthritis development. *Nat. Med.* **2010**, *16*, 678–686. [CrossRef] [PubMed]
40. Yang, S.; Kim, J.; Ryu, J.H.; Oh, H.; Chun, C.H.; Kim, B.J.; Min, B.H.; Chun, J.S. Hypoxia-inducible factor-2alpha is a catabolic regulator of osteoarthritic cartilage destruction. *Nat. Med.* **2010**, *16*, 687–693. [CrossRef] [PubMed]

41. Rigoglou, S.; Papavassiliou, A.G. The NF-kappaB signalling pathway in osteoarthritis. *Int. J. Biochem. Cell Biol.* **2013**, *45*, 2580–2584. [CrossRef] [PubMed]

42. Chen, L.X.; Lin, L.; Wang, H.J.; Wei, X.L.; Fu, X.; Zhang, J.Y.; Yu, C.L. Suppression of early experimental osteoarthritis by in vivo delivery of the adenoviral vector-mediated NF-kappaBp65-specific siRNA. *Osteoarthr. Cartil.* **2008**, *16*, 174–184. [CrossRef] [PubMed]

43. Bondeson, J.; Lauder, S.; Wainwright, S.; Amos, N.; Evans, A.; Hughes, C.; Feldmann, M.; Caterson, B. Adenoviral gene transfer of the endogenous inhibitor IκBα into human osteoarthritis synovial fibroblasts demonstrates that several matrix metalloproteinases and aggrecanases are nuclear factor-κB-dependent. *J. Rheumatol.* **2007**, *34*, 523–533. [PubMed]

44. Amos, N.; Lauder, S.; Evans, A.; Feldmann, M.; Bondeson, J. Adenoviral gene transfer into osteoarthritis synovial cells using the endogenous inhibitor IkappaBalpha reveals that most, but not all, inflammatory and destructive mediators are NFkappaB dependent. *Rheumatology* **2006**, *45*, 1201–1209. [CrossRef] [PubMed]

45. Kim, J.H.; Jeon, J.; Shin, M.; Won, Y.; Lee, M.; Kwak, J.S.; Lee, G.; Rhee, J.; Ryu, J.H.; Chun, C.H.; et al. Regulation of the catabolic cascade in osteoarthritis by the zinc-ZIP8-MTF1 axis. *Cell* **2014**, *156*, 730–743. [CrossRef] [PubMed]

46. McCulloch, K.; Litherland, G.J.; Rai, T.S. Cellular senescence in osteoarthritis pathology. *Aging Cell* **2017**, *16*, 210–218. [CrossRef] [PubMed]

47. Campisi, J. Aging, cellular senescence, and cancer. *Annu. Rev. Physiol.* **2013**, *75*, 685–705. [CrossRef] [PubMed]

48. Van Deursen, J.M. The role of senescent cells in ageing. *Nature* **2014**, *509*, 439–446. [CrossRef] [PubMed]

49. Carlo, M.D., Jr.; Loeser, R.F. Increased oxidative stress with aging reduces chondrocyte survival: Correlation with intracellular glutathione levels. *Arthritis Rheum.* **2003**, *48*, 3419–3430. [CrossRef] [PubMed]

50. Forsyth, C.B.; Cole, A.; Murphy, G.; Bienias, J.L.; Im, H.J.; Loeser, R.F., Jr. Increased matrix metalloproteinase-13 production with aging by human articular chondrocytes in response to catabolic stimuli. *J. Gerontol. A Biol. Sci. Med. Sci.* **2005**, *60*, 1118–1124. [CrossRef] [PubMed]

51. Long, D.; Blake, S.; Song, X.Y.; Lark, M.; Loeser, R.F. Human articular chondrocytes produce IL-7 and respond to IL-7 with increased production of matrix metalloproteinase-13. *Arthritis Res. Ther.* **2008**, *10*, R23. [CrossRef] [PubMed]

52. Jeon, O.H.; Kim, C.; Laberge, R.M.; Demaria, M.; Rathod, S.; Vasserot, A.P.; Chung, J.W.; Kim, D.H.; Poon, Y.; David, N.; et al. Local clearance of senescent cells attenuates the development of post-traumatic osteoarthritis and creates a pro-regenerative environment. *Nat. Med.* **2017**, *23*, 775–781. [CrossRef] [PubMed]

53. Heraud, F.; Heraud, A.; Harmand, M.F. Apoptosis in normal and osteoarthritic human articular cartilage. *Ann. Rheum. Dis.* **2000**, *59*, 959–965. [CrossRef] [PubMed]

54. Hwang, H.S.; Kim, H.A. Chondrocyte Apoptosis in the Pathogenesis of Osteoarthritis. *Int. J. Mol. Sci.* **2015**, *16*, 26035–26054. [CrossRef] [PubMed]

55. Kim, H.A.; Suh, D.I.; Song, Y.W. Relationship between chondrocyte apoptosis and matrix depletion in human articular cartilage. *J. Rheumatol.* **2001**, *28*, 2038–2045. [PubMed]

56. Pelletier, J.P.; Fernandes, J.C.; Jovanovic, D.V.; Reboul, P.; Martel-Pelletier, J. Chondrocyte death in experimental osteoarthritis is mediated by MEK 1/2 and p38 pathways: Role of cyclooxygenase-2 and inducible nitric oxide synthase. *J. Rheumatol.* **2001**, *28*, 2509–2519. [PubMed]

57. Loening, A.M.; James, I.E.; Levenston, M.E.; Badger, A.M.; Frank, E.H.; Kurz, B.; Nuttall, M.E.; Hung, H.H.; Blake, S.M.; Grodzinsky, A.J.; et al. Injurious mechanical compression of bovine articular cartilage induces chondrocyte apoptosis. *Arch. Biochem. Biophys.* **2000**, *381*, 205–212. [CrossRef] [PubMed]

58. D'Lima, D.; Hermida, J.; Hashimoto, S.; Colwell, C.; Lotz, M. Caspase inhibitors reduce severity of cartilage lesions in experimental osteoarthritis. *Arthritis Rheum.* **2006**, *54*, 1814–1821. [CrossRef] [PubMed]

59. Sasaki, H.; Takayama, K.; Matsushita, T.; Ishida, K.; Kubo, S.; Matsumoto, T.; Fujita, N.; Oka, S.; Kurosaka, M.; Kuroda, R. Autophagy modulates osteoarthritis-related gene expression in human chondrocytes. *Arthritis Rheum.* **2012**, *64*, 1920–1928. [CrossRef] [PubMed]

60. Mizushima, N.; Komatsu, M. Autophagy: Renovation of cells and tissues. *Cell* **2011**, *147*, 728–741. [CrossRef] [PubMed]

61. Carames, B.; Hasegawa, A.; Taniguchi, N.; Miyaki, S.; Blanco, F.J.; Lotz, M. Autophagy activation by rapamycin reduces severity of experimental osteoarthritis. *Ann. Rheum. Dis.* **2012**, *71*, 575–581. [CrossRef] [PubMed]

62. Bohensky, J.; Terkhorn, S.P.; Freeman, T.A.; Adams, C.S.; Garcia, J.A.; Shapiro, I.M.; Srinivas, V. Regulation of autophagy in human and murine cartilage: Hypoxia-inducible factor 2 suppresses chondrocyte autophagy. *Arthritis Rheum.* **2009**, *60*, 1406–1415. [CrossRef] [PubMed]

63. Qin, N.; Wei, L.; Li, W.; Yang, W.; Cai, L.; Qian, Z.; Wu, S. Local intra-articular injection of resveratrol delays cartilage degeneration in C57BL/6 mice by inducing autophagy via AMPK/mTOR pathway. *J. Pharmacol. Sci.* **2017**, *134*, 166–174. [CrossRef] [PubMed]

64. Li, W.; Cai, L.; Zhang, Y.; Cui, L.; Shen, G. Intra-articular resveratrol injection prevents osteoarthritis progression in a mouse model by activating SIRT1 and thereby silencing HIF-2alpha. *J. Orthop. Res.* **2015**, *33*, 1061–1070. [CrossRef] [PubMed]

65. Goldring, S.R. Role of bone in osteoarthritis pathogenesis. *Med. Clin. N. Am.* **2009**, *93*, 25–35. [CrossRef] [PubMed]

66. Hwang, J.; Bae, W.C.; Shieu, W.; Lewis, C.W.; Bugbee, W.D.; Sah, R.L. Increased hydraulic conductance of human articular cartilage and subchondral bone plate with progression of osteoarthritis. *Arthritis Rheum.* **2008**, *58*, 3831–3842. [CrossRef] [PubMed]

67. Day, J.S.; Ding, M.; van der Linden, J.C.; Hvid, I.; Sumner, D.R.; Weinans, H. A decreased subchondral trabecular bone tissue elastic modulus is associated with pre-arthritic cartilage damage. *J. Orthop. Res.* **2001**, *19*, 914–918. [CrossRef]

68. Felson, D.T.; Gale, D.R.; Elon Gale, M.; Niu, J.; Hunter, D.J.; Goggins, J.; Lavalley, M.P. Osteophytes and progression of knee osteoarthritis. *Rheumatology* **2005**, *44*, 100–104. [CrossRef] [PubMed]

69. Yuan, X.L.; Meng, H.Y.; Wang, Y.C.; Peng, J.; Guo, Q.Y.; Wang, A.Y.; Lu, S.B. Bone-cartilage interface crosstalk in osteoarthritis: Potential pathways and future therapeutic strategies. *Osteoarthr. Cartil.* **2014**, *22*, 1077–1089. [CrossRef] [PubMed]

70. Wang, Y.; Wluka, A.E.; Pelletier, J.P.; Martel-Pelletier, J.; Abram, F.; Ding, C.; Cicuttini, F.M. Meniscal extrusion predicts increases in subchondral bone marrow lesions and bone cysts and expansion of subchondral bone in osteoarthritic knees. *Rheumatology* **2010**, *49*, 997–1004. [CrossRef] [PubMed]

71. Wei, Y.; Bai, L. Recent advances in the understanding of molecular mechanisms of cartilage degeneration, synovitis and subchondral bone changes in osteoarthritis. *Connect. Tissue Res.* **2016**, *57*, 245–261. [CrossRef] [PubMed]

72. Baron, R.; Kneissel, M. WNT signaling in bone homeostasis and disease: From human mutations to treatments. *Nat. Med.* **2013**, *19*, 179–192. [CrossRef] [PubMed]

73. Lories, R.J.; Peeters, J.; Bakker, A.; Tylzanowski, P.; Derese, I.; Schrooten, J.; Thomas, J.T.; Luyten, F.P. Articular cartilage and biomechanical properties of the long bones in Frzb-knockout mice. *Arthritis Rheum.* **2007**, *56*, 4095–4103. [CrossRef] [PubMed]

74. Zhu, M.; Tang, D.; Wu, Q.; Hao, S.; Chen, M.; Xie, C.; Rosier, R.N.; O'Keefe, R.J.; Zuscik, M.; Chen, D. Activation of beta-catenin signaling in articular chondrocytes leads to osteoarthritis-like phenotype in adult beta-catenin conditional activation mice. *J. Bone Miner. Res.* **2009**, *24*, 12–21. [CrossRef] [PubMed]

75. Zhong, L.; Schivo, S.; Huang, X.; Leijten, J.; Karperien, M.; Post, J.N. Nitric Oxide Mediates Crosstalk between Interleukin 1beta and WNT Signaling in Primary Human Chondrocytes by Reducing DKK1 and FRZB Expression. *Int. J. Mol. Sci.* **2017**, *18*, 2491. [CrossRef] [PubMed]

76. Bennell, K.L.; Hunt, M.A.; Wrigley, T.V.; Lim, B.W.; Hinman, R.S. Role of muscle in the genesis and management of knee osteoarthritis. *Rheum. Dis. Clin. N. Am.* **2008**, *34*, 731–754. [CrossRef] [PubMed]

77. Hurley, M.V.; Scott, D.L.; Rees, J.; Newham, D.J. Sensorimotor changes and functional performance in patients with knee osteoarthritis. *Ann. Rheum. Dis.* **1997**, *56*, 641–648. [CrossRef] [PubMed]

78. Liikavainio, T.; Lyytinen, T.; Tyrvainen, E.; Sipila, S.; Arokoski, J.P. Physical function and properties of quadriceps femoris muscle in men with knee osteoarthritis. *Arch. Phys. Med. Rehabil.* **2008**, *89*, 2185–2194. [CrossRef] [PubMed]

79. Alnahdi, A.H.; Zeni, J.A.; Snyder-Mackler, L. Muscle impairments in patients with knee osteoarthritis. *Sports Health* **2012**, *4*, 284–292. [CrossRef] [PubMed]

80. De Ceuninck, F.; Fradin, A.; Pastoureau, P. Bearing arms against osteoarthritis and sarcopenia: When cartilage and skeletal muscle find common interest in talking together. *Drug Discov. Today* **2014**, *19*, 305–311. [CrossRef] [PubMed]

81. Rehan Youssef, A.; Longino, D.; Seerattan, R.; Leonard, T.; Herzog, W. Muscle weakness causes joint degeneration in rabbits. *Osteoarthr. Cartil.* **2009**, *17*, 1228–1235. [CrossRef] [PubMed]

82. Isaac, C.; Wright, A.; Usas, A.; Li, H.; Tang, Y.; Mu, X.; Greco, N.; Dong, Q.; Vo, N.; Kang, J.; et al. Dystrophin and utrophin "double knockout" dystrophic mice exhibit a spectrum of degenerative musculoskeletal abnormalities. *J. Orthop. Res.* **2013**, *31*, 343–349. [CrossRef] [PubMed]

83. van der Poel, C.; Levinger, P.; Tonkin, B.A.; Levinger, I.; Walsh, N.C. Impaired muscle function in a mouse surgical model of post-traumatic osteoarthritis. *Osteoarthr. Cartil.* **2016**, *24*, 1047–1053. [CrossRef] [PubMed]

84. Peake, J.; Della Gatta, P.; Cameron-Smith, D. Aging and its effects on inflammation in skeletal muscle at rest and following exercise-induced muscle injury. *Am. J. Physiol. Regul. Integr. Comp. Physiol.* **2010**, *298*, R1485–R1495. [CrossRef] [PubMed]

85. Russell, A.P. Molecular regulation of skeletal muscle mass. *Clin. Exp. Pharmacol. Physiol.* **2010**, *37*, 378–384. [CrossRef] [PubMed]

86. Sarkar, D.; Fisher, P.B. Molecular mechanisms of aging-associated inflammation. *Cancer Lett.* **2006**, *236*, 13–23. [CrossRef] [PubMed]

87. Levinger, I.; Levinger, P.; Trenerry, M.K.; Feller, J.A.; Bartlett, J.R.; Bergman, N.; McKenna, M.J.; Cameron-Smith, D. Increased inflammatory cytokine expression in the vastus lateralis of patients with knee osteoarthritis. *Arthritis Rheum.* **2011**, *63*, 1343–1348. [CrossRef] [PubMed]

88. Rau, R. Adalimumab (a fully human anti-tumour necrosis factor alpha monoclonal antibody) in the treatment of active rheumatoid arthritis: The initial results of five trials. *Ann. Rheum. Dis.* **2002**, *61* (Suppl. S2), ii70–ii73. [CrossRef] [PubMed]

89. Verbruggen, G.; Wittoek, R.; Vander Cruyssen, B.; Elewaut, D. Tumour necrosis factor blockade for the treatment of erosive osteoarthritis of the interphalangeal finger joints: A double blind, randomised trial on structure modification. *Ann. Rheum. Dis.* **2012**, *71*, 891–898. [CrossRef] [PubMed]

90. Chevalier, X.; Ravaud, P.; Maheu, E.; Baron, G.; Rialland, A.; Vergnaud, P.; Roux, C.; Maugars, Y.; Mulleman, D.; Lukas, C.; et al. Adalimumab in patients with hand osteoarthritis refractory to analgesics and NSAIDs: A randomised, multicentre, double-blind, placebo-controlled trial. *Ann. Rheum. Dis.* **2015**, *74*, 1697–1705. [CrossRef] [PubMed]

91. Guler-Yuksel, M.; Allaart, C.F.; Watt, I.; Goekoop-Ruiterman, Y.P.; de Vries-Bouwstra, J.K.; van Schaardenburg, D.; van Krugten, M.V.; Dijkmans, B.A.; Huizinga, T.W.; Lems, W.F.; et al. Treatment with TNF-alpha inhibitor infliximab might reduce hand osteoarthritis in patients with rheumatoid arthritis. *Osteoarthr. Cartil.* **2010**, *18*, 1256–1262. [CrossRef] [PubMed]

92. Wang, J. Efficacy and safety of adalimumab by intra-articular injection for moderate to severe knee osteoarthritis: An open-label randomized controlled trial. *J. Int. Med. Res.* **2018**, *46*, 326–334. [CrossRef] [PubMed]

93. Haywood, L.; McWilliams, D.F.; Pearson, C.I.; Gill, S.E.; Ganesan, A.; Wilson, D.; Walsh, D.A. Inflammation and angiogenesis in osteoarthritis. *Arthritis Rheum.* **2003**, *48*, 2173–2177. [CrossRef] [PubMed]

94. Clinicaltrials.gov. Osteoarthritis of the Knee, Inflammation, and the Effect of Adalimumab (OKINADA) (OKINADA). Canadian Research & Education in Arthritis. 2017. Available online: https://clinicaltrials.gov/ct2/show/NCT02471118 (accessed on 11 April 2017).

95. Martel-Pelletier, J.; Pelletier, J.P. Effects of diacerein at the molecular level in the osteoarthritis disease process. *Ther. Adv. Musculoskelet. Dis.* **2010**, *2*, 95–104. [CrossRef] [PubMed]

96. Dougados, M.; Nguyen, M.; Berdah, L.; Mazieres, B.; Vignon, E.; Lequesne, M.; Group, E.I.S. Evaluation of the structure-modifying effects of diacerein in hip osteoarthritis: ECHODIAH, a three-year, placebo-controlled trial. Evaluation of the Chondromodulating Effect of Diacerein in OA of the Hip. *Arthritis Rheum.* **2001**, *44*, 2539–2547. [CrossRef]

97. Fidelix, T.S.; Macedo, C.R.; Maxwell, L.J.; Fernandes Moca Trevisani, V. Diacerein for osteoarthritis. *Cochrane Database Syst. Rev.* **2014**, CD005117. [CrossRef] [PubMed]

98. Calich, A.L.; Domiciano, D.S.; Fuller, R. Osteoarthritis: Can anti-cytokine therapy play a role in treatment? *Clin. Rheumatol.* **2010**, *29*, 451–455. [CrossRef] [PubMed]

99. Bacconnier, L.; Jorgensen, C.; Fabre, S. Erosive osteoarthritis of the hand: Clinical experience with anakinra. *Ann. Rheum. Dis.* **2009**, *68*, 1078–1079. [CrossRef] [PubMed]

100. Chevalier, X.; Goupille, P.; Beaulieu, A.D.; Burch, F.X.; Bensen, W.G.; Conrozier, T.; Loeuille, D.; Kivitz, A.J.; Silver, D.; Appleton, B.E. Intraarticular injection of anakinra in osteoarthritis of the knee: A multicenter, randomized, double-blind, placebo-controlled study. *Arthritis Rheum.* **2009**, *61*, 344–352. [CrossRef] [PubMed]

101. Salerno, L.; Sorrenti, V.; Di Giacomo, C.; Romeo, G.; Siracusa, M.A. Progress in the development of selective nitric oxide synthase (NOS) inhibitors. *Curr. Pharm. Des.* **2002**, *8*, 177–200. [CrossRef] [PubMed]

102. More, A.S.; Kumari, R.R.; Gupta, G.; Lingaraju, M.C.; Balaganur, V.; Pathak, N.N.; Kumar, D.; Kumar, D.; Sharma, A.K.; Tandan, S.K. Effect of iNOS inhibitor S-methylisothiourea in monosodium iodoacetate-induced osteoarthritic pain: Implication for osteoarthritis therapy. *Pharmacol. Biochem. Behav.* **2013**, *103*, 764–772. [CrossRef] [PubMed]

103. Hellio le Graverand, M.P.; Clemmer, R.S.; Redifer, P.; Brunell, R.M.; Hayes, C.W.; Brandt, K.D.; Abramson, S.B.; Manning, P.T.; Miller, C.G.; Vignon, E. A 2-year randomised, double-blind, placebo-controlled, multicentre study of oral selective iNOS inhibitor, cindunistat (SD-6010), in patients with symptomatic osteoarthritis of the knee. *Ann. Rheum. Dis.* **2013**, *72*, 187–195. [CrossRef] [PubMed]

104. Davis, A.J.; Smith, T.O.; Hing, C.B.; Sofat, N. Are bisphosphonates effective in the treatment of osteoarthritis pain? A meta-analysis and systematic review. *PLoS ONE* **2013**, *8*, e72714. [CrossRef] [PubMed]

105. Zhu, S.; Chen, K.; Lan, Y.; Zhang, N.; Jiang, R.; Hu, J. Alendronate protects against articular cartilage erosion by inhibiting subchondral bone loss in ovariectomized rats. *Bone* **2013**, *53*, 340–349. [CrossRef] [PubMed]

106. Strassle, B.W.; Mark, L.; Leventhal, L.; Piesla, M.J.; Jian Li, X.; Kennedy, J.D.; Glasson, S.S.; Whiteside, G.T. Inhibition of osteoclasts prevents cartilage loss and pain in a rat model of degenerative joint disease. *Osteoarthr. Cartil.* **2010**, *18*, 1319–1328. [CrossRef] [PubMed]

107. Bingham, C.O., III; Buckland-Wright, J.C.; Garnero, P.; Cohen, S.B.; Dougados, M.; Adami, S.; Clauw, D.J.; Spector, T.D.; Pelletier, J.P.; Raynauld, J.P.; et al. Risedronate decreases biochemical markers of cartilage degradation but does not decrease symptoms or slow radiographic progression in patients with medial compartment osteoarthritis of the knee: Results of the two-year multinational knee osteoarthritis structural arthritis study. *Arthritis Rheum.* **2006**, *54*, 3494–3507. [PubMed]

108. Laslett, L.L.; Dore, D.A.; Quinn, S.J.; Boon, P.; Ryan, E.; Winzenberg, T.M.; Jones, G. Zoledronic acid reduces knee pain and bone marrow lesions over 1 year: A randomised controlled trial. *Ann. Rheum. Dis.* **2012**, *71*, 1322–1328. [CrossRef] [PubMed]

109. Xing, R.L.; Zhao, L.R.; Wang, P.M. Bisphosphonates therapy for osteoarthritis: A meta-analysis of randomized controlled trials. *SpringerPlus* **2016**, *5*, 1704. [CrossRef] [PubMed]

110. Valenti, M.T.; Mottes, M.; Biotti, A.; Perduca, M.; Pisani, A.; Bovi, M.; Deiana, M.; Cheri, S.; Dalle Carbonare, L. Clodronate as a Therapeutic Strategy against Osteoarthritis. *Int. J. Mol. Sci.* **2017**, *18*, 2696. [CrossRef] [PubMed]

111. Rossini, M.; Adami, S.; Fracassi, E.; Viapiana, O.; Orsolini, G.; Povino, M.R.; Idolazzi, L.; Gatti, D. Effects of intra-articular clodronate in the treatment of knee osteoarthritis: Results of a double-blind, randomized placebo-controlled trial. *Rheumatol. Int.* **2015**, *35*, 255–263. [CrossRef] [PubMed]

112. Saviola, G.; Abdi-Ali, L.; Povino, M.R.; Campostrini, L.; Sacco, S.; Carbonare, L.D. Intramuscular clodronate in erosive osteoarthritis of the hand is effective on pain and reduces serum COMP: A randomized pilot trial—The ER.O.D.E. study (ERosive Osteoarthritis and Disodium-clodronate Evaluation). *Clin. Rheumatol.* **2017**, *36*, 2343–2350. [CrossRef] [PubMed]

113. Meunier, P.J.; Roux, C.; Seeman, E.; Ortolani, S.; Badurski, J.E.; Spector, T.D.; Cannata, J.; Balogh, A.; Lemmel, E.M.; Pors-Nielsen, S.; et al. The effects of strontium ranelate on the risk of vertebral fracture in women with postmenopausal osteoporosis. *N. Engl. J. Med.* **2004**, *350*, 459–468. [CrossRef] [PubMed]

114. Delmas, P.D. Clinical effects of strontium ranelate in women with postmenopausal osteoporosis. *Osteoporos. Int.* **2005**, *16* (Suppl. S1), S16–S19. [CrossRef] [PubMed]

115. Reginster, J.Y.; Badurski, J.; Bellamy, N.; Bensen, W.; Chapurlat, R.; Chevalier, X.; Christiansen, C.; Genant, H.; Navarro, F.; Nasonov, E.; et al. Efficacy and safety of strontium ranelate in the treatment of knee osteoarthritis: Results of a double-blind, randomised placebo-controlled trial. *Ann. Rheum. Dis.* **2013**, *72*, 179–186. [CrossRef] [PubMed]

116. Yu, D.G.; Ding, H.F.; Mao, Y.Q.; Liu, M.; Yu, B.; Zhao, X.; Wang, X.Q.; Li, Y.; Liu, G.W.; Nie, S.B.; et al. Strontium ranelate reduces cartilage degeneration and subchondral bone remodeling in rat osteoarthritis model. *Acta Pharmacol. Sin.* **2013**, *34*, 393–402. [CrossRef] [PubMed]

117. Pelletier, J.P.; Roubille, C.; Raynauld, J.P.; Abram, F.; Dorais, M.; Delorme, P.; Martel-Pelletier, J. Disease-modifying effect of strontium ranelate in a subset of patients from the Phase III knee osteoarthritis study SEKOIA using quantitative MRI: Reduction in bone marrow lesions protects against cartilage loss. *Ann. Rheum. Dis.* **2015**, *74*, 422–429. [CrossRef] [PubMed]

118. Schnitzer, T.J.; Ekman, E.F.; Spierings, E.L.; Greenberg, H.S.; Smith, M.D.; Brown, M.T.; West, C.R.; Verburg, K.M. Efficacy and safety of tanezumab monotherapy or combined with non-steroidal anti-inflammatory drugs in the treatment of knee or hip osteoarthritis pain. *Ann. Rheum. Dis.* **2015**, *74*, 1202–1211. [CrossRef] [PubMed]

119. Hochberg, M.C.; Tive, L.A.; Abramson, S.B.; Vignon, E.; Verburg, K.M.; West, C.R.; Smith, M.D.; Hungerford, D.S. When Is Osteonecrosis Not Osteonecrosis?: Adjudication of Reported Serious Adverse Joint Events in the Tanezumab Clinical Development Program. *Arthritis Rheumatol.* **2016**, *68*, 382–391. [CrossRef] [PubMed]

120. Clinicaltrials.gov. A Study to Determine the Safety and the Efficacy of Fasinumab Compared to Placebo and Naproxen for Treatment of Adults with Pain From Osteoarthritis of the Knee or Hip (FACT OA1). Regeneron Pharmaceuticals. 2018. Available online: https://clinicaltrials.gov/ct2/show/NCT03161093 (accessed on 29 August 2017).

121. Clinicaltrials.gov. Long-Term Safety and Efficacy Study of Fasinumab in Patients with Pain Due to Osteoarthritis (OA) of the Knee or Hip (FACT LTS & OA). Regeneron Pharmaceuticals. 2018. Available online: https://clinicaltrials.gov/ct2/show/NCT02683239 (accessed on 18 May 2017).

122. Clinicaltrials.gov. Study to Determine the Safety and the Efficacy of Fasinumab Compared to Placebo and Nonsteroidal Anti-Inflammatory Drugs (NSAIDs) for Treatment of Adults with Pain from Osteoarthritis of the Knee or Hip (FACT OA2). Regeneron Pharmaceuticals. 2018. Available online: https://clinicaltrials.gov/ct2/show/NCT03304379 (accessed on 6 December 2017).

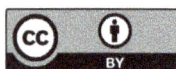

International Journal of
Molecular Sciences

MDPI

Review

Human MHC-II with Shared Epitope Motifs Are Optimal Epstein-Barr Virus Glycoprotein 42 Ligands—Relation to Rheumatoid Arthritis

Nicole Trier [1,*], Jose Izarzugaza [2], Anna Chailyan [3], Paolo Marcatili [2] and Gunnar Houen [1,*]

[1] Department of Autoimmunology and Biomarkers, Statens Serum Institute, Artillerivej 5, 2300 Copenhagen, Denmark
[2] Department of Bioinformatics, Technical University of Denmark, Anker Engelundsvej 1, 2800 Kongens Lyngby, Denmark; txema@bioinformatics.dtu.dk (J.I.); pamar@bioinformatics.dtu.dk (P.M.)
[3] Carlsberg Research Laboratory, J. C. Jacobsens Gade, 1799 Copenhagen, Denmark; anna.chailyan@gmail.com
* Correspondence: nhp@ssi.dk (N.T.); gh@ssi.dk (G.H.); Tel.: +45-3268-3268 (N.T. & G.H.)

Received: 30 December 2017; Accepted: 17 January 2018; Published: 21 January 2018

Abstract: Rheumatoid arthritis (RA) is a chronic systemic autoimmune disorder of unknown etiology, which is characterized by inflammation in the synovium and joint damage. Although the pathogenesis of RA remains to be determined, a combination of environmental (e.g., viral infections) and genetic factors influence disease onset. Especially genetic factors play a vital role in the onset of disease, as the heritability of RA is 50–60%, with the human leukocyte antigen (HLA) alleles accounting for at least 30% of the overall genetic risk. Some HLA-DR alleles encode a conserved sequence of amino acids, referred to as the shared epitope (SE) structure. By analyzing the structure of a HLA-DR molecule in complex with Epstein-Barr virus (EBV), the SE motif is suggested to play a vital role in the interaction of MHC II with the viral glycoprotein (gp) 42, an essential entry factor for EBV. EBV has been repeatedly linked to RA by several lines of evidence and, based on several findings, we suggest that EBV is able to induce the onset of RA in predisposed SE-positive individuals, by promoting entry of B-cells through direct contact between SE and gp42 in the entry complex.

Keywords: Epstein-Barr virus; glycoprotein 42; rheumatoid arthritis; shared epitope

---

1. Introduction

1.1. Rheumatoid Arthritis

Rheumatoid arthritis (RA) is a chronic systemic autoimmune disease of unknown etiology. If left untreated, the disease manifests as sustained synovitis and erosions of articular cartilage and surrounding bone, which causes joint damage, reduced mobility and decreased quality of life, as well as cardiovascular and other extra-articular complications [1,2]. The typical clinical presentation of RA is a symmetrical peripheral joint arthritis and progressive erosions of the affected joints [1,2]. The disease course of RA is highly variable; the course and the severity of the arthritis may vary from quite mild to extremely destructive, resulting in severe disability. Thus, in a limited group of RA individuals, the arthritis is self-limiting, however, most patients suffer from chronic arthritis. Besides causing significant clinical problems, RA is also responsible for substantial economic and social costs, particularly from work-related disability [3].

RA affects approximately 1–2% of the world's population with 5–50 new cases per 100,000 individuals annually [4,5]. The disorder is most typical in elderly people and women, with a female preponderance of 3:1 [6,7], and onset of the disease is most frequent between the ages of 40–50 [5], suggesting that hormonal factors could have a pathogenic role [7].

RA is diagnosed according to clinical manifestations supported by detection of the autoantibodies IgM/IgA rheumatoid factor (RF) and anti-citrullinated protein antibodies (ACPA) [8]. Being specific for the Fc region of IgGs, RFs are detected in approximately 50–90% of RA individuals, dependent on age [9–11]. Approximately 70–80% of RA individuals are ACPA positive, and as with RF, these antibodies are present early in the course of the disease and precede clinical onset [12–15]. Compared to RFs, ACPA are more RA-specific, as RFs also may be detected in individuals affected by infections, other autoimmune diseases, e.g., such as systemic lupus erythematosus (SLE), mixed connective tissue disease, Sjögren's syndrome, and occasionally in healthy individuals [16,17].

Antibodies recognizing epitopes with the modified amino acid residue citrulline (Cit), are referred to as ACPAs. These antibodies are primarily directed to citrullinated proteins located in the joints [18,19]. Citrullination, catalyzed by the calcium-dependent peptidyl arginine deiminase (PAD) enzymes, is a post-translational modification of arginine generated as a result of deimination [20], which physiologically occurs during apoptosis, inflammation or keratinization [21]. Under pathological conditions, where cell death may overwhelm the phagocytic capacity of phagocytes, necrotic cells may release PAD into the extracellular space, where higher calcium concentrations allow citrullination of other proteins located outside the cell [21]. Therefore, when the apoptotic cells are not cleared efficiently, such as in an inflammatory environment, intracellular proteins and/or PAD are released into the extracellular space, where the former are taken up by antigen-presenting cells and the latter induces citrullination of synovial joint proteins. Consequently, antibodies to various citrullinated proteins are locally produced in affected joints, where proteins are citrullinated during the inflammatory process [22]. Interestingly, ACPAs have been proposed to be involved in the pathogenesis of RA, although no exact mechanism has been determined [12,23].

Through the identification and characterization of ACPAs, and by novel insights into RA-diagnosis and etiopathology, it has become clear that RA is of heterogeneous nature, consisting of clinical subsets of ACPA-positive and ACPA-negative RA. These subsets share many clinical features, but differ with respect to genetic background, predisposing environmental factors and clinical progression/remission [14,24–26]. Consequently, individuals with ACPA-positive RA typically have severe symptoms and disease course, whereas individuals with ACPA-negative RA often experience a mild disease course [24,27–29].

1.2. Rheumatoid Arthritis and Genetic Risk Factors

Based on twin studies, it has been proposed that the relative contribution of genetic variation to the liability of developing RA is around 60% [2,30]. The strongest evidence for the influence of genetic factors on RA onset relates to major histocompability complex (MHC) class II antigens, and, in particular to various human leukocyte antigen (HLA) alleles, e.g., HLA-DR. HLA-DR is a MHC cell-surface receptor, which interacts with T-cell receptors through presentation of internalized antigens, which ultimately results in stimulation of T-cells and antibody-producing B-cells. Widely recognized alleles that are major contributors to RA risk at the DRB1 locus are DRB1*04:01, *04:04, *04:05, *04:08, 04:09, *01:01, *01:02, *10:01 and *14:02 (Table 1) [31].

Table 1. Classification of HLA-DRB1 alleles and their role relative to onset of rheumatoid arthritis. Highlighted alleles constitute the most frequently reported alleles associated with rheumatoid arthritis. The risk of developing rheumatoid arthritis is among others associated with the presence of specific amino acids in the amino acid positions 70–74. Crucial is the RAA motif in positions 72–74, but the effect is modulated by the amino acids in positions 71 and 70 as well, where K in position 71 confers the highest risk, R an intermediate risk, and A and E a lower risk. Similarly, the amino acids Q and R in position 70 confer a higher risk than D. Bold alleles represent the most common alleles detected in individuals with rheumatoid arthritis.

Sequence	SE Motif	Alleles	Relative Genotype Risk *	References
QKRAA	+	***04:01**, ***04:09**, *04:13, *04:16, *04:19, *04:21,*14:21	5.9	[32]
DKRAA	-	*13:03	5.9	[32]
QRRAA	+	***01:01**, ***01:02**, *01:05, ***04:04**, ***04:05**, ***04:08**, *04:10, *04:19, ***14:02**, 14:06, *14:09, *14:13, *14:17, *14:20	3.3	[31,32]
RRRAA	+	***10:01**	3.3	[32]
QRRAE	-	*04:03, *04:06, *04:07, *04:11, *04:17, *04:20	1	[33]
RRRAE	-	*09:01, *14:01, *14:04, *14:05, *14:07, *14:08, *14:10, *14:11, *14:14, *14:18	1	[33]
QARAA	-	*13:09, *15:01	1	[33]
QKRGR	-	*03:01, *04:22, *11:07	1	[33]
DRRGQ	-	*07:01	1	[33]
DRRAL	-	*08:01	1	[32]
DRRAA	-	*04:15, *08:05, *11:01, *11:04, *11:05, *11:06, *11:09, *11:10, *11:12, *11:15, *11:18, *11:19, *11:22, *12:01, *13:05, *13:06, *13:07, *13:11, *13:12, *13:14, *13:21, *13:25, *14:22, *16:01, *16:05	1	[31,32]
DERAA	-	*01:03, *04:02, *11:02, *11:03, *11:16, *11:20, *11:21, *13:01, *13:02, *13:04, *13:08, *13:15, *13:17, *13:19, *13:22, *13:23, *14:16, *15:01	1	[31,32]

* Relative to model proposed by Du Montcel et al. [33] when expressing two of the same HLA-DR1 alleles.

All of these HLA-DRB1 alleles share a common amino acid motif, referred to as the shared epitope (SE) [34]. In fact, it has been estimated that up to 50% of RA patients are positive for this amino acid motif [35]. Stastny originally documented an association between HLA-DR4 and the risk of developing RA [34]. Discrepancy in the association of different HLA-DRB1 genes revealed the presence of a conserved hexameric amino acid sequence in the third hypervariable regions of all RA-associated HLA-DRB1 alleles, involving amino acid positions 70–74 and consisting of glutamine (arginine), lysine (arginine), arginine, alanine and alanine "R/QK/RRAA", also referred to as the SE structure [34,35], although the most common sequence of amino acids in these positions is QKRAA. These residues constitute an α-helix (Figure 1), forming one side of the antigen-binding cleft, a site likely to affect antigen presentation. Especially position 70 of the SE has received attention, as glutamine or arginine in position 70 are critical for the risk of developing RA, whereas aspartic acid in that position appears to have a protective effect [36]. Although the SE structure is conserved in some alleles, further differentiations in the third hyper-variable region have been proposed. For example, HLA-DRB1 alleles can be discriminated in the amino acid region from 71 to 86 [37]. Other studies propose another classification focusing primarily on the positions 72–74 (RAA), which is modulated by the amino acid in position 71 (K confers the highest risk, R an intermediate risk, E and A a lower risk) and by the amino acid in position 70 (R or Q confers a higher risk than D) [33,38].

In addition to prior indications that aspartic acid in position 70 may reduce RA risk, it also appears to reduce disease severity. By analyzing the effect of the DERAA sequence (residues 70–74 encoded by several HLA-DRB1 alleles, including the RA-protective HLA-DRB1*04:02 allele) on disease outcomes in individuals with early arthritis, it has been found that in RA patients without early erosions, DERAA-coding DRB1 alleles are strongly protective against severe disease [39]. Similarly, alleles carrying Ile in position 67 appear to have a protective effect [40], whereas variants at position 11 and 13 in DRB1 have been proposed to predispose strongly to RA as well [41,42]. Furthermore, alleles such as HLA-DRB1*11:01, *11:04, *12:01 and *16:01 have been reported to be correlated with benign forms of RA [32].

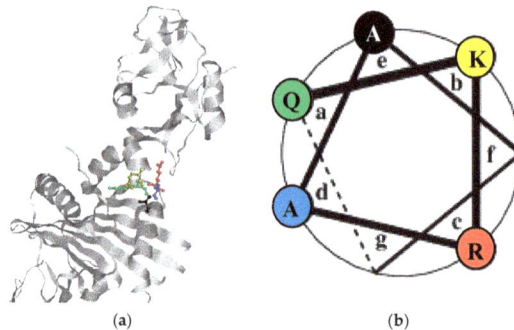

(a)   (b)

Figure 1. Structure analysis of the shared epitope motif in the HLA-DR1-gp42 complex. (**a**) The SE motif (amino acids 70–71) is located in an α-helix structure. The individual amino acids and their orientation is visualized by the following colors Q70 (green), K71 (yellow), R72 (red), A73 (blue), A74 black. A, K, Q, R represent the amino acids Ala, Lys, Gln and Arg. (**b**) Helical wheel of the SE motif. The left side of the wheel faces the peptide groove, the right side is on the "outside" of the helix. The heptad positions of the helix are labeled a–g, by convention.

Among the SE alleles, DRB*04:01 and *04:04 confer a stronger disposition to RA than DRB1*01:01 and *10:01 [40,42]. Similarly, DRB1*04:01 homozygosity and DRB1*04:01/*04:04 heterozygosity are associated with increased risk for RA [40]. The associations between HLA and RA have been analyzed mainly for the DR loci. However, the strong linkage disequilibrium between DR and DQ suggests that both DR and DQ may contribute to predisposition to RA.

Besides causing a predisposition to RA, the SE motif has been proposed to promote joint destruction and extra-articular involvement and even early mortality [43,44]. Interestingly, in Europeans, the association between DRB1 and RA is stronger in ACPA-positive RA than in ACPA-negative RA [15,40,41]. Thus, in RA individuals with heterozygosity and homozygosity of HLA-DRB1 SE alleles, ACPA production has been found to be significantly increased [15,40,41]. Similarly, the risk of developing RA is reduced in SE-negative individuals, although it has been proposed that exposure to maternal antigens (e.g., HLA molecules) in utero could contribute to RA development in SE-negative women [35].

The mechanism underlying SE-positive RA remains unclear [45–49]. It has been hypothesized that SE-positive DRB1 alleles confer disease susceptibility through a mechanism that involves alteration of the peripheral T-cell repertoire or through the selective presentation of arthritogenic self or foreign peptides [45–49]. In addition, it has been described that the DRB1*04:01 protein interacts with citrullinated peptides with higher affinity than with non-citrullinated peptides, which may indicate that the SE alleles exert pathogenic effects through the presentation of citrullinated peptides, which are recognized as non-self by T-cells [50]. Similarly, it has been found that the citrullinated DERAA motif, which is found in DRB1 alleles, including DRB1*13 may have a protective function [51]. This protective effect is, among others, ascribed to the cross-reactivity of self-reactive T-cells to the citrullinated motif [51]. Finally, it has been proposed that the SE, analogous to certain domains of class I MHC-molecules [52,53], acts as a ligand that interacts with cell surface calreticulin and activates innate immune signaling [54]. However, the exact role of SE in the onset of RA remains to be determined.

The second major polymorphism occurs in the *PTPN22* gene, which encodes the protein tyrosine phosphatase, non-receptor type 22, a tyrosine phosphatase of importance in T-cell signaling [55,56]. Interestingly, this gene is a genetic risk factor in other autoimmune diseases as well, e.g., the onset of type 1 diabetes, which correlates with an increased risk of developing type 1 diabetes in ACPA-positive RA individuals.

In general, the currently known genetic risk factors associated with RA are thought to be specifically associated with either ACPA-positive or ACPA-negative disease. Thus, ACPA-positive RA has been found to be closely linked to the presence of HLA-DRB1 alleles containing SE motifs [57,58] and polymorphisms in the *PTPN22* gene [56,57,59]. Moreover, ACPA-positive status has been suggested to be associated with the recently identified, but modest genetic risk factor tumor necrosis factor receptor-associated factor 1 (TRAF1)-C5 [60]. Other genetic factors such as variations in the interferon-regulating factor (IRF)-5 and polymorphisms in a newly identified risk gene in the C-type lectin complex have been suggested to be associated with ACPA-negative RA disease [61,62].

Additional genetic risk factors have been proposed, including PAD4, signal transducer and activator of transcription (STAT4), cluster of differentiation 244 (CD244) and cytotoxic T lymphocyte-associated antigen 4 (CTLA4), located outside the MHC [63].

1.3. Rheumatoid Arthritis and Environmental Risk Factors

Various environmental factors have been linked to the onset of RA, e.g., infectious agents and smoking [64–66]. Among several environmental factors, which are implicated in the onset of RA, infectious agents have been suggested to be the most likely culprits [65]. A variety of viral candidates has been proposed, e.g., Epstein-Barr virus (EBV), Parvovirus B19 and Rubella virus. Moreover, some bacterial candidates have been linked to the onset of RA as well, e.g., *Proteus mirabillis* [65] and *Porphyromonas gingivalis* [67]. The latter are both gram-negative anaerobic bacteria, but *Proteus mirabillis* is primarily associated with urinary tract infection, whereas *P. gingivalis* primarily is associated with periodontal disease. Interestingly, *P. gingivalis* is the only bacterium known so far to contain a PAD enzyme, which is involved in citrullination of both bacterial and human proteins in periodontal tissue [68,69]. Moreover, RA is prevalent in individuals with chronic periodontitis [70]. Based on these findings it has been suggested that *P. gingivalis* can potentially contribute to the generation of de novo epitopes that may trigger the formation of ACPA. Several reviews nicely illustrate the connection between RA, ACPA and bacterial PAD [71,72]. Nevertheless, contradictory data have been published regarding the correlation between the levels of antibodies against *P. gingivalis* and ACPA in RA individuals [69,73,74]. ACPA might be produced outside the joint in mucosal sites such as the lung and gingiva. Consequently, ACPA might cross-react through molecular mimicry with citrullinated epitopes in the joint initiating an inflammatory response in genetically susceptible individuals. Cigarette smoking constitutes the main environmental risk for development of RA. It is well established that cigarette smoking significantly increases the risk of RA [75–77]. Although it remains to be determined exactly how cigarette smoking induces the onset of RA and the pathogenic effect of smoking, several mechanisms have been proposed to understand the role of cigarette smoking in RA [75–77]. Smoking is known to modulate the immune system through many mechanisms, including the induction of the inflammatory response, immune suppression, alteration of cytokine balances and induction of apoptosis. In addition, recent studies ascribe an inhibitory effect of smoking on RA treatment, as the response and drug survival in RA patients treated with anti-tumor necrosis factor therapy is reduced in heavy smokers [78]. No sole mechanism, however, has been linked to RA, which therefore complicates full comprehension of the smoking effect [75]. A profound gene-environment interaction between smoking and HLA-DR SE genes as risk factors is evident. In individuals who are HLA-DR SE-negative, smoking is a relatively modest risk factor, however, in individuals who carry one or two sets of the SE genes, smoking dramatically increases the risk of developing RA [71,79]. A similar picture applies to the risk of developing ACPA-positive RA, although the risk primarily applies to individuals having two sets of the SE alleles [80]. A report from the Swedish population-based case-control study Epidemiologic Investigation of Rheumatoid Arthritis (EIRA), in which RA cases are recruited within one year of disease onset, found that smokers, who do not carry the SE, have a 1.5-fold elevated risk of developing ACPA-positive RA over non-smokers, who also do not carry the SE. The risk of developing

ACPA and RA for an individual who smokes and carries two copies of the SE is 21-fold higher than for non-smokers who do not carry the SE [80]. Based on these findings, it has been hypothesized that the influence of genes on the susceptibility of RA might be highly dependent on which environmental factors are present [71,79,80].

Other potential environmental risk factors proposed include alcohol intake, coffee intake, vitamin D status, oral contraceptive use and low socioeconomic status, although supporting evidence for these other factors is weak [81].

1.4. Epstein-Barr Virus

EBV has been proposed to be involved in the onset of numerous diseases, e.g., mononucleosis and connective tissue diseases such as SLE and RA [82–84].

EBV is a member of the human herpes virus family. It is an enveloped virus with a 172 kB double-stranded DNA genome coding for 87 proteins and a number of non-coding RNAs. EBV infects pharyngeal epithelial cells upon the first encounter with a host, whereafter it establishes a latent infection in (memory) B-cells [84]. EBV has an elaborate set of glycoproteins (gPs) in its host-derived lipid envelope together with a set of host-derived cellular membrane proteins, which depends on the infected cell. The viral set of gPs constitutes an efficient entry complex and the combination of viral gPs and host-derived envelope proteins enables EBV to switch between B-cells and epithelial cells and to infect several other cell types, including T cells, NK cells and others. EBV furthermore has very efficient immune evasion and exhaustion abilities, including its ability to switch between latent infection, with minimal viral gene expression and lytic infection, with extensive viral gene expression and active virus production. These properties make EBV a constant challenge for the host immune system and it plays an important role in several related diseases, including autoimmune rheumatic diseases. In these diseases, the viral gPs play several roles, notably during entry of target cells, which occurs by an ordered sequence of events. Initially, viral envelope proteins interact with target cell receptors and the viral envelope may then fuse with the plasma membrane (e.g., epithelial cells) or the virus may be endocytosed followed by (pH induced) fusion of the viral envelope with the endosome membrane (e.g., B-cells). In the case of B-cell infection, 5 viral gPs play a major role; gP350/220 interacts with CD21 and gp42 interacts with MHCII, while gB and gH/gL promote membrane fusion (Figure 2). In addition, complement activation products (e.g., C3d) bound to the viral surface may promote interaction by binding to B-cell CR2 (CD21) and the B-cell receptor of memory B-cells may increase interaction, if it has affinity for a viral envelope protein. All this equips EBV with a high tropism for (memory) B-cells and gp42 plays a central role by its interaction with MHCII on B-cells [85–90].

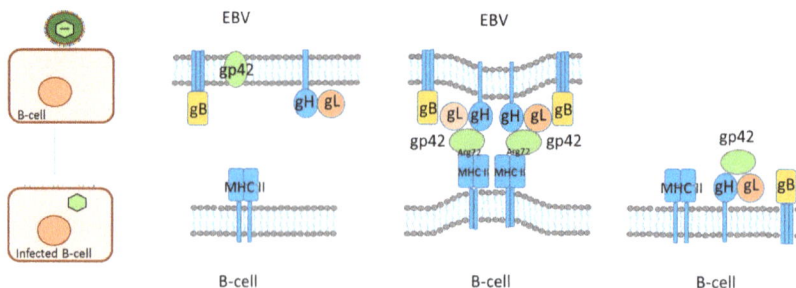

Figure 2. Epstein-Barr B-cell fusion model. Rough sketch of EBV fusing with the cellular lipid bilayer of B-cells. For gp42 to become active, the protein is cleaved N-terminally. Gp42 interacts with gH/gL, and the complex interacts with gB. Gp42 interacts with the β1 domain of MHC-II, which ultimately results in membrane fusion.

1.4.1. Glycoprotein 42, Characteristics and Interactions

EBV gp42 is one of the smallest gPs (223 amino acids) involved in EBV attachment to host B-cells. Although of limited size, this protein is extremely important for B-cell infection, as EBV entry into B-cells requires binding of gp42 to HLA class II. Consequently, virus lacking gp42 can only interact with human B-cells, but cannot infect them [91,92]. Similarly, the amount of gp42 present on the virion determines the cell type that EBV infects [91,92].

EBV gp42 is unique to EBV, but sequence homologs among the closely related primate lymphocryptoviruses and homologs in other herpesviruses exist [93]. The protein contains an N-terminal domain of approximately 100 amino acids and a C-terminal C-type lectin domain (CTLD) [94,95]. While the relatively small, but flexible, N-terminal region interacts with gH/gL, the CTLD interacts with HLA class II. A hydrophobic pocket is located in the CTLD, which appears to be important for its ability to trigger membrane fusion subsequent to HLA class II binding. Mutations in the pocket appear to inhibit fusion, but not binding to gH/gL or HLA, confirming its functional importance in B-cell fusion [96]. Findings by Janz and Haan indicate that the pocket undergoes small structural changes upon interaction with HLA, which could be important for triggering membrane fusion [97,98]. In addition, gp42 contains a transmembrane domain spanning residues 9–29, with its C-terminus on the external side of the membrane [93,99].

EBV gp42 occurs in two forms in infected cells, a full-length membrane-bound form and a soluble form, generated by proteolytic cleavage, that is secreted from infected cells due to loss of the N-terminal transmembrane domain. Both the full-length and the secreted gp42 forms bind to gH/g and HLA class II, however, the functional significance of gp42 cleavage is currently unclear [100,101].

Interestingly, gp42 appears to act as a tropism switch that directs fusion with B-cells and inhibits fusion with epithelial cells, a process mediated through its interactions with gH/gL [91]. Similarly, infected B-cells have reduced amounts of gp42 due to sequestration by cellular HLA class II, whereas infected epithelial cells have higher amounts of gp42, as these cells normally do not contain HLA class II [91]. Consequently, virus originating in epithelial cells efficiently infects B-cells, whereas B-cell-derived EBV more efficiently infects epithelial cells [91].

EBV gp42 plays multiple roles during infection, including acting as a co-receptor for viral entry into B-cells by interacting with HLA class II, and binding to EBV gPs gH and gL during the process of membrane fusion, which together with gB constitute the core proteins for EBV entry into cells. gp42 forms a stable, high affinity complex with gH/gL [102]. The residues 36–81 of the N-terminal region of gp42 are critical for the interaction between gp42 and gH/gL. Studies by Kirschner and colleagues have proposed that the N-terminal region interacts with gH/gL by contact through amino acids 44–61 and 67–81 with high molecular affinity in a hairpin-like conformation [103,104]. A current theory is that the gH/gL complex primarily acts as a regulator of gB activation rather than having a direct function in driving membrane fusion [105], which ultimately leads to initiation of membrane fusion.

In contrast to the gH/gL complex, which primarily interacts with the N-terminal domain of gp42, the β-chain of HLA class II binds to the CTLD, more specifically to amino acids 94–221. HLA class II consists of two distinct peptide chains, which non-covalently hetero-dimerize. As a result of this 1:1 interaction, a peptide binding groove is formed by an eight-stranded pleated sheet supporting two helices. However, the interaction between HLA class II and gp42 is not restricted to this binding groove, but to the β-chain of HLA. In fact, gp42 interacts exclusively with the β-1 domain to one side of the peptide binding groove [106]. Studies by McShane and colleagues showed that a soluble form of gp42 generated stable interactions with HLA class II and that especially glutamic acid 46 and arginine 72 in HLA class II were essential for reactivity, which is in accordance to crystal structure analyses of the gp42: HLA-DR1 complex [106,107].

1.4.2. Epstein-Barr Virus as a Contributor to Initiation of Rheumatoid Arthritis

Several studies point to an association between EBV and RA [108–112], thus EBV infection has been considered to be one of the environmental factors that contribute to the onset of RA.

It has been demonstrated that individuals with RA display serological signs of EBV infections, e.g., have elevated antibody levels to latent and replicative EBV proteins, e.g., Epstein-Barr viral capsid antigen, early antigen, EBNA-1 and EBNA-2 [109,112–115]. Moreover, it has been shown that individuals with RA are less efficient in neutralizing autologous EBV-infected cells and prone to have significantly higher numbers of circulating EBV-infected B-cells [108,116,117] and that individuals with RA have elevated viral EBV DNA load compared to controls [109,118–120]. Other studies indicate the EBV is associated with RA through molecular mimicry, where antibodies to an EBV-encoded protein (gp110) has sequence homology with the QKRAA motif of the HLA-DR4 [108,121,122]. In addition, individuals with RA have an increased risk of experiencing EBV-associated lymphoma, due to the presence of EBV in a latent stage in the B-cells of RA individuals, supporting the hypothesis that EBV is associated with RA [123,124].

Nevertheless, other studies claim that no association between EBV infection and onset of RA is evident [110,125,126]. For example, findings by Sherina and colleagues, analyzing anti-viral antibodies in relation of ACPAs, smoking HLA-DRB1 alleles and clinical parameters, do not support the hypothesis of EBV involvement in RA onset [126]. These findings are supported by similar studies analyzing antibody levels to several viral proteins [110]. Other findings do not support the hypothesis that EBV infection predisposes to the development of RA, but indicate that EBV infection is associates with other autoimmune diseases such as SLE [125].

These differences between studies describing whether EBV is involved in the onset of RA may be related to differences in cohorts applied and assays used for analysis. Furthermore, the presented studies are conducted using sera from individuals infected with EBV, as up to 99% of humans are infected with EBV, making it very difficult to analyze EBV-negative RA individuals.

2. Discussion

HLA-DR1 and Gp42 Interaction as a Mediator or EBV Entry and Ultimately Onset of SE-Positive Rheumatoid Arthritis

HLA-DR was originally shown to interact with gp42 in an expression library screen for proteins binding to a soluble gp42Fc construct [127]. Subsequent studies demonstrated that the interaction between gp42 and HLA-DR is crucial for EBV infection in B-cells, since monoclonal antibodies to gp42 as well as HLA-DR inhibited B-cell infection in vitro [128]. EBV infects B-cells in vivo through an entry complex, which among others involves the viral gPs, gH, gL, gB and gp42, with gp42 constituting a key factor in activating membrane fusion and hence triggering virus entry (Figure 2) [89,129]. In this process, gp42 interacts with both the viral gH/gL complex and MHC II, which is crucial for EBV entry [127,129–131]. Gp42 binds to the β1 domain of the HLA molecule to one side of the peptide binding groove [106]. The specific interaction buries a total surface area of 1002 Å^2 and constitutes primarily hydrophilic and charged residues. Thorough analysis of the crystal structure of gp42 in complex with HLA-DR1 reveals specific key amino acids (Figure 3), which are characterized as crucial for this interaction. R72 and E46 of HLA-DR1 make extensive interactions with gp42 and substitution analyses confirm that these amino acids are essential for reactivity [107]. E46 is located in the N-terminal end of a strand in the β1 domain at the outer base of the MHC peptide binding groove, whereas R72 is located on the outer face of the second β1 domain α-helix (Figure 3). The crystal structure of the gp42: HLA-DR1 complex reveals that E46 of HLA is directly in contact with R220 and Y107 of gp42 through a salt bridge and a hydrogen bond, respectively, whereas R72 interacts with T104 and Y107 of gp42 through hydrogen bonding [106]. The interaction of R72 with T104 and Y107 forms part of the binding site for E46, which cooperatively link gp42 recognition of E46 and R72, thus a precise positioning of R72 is essential for generating a stable interaction between E46 and R220 of gp42, which has been confirmed by substitution studies [107].

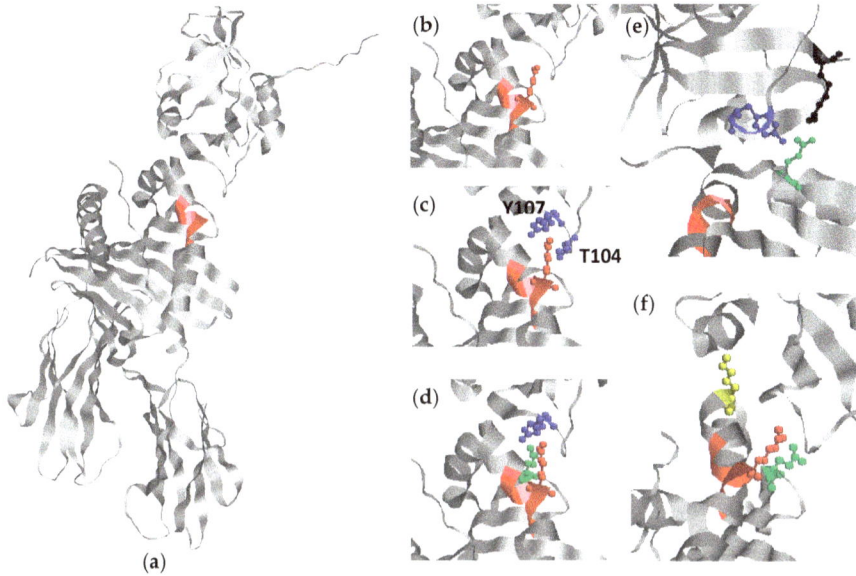

Figure 3. Interactions between gp42 and HLA-DR1: (**a**) crystal structure of the HLA-DR1 and gp42 complex. The shared epitope backbone structure (amino acids 70–74) is colored in red; (**b**) location of Arg72 in the shared epitope; (**c**) interaction between Arg72 (HLA-DR1) and T104 (blue) and Y107 (blue) of gp42; (**d**) interaction between E46 (green) and Arg72 (red) (HLA-DR1) and Y107 (blue) (gp42) through a salt bridge and hydrogen bonding, respectively; (**e**) interaction between E46 (green) (HLA-DRB1) and R220 (black) and Y107 (blue) (gp42); and (**f**) location of E46 (green), I67 (yellow), R72 (red) in HLA-DRB1.

Based on the current description of the EBV gp42-HLA-DRB1 interaction, we hypothesize that R72, which is part of the SE structure located at amino acid positions 70–74 of HLA-DRB1, is directly related to EBV entry. Hence, EBV infection, through specific interactions between gp42 and HLA alleles, might ultimately contribute to the onset of RA. This hypothesis is supported by several findings.

Although the amino acid E46 is not directly related to the SE motif, are the amino acids E46 and R72 of HLA crucial for a stable interaction to gp42 [106,107]. Site-directed mutations of E46 to V, Q or K, reveal that nonfunctional HLA molecules are generated which do not promote EBV entry [130]. Nevertheless, substitution of E46 to aspartic acid does not appear to affect the ability to induce entry, indicating that a negative charge in this position, and hence the presence of a salt bridge, is crucial for interaction in this position. Similarly, R72A and R72E mutants are not able to interact with gp42, which confirm the importance of the extensive interaction of R72 with gp42 in the gp42:HLA-DR1 crystal structure and establish this residue as crucial in mediating interaction and ultimately EBV entry [107]. This may be explained by that in the absence of R72 (or the lack of a precise presentation of R72) no scaffold for E46 is generated, as previously mentioned, and hence the crucial ionic bond between E46 and R220 of gp42 is not established (Figure 3).

The importance of the E46 and R72 for a stable interaction is confirmed when analyzing HLA alleles, which shows that E46 is completely conserved in HLA-DP sequences and only a single allelic change of E46 is found within DR sequences (to aspartic acid), which has very little effect on EBV entry [130]. Likewise, R72 is predominantly conserved in HLA-DR and completely conserved in HLA-DQ and -DP sequences [106]. These findings are in accordance to that EBV also can use the other two HLA class II isotypes-DP and DQ to gain entry into B-cells [97].

Especially R72, being part of the SE structure, has been found to be essential in predisposing to RA, as illustrated in Table 1. Nevertheless, the residues surrounding R72 are not conserved, but have a profound influence on the MHC II-gp42 interaction by influencing the geometry of R72 and also the stability of the MHC molecule. Studies illustrate that a double mutation of residues 71 and 74 still mediated entry [130]. These findings are in accordance to analyses of the crystal structure of the MHC II: gp42 complex, where no specific interaction between amino acids 70–71 and 73–74 of HLA and gp42 has been identified [106]. Modifying the surrounding amino acids may also affect the peptide structure and ultimately the peptide binding groove. Some studies have suggested that these structural modifications are based more on the charge of the relevant amino acid than on the amino acid sequences and in particular on the charge of the amino acids at positions 70, 71 and 74 [132]. Further studies by Rosloniec and colleagues showed that alleles, which share the RRAA and the KRAA motif, have different binding affinities, although they have the same charge [133]. Thus, physico-chemical properties rather than the specific electric charge appear to be essential for interactions. These findings are in accordance to that the mere presence of R72 not is sufficient for predisposing RA, as HLA-alleles that are negative for the SE motif, but positive for R72, do not predispose to RA. Based on the findings by Ou and Rosloniec, we propose that the crucial amino acids found in the SE motif most likely contribute to ensure a stable α-helix structure, favoring optimal presentation of R72 protruding into the gp42 binding pocket composed by amino acid positions 104–107 of gp42, in combination with providing a peptide scaffold, which is essential for E46 presentation and binding as well (Figure 3). If one or more of these interactions is absent, the HLA allele interacts more weakly with gp42 and supports EBV entry less efficiently [106,107]. This has been proposed by Mullen and colleagues, although it remains to be verified [106]. Moreover, the proposed theory may explain why e.g., the motif DKRAA predisposes to RA, whereas the DRRAA motif does not, as physico-chemical interactions between the amino acids in positions 70 and 71 in the latter are different from the DKRAA motif; although R and K provide the same electric charge, do they contribute differently to the physico-chemical interaction, as the positive charge in R is arranged differently from K due to the specific side chains. Modification in the physico-chemical interactions within the motif may crook the α-helix structure of the SE motif (Figure 1), which may change the protruding presentation of R72 and ultimately reduce the interaction between R72 and gp42. However, structural studies alone may be insufficient to explain completely the role of gp42 and the various RA-promoting and -protecting MHC II forms, since EBV tethering and infection is a highly dynamic process. This view is supported by preliminary molecular dynamics calculations, which indicate that the physical stability of gp42-MHC II complexes cannot alone account for the observed RA susceptibility (unpublished results), although SE residues are clearly crucial for the interaction.

Based on the current findings described in this article, the mentioned studies and observations support the hypothesis that HLA-gp42 interaction in predisposed SE-positive individuals facilitates EBV entry and infection, which ultimately may result in uncontrolled EBV infection (especially in joints, where EBV may drive processes normally restricted to lymph nodes, i.e., antigen uptake and presentation, cytokine release and lymphocyte interactions) and thus in the onset of RA. EBV infects all individuals, as all natural MHC II variants (human) can interact with gp42. However, the interaction with SE-positive MHC II, seems to support EBV entry more efficiently.

The exact mechanism underlying SE-positive RA remains unclear [45–49]. It has been proposed that SE-positive DRB1 alleles confer disease susceptibility through a mechanism that involves alteration of the peripheral T-cell repertoire or through the selective presentation of arthritogenic self or foreign peptides [45–49]. Moreover, it has been proposed that SE-positive HLA alleles exert pathogenic effects through the presentation of citrullinated peptides, which are recognized as non-self by T-cells [50]. Finally, it has been proposed that the SE, analogous to certain domains of class I MHC-molecules [52,53], acts as a ligand that interacts with cell surface calreticulin and activates innate immune signaling [54]. None of the mentioned mechanisms are contradictory in relation to the current hypothesis proposed, and the onset of RA may turn out to involve an interplay between several of these mechanisms.

Author Contributions: Anna Chailyan, Paolo Marcatili and Jose Izarzugaza conducted the energy calculations for the HLA-DRB1 and gp42 interaction. Nicole Trier and Gunnar Houen wrote the manuscript.

Conflicts of Interest: The authors declare no conflict of interest.

Abbreviations

ACPA	Anti-citrullinated protein antibodies
CD	Cluster of differentiation
CTLA	Cytotoxic T lymphocyte-associated antigen
CTLD	C-type lectin domain
EBV	Epstein-Barr virus
Gp	Glycoprotein
HLA	Human leukocyte antigen
IRF	Interferon-regulating factor
MHC	Major histocompability complex
PTPN22	Protein tyrosine phosphatase, non-receptor type 22
PAD	Peptidyl arginine deiminase
RA	Rheumatoid arthritis
RF	Rheumatoid factor
SE	Shared epitope
SLE	Systemic lupus erythematosus
STAT	Signal transducer and activator of transcription
TRAF	Tumor necrosis factor receptor-associated factor

References

1. Cooles, F.A.; Isaacs, J.D. Pathophysiology of rheumatoid arthritis. *Curr. Opin. Rheumatol.* **2011**, *23*, 233–240. [CrossRef] [PubMed]
2. Scott, D.L.; Wolfe, F.; Huizinga, T.W. Rheumatoid arthritis. *Lancet* **2010**, *376*, 1094–1108. [CrossRef]
3. Cooper, N.J. Economic burden of rheumatoid arthritis: A systematic review. *Rheumatology* **2000**, *39*, 28–33. [CrossRef] [PubMed]
4. Carbonell, J.; Cobo, T.; Balsa, A.; Descalzo, M.A.; Carmona, L.; Group, S.S. The incidence of rheumatoid arthritis in spain: Results from a nationwide primary care registry. *Rheumatology* **2008**, *47*, 1088–1092. [CrossRef] [PubMed]
5. Pedersen, J.K.; Kjaer, N.K.; Svendsen, A.J.; Horslev-Petersen, K. Incidence of rheumatoid arthritis from 1995 to 2001: Impact of ascertainment from multiple sources. *Rheumatol. Int.* **2009**, *29*, 411–415. [CrossRef] [PubMed]
6. Sangha, O. Epidemiology of rheumatic diseases. *Rheumatology* **2000**, *39*, 3–12. [CrossRef] [PubMed]
7. Symmons, D.; Turner, G.; Webb, R.; Asten, P.; Barrett, E.; Lunt, M.; Scott, D.; Silman, A. The prevalence of rheumatoid arthritis in the united kingdom: New estimates for a new century. *Rheumatology* **2002**, *41*, 793–800. [CrossRef] [PubMed]
8. Aletaha, D.; Neogi, T.; Silman, A.J.; Funovits, J.; Felson, D.T.; Bingham, C.O., 3rd; Birnbaum, N.S.; Burmester, G.R.; Bykerk, V.P.; Cohen, M.D.; et al. 2010 rheumatoid arthritis classification criteria: An American college of rheumatology/european league against rheumatism collaborative initiative. *Arthritis Rheumatol.* **2010**, *62*, 2569–2581. [CrossRef] [PubMed]
9. Dorner, T.; Egerer, K.; Feist, E.; Burmester, G.R. Rheumatoid factor revisited. *Curr. Opin. Rheumatol.* **2004**, *16*, 246–253. [CrossRef] [PubMed]
10. Nishimura, K.; Sugiyama, D.; Kogata, Y.; Tsuji, G.; Nakazawa, T.; Kawano, S.; Saigo, K.; Morinobu, A.; Koshiba, M.; Kuntz, K.M.; et al. Meta-analysis: Diagnostic accuracy of anti-cyclic citrullinated peptide antibody and rheumatoid factor for rheumatoid arthritis. *Ann. Intern. Med.* **2007**, *146*, 797–808. [CrossRef] [PubMed]
11. Shmerling, R.H.; Delbanco, T.L. The rheumatoid factor: An analysis of clinical utility. *Am. J. Med.* **1991**, *91*, 528–534. [CrossRef]

12. Rantapaa-Dahlqvist, S.; de Jong, B.A.; Berglin, E.; Hallmans, G.; Wadell, G.; Stenlund, H.; Sundin, U.; van Venrooij, W.J. Antibodies against cyclic citrullinated peptide and IgA rheumatoid factor predict the development of rheumatoid arthritis. *Arthritis Rheumatol.* **2003**, *48*, 2741–2749. [CrossRef] [PubMed]

13. Ronnelid, J.; Wick, M.C.; Lampa, J.; Lindblad, S.; Nordmark, B.; Klareskog, L.; van Vollenhoven, R.F. Longitudinal analysis of citrullinated protein/peptide antibodies (anti-cp) during 5 year follow up in early rheumatoid arthritis: Anti-cp status predicts worse disease activity and greater radiological progression. *Ann. Rheum. Dis.* **2005**, *64*, 1744–1749. [CrossRef] [PubMed]

14. Schellekens, G.A.; Visser, H.; de Jong, B.A.; van den Hoogen, F.H.; Hazes, J.M.; Breedveld, F.C.; van Venrooij, W.J. The diagnostic properties of rheumatoid arthritis antibodies recognizing a cyclic citrullinated peptide. *Arthritis Rheumatol.* **2000**, *43*, 155–163. [CrossRef]

15. Van Gaalen, F.A.; Linn-Rasker, S.P.; van Venrooij, W.J.; de Jong, B.A.; Breedveld, F.C.; Verweij, C.L.; Toes, R.E.; Huizinga, T.W. Autoantibodies to cyclic citrullinated peptides predict progression to rheumatoid arthritis in patients with undifferentiated arthritis: A prospective cohort study. *Arthritis Rheumatol.* **2004**, *50*, 709–715. [CrossRef] [PubMed]

16. Nell, V.P.; Machold, K.P.; Stamm, T.A.; Eberl, G.; Heinzl, H.; Uffmann, M.; Smolen, J.S.; Steiner, G. Autoantibody profiling as early diagnostic and prognostic tool for rheumatoid arthritis. *Ann. Rheum. Dis.* **2005**, *64*, 1731–1736. [CrossRef] [PubMed]

17. Payet, J.; Goulvestre, C.; Biale, L.; Avouac, J.; Wipff, J.; Job-Deslandre, C.; Batteux, F.; Dougados, M.; Kahan, A.; Allanore, Y. Anticyclic citrullinated peptide antibodies in rheumatoid and nonrheumatoid rheumatic disorders: Experience with 1162 patients. *J. Rheumatol.* **2014**, *41*, 2395–2402. [CrossRef] [PubMed]

18. Baeten, D.; Peene, I.; Union, A.; Meheus, L.; Sebbag, M.; Serre, G.; Veys, E.M.; de Keyser, F. Specific presence of intracellular citrullinated proteins in rheumatoid arthritis synovium: Relevance to antifilaggrin autoantibodies. *Arthritis Rheumatol.* **2001**, *44*, 2255–2262. [CrossRef]

19. Snir, O.; Widhe, M.; Hermansson, M.; von Spee, C.; Lindberg, J.; Hensen, S.; Lundberg, K.; Engstrom, A.; Venables, P.J.; Toes, R.E.; et al. Antibodies to several citrullinated antigens are enriched in the joints of rheumatoid arthritis patients. *Arthritis Rheumatol.* **2010**, *62*, 44–52. [CrossRef] [PubMed]

20. Tarcsa, E.; Marekov, L.N.; Mei, G.; Melino, G.; Lee, S.C.; Steinert, P.M. Protein unfolding by peptidylarginine deiminase. Substrate specificity and structural relationships of the natural substrates trichohyalin and filaggrin. *J. Biol. Chem.* **1996**, *271*, 30709–30716. [CrossRef] [PubMed]

21. Gyorgy, B.; Toth, E.; Tarcsa, E.; Falus, A.; Buzas, E.I. Citrullination: A posttranslational modification in health and disease. *Int. J. Biochem. Cell Biol.* **2006**, *38*, 1662–1677. [CrossRef] [PubMed]

22. Reparon-Schuijt, C.C.; van Esch, W.J.; van Kooten, C.; Schellekens, G.A.; de Jong, B.A.; van Venrooij, W.J.; Breedveld, F.C.; Verweij, C.L. Secretion of anti-citrulline-containing peptide antibody by b lymphocytes in rheumatoid arthritis. *Arthritis Rheumatol.* **2001**, *44*, 41–47. [CrossRef]

23. Kuhn, K.A.; Kulik, L.; Tomooka, B.; Braschler, K.J.; Arend, W.P.; Robinson, W.H.; Holers, V.M. Antibodies against citrullinated proteins enhance tissue injury in experimental autoimmune arthritis. *J. Clin. Investig.* **2006**, *116*, 961–973. [CrossRef] [PubMed]

24. Van der Helm-van Mil, A.H.; Verpoort, K.N.; Breedveld, F.C.; Toes, R.E.; Huizinga, T.W. Antibodies to citrullinated proteins and differences in clinical progression of rheumatoid arthritis. *Arthritis Res. Ther.* **2005**, *7*, R949–R958. [CrossRef] [PubMed]

25. Van der Woude, D.; Young, A.; Jayakumar, K.; Mertens, B.J.; Toes, R.E.; van der Heijde, D.; Huizinga, T.W.; van der Helm-van Mil, A.H. Prevalence of and predictive factors for sustained disease-modifying antirheumatic drug-free remission in rheumatoid arthritis: Results from two large early arthritis cohorts. *Arthritis Rheumatol.* **2009**, *60*, 2262–2271. [CrossRef] [PubMed]

26. Verpoort, K.N.; van Gaalen, F.A.; van der Helm-van Mil, A.H.; Schreuder, G.M.; Breedveld, F.C.; Huizinga, T.W.; de Vries, R.R.; Toes, R.E. Association of HLA-DR3 with anti-cyclic citrullinated peptide antibody-negative rheumatoid arthritis. *Arthritis Rheumatol.* **2005**, *52*, 3058–3062. [CrossRef] [PubMed]

27. Berglin, E.; Johansson, T.; Sundin, U.; Jidell, E.; Wadell, G.; Hallmans, G.; Rantapaa-Dahlqvist, S. Radiological outcome in rheumatoid arthritis is predicted by presence of antibodies against cyclic citrullinated peptide before and at disease onset, and by iga-rf at disease onset. *Ann. Rheum. Dis.* **2006**, *65*, 453–458. [CrossRef] [PubMed]

28. Machold, K.P.; Stamm, T.A.; Nell, V.P.; Pflugbeil, S.; Aletaha, D.; Steiner, G.; Uffmann, M.; Smolen, J.S. Very recent onset rheumatoid arthritis: Clinical and serological patient characteristics associated with radiographic progression over the first years of disease. *Rheumatology* **2007**, *46*, 342–349. [CrossRef] [PubMed]

29. Quinn, M.A.; Gough, A.K.; Green, M.J.; Devlin, J.; Hensor, E.M.; Greenstein, A.; Fraser, A.; Emery, P. Anti-ccp antibodies measured at disease onset help identify seronegative rheumatoid arthritis and predict radiological and functional outcome. *Rheumatology* **2006**, *45*, 478–480. [CrossRef] [PubMed]

30. MacGregor, A.J.; Snieder, H.; Rigby, A.S.; Koskenvuo, M.; Kaprio, J.; Aho, K.; Silman, A.J. Characterizing the quantitative genetic contribution to rheumatoid arthritis using data from twins. *Arthritis Rheumatol.* **2000**, *43*, 30–37. [CrossRef]

31. Zanelli, E.; Breedveld, F.C.; de Vries, R.R. Hla class II association with rheumatoid arthritis: Facts and interpretations. *Hum. Immunol.* **2000**, *61*, 1254–1261. [CrossRef]

32. Gourraud, P.A.; Boyer, J.F.; Barnetche, T.; Abbal, M.; Cambon-Thomsen, A.; Cantagrel, A.; Constantin, A. A new classification of HLA-DRB1 alleles differentiates predisposing and protective alleles for rheumatoid arthritis structural severity. *Arthritis Rheumatol.* **2006**, *54*, 593–599. [CrossRef] [PubMed]

33. Du Montcel, S.T.; Michou, L.; Petit-Teixeira, E.; Osorio, J.; Lemaire, I.; Lasbleiz, S.; Pierlot, C.; Quillet, P.; Bardin, T.; Prum, B.; et al. New classification of HLA-DRB1 alleles supports the shared epitope hypothesis of rheumatoid arthritis susceptibility. *Arthritis Rheumatol.* **2005**, *52*, 1063–1068. [CrossRef] [PubMed]

34. Stastny, P. Mixed lymphocyte cultures in rheumatoid arthritis. *J. Clin. Investig.* **1976**, *57*, 1148–1157. [CrossRef] [PubMed]

35. Holoshitz, J. The rheumatoid arthritis HLA-DRB1 shared epitope. *Curr. Opin. Rheumatol.* **2010**, *22*, 293–298. [CrossRef] [PubMed]

36. Mattey, D.L.; Dawes, P.T.; Gonzalez-Gay, M.A.; Garcia-Porrua, C.; Thomson, W.; Hajeer, A.H.; Ollier, W.E. HLA-DRB1 alleles encoding an aspartic acid at position 70 protect against development of rheumatoid arthritis. *J. Rheumatol.* **2001**, *28*, 232–239. [PubMed]

37. Gao, X.; Gazit, E.; Livneh, A.; Stastny, P. Rheumatoid arthritis in Israeli Jews: Shared sequences in the third hypervariable region of DRB1 alleles are associated with susceptibility. *J. Rheumatol.* **1991**, *18*, 801–803. [PubMed]

38. Michou, L.; Croiseau, P.; Petit-Teixeira, E.; du Montcel, S.T.; Lemaire, I.; Pierlot, C.; Osorio, J.; Frigui, W.; Lasbleiz, S.; Quillet, P.; et al. Validation of the reshaped shared epitope HLA-DRB1 classification in rheumatoid arthritis. *Arthritis Res. Ther.* **2006**, *8*, R79. [CrossRef] [PubMed]

39. Carrier, N.; Cossette, P.; Daniel, C.; de Brum-Fernandes, A.; Liang, P.; Menard, H.A.; Boire, G. The deraa HLA-DR alleles in patients with early polyarthritis: Protection against severe disease and lack of association with rheumatoid arthritis autoantibodies. *Arthritis Rheumatol.* **2009**, *60*, 698–707. [CrossRef] [PubMed]

40. Mackie, S.L.; Taylor, J.C.; Martin, S.G.; Consortium, Y.; Consortium, U.; Wordsworth, P.; Steer, S.; Wilson, A.G.; Worthington, J.; Emery, P.; et al. A spectrum of susceptibility to rheumatoid arthritis within HLA-DRB1: Stratification by autoantibody status in a large UK population. *Genes Immun.* **2012**, *13*, 120–128. [CrossRef] [PubMed]

41. Morgan, A.W.; Thomson, W.; Martin, S.G.; Yorkshire Early Arthritis Register Consortium; Carter, A.M.; Consortium, U.K.R.A.G.; Erlich, H.A.; Barton, A.; Hocking, L.; Reid, D.M.; et al. Reevaluation of the interaction between HLA-DRB1 shared epitope alleles, PTPN22, and smoking in determining susceptibility to autoantibody-positive and autoantibody-negative rheumatoid arthritis in a large UK caucasian population. *Arthritis Rheumatol.* **2009**, *60*, 2565–2576. [CrossRef] [PubMed]

42. Raychaudhuri, S.; Sandor, C.; Stahl, E.A.; Freudenberg, J.; Lee, H.S.; Jia, X.; Alfredsson, L.; Padyukov, L.; Klareskog, L.; Worthington, J.; et al. Five amino acids in three HLA proteins explain most of the association between MHC and seropositive rheumatoid arthritis. *Nat. Genet.* **2012**, *44*, 291–296. [CrossRef] [PubMed]

43. Mattey, D.L.; Thomson, W.; Ollier, W.E.; Batley, M.; Davies, P.G.; Gough, A.K.; Devlin, J.; Prouse, P.; James, D.W.; Williams, P.L.; et al. Association of drb1 shared epitope genotypes with early mortality in rheumatoid arthritis: Results of eighteen years of followup from the early rheumatoid arthritis study. *Arthritis Rheumatol.* **2007**, *56*, 1408–1416. [CrossRef] [PubMed]

44. Wagner, U.; Kaltenhauser, S.; Sauer, H.; Arnold, S.; Seidel, W.; Hantzschel, H.; Kalden, J.R.; Wassmuth, R. HLA markers and prediction of clinical course and outcome in rheumatoid arthritis. *Arthritis Rheumatol.* **1997**, *40*, 341–351. [CrossRef]

45. Auger, I.; Toussirot, E.; Roudier, J. Molecular mechanisms involved in the association of HLA-DR4 and rheumatoid arthritis. *Immunol. Res.* **1997**, *16*, 121–126. [CrossRef] [PubMed]

46. Bhayani, H.R.; Hedrick, S.M. The role of polymorphic amino acids of the MHC molecule in the selection of the t cell repertoire. *J. Immunol.* **1991**, *146*, 1093–1098. [PubMed]

47. Hammer, J.; Gallazzi, F.; Bono, E.; Karr, R.W.; Guenot, J.; Valsasnini, P.; Nagy, Z.A.; Sinigaglia, F. Peptide binding specificity of HLA-DR4 molecules: Correlation with rheumatoid arthritis association. *J. Exp. Med.* **1995**, *181*, 1847–1855. [CrossRef] [PubMed]

48. Roudier, J. Association of MHC and rheumatoid arthritis. Association of RA with HLA-DR4: The role of repertoire selection. *Arthritis Res.* **2000**, *2*, 217–220. [CrossRef] [PubMed]

49. Wucherpfennig, K.W.; Strominger, J.L. Selective binding of self peptides to disease-associated major histocompatibility complex (MHC) molecules: A mechanism for MHC-linked susceptibility to human autoimmune diseases. *J. Exp. Med.* **1995**, *181*, 1597–1601. [CrossRef] [PubMed]

50. Hill, J.A.; Southwood, S.; Sette, A.; Jevnikar, A.M.; Bell, D.A.; Cairns, E. Cutting edge: The conversion of arginine to citrulline allows for a high-affinity peptide interaction with the rheumatoid arthritis-associated HLA-DRB1*0401 MHC class ii molecule. *J. Immunol.* **2003**, *171*, 538–541. [CrossRef] [PubMed]

51. Van Heemst, J.; Jansen, D.T.; Polydorides, S.; Moustakas, A.K.; Bax, M.; Feitsma, A.L.; Bontrop-Elferink, D.G.; Baarse, M.; van der Woude, D.; Wolbink, G.J.; et al. Crossreactivity to vinculin and microbes provides a molecular basis for HLA-based protection against rheumatoid arthritis. *Nat. Commun.* **2015**, *6*, 6681. [CrossRef] [PubMed]

52. Bauer, S.; Groh, V.; Wu, J.; Steinle, A.; Phillips, J.H.; Lanier, L.L.; Spies, T. Activation of NK cells and T cells by NKG2D, a receptor for stress-inducible mica. *Science* **1999**, *285*, 727–729. [CrossRef] [PubMed]

53. Radaev, S.; Sun, P.D. Structure and function of natural killer cell surface receptors. *Annu. Rev. Biophys. Biomol. Struct.* **2003**, *32*, 93–114. [CrossRef] [PubMed]

54. Ling, S.; Cheng, A.; Pumpens, P.; Michalak, M.; Holoshitz, J. Identification of the rheumatoid arthritis shared epitope binding site on calreticulin. *PLoS ONE* **2010**, *5*, e11703. [CrossRef] [PubMed]

55. Begovich, A.B.; Carlton, V.E.; Honigberg, L.A.; Schrodi, S.J.; Chokkalingam, A.P.; Alexander, H.C.; Ardlie, K.G.; Huang, Q.; Smith, A.M.; Spoerke, J.M.; et al. A missense single-nucleotide polymorphism in a gene encoding a protein tyrosine phosphatase (PTPN22) is associated with rheumatoid arthritis. *Am. J. Hum. Genet.* **2004**, *75*, 330–337. [CrossRef] [PubMed]

56. Plenge, R.M.; Padyukov, L.; Remmers, E.F.; Purcell, S.; Lee, A.T.; Karlson, E.W.; Wolfe, F.; Kastner, D.L.; Alfredsson, L.; Altshuler, D.; et al. Replication of putative candidate-gene associations with rheumatoid arthritis in >4000 samples from north america and sweden: Association of susceptibility with PTPN22, CTLA4, and PADI4. *Am. J. Hum. Genet.* **2005**, *77*, 1044–1060. [CrossRef] [PubMed]

57. Klareskog, L.; Stolt, P.; Lundberg, K.; Kallberg, H.; Bengtsson, C.; Grunewald, J.; Ronnelid, J.; Harris, H.E.; Ulfgren, A.K.; Rantapaa-Dahlqvist, S.; et al. A new model for an etiology of rheumatoid arthritis: Smoking may trigger HLA-DR (shared epitope)-restricted immune reactions to autoantigens modified by citrullination. *Arthritis Rheumatol.* **2006**, *54*, 38–46. [CrossRef] [PubMed]

58. Van der Helm-van Mil, A.H.; Verpoort, K.N.; le Cessie, S.; Huizinga, T.W.; de Vries, R.R.; Toes, R.E. The HLA-DRB1 shared epitope alleles differ in the interaction with smoking and predisposition to antibodies to cyclic citrullinated peptide. *Arthritis Rheumatol.* **2007**, *56*, 425–432. [CrossRef] [PubMed]

59. Wesoly, J.; van der Helm-van Mil, A.H.; Toes, R.E.; Chokkalingam, A.P.; Carlton, V.E.; Begovich, A.B.; Huizinga, T.W. Association of the PTPN22 C1858T single-nucleotide polymorphism with rheumatoid arthritis phenotypes in an inception cohort. *Arthritis Rheumatol.* **2005**, *52*, 2948–2950. [CrossRef] [PubMed]

60. Plenge, R.M.; Seielstad, M.; Padyukov, L.; Lee, A.T.; Remmers, E.F.; Ding, B.; Liew, A.; Khalili, H.; Chandrasekaran, A.; Davies, L.R.; et al. TRAF1-C5 as a risk locus for rheumatoid arthritis—A genomewide study. *N. Engl. J. Med.* **2007**, *357*, 1199–1209. [CrossRef] [PubMed]

61. Lorentzen, J.C.; Flornes, L.; Eklow, C.; Backdahl, L.; Ribbhammar, U.; Guo, J.P.; Smolnikova, M.; Dissen, E.; Seddighzadeh, M.; Brookes, A.J.; et al. Association of arthritis with a gene complex encoding C-type lectin-like receptors. *Arthritis Rheumatol.* **2007**, *56*, 2620–2632. [CrossRef] [PubMed]

62. Sigurdsson, S.; Padyukov, L.; Kurreeman, F.A.; Liljedahl, U.; Wiman, A.C.; Alfredsson, L.; Toes, R.; Ronnelid, J.; Klareskog, L.; Huizinga, T.W.; et al. Association of a haplotype in the promoter region of the interferon regulatory factor 5 gene with rheumatoid arthritis. *Arthritis Rheumatol.* **2007**, *56*, 2202–2210. [CrossRef] [PubMed]

63. Mohan, V.K.; Ganesan, N.; Gopalakrishnan, R. Association of susceptible genetic markers and autoantibodies in rheumatoid arthritis. *J. Genet.* **2014**, *93*, 597–605. [CrossRef] [PubMed]

64. Di Giuseppe, D.; Discacciati, A.; Orsini, N.; Wolk, A. Cigarette smoking and risk of rheumatoid arthritis: A dose-response meta-analysis. *Arthritis Res. Ther.* **2014**, *16*, R61. [CrossRef] [PubMed]

65. Rashid, T.; Ebringer, A. Rheumatoid arthritis is linked to proteus—The evidence. *Clin. Rheumatol.* **2007**, *26*, 1036–1043. [CrossRef] [PubMed]

66. Stolt, P.; Bengtsson, C.; Nordmark, B.; Lindblad, S.; Lundberg, I.; Klareskog, L.; Alfredsson, L.; EIRA Study Group. Quantification of the influence of cigarette smoking on rheumatoid arthritis: Results from a population based case-control study, using incident cases. *Ann. Rheum. Dis.* **2003**, *62*, 835–841. [CrossRef] [PubMed]

67. Bartold, P.M.; Marino, V.; Cantley, M.; Haynes, D.R. Effect of porphyromonas gingivalis-induced inflammation on the development of rheumatoid arthritis. *J. Clin. Periodontol.* **2010**, *37*, 405–411. [CrossRef] [PubMed]

68. Mikuls, T.R.; Payne, J.B.; Yu, F.; Thiele, G.M.; Reynolds, R.J.; Cannon, G.W.; Markt, J.; McGowan, D.; Kerr, G.S.; Redman, R.S.; et al. Periodontitis and porphyromonas gingivalis in patients with rheumatoid arthritis. *Arthritis Rheumatol.* **2014**, *66*, 1090–1100. [CrossRef] [PubMed]

69. Seror, R.; le Gall-David, S.; Bonnaure-Mallet, M.; Schaeverbeke, T.; Cantagrel, A.; Minet, J.; Gottenberg, J.E.; Chanson, P.; Ravaud, P.; Mariette, X. Association of anti-porphyromonas gingivalis antibody titers with nonsmoking status in early rheumatoid arthritis: Results from the prospective french cohort of patients with early rheumatoid arthritis. *Arthritis Rheumatol.* **2015**, *67*, 1729–1737. [CrossRef] [PubMed]

70. De Pablo, P.; Dietrich, T.; McAlindon, T.E. Association of periodontal disease and tooth loss with rheumatoid arthritis in the us population. *J. Rheumatol.* **2008**, *35*, 70–76. [PubMed]

71. Klareskog, L.; Padyukov, L.; Lorentzen, J.; Alfredsson, L. Mechanisms of disease: Genetic susceptibility and environmental triggers in the development of rheumatoid arthritis. *Nat. Clin. Pract. Rheumatol.* **2006**, *2*, 425–433. [CrossRef] [PubMed]

72. Sakkas, L.I.; Daoussis, D.; Liossis, S.N.; Bogdanos, D.P. The infectious basis of ACPA-positive rheumatoid arthritis. *Front. Microbiol.* **2017**, *8*, 1853. [CrossRef] [PubMed]

73. Kharlamova, N.; Jiang, X.; Sherina, N.; Potempa, B.; Israelsson, L.; Quirke, A.M.; Eriksson, K.; Yucel-Lindberg, T.; Venables, P.J.; Potempa, J.; et al. Antibodies to porphyromonas gingivalis indicate interaction between oral infection, smoking, and risk genes in rheumatoid arthritis etiology. *Arthritis Rheumatol.* **2016**, *68*, 604–613. [CrossRef] [PubMed]

74. Wegner, N.; Wait, R.; Sroka, A.; Eick, S.; Nguyen, K.A.; Lundberg, K.; Kinloch, A.; Culshaw, S.; Potempa, J.; Venables, P.J. Peptidylarginine deiminase from porphyromonas gingivalis citrullinates human fibrinogen and α-enolase: Implications for autoimmunity in rheumatoid arthritis. *Arthritis Rheumatol.* **2010**, *62*, 2662–2672. [CrossRef] [PubMed]

75. Harel-Meir, M.; Sherer, Y.; Shoenfeld, Y. Tobacco smoking and autoimmune rheumatic diseases. *Nat. Clin. Pract. Rheumatol.* **2007**, *3*, 707–715. [CrossRef] [PubMed]

76. Hoovestol, R.A.; Mikuls, T.R. Environmental exposures and rheumatoid arthritis risk. *Curr. Rheumatol. Rep.* **2011**, *13*, 431–439. [CrossRef] [PubMed]

77. Onozaki, K. Etiological and biological aspects of cigarette smoking in rheumatoid arthritis. *Inflamm. Allergy Drug Targets* **2009**, *8*, 364–368. [CrossRef] [PubMed]

78. Chang, K.; Yang, S.M.; Kim, S.H.; Han, K.H.; Park, S.J.; Shin, J.I. Smoking and rheumatoid arthritis. *Int. J. Mol. Sci.* **2014**, *15*, 22279–22295. [CrossRef] [PubMed]

79. Padyukov, L.; Silva, C.; Stolt, P.; Alfredsson, L.; Klareskog, L. A gene-environment interaction between smoking and shared epitope genes in HLA-DR provides a high risk of seropositive rheumatoid arthritis. *Arthritis Rheumatol.* **2004**, *50*, 3085–3092. [CrossRef] [PubMed]

80. Linn-Rasker, S.P.; van der Helm-van Mil, A.H.; van Gaalen, F.A.; Kloppenburg, M.; de Vries, R.R.; le Cessie, S.; Breedveld, F.C.; Toes, R.E.; Huizinga, T.W. Smoking is a risk factor for anti-CCP antibodies only in rheumatoid arthritis patients who carry HLA-DRB1 shared epitope alleles. *Ann. Rheum. Dis.* **2006**, *65*, 366–371. [CrossRef] [PubMed]

81. Liao, K.P.; Alfredsson, L.; Karlson, E.W. Environmental influences on risk for rheumatoid arthritis. *Curr. Opin. Rheumatol.* **2009**, *21*, 279–283. [CrossRef] [PubMed]

82. Draborg, A.; Izarzugaza, J.M.; Houen, G. How compelling are the data for Epstein-Barr virus being a trigger for systemic lupus and other autoimmune diseases? *Curr. Opin. Rheumatol.* **2016**, *28*, 398–404. [CrossRef] [PubMed]

83. Draborg, A.H.; Duus, K.; Houen, G. Epstein-Barr virus and systemic lupus erythematosus. *Clin. Dev. Immunol.* **2012**, *2012*, 370516. [CrossRef] [PubMed]

84. Draborg, A.H.; Duus, K.; Houen, G. Epstein-Barr virus in systemic autoimmune diseases. *Clin. Dev. Immunol.* **2013**, *2013*, 535738. [CrossRef] [PubMed]

85. Connolly, S.A.; Jackson, J.O.; Jardetzky, T.S.; Longnecker, R. Fusing structure and function: A structural view of the herpesvirus entry machinery. *Nat. Rev. Microbiol.* **2011**, *9*, 369–381. [CrossRef] [PubMed]

86. Mohl, B.S.; Chen, J.; Sathiyamoorthy, K.; Jardetzky, T.S.; Longnecker, R. Structural and mechanistic insights into the tropism of Epstein-Barr virus. *Mol. Cell* **2016**, *39*, 286–291.

87. Sathiyamoorthy, K.; Chen, J.; Longnecker, R.; Jardetzky, T.S. The complexity in herpesvirus entry. *Curr. Opin. Virol.* **2017**, *24*, 97–104. [CrossRef] [PubMed]

88. Sathiyamoorthy, K.; Hu, Y.X.; Mohl, B.S.; Chen, J.; Longnecker, R.; Jardetzky, T.S. Structural basis for Epstein-Barr virus host cell tropism mediated by gp42 and gHgL entry glycoproteins. *Nat. Commun.* **2016**, *7*, 13557. [CrossRef] [PubMed]

89. Sathiyamoorthy, K.; Jiang, J.; Hu, Y.X.; Rowe, C.L.; Mohl, B.S.; Chen, J.; Jiang, W.; Mellins, E.D.; Longnecker, R.; Zhou, Z.H.; et al. Assembly and architecture of the EBV B cell entry triggering complex. *PLoS Pathog.* **2014**, *10*, e1004309. [CrossRef] [PubMed]

90. Shannon-Lowe, C.; Rowe, M. Epstein barr virus entry; kissing and conjugation. *Curr. Opin. Virol.* **2014**, *4*, 78–84. [CrossRef] [PubMed]

91. Borza, C.M.; Hutt-Fletcher, L.M. Alternate replication in B cells and epithelial cells switches tropism of Epstein-Barr virus. *Nat. Med.* **2002**, *8*, 594–599. [CrossRef] [PubMed]

92. Wang, X.; Hutt-Fletcher, L.M. Epstein-Barr virus lacking glycoprotein gp42 can bind to B cells but is not able to infect. *J. Virol.* **1998**, *72*, 158–163. [PubMed]

93. Shaw, P.L.; Kirschner, A.N.; Jardetzky, T.S.; Longnecker, R. Characteristics of Epstein-Barr virus envelope protein gp42. *Virus Genes* **2010**, *40*, 307–319. [CrossRef] [PubMed]

94. Drickamer, K. C-type lectin-like domains. *Curr. Opin. Struct. Biol.* **1999**, *9*, 585–590. [CrossRef]

95. Weis, W.I.; Taylor, M.E.; Drickamer, K. The C-type lectin superfamily in the immune system. *Immunol. Rev.* **1998**, *163*, 19–34. [CrossRef] [PubMed]

96. Silva, A.L.; Omerovic, J.; Jardetzky, T.S.; Longnecker, R. Mutational analyses of Epstein-Barr virus glycoprotein 42 reveal functional domains not involved in receptor binding but required for membrane fusion. *J. Virol.* **2004**, *78*, 5946–5956. [CrossRef] [PubMed]

97. Haan, K.M.; Kwok, W.W.; Longnecker, R.; Speck, P. Epstein-Barr virus entry utilizing HLA-DP or HLA-DQ as a coreceptor. *J. Virol.* **2000**, *74*, 2451–2454. [CrossRef] [PubMed]

98. Janz, A.; Oezel, M.; Kurzeder, C.; Mautner, J.; Pich, D.; Kost, M.; Hammerschmidt, W.; Delecluse, H.J. Infectious Epstein-Barr virus lacking major glycoprotein BLLF1 (gp350/220) demonstrates the existence of additional viral ligands. *J. Virol.* **2000**, *74*, 10142–10152. [CrossRef] [PubMed]

99. Kirschner, A.N.; Sorem, J.; Longnecker, R.; Jardetzky, T.S. Structure of Epstein-Barr virus glycoprotein 42 suggests a mechanism for triggering receptor-activated virus entry. *Structure* **2009**, *17*, 223–233. [CrossRef] [PubMed]

100. Rowe, C.L.; Connolly, S.A.; Chen, J.; Jardetzky, T.S.; Longnecker, R. A soluble form of Epstein-Barr virus gH/gL inhibits EBV-induced membrane fusion and does not function in fusion. *Virology* **2013**, *436*, 118–126. [CrossRef] [PubMed]

101. Sorem, J.; Jardetzky, T.S.; Longnecker, R. Cleavage and secretion of Epstein-Barr virus glycoprotein 42 promote membrane fusion with B lymphocytes. *J. Virol.* **2009**, *83*, 6664–6672. [CrossRef] [PubMed]

102. Spear, P.G.; Longnecker, R. Herpesvirus entry: An update. *J. Virol.* **2003**, *77*, 10179–10185. [CrossRef] [PubMed]

103. Kirschner, A.N.; Lowrey, A.S.; Longnecker, R.; Jardetzky, T.S. Binding-site interactions between Epstein-Barr virus fusion proteins gp42 and gH/gL reveal a peptide that inhibits both epithelial and B-cell membrane fusion. *J. Virol.* **2007**, *81*, 9216–9229. [CrossRef] [PubMed]

104. Liu, F.; Marquardt, G.; Kirschner, A.N.; Longnecker, R.; Jardetzky, T.S. Mapping the n-terminal residues of Epstein-Barr virus gp42 that bind gH/gL by using fluorescence polarization and cell-based fusion assays. *J. Virol.* **2010**, *84*, 10375–10385. [CrossRef] [PubMed]

105. Backovic, M.; Jardetzky, T.S.; Longnecker, R. Hydrophobic residues that form putative fusion loops of Epstein-Barr virus glycoprotein b are critical for fusion activity. *J. Virol.* **2007**, *81*, 9596–9600. [CrossRef] [PubMed]

106. Mullen, M.M.; Haan, K.M.; Longnecker, R.; Jardetzky, T.S. Structure of the Epstein-Barr virus gp42 protein bound to the MHC class II receptor HLA-DR1. *Mol. Cell* **2002**, *9*, 375–385. [CrossRef]

107. McShane, M.P.; Mullen, M.M.; Haan, K.M.; Jardetzky, T.S.; Longnecker, R. Mutational analysis of the HLA class II interaction with Epstein-Barr virus glycoprotein 42. *J. Virol.* **2003**, *77*, 7655–7662. [CrossRef] [PubMed]

108. Costenbader, K.H.; Karlson, E.W. Epstein-Barr virus and rheumatoid arthritis: Is there a link? *Arthritis Res. Ther.* **2006**, *8*, 204. [CrossRef] [PubMed]

109. Erre, G.L.; Mameli, G.; Cossu, D.; Muzzeddu, B.; Piras, C.; Paccagnini, D.; Passiu, G.; Sechi, L.A. Increased Epstein-Barr virus DNA load and antibodies against EBNA1 and EA in sardinian patients with rheumatoid arthritis. *Viral Immunol.* **2015**, *28*, 385–390. [CrossRef] [PubMed]

110. Goldstein, B.L.; Chibnik, L.B.; Karlson, E.W.; Costenbader, K.H. Epstein-Barr virus serologic abnormalities and risk of rheumatoid arthritis among women. *Autoimmunity* **2012**, *45*, 161–168. [CrossRef] [PubMed]

111. Toussirot, E.; Roudier, J. Pathophysiological links between rheumatoid arthritis and the Epstein-Barr virus: An update. *Jt. Bone Spine* **2007**, *74*, 418–426. [CrossRef] [PubMed]

112. Westergaard, M.W.; Draborg, A.H.; Troelsen, L.; Jacobsen, S.; Houen, G. Isotypes of Epstein-Barr virus antibodies in rheumatoid arthritis: Association with rheumatoid factors and citrulline-dependent antibodies. *BioMed Res. Int.* **2015**, *2015*, 472174. [CrossRef] [PubMed]

113. Alspaugh, M.A.; Henle, G.; Lennette, E.T.; Henle, W. Elevated levels of antibodies to Epstein-Barr virus antigens in sera and synovial fluids of patients with rheumatoid arthritis. *J. Clin. Investig.* **1981**, *67*, 1134–1140. [CrossRef] [PubMed]

114. Billings, P.B.; Hoch, S.O.; White, P.J.; Carson, D.A.; Vaughan, J.H. Antibodies to the Epstein-Barr virus nuclear antigen and to rheumatoid arthritis nuclear antigen identify the same polypeptide. *Proc. Natl. Acad. Sci. USA* **1983**, *80*, 7104–7108. [CrossRef] [PubMed]

115. Venables, P.J.; Pawlowski, T.; Mumford, P.A.; Brown, C.; Crawford, D.H.; Maini, R.N. Reaction of antibodies to rheumatoid arthritis nuclear antigen with a synthetic peptide corresponding to part of Epstein-Barr nuclear antigen 1. *Ann. Rheum. Dis.* **1988**, *47*, 270–279. [CrossRef] [PubMed]

116. Tosato, G.; Steinberg, A.D.; Blaese, R.M. Defective EBV-specific suppressor T-cell function in rheumatoid arthritis. *N. Engl. J. Med.* **1981**, *305*, 1238–1243. [CrossRef] [PubMed]

117. Tosato, G.; Steinberg, A.D.; Yarchoan, R.; Heilman, C.A.; Pike, S.E.; de Seau, V.; Blaese, R.M. Abnormally elevated frequency of Epstein-Barr virus-infected B cells in the blood of patients with rheumatoid arthritis. *J. Clin. Investig.* **1984**, *73*, 1789–1795. [CrossRef] [PubMed]

118. Balandraud, N.; Meynard, J.B.; Auger, I.; Sovran, H.; Mugnier, B.; Reviron, D.; Roudier, J.; Roudier, C. Epstein-Barr virus load in the peripheral blood of patients with rheumatoid arthritis: Accurate quantification using real-time polymerase chain reaction. *Arthritis Rheumatol.* **2003**, *48*, 1223–1228. [CrossRef] [PubMed]

119. Blaschke, S.; Schwarz, G.; Moneke, D.; Binder, L.; Muller, G.; Reuss-Borst, M. Epstein-Barr virus infection in peripheral blood mononuclear cells, synovial fluid cells, and synovial membranes of patients with rheumatoid arthritis. *J. Rheumatol.* **2000**, *27*, 866–873. [PubMed]

120. Takeda, T.; Mizugaki, Y.; Matsubara, L.; Imai, S.; Koike, T.; Takada, K. Lytic Epstein-Barr virus infection in the synovial tissue of patients with rheumatoid arthritis. *Arthritis Rheumatol.* **2000**, *43*, 1218–1225. [CrossRef]

121. Lotz, M.; Roudier, J. Epstein-Barr virus and rheumatoid arthritis: Cellular and molecular aspects. *Rheumatol. Int.* **1989**, *9*, 147–152. [PubMed]

122. Roudier, J.; Petersen, J.; Rhodes, G.H.; Luka, J.; Carson, D.A. Susceptibility to rheumatoid arthritis maps to a T-cell epitope shared by the HLA-DW4 DR β-1 chain and the Epstein-Barr virus glycoprotein gp110. *Proc. Natl. Acad. Sci. USA* **1989**, *86*, 5104–5108. [CrossRef] [PubMed]

123. Callan, M.F. Epstein-Barr virus, arthritis, and the development of lymphoma in arthritis patients. *Curr. Opin. Rheumatol.* **2004**, *16*, 399–405. [CrossRef] [PubMed]

124. Cohen, J.I. Epstein-Barr virus infection. *N. Engl. J. Med.* **2000**, *343*, 481–492. [CrossRef] [PubMed]

125. Ball, R.J.; Avenell, A.; Aucott, L.; Hanlon, P.; Vickers, M.A. Systematic review and meta-analysis of the sero-epidemiological association between Epstein-Barr virus and rheumatoid arthritis. *Arthritis Res. Ther.* **2015**, *17*, 274. [CrossRef] [PubMed]
126. Sherina, N.; Hreggvidsdottir, H.S.; Bengtsson, C.; Hansson, M.; Israelsson, L.; Alfredsson, L.; Lundberg, K. Low levels of antibodies against common viruses associate with anti-citrullinated protein antibody-positive rheumatoid arthritis; implications for disease aetiology. *Arthritis Res. Ther.* **2017**, *19*, 219. [CrossRef] [PubMed]
127. Spriggs, M.K.; Armitage, R.J.; Comeau, M.R.; Strockbine, L.; Farrah, T.; Macduff, B.; Ulrich, D.; Alderson, M.R.; Mullberg, J.; Cohen, J.I. The extracellular domain of the Epstein-Barr virus BZLF2 protein binds the HLA-DR β chain and inhibits antigen presentation. *J. Virol.* **1996**, *70*, 5557–5563. [PubMed]
128. Li, Q.; Spriggs, M.K.; Kovats, S.; Turk, S.M.; Comeau, M.R.; Nepom, B.; Hutt-Fletcher, L.M. Epstein-Barr virus uses HLA class II as a cofactor for infection of B lymphocytes. *J. Virol.* **1997**, *71*, 4657–4662. [PubMed]
129. Li, Q.; Turk, S.M.; Hutt-Fletcher, L.M. The Epstein-Barr virus (EBV) *BZLF2* gene product associates with the gH and gL homologs of ebv and carries an epitope critical to infection of B cells but not of epithelial cells. *J. Virol.* **1995**, *69*, 3987–3994. [PubMed]
130. Haan, K.M.; Longnecker, R. Coreceptor restriction within the HLA-DQ locus for Epstein-Barr virus infection. *Proc. Natl. Acad. Sci. USA* **2000**, *97*, 9252–9257. [CrossRef] [PubMed]
131. Speck, P.; Haan, K.M.; Longnecker, R. Epstein-Barr virus entry into cells. *Virology* **2000**, *277*, 1–5. [CrossRef] [PubMed]
132. Ou, D.; Mitchell, L.A.; Tingle, A.J. A new categorization of HLA DR alleles on a functional basis. *Hum. Immunol.* **1998**, *59*, 665–676. [CrossRef]
133. Rosloniec, E.F.; Whittington, K.B.; Zaller, D.M.; Kang, A.H. HLA-DR1 (DRB1*0101) and DR4 (DRB1*0401) use the same anchor residues for binding an immunodominant peptide derived from human type II collagen. *J. Immunol.* **2002**, *168*, 253–259. [CrossRef] [PubMed]

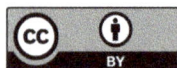

International Journal of
Molecular Sciences

MDPI

Review

Role of Stem Cells in Pathophysiology and Therapy of Spondyloarthropathies— New Therapeutic Possibilities?

Magdalena Krajewska-Włodarczyk [1,2,*], Agnieszka Owczarczyk-Saczonek [3,*], Waldemar Placek [3], Adam Osowski [2], Piotr Engelgardt [4] and Joanna Wojtkiewicz [2,5,6,*]

[1]   Department of Rheumatology, Municipal Hospital in Olsztyn, 10-900 Olsztyn, Poland
[2]   Department of Pathophysiology, Faculty of Medicine, University of Warmia and Mazury, 10-900 Olsztyn, Poland; adam.osowski@uwm.edu.pl
[3]   Department of Dermatology, Sexually Transmitted Diseases and Clinical Immunology, Faculty of Medicine, University of Warmia and Mazury, 10-900 Olsztyn, Poland; w.placek@wp.pl
[4]   Department of Forensic Medicine, Faculty of Medicine, University of Warmia and Mazury, 10-900 Olsztyn, Poland; ra-bit@wp.pl
[5]   Laboratory for Regenerative Medicine, Faculty of Medicine, University of Warmia and Mazury, 10-900 Olsztyn, Poland
[6]   Foundation for Nerve Cell Regeneration, University of Warmia and Mazury in Olsztyn, 10-900 Olsztyn, Poland
*   Correspondence: magdalenakw@op.pl (M. K.-W.); aganek@wp.pl (A.O.-S.); joanna.wojtkiewicz@uwm.edu.pl (J.W.)

Received: 26 November 2017; Accepted: 25 December 2017; Published: 28 December 2017

Abstract: Considerable progress has been made recently in understanding the complex pathogenesis and treatment of spondyloarthropathies (SpA). Currently, along with traditional disease modifying anti-rheumatic drugs (DMARDs), TNF-α, IL-12/23 and IL-17 are available for treatment of such diseases as ankylosing spondylitis (AS) and psoriatic arthritis (PsA). Although they adequately control inflammatory symptoms, they do not affect the abnormal bone formation processes associated with SpA. However, the traditional therapeutic approach does not cover the regenerative treatment of damaged tissues. In this regards, stem cells may offer a promising, safe and effective therapeutic option. The aim of this paper is to present the role of mesenchymal stromal cells (MSC) in pathogenesis of SpA and to highlight the opportunities for using stem cells in regenerative processes and in the treatment of inflammatory changes in articular structures.

Keywords: spondyloarthropathies; inflammation; mesenchymal stem cells

---

1. Introduction

Spondyloarthropathies (SpA) are a group of inflammatory rheumatoid diseases which traditionally include ankylosing spondylitis (AS), psoriatic arthritis (PsA), reactive arthritis (ReA), arthritis associated with Crohn's disease and ulcerative colitis as well as undifferentiated spondyloarthropathies. Apart from typical symptoms within the locomotor system, such as chronic inflammation of spinal joints, inflammation of entheses and inflammation of peripheral joints, the very complex clinical picture of SpA includes numerous non-articular manifestations, including the skin, intestines and eyes [1]. Local inflammatory changes in the skeletal system in the course of SpA result in local loss of bone tissue and the formation of erosions with simultaneous bone formation, which leads to profound destruction and impairment of the affected joints. Considerable progress has been made in recent years in the treatment of SpA thanks to the introduction of the tumor necrosis factor-α (TNF-α) inhibitors as well as interleukin 17 (IL-17) and interleukin 12/23 (IL-12/23) inhibitors [2–4].

Although non-articular symptoms can be well-controlled thanks to modern biological therapies, which considerably slow down the progression of destructive processes in the locomotory system, they do not affect changes in the osteo-articular system already present, nor do they inhibit the SpA-related bone-formation processes. Therefore, mesenchymal stromal cells, mesenchymal stromal cells (MSC), with their immunomodulatory and regenerative potential [5] (Figure 1), may represent a promising tool in long-term treatment of SpA, changing the present therapeutic approach.

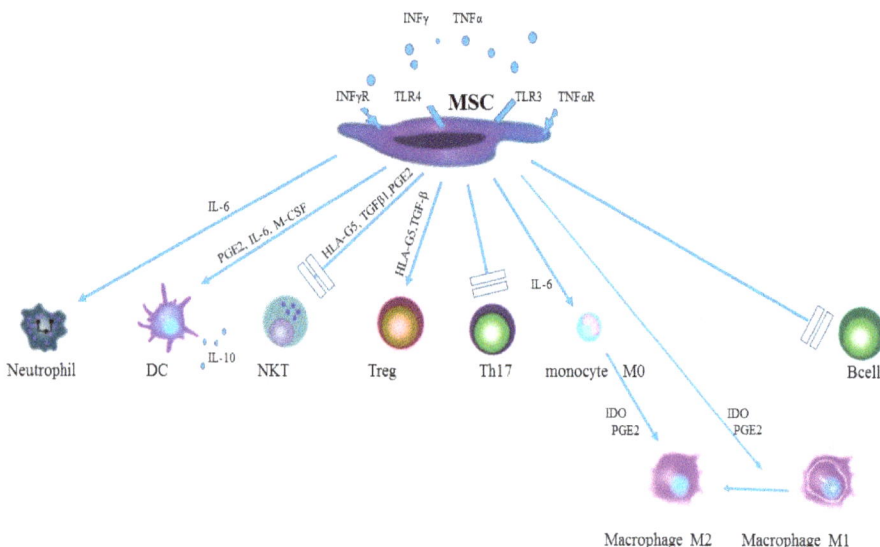

Figure 1. Immunomodulatory effect of MSC on elements of the innate and adaptive immunity systems in spondyloarthropathies. IFN-γ, interferon γ; TNF-α, tumor necrosis factor α; TLR, Toll-like receptor; MSC, mesenchymal stem cell; IL, interleukin; PGE2, prostaglandin E2; M-CSF, macrophage colony-stimulating factor; TGFβ1, transforming growth factor β1;HLA-G5, human leukocyte antigen G5; DC, dendritic cell; NKT, natural killers; Treg, regulatory T cell, IDO, indolamine.

2. The Role of Mesenchymal Stromal Cells in the Inflammatory Process and in the Pathogenesis of Spondyloarthropathies

2.1. Origin of Stromal Cells

MSC are able to form clones, to differentiate in multiple directions and to self-regenerate [6]. In early cultures, MSC resemble fibroblast (MSC type I) in their appearance and in the way they grow; round, small, self-regenerating cells are observed less frequently [7]; in later phases, MSC can be bigger and flatter (MSC type II) [8]. Unexpectedly, MSC are not immortal—they age and die after several passages [9]. Since MSC are present in many embryonic tissues (embryonic stem cells, ESC) and in adult individuals (adult stem cells, ASC), there are many methods of acquiring them. Embryonic stem cells can be collected after delivery from the umbilical cord blood, from Wharton's jelly, from the placenta, amniotic fluid and as well as from subamniotic membrane and perivascular area of the umbilical cord. MSC has been identified in the following tissues in adult individuals: In marrow, in adipose tissue, in the skin, lungs, dental pulp, periosteum, skeletal muscles, tendons and synovial membrane [10], but clinical application of "adult" MSC is limited mainly to bone marrow-derived mesenchymal stromal cells (BM-MSC) and adipose-derived stem cells (ADSC, ASC) [11]. The International Society for Cellular Therapy (ISCT) has developed the minimum criteria to be used in identifying mesenchymal cells. By these assumptions, characteristic features of mesenchymal cells include the ability to adhere to a plastic base, the presence of three surface antigens: CD105 (endoglin), CD90 (Thy-1), CD73 (ecto-5′-nucleotidase) and concomitant absence of antigens CD45, CD34, CD14 or CD11a, CD79a, or CD19 and class II HLA, and the capability of in vitro differentiation towards three cellular lines: osteoblasts, chondroblasts and adipocytes [12]. A detailed description of stem cells includes additional information, such as the cell origin (tissue, organ, systemic), culture conditions, medium composition, presence of other antigens of positive identification and absence of negative markers, potential for differentiation, cloning, proteomes, secretomes and transcriptone data [13]. In vivo, MSC probably constitute a significant element of a niche of hematopoietic stem cells (HSC) [14], they take part in angiogenesis and regulation of blood vessel function [15] as well in controlling inflammatory processes [16].

2.2. The Role of Toll-Like Receptors in Activity of Stem Cells

Signal transfer in the inflammatory response of the innate immune system is effected, inter alia, by means of Toll-like receptors (TLR), which activate phagocytes. In cell culture studies, expression of various Toll-like receptors has been observed, including TLR3 (virus dsRNA receptor) and TLR4 (lipopolysaccharide receptor, LPS) [17]. In in vitro studies, under hypoxic conditions, short-term stimulation of human MSC by pro-inflammatory cytokines, such as interferon-γ (INF-γ), TNF-α, INF-α, IL-1β, increased expression of TLR1, TLR2, TLR3, TLR4, TLR5 [18], whereas prolonged stimulation resulted in a decreasing the number of TLR2 and TLR4 [19] and decreasing the inflammatory response. An increase in the expression of TLR3 and TLR4 on MSC observed in a study by Raicevic et al. boosted the response to LPS and poly(I:C) (polyinosinic-polycytidylic acid), which resulted in a decrease in the immunosuppressive properties of MSC [18]. It has also been suggested that MSC can acquire a pro-inflammatory phenotype (MSC1) when stimulated by TLR4 and undergo anti-inflammatory polarization (MSC2) when activated by TLR3 [20], which could partly explain the apparently conflicting roles of MSC in the inflammatory process. There is data which indicates the importance of TLR dysregulation in intensifying the inflammatory condition in spondyloarthropathy. Heuschen et al. examined patients with ulcerative colitis and described an increase in expression of TLR5 in patients with intensified inflammation of the intestinal mucosal membrane and a decrease in the number of TLR3 receptors in a healthy mucosal membrane with local suppression of the inflammatory condition [21]. An increase in TLR4 expression on peripheral blood mononuclear cells (PBMCs) in AS patients has been reported by de Rycke et al. [22] and by Yang et al. [23]. An increase in expression of TLR2 and TLR4 has also been observed in the synovial membrane collected from patients with other SpAs, including with PsA and undifferentiated SpA, compared to patients with rheumatoid arthritis (RA) and osteoarthritis (OA) [22]. Treatment with TNF-α inhibitors decreased the number of TLR2 and TLR4 receptors, both on peripheral mononuclear cells and on synoviocytes [22]. A small study by Candia et al. on PsA patients showed a temporary increase in the number of TLR2 on immature dendritic cells in vitro [24], whereas Myles et al. examined patients with juvenile chronic arthritis associated with enthesitis, and observed an increased expression of TLR2 and TLR4 on monocytes in peripheral blood and in articular fluid, which was associated with increased production of IL-6 and metalloproteinase 3 (MMP-3) following stimulation with LPS [25]. These studies indicate that there is a link between high expression of TLR in SpA, but they do not confirm a causal relationship between them. Expression of TLR in SpA may intensify the inflammatory response or be a specific indicator of chronic inflammation.

2.3. Stem Cells at an Early Phase of Inflammation

The immunomodulatory activity of MSC in an early phase of the inflammatory process seems to favor the development of an effective immune response. In a study on mice, a MSC response associated with recognition of bacterial proteins resulted in an increased secretion of IL-6, IL-8, GM-CSF (granulocyte-macrophage colony-stimulating factor) and MIF (macrophage migration inhibitory factor)—which are factors stimulating influx and activity of neutrocytes [26]. In a study conducted by Mantovani et al., BM-MSC activated through the TLR3 receptor extended the survival period of neutrophils—inactive and activated by IL-6, INF-γ and GM-CSF [27]. In addition, MSC can produce chemokines (CXCL-9, CXCL-10 and CXCL-11) by stimulating recruitment of lymphocytes to the inflammation sites [28]. Such an effect has been observed in in vitro studies in mouse and human MSC cultures at low concentrations of TNF-α and INF-γ, where human MSC reduced secretion of IDO in these conditions, and mouse MSC produced decreased amounts of iNOS, which was associated with decreased inhibition of T cell proliferation [29,30]. The findings of these studies may suggest an effect of concentrations of IDO and iNOS on the pro- and anti-inflammatory activity of human and murine MSC, respectively. Through expression of ligands (C-C motif) of chemokines CCL2, CCL3, CCL12, human and murine BM-MSC can boost influx of monocytes to the inflammation sites, thereby supporting local regenerative processes [31].

2.4. Monocytes and Macrophages

Apart from recruiting circulating monocytes, MSC can affect the function of macrophages at inflammation sites. It seems that polarization of macrophages towards a pro-inflammatory M1 phenotype and an anti-inflammatory M2 phenotype can depend on the immunomodulatory properties of MSC [32,33]. MSC polarize M0 macrophages to the M1 phenotype at low concentrations of IL-6. Increased production and secretion of pro-inflammatory cytokines by M1 macrophages and activated T cells stimulate MSC to produce mediators, including immunosuppressive agents, such as iNOS (inducible NO synthase) in cultures of murine MSC and IDO (indolamines) [34] (Figure 2). In studies of joint cultures of monocytes and human or murine BM-MSC, polarization of macrophages to the anti-inflammatory M2 phenotype depended on the cellular interactions and on E2 prostaglandin (PGE2) concentrations and on products of IDO activity, including kynurenine (a product of tryptophan degradation) and other catabolites [35]. Activation of MSC by TNF-α and IFN-γ as well as LPS boosts expression of cyclooxygenase 2 (COX2) and IDO in BM-MSC, additionally stimulating macrophage activation to the M2 phenotype [36]. M2 macrophages produce mainly anti-inflammatory cytokines IL-10 and TGF-β and small amounts of pro-inflammatory cytokines IL-1, IL-6, TNF-α and IFN-γ, thereby inhibiting the inflammatory process and helping to regenerate damaged tissues [27]. Polarization of monocytes and macrophages to the pro- or anti-inflammatory phenotype in SpA may be responsible for an active inflammatory process, regeneration processes and rebuilding the affected tissues. Zhao et al. examined peripheral blood in patients with advanced AS and detected significant polarization of monocytes to the M2 type, with the M2/M1 ratio being correlated positively with the damage to the affected structures, and negatively with inflammation indicators (ESR, CRP) and BASDAI (Bath Ankylosing Spondylitis Disease Activity Index) [37]. Other researchers have also described polarization of histiocytes to the M2 type at sites affected by inflammation in AS [38] and PsA [39]. Interestingly, a therapy with TNF-α inhibitors in SpA is linked with an increase in the M2/M1 ratio, which could be attributed to a decrease in the number of M1 monocytes [37], but it does not prevent progressive bone formation, typical of SpA [40]. Guihard et al. found stimulation of MSC differentiation towards osteoblasts by activated monocytes is effected in the presence of OSM (oncostatin M), an IL-6 cytokine, and is mediated through a type II receptor on MSC, which activates the transcriptive agent STA3 [41].

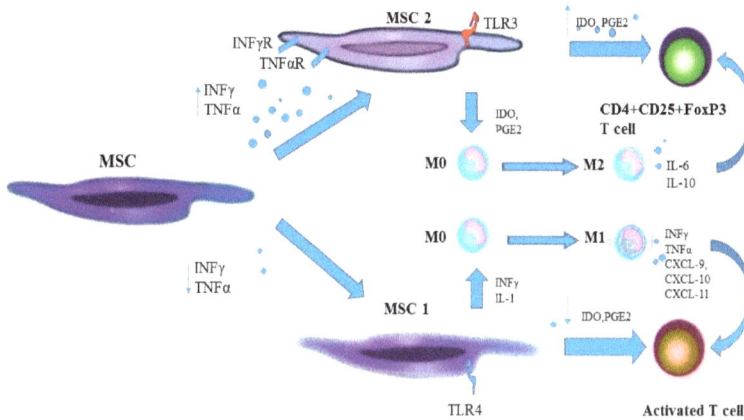

Figure 2. Polarization of MSC into an anti-inflammatory and pro-inflammatory phenotype and impact of anti-inflammatory and pro-inflammatory MSC on T cells activity. IFN-γ, interferon γ; TNF-α, tumor necrosis factor α; TLR, Toll-like receptor; MSC, mesenchymal stem cell; IL, interleukin; PGE2, prostaglandin E2; IDO, indolamine M, monocyte; CXCL, chemokine.

2.5. Dendritic Cells

Studies of animal models and human dendritic cells (DC) in SpA provide data which indicates a contribution of DC in the development of SpA. DC HLA-B27+ are capable of synthesis of IL-23, which is one of the main pro-inflammatory cytokines in SpA [42,43]. IL-23 exerts a systemic effect through induction of differentiation of naive T cells in lymph nodes to pro-inflammatory Th17 [44] and through stimulation of lymphocytes IL-23R+ residing in entheses to secrete IL-22 and to stimulate osteoblasts, leading to local bone formation [45]. MSC inhibit differentiation of CD14+CD1a precursors originating in peripheral and umbilical blood to dendritic cells [46]. Zhang et al. found the presence of MSC to be associated with reduced expression of presenting and co-stimulating cells, including CD1a, CD40, CD80, CD86 and HLA-DR during the process of DC differentiation and limited expression of CD40, CD86 and CD83 during DC maturation [47]. Similar findings have been presented by Jiang et al., where the presence of MSC additionally decreased expression of CD83 on already-matured DC, which suggested the loss of maturity features by dendritic cells [48]. Through secreted PGE2, MSC can also inhibit maturation of DC stimulated by CSF and IL-4 without disrupting the process of DC maturation stimulated by LPS [49]. An effect has been described of MSC resulting in a decrease in DC activity in antigen transformation and presentation to T cells, related to inhibiting of MAPKs (mitogen-activated protein kinases) activity following stimulation of by TLR4 [50]. In a recently published study, MSC in a cell culture polarized DC to a regulatory phenotype with expression of IL-6 and IL-10 [51].

2.6. Neutrophils

Neutrophils are a valuable source of IL-17, which is another pro-inflammatory cytokine of key importance in the pathogenesis of SpA. Appel et al. examined facet joints in patients with axial SpA and noted that it was mainly neutrophils that were responsible for local synthesis of IL-17 [52]. It seems that neutrophils are stimulated by MSC, which may maintain the inflammation. Maqbool et al. presented the findings of a study in which MSC extended the survival period of neutrophils deprived of nutrients or plasma [53]. In a study conducted by Raffaghello et al., MSC secreted IL-6, whereby they were able to inhibit apoptosis of resting neutrophils and those activated with IL-8 [54]. In another study, MSC activated by TLR3 significantly boosted the vitality and activity of neutrophils through IL-6, IFN-γ and GM-CSF [28].

2.7. NK Cells

Natural killer cells are one of the main parts of the innate immune system. The discovery that the HLA-B27 antigen is specifically recognized by the inhibitory KIR3DL1 receptor of NK cells and identifying the link between the expression of KIR activating and inhibitory receptors with the activity of AS indicates that NK may play a significant role in pathogenesis of SpA [55]. MSC can change the NK phenotype and inhibit their proliferation, as well as the secretion of cytokines and cytotoxicity against T cells with expression of class I HLA. This activity is exerted through intercellular interactions or soluble mediators, such as TGF-β1 and PGE2 [56]. MSC can inhibit IL-2-stimulated proliferation of inactive NK [57]. Through HLA-G5, MSC have an inhibitory effect on NK-dependent cytolysis and on INF-γ secretion [58]. In a study by Prigione et al., MSC inhibited INF-γ production through activated NK with no effect on their cytotoxic activity [59].

2.8. T Cells

MSC have a modulatory effect on proliferation of T cells by the production and secretion of TGF-β, hepatocyte growth factor (HGF), PGE2, IDO and HO (hemoxygenase) [60]. Human MSC inhibit the proliferation of T cells, both CD4$^+$ and CD8$^+$ also with IDO, while at the same time inducing proliferation of regulatory T cells (Treg) [61]. The inhibitory effect of MSC on T cells decreases when there are no monocytes present, which indicates not only an effect of soluble factors secreted by MSC, but it also suggests cellular interdependence of MSC and monocytes in inhibiting lymphocyte proliferation [62]. It appears that MSC inhibit differentiation of effector Th17 [63], although the mechanisms affecting it are not clear [64,65]. Huang et al. described an inhibitory effect of human umbilical cord derived MSC (hUCMSC) on T cells in SpA patients. In a culture with mononuclear cells from peripheral blood, hUCMSC considerably reduced IL-17 production, which may suggest a therapeutic potential of MSC [66]. Th17 cells play a key role in development of an inflammatory condition which accompany SpA, they recruit circulating monocytes and neutrophils to the sites affected by the disease, stimulate maturation of osteoclasts, and, in consequence, resorption of bone tissue [67,68]. The ability of MSC to convert mature Th17 into Treg is very important in the context of chronic inflammation in SpA [69,70]. Treg cells are mediators of immune tolerance which exert their effect through suppression of effector T cells and inhibition of tissue destruction induced by an immune process. Examination of peripheral blood and articular fluid of patients reveals a relative reduction in the number of Treg cells [71,72] and recent studies have shown a link between functional defects of CD4$^+$CD25^{high}FoxP3$^+$ [73] and the Treg/Th17 balance being disturbed with the development of SpA [74]. An ability to induce proliferation of Treg, which has been confirmed in numerous studies, is one of the key mechanisms of limiting inflammation by MSC. Joint culturing of MSC and peripheral blood mononuclear cells (PBMC) stimulated differentiation of CD4$^+$ cells towards Treg cells with the expression of CD25^{high}FoxP3$^+$ [75]. In cultures of MSC and washed CD4$^+$ cells or PBMC with monocyte depletion did not show any differentiation of lymphocytes towards Treg cells, whereas proliferation of CD4$^+$CD25^{high}FoxP3$^+$ cells in cultures took place after monocytes were added [76]. Induction of Treg cells dependent on MSC may be linked to the secretion by MSC of the soluble human leukocyte antigen G5 (sHLA-G5). The HLA-G5 molecule inhibits the proliferation of alloreactive T cells and stimulates differentiation of immature T cells towards suppressor Treg cells [77] and is linked to the induction of proliferation of CD4$^+$CD25^{high}Fox P3$^+$ cells [78]. In a study conducted by Wu et al., BM MSC in AS patients had decreased immunomodulatory potential; in addition, an increased amount of Treg and Fox P3$^+$ cells was found, as well as an increased amount of T cells with CCR4$^+$CCR6$^+$ receptors compared to healthy people. This may suggest a decreased immunomodulatory potential of MSC as a factor which plays a role in the development of AS [74].

2.9. B Cells

There is currently no proof of the participation of specific antibodies in the pathogenesis of spondyloarthropathy, but one must bear in mind that B cells have chemotactic properties, they produce cytokines and can be very effective antigen-presenting cells [79]. With their immunomodulatory potential, regulatory B cells (Breg) can also inhibit Th1 response and differentiation of Th17 cells [80]. An increased number of circulating Breg cells in SpA has been reported [81] and, although no link has been found with disease activity, the number of Breg cells has been reported to decrease in patients treated with anti-TNF-α [82]. MCS regulate a number of functions of B-cells. In a study conducted by Corcione et al., MSC inhibited proliferation of B-cells by arresting the cellular cycle at the G0/G1 phase and secretion of immunoglobulins (Ig) IgM, IgG and IgA, which was reflected by inhibited differentiation of lymphocytes. In the same study, expression of chemokine receptors (C-X-C motif) CXCR4 and CXCR5 as well as CCR7 on B-cells decreased considerably in the presence of MSC, which may suggest an effect of MSC on the chemotactic properties of B cells [83]. Lee et al. described inhibition of IgG production by a C3 component of the complement secreted by MSC following infection by a strain of *Mycoplasma arginini* [84]. In a different study, MSC, following stimulation by TLR4, exhibited increased expression of the B-cell activating factor (BAFF), thereby affecting immunoglobin production [85]. In another study, excitation of MSC by INF-γ stimulated cells to secrete galectin 9 (Gal-9), an inhibitor of T- and B-cell proliferation and production and secretion of antigen-specific antibodies [86]. However, different findings were reported by Rosado et al. and by Ji et al., who described increased proliferation and differentiation of B cells in the presence of BM-MSC and umbilical cord MSC (UC-MSC), respectively [87,88]. These discrepancies can probably be attributed to an indirect effect of other factors present in the cultures, which were not covered by those studies.

3. The Role of Stem Cells of Irregular Ossification in Spondyloarthropathy

It appears that MSC in SpA are involved in processes of irregular ossification. MSC can affect the process of bone mineralization by regulating the activity of TNAP (tissue-nonspecific alkaline phosphatase). In a study which sought to provide a probable explanation of the differences between changes in bones observed in RA and SpA, Ding et al., treated cultured human MSC (hMSC) with TNF-α and IL-1β. The action of these cytokines resulted in decreased expression of collagen and increased activity of TNAP. Differences in the effect of TNF-α and IL-1β on expression of collagen and the activity of TNAP can partially explain why bone changes in SpA are linked to bone loss and accompanying bone formation, whereas they are linked to the formation of corrosions in RA [89]. In another study, stimulation of osteoblast activity with Wnt5a was observed in response to the action of TNF-α. The concentration of Wnt5a was significantly increased by TNF-α and it was linked to an increase in the activity of TNAP and intensified mineralization. The findings of this study indicate a connection between inflammation in SpA and bone formation by activation of the cannonical Wnt/β-catenin pathway by Wnt5a. Stimulation of ossification by MSC could explain the lack of, or weak, effect of an anti-TNF-α therapy in inhibiting bone formation in SpA [90]. Characteristic features of all SpAs include inflammatory changes in entheses, which are independent of inflammation of synovial membrane in joints. MSC in places where ligaments, tendons and articular capsules are attached to bones can be a reservoir of cells responsible for the repair of articular cartilage—which is a tissue of a low regenerative potential—damaged by inflammation [91]. In a study on a rat model of the degenerative joint disease, regeneration of articular cartilage was faster and of a better quality following intra-articular injections of MSC compared to the administration of mature chondrocytes [92]. Differentiation of MSC in entheses towards tenocytes, chondrocytes or osteoblasts depends, inter alia, on the tensile force [93]. Under the influence of mechanical stimulae, mechanosensitive calcium permeable channels become involved in changes in intracellular calcium concentrations [94,95]. Stimulation of these channels in the MSC membrane, which results in MSC activation, can trigger inflammatory processes and ossification in entheses, which confirms the hypothesis of the role of physical damage in the development of SpA [96,97]. Apart from the mechanical load of the structures of entheses, osteogenic differentiation of MSC is stimulated by fibronectin, whereas a high concentration of type I collagen inhibits osteoblastogenesis and promotes differentiation towards tenocytes [93]. In a recently published study by Xie et al., differentiation of MSC towards osteoblasts in AS patients was linked to disturbed balance between bone morphogenic protein-2 (BMP-2) and Noggin protein. The discovery of this mechanism, which leads to intensified osteogenesis in entheses, suggests that restoring the BMP-2/Noggin balance or local suppression of MSC could inhibit excessive bone formation in SpA [98].

Numerous publications have confirmed the immunomodulatory effect of MSC on elements of the inflammatory process. There is plenty of data which may indicate the role of MSC in spondyloarthropathies (Table 1), which encourages further studies on applications of MSC in the treatment of SpA.

Table 1. An analysis of a potential role of stem cells in the development of spondyloarthropathy.

Elements of Pathogenesis of Spondyloarthropathy	Results of Stem Cell Action
Dysregulation of TLR. Increase in expression of TLR2 and TLR 4 on mononuclear cells of peripheral blood and in articular synovial membrane [21–24].	Acquisition of the pro-inflammatory phenotype by MSC following stimulation by TLR4 and the anti-inflammatory phenotype following stimulation by TLR3 [18–20].
Increased production of pro-inflammatory TNF-α and IFN-γ by activated monocytes and macrophages.	Activation of MSC with TNF-α and IFN-γ boosts expression of iNOS, COX2 and IDO and favours polarisation of monocytes and macrophages to the anti-inflammatory M2 phenotype M2 [34–36].
Increase in production of inflammatory cytokines, e.g., IL-12, IL-23, IL-6 by dendritic cells [42,43].	Inhibition of differentiation of precursors of CD40CD1a into DC, inhibition of the ability to present antigen by DC, induction of the loss of maturity features by DC [46,48,49].
Increase in local production of IL-17 in joints by neutrophils [52].	Inhibition of apoptosis and stimulation of activity of activity of neutrophils by IL-6, IL-8 IFN-β and GM-CSF [28,54].
A link between expression of activating KIR receptors on NK cells with the disease activity. Recognising of HLA B27 antigen by the KIR3DL1 receptor [55].	Inhibition of proliferation, cytokine secretion and cytotoxicity of NK cells [56–59].
The key role of Th17 cells in development of SpA [67,68]	Ability of mature Th17 to convert into Treg [69,70].
Decrease in the amount of Treg. Upsetting the Treg/Th17 balance. Functional defects of CD4+CD25+FOXP3 [71–74].	Induction of Treg proliferation. Stimulation of differentiation of CD4 towards CD4+CD25+FOXP3 [75].
Ossification of entheses, formation of new bone tissue on marginal surfaces of joints [1].	Regulation of ossification with TNAP. Increased bone formation by activation of Wnt/β-catenin pathway with Wnt5a. Ossification of entheses following stimulation of calcium channels in MSC by mechanical stimul [89,90,97].

TLR, Toll-like receptor; TNF-α, tumor necrosis factor-α; IFN-γ, interferon γ; iNOS, inducible NO synthase; COX2, cyclooxygenase 2; IDO, indolamine; IL, interleukin; GM-CSF, granulocyte-macrophage colony-stimulating factor; DC, dendritic cells; NK, natural killers; TNAP, tissue-nonspecific alkaline phosphatase.

4. The Role of MSC in the Treatment of Spondyloarthropathies

The available data on the immunomodulatory effect of MSC comes mainly from in vitro studies. However, there has been a lot of data from in vivo studies which confirms such an effect of MSC. Adipose-tissue-derived MSCs (AT-MSC) effectively suppressed the T1-dependent immune response and stimulated the proliferation of Treg in transgenic diabetic NOD/SCID mice, in effect maintaining the function of β cells in the pancreas [99]. Monocytes incubated in the presence of AT-MSC administered by infusion decreased the activity of chronic intestine inflammation and protected against the development of severe sepsis by inducing immunomodulatory macrophages secreting IL-10 and inhibiting uncontrolled production of inflammatory mediators [100]. Improvement of survival and mitigation of the course of sepsis following IV administration of MSC and their interaction with monocytes and macrophages was also described in the paper by Nemeth et al., which was linked to the production of IL-10 by monocytes and macrophages and decreased serum concentrations of pro-inflammatory TNF-α and IL-6 [36]. In other studies, MSC improved the survival of skin grafts [101], allogenic corneal transplants [102] and alleviated symptoms of experimental encephalomyelitis in mice [103]. Administration of human BM-MSC, UC-MSC and AT-MSC in asthma increased the pool of macrophages in pulmonary alveoli, mitigated bronchial hyper-reactivity, reduced eosinophil counts in bronchi and the production of Th2-dependent cytokines. Depletion of macrophages in pulmonary alveoli resulted in intensification of bronchial hyper-reactivity [104]. The immunomodulatory effect of MSC seems not to result from direct intercellular interactions or cells colonizing specific organs, but from secreted soluble mediators, which affects the systemic effect of MSC. This was confirmed in a study conducted by Zanotti et al., in which polymer encapsulated MSC (E-MSC) exerted an immunosuppressive and anti-inflammatory effect, probably by means of secreted soluble agents [105].

The potentially regenerative and immunomodulatory properties of MSC in arthritis and in degenerative joint disease have also been studied [106,107]. The first reports of the effectiveness of treatment of autoimmune diseases come from a description of bone marrow transplants in patients with comorbidities, such as proliferative diseases of the hematopoietic system and autoimmune diseases [108]. A positive outcome of bone marrow transplant on the course of immune diseases encouraged researchers to make numerous attempts to apply HSC and MSC in RA, systemic lupus erythematosus (SLE), scleroderma and sclerosis multiplex [108]. Unfortunately, no studies have been conducted of the efficacy of SpA treatment with stem cells. There have been several reports in the literature on bone marrow transplants for hematological reasons in patients with psoriatic arthritis and ankylosing spondylitis. Remission and even a reduction of radiographic changes has been achieved in the patients [109–113]. In 2012, the first autologous HSC transplant was carried out following chemotherapy in a male patient with AS and with the HLA-B27 antigen, with the intent to treat ankylosing spondylitis. A complete remission was achieved, which lasted throughout the two-year follow-up period [114]. In another study, Wang et al. described the effectiveness of IV administration of allogenic MSC in 31 AS patients, following ineffective treatment with NSAIDs. The study lasted 20 weeks, MSC infusions were carried out four times, on days 0, 7, 17 and 21. At the end of the fourth week, a response to treatment was achieved, as assessed by ASAS 20 (Assessment in Ankylosing Spondylitis Response Criteria 20), in approx. 75% of the patients, a reduction of ASDAS-CRP (Ankylosing Spondylitis Disease Activity Score Containing C-Reactive Protein) from 3.6 ± 0.6 to 2.4 ± 0.5 was recorded with an increase to 3.2 ± 0.8 in the 20th week. The response to treatment lasted 7.1 weeks on average. No adverse effects were reported in the study [115]. There are several clinical trials currently underway to assess the efficacy and safety of stem cell transfusions in AS [116–119] (Table 2).

Table 2. Use of stem cells in patients with spondyloarthropathies in published literature and registered clinical trials.

SpA	Stem Cells	Description	Reference
Psoriatic arthritis	Allogenic blood stem cell transplantation (myeloablative)	Concomitant chronic myelogenous leukemia. Graft versus autoimmunity effect.	Slavin et al. [109]
Psoriatic arthritis	Allogenic hematopoetic stem cell transplantation	Concomitant aplastic anemia. Short remission with long chronic disability-free period	Woods et al. [110]
Psoriatic arthritis	Autologous hematopoetic stem cell transplantation (myeloablative)	Concomitant multiple myeloma. Complete remission of arthritis and skin lesions	Braiteh et al. [111]
Ankylosing spondylitis	Autologous hematopoetic stem cell transplantation	Concomitant lymphoma. The patient underwent chemotherapy. Clinical remission for both AS and lymphoma	Jantunen et al. [112]
Ankylosing spondylitis	Allogenic blood stem cell transplantation	Concomitant acute myeloid leukemia. The patient underwent chemotherapy and body irradiation. Clinical remission. Partial radiological regression of syndesophytes	Britanova et al. [114]
Ankylosing spondylitis	Autologus hematopoetic stem cell transplant	The first reported intentional stem cell transplant for AS. The patient underwent chemotherapy. Complete remission for AS for two-year follow up period	Yang et al. [113]
Ankylosing spondylitis	Allogenic mesenchymal stem cells intravenous infusion	Clinical trial. Phase 1. Trial involving 31 AS patients. No adverse effects noted. Reduction of ASDAS-CRP from 3.6 ± 0.6 to 2.4 ± 0.5 at the 4th week. The percentage of ASAS 20 responders reached 77.4%	Wanga et al. [115]
Ankylosing spondylitis	Human umbilical cord-derived mesenchymal stem cells	Clinical trial. Human umbilical cord-derived MSCs at a dose of 1.0×10^6 MSC/kg, repeated after three months and DMARDs such as sulfasalazine, methotrexate, thalidomide for 12 months	Clinical Trials. gov Identifier: NCT01420432 [116]
Ankylosing spondylitis	Human mesenchymal stem cells	Clinical trial. human mesenchymal stem cells: $1.0 \times 10^{+6}$ cells/kg, IV on day 1 of each 14–60 day cycle, 1–6 times treatment, plus NSAIDs.	ClinicalTrials.gov Identifier: NCT01709656 [117]
Ankylosing spondylitis	Human bone marrow-derived MSCs	Recruiting clinical trial. Phase 2. hBM-MSCs at a dose of 1.0×10^6 MSC/kg, receive infusion per week in the first 4 weeks and every two weeks in the second 8 weeks. Study Start Date: June 2016 Estimated Study Completion Date: December 2018	ClinicalTrials.gov Identifier: NCT02809781 [118]
Ankylosing spondylitis	Mesenchymal stem cells	Clinical trial. Phase I/II. To observe the safety and clinical effect of MSC transplantation in AS	Clinical trial. Registration number: ChiCTR-TRC-11001417 [119]

AS, ankylosing spondylitis; ASDAS-CRP, Ankylosing Spondylitis Disease Activity Score Containing C-Reactive Protein; ASAS 20, Assessment in Ankylosing Spondylitis Response Criteria 20; hBM-MSCs, human bone marrow-derived mesenchymal stem cells, DMARDs, disease-modifying anti-rheumatic drugs; NSAIDs, on steroidal anti-inflammatory drugs.

5. Conclusions

Promising results of studies into the application of stem cells in autoimmune diseases may be indicative of the therapeutic potential of MSC in SpAs. Depending on conditions in joints, MSC can exhibit anti-inflammatory or pro-inflammatory activity and can speed up regeneration in entheses or contribute to their ossification, which is typical of SpA. Local modification of MSC activity in the anti-inflammatory direction by appropriate agents or the administration of selected MSC may prove a highly affective option in the treatment of severe forms, especially in ankylosing spondylitis and psoriatic arthritis. However, it is still uncertain whether MSC used in SpA therapy should be autologous or allogenic and which tissue origin of cells is the most beneficial. It is also unclear whether treatment should be applied in early stages of a disease or rather as a regenerative therapy and which route of administration should be chosen, the number of cells and the therapeutic regimen. Obviously, further studies will be needed before the use of MSC in SpA could become the treatment of choice.

Acknowledgments: This study is supported by the National Centre for Research and Development Grant STRATEGMED1/234261/2NCBR/2014 and by the statutory grant Faculty of Medical Sciences, the University of Warmia and Mazury in Olsztyn, Poland.

Conflicts of Interest: The authors declare no conflict of interest.

References

1. Rutwaleit, M. New approaches to diagnosis and classification of axial and peripheral spondyloarthritis. *Curr. Opin. Rheumatol.* **2010**, *22*, 375–380. [CrossRef] [PubMed]
2. Callhoff, J.; Sieper, J.; Weiß, A.; Zink, A.; Listing, J. Efficacy of TNF-α blockers in patients with ankylosing spondylitis and non-radiographic axial spondyloarthritis: A meta-analysis. *Ann. Rheum. Dis.* **2015**, *74*, 1241–1248. [CrossRef] [PubMed]
3. Poddubnyy, D.; Hermann, K.G.; Callhoff, J.; Listing, J.; Sieper, J. Ustekinumab for the treatment of patients with active ankylosing spondylitis: Results of a 28-week, prospective, open-label, proof-of-concept study (TOPAS). *Ann. Rheum. Dis.* **2014**, *73*, 817–823. [CrossRef] [PubMed]
4. Baeten, D.; Baraliakos, X.; Braun, J.; Sieper, J.; Emery, P.; van der Heijde, D.; McInnes, I.; van Laar, J.M.; Landewé, R.; Wordsworth, P.; et al. Anti-interleukin-17A monoclonal antibody secukinumab in treatment of ankylosing spondylitis: A randomised, double-blind, placebocontrolled trial. *Lancet* **2013**, *382*, 1705–1713. [CrossRef]
5. Glenn, J.D.; Whartenby, K.A. Mesenchymal stem cells: Emerging mechanisms of immunomodulation and therapy. *World J. Stem Cells* **2014**, *6*, 526–539. [CrossRef] [PubMed]
6. Horwitz, E.M.; Le Blanc, K.; Dominici, M.; Mueller, I.; Slaper-Cortenbach, I.; Marini, F.C.; Deans, R.J.; Krause, D.S.; Keating, A. International Society for Cellular Therapy. Clarification of the nomenclature for MSC: The International Society for Cellular Therapy position statement. *Cytotherapy* **2005**, *7*, 393–395. [CrossRef] [PubMed]
7. Colter, D.C.; Sekiya, I.; Prockop, D.J. Identification of a subpopulation of rapidly self-renewing and multipotential adult stem cells in colonies of human marrow stromal cells. *Proc. Natl. Acad. Sci. USA* **2001**, *98*, 7841–7845. [CrossRef] [PubMed]
8. Braun, J.; Kurtz, A.; Barutcu, N.; Bodo, J.; Thiel, A.; Dong, J. Concerted regulation of CD34 and CD105 accompanies mesenchymal stromal cell derivation from human adventitial stromal cell. *Stem Cells Dev.* **2013**, *22*, 815–827. [CrossRef] [PubMed]
9. Ho, A.D.; Wagner, W.; Franke, W. Heterogeneity of mesenchymal stromal cell preparations. *Cytotherapy* **2008**, *10*, 320–330. [CrossRef] [PubMed]
10. Girlovanu, M.; Susman, S.; Soritau, O.; Rus-Ciuca, D.; Melincovici, C.; Constantin, A.M.; Mihu, C.M. Stem cells—Biological update and cell therapy progress. *Clujul Med.* **2015**, *88*, 265–271. [CrossRef] [PubMed]
11. Im, G.I. Bone marrow-derived stem/stromal cells and adipose tissue-derived stem/stromal cells: Their comparative efficacies and synergistic effects. *J. Biomed. Mater. Res. A* **2017**, *105*, 2640–2648. [CrossRef] [PubMed]

12. Dominici, M.; Le Blanc, K.; Mueller, I.; Slaper-Cortenbach, I.; Marini, F.; Krause, D.; Deans, R.; Keating, A.; Prockop, D.J.; Horwitz, E. Minimal criteria for defining multipotent mesenchymal stromal cells. The International Society for Cellular Therapy position statement. *Cytotherapy* **2006**, *8*, 315–317. [CrossRef] [PubMed]

13. Keating, A. Mesenchymal stromal cells: New directions. *Cell Stem Cell* **2012**, *10*, 709–716. [CrossRef] [PubMed]

14. Frenette, P.S.; Pinho, S.; Lucas, D.; Scheiermann, C. Mesenchymal stem cell: Keystone of the hematopoietic stem cell niche and a stepping-stone for regenerative medicine. *Annu. Rev. Immunol.* **2013**, *31*, 285–316. [CrossRef] [PubMed]

15. Bronckaers, A.; Hilkens, P.; Martens, W.; Gervois, P.; Ratajczak, J.; Struys, T.; Lambrichts, I. Mesenchymal stem/stromal cells as a pharmacological and therapeutic approach to accelerate angiogenesis. *Pharmacol. Ther.* **2014**, *143*, 181–196. [CrossRef] [PubMed]

16. Prockop, D.J. Concise review: Two negative feedback loops place mesenchymal stem/stromal cells at the center of early regulators of inflammation. *Stem Cells* **2013**, *31*, 2042–2046. [CrossRef] [PubMed]

17. Delarosa, O.; Dalemans, W.; Lombardo, E. Toll-like receptors as modulators of mesenchymal stem cells. *Front. Immunol.* **2012**, *3*, 182. [CrossRef] [PubMed]

18. Raicevic, G.; Rouas, R.; Najar, M.; Stordeur, P.; Boufker, H.I.; Bron, D.; Martiat, P.; Goldman, M.; Nevessignsky, M.T.; Lagneaux, L. Inflammation modifies the pattern and the function of Toll-like receptors expressed by human mesenchymal stromal cells. *Hum. Immunol.* **2010**, *71*, 235–244. [CrossRef] [PubMed]

19. Mo, I.F.; Yip, K.H.; Chan, W.K.; Law, H.K.; Lau, Y.L.; Chan, G.C. Prolonged exposure to bacterial toxins downregulated expression of toll-like receptors in mesenchymal stromal cell-derived osteoprogenitors. *BMC Cell Biol.* **2008**, *9*, 52. [CrossRef] [PubMed]

20. Waterman, R.S.; Tomchuck, S.L.; Henkle, S.L.; Betancourt, A.M. A new mesenchymal stem cell (MSC) paradigm: Polarization into a pro-inflammatory MSC1 or an immunosuppressive MSC2 phenotype. *PLoS ONE* **2010**, *5*, e10088. [CrossRef] [PubMed]

21. Heuschen, G.; Leowardi, C.; Hinz, U.; Autschbach, F.; Stallmach, A.; Herfarth, C.; Heuschen, U.A. Differential expression of toll-like receptor 3 and 5 in ileal pouch mucosa of ulcerative colitis patients. *Int. J. Colorectal Dis.* **2007**, *22*, 293–301. [CrossRef] [PubMed]

22. De Rycke, L.; Vandooren, B.; Kruithof, E.; De Keyser, F.; Veys, E.M.; Baeten, D. Tumor necrosis factor alpha blockade treatment down-modulates the increased systemic and local expression of Toll-like receptor 2 and Toll-like receptor 4 in spondylarthropathy. *Arthritis Rheum.* **2005**, *52*, 2146–2158. [CrossRef] [PubMed]

23. Yang, Z.X.; Liang, Y.; Zhu, Y.; Li, C.; Zhang, L.Z.; Zeng, X.M.; Zhong, R.Q. Increased expression of Toll-like receptor 4 in peripheral blood leucocytes and serum levels of some cytokines in patients with ankylosing spondylitis. *Clin. Exp. Immunol.* **2007**, *149*, 48–55. [CrossRef] [PubMed]

24. Candia, L.; Marquez, J.; Hernandez, C.; Zea, A.H.; Espinoza, L.R. Toll-like receptor-2 expression is upregulated in antigen-presenting cells from patients with psoriatic arthritis: A pathogenic role for innate immunity. *J. Rheumatol.* **2007**, *34*, 374–379. [PubMed]

25. Myles, A.; Aggarwal, A. Expression of Toll-like receptors 2 and 4 is increased in peripheral blood and synovial fluid monocytes of patients with enthesitis-related arthritis subtype of juvenile idiopathic arthritis. *Rheumatology* **2011**, *50*, 481–488. [CrossRef] [PubMed]

26. Brandau, S.; Jakob, M.; Hemeda, H.; Bruderek, K.; Janeschik, S.; Bootz, F.; Lang, S. Tissue-resident mesenchymal stem cells attract peripheral blood neutrophils and enhance their inflammatory activity in response to microbial challenge. *J. Leukoc. Biol.* **2010**, *88*, 1005–1015. [CrossRef] [PubMed]

27. Mantovani, A.; Biswas, S.K.; Galdiero, M.R.; Sica, A.; Locati, M. Macrophage plasticity and polarization in tissue repair and remodelling. *J. Pathol.* **2013**, *229*, 176–185. [CrossRef] [PubMed]

28. Cassatella, M.A.; Mosna, F.; Micheletti, A.; Lisi, V.; Tamassia, N.; Cont, C.; Calzetti, F.; Pelletier, M.; Pizzolo, G.; Krampera, M. Toll-like receptor-3-activated human mesenchymal stromal cells significantly prolong the survival and function of neutrophils. *Stem Cells* **2011**, *29*, 1001–1011. [CrossRef] [PubMed]

29. Li, W.; Ren, G.; Huang, Y.; Su, J.; Han, Y.; Li, J.; Chen, X.; Cao, K.; Chen, Q.; Shou, P.; et al. Mesenchymal stem cells: A double-edged sword in regulating immune responses. *Cell Death Differ.* **2012**, *19*, 1505–1513. [CrossRef] [PubMed]

30. Shi, C.; Jia, T.; Mendez-Ferrer, S.; Hohl, T.M.; Serbina, N.V.; Lipuma, L.; Leiner, I.; Li, M.O.; Frenette, P.S.; Pamer, E.G. Bone marrow mesenchymal stem and progenitor cells induce monocyte emigration in response to circulating toll-like receptor ligands. *Immunity* **2011**, *34*, 590–601. [CrossRef] [PubMed]

31. Chen, L.; Tredget, E.E.; Wu, P.Y.; Wu, Y. Paracrine factors of mesenchymal stem cells recruit macrophages and endothelial lineage cells and enhance wound healing. *PLoS ONE* **2008**, *3*, e1886. [CrossRef] [PubMed]

32. Abumaree, M.H.; Al Jumah, M.A.; Kalionis, B.; Jawdat, D.; Al Khaldi, A.; Abomaray, F.M.; Fatani, A.S.; Chamley, L.W.; Knawy, B.A. Human placental mesenchymal stem cells (pMSCs) play a role as immune suppressive cells by shifting macrophage differentiation from inflammatory M1 to anti-inflammatory M2 macrophages. *Stem Cell Rev.* **2013**, *9*, 620–641. Available online: https://www.ncbi.nlm.nih.gov/pubmed/23812784 (accessed on 25 November 2017). [CrossRef] [PubMed]

33. Cho, D.I.; Kim, M.R.; Jeong, H.Y.; Jeong, H.C.; Jeong, M.H.; Yoon, S.H.; Kim, Y.S.; Ahn, Y. Mesenchymal stem cells reciprocally regulate the M1/M2 balance in mouse bone marrow-derived macrophages. *Exp. Mol. Med.* **2014**, *46*, e70. [CrossRef] [PubMed]

34. Dayan, V.; Yannarelli, G.; Billia, F.; Filomeno, P.; Wang, X.H.; Davies, J.E.; Keating, A. Mesenchymal stromal cells mediate a switch to alternatively activated monocytes/macrophages after acute myocardial infarction. *Basic Res. Cardiol.* **2011**, *106*, 1299–1310. [CrossRef] [PubMed]

35. Eggenhofer, E.; Hoogduijn, M.J. Mesenchymal stem cell-educated macrophages. *Transp. Res.* **2012**, *1*, 12. [CrossRef] [PubMed]

36. Nemeth, K.; Leelahavanichkul, A.; Yuen, P.S.; Mayer, B.; Parmelee, A.; Doi, K.; Robey, P.G.; Leelahavanichkul, K.; Koller, B.H.; Brown, J.M.; et al. Bone marrow stromal cells attenuate sepsis via prostaglandin E(2)-dependent reprogramming of host macrophages to increase their interleukin-10 production. *Nat. Med.* **2009**, *15*, 42–49. [CrossRef] [PubMed]

37. Zhao, J.; Yuan, W.; Tao, C.; Sun, P.; Yang, Z.; Xu, W. M2 polarization of monocytes in ankylosing spondylitis and relationship with inflammation and structural damage. *APMIS* **2017**. [CrossRef] [PubMed]

38. Ciccia, F.; Alessandro, R.; Rizzo, A.; Accardo-Palumbo, A.; Raimondo, S.; Raiata, F.; Guggino, G.; Giardina, A.; De Leo, G.; Sireci, G.; et al. Macrophage phenotype in the subclinical gut inflammation of patients with ankylosing spondylitis. *Rheumatology* **2014**, *53*, 104–113. [CrossRef] [PubMed]

39. Van Kuijk, A.W.; Reinders-Blankert, P.; Smeets, T.J.; Dijkmans, B.A.; Tak, P.P. Detailed analysis of the cell infiltrate and the expression of mediators of synovial inflammation and joint destruction in the synovium of patients with psoriatic arthritis: Implications for treatment. *Ann. Rheum Dis.* **2006**, *65*, 1551–1557. [CrossRef] [PubMed]

40. Kang, K.Y.; Ju, J.H.; Park, S.H.; Kim, H.Y. The paradoxical effects of TNF inhibitors on bone mineral density and radiographic progression in patients with ankylosing spondylitis. *Rheumatology* **2013**, *52*, 718–726. [CrossRef] [PubMed]

41. Guihard, P.; Danger, Y.; Brounais, B.; David, E.; Brion, R.; Delecrin, J.; Richards, C.D.; Chevalier, S.; Rédini, F.; Heymann, D.; et al. Induction of Osteogenesis in mesenchymal stem cells by activated monocytes/macrophages depends on oncostatin M signaling. *Stem Cells* **2012**, *30*, 762–772. [CrossRef] [PubMed]

42. Dillon, S.M.; Rogers, L.M.; Howe, R.; Hostetler, L.A.; Buhrman, J.; McCarter, M.D.; Wilson, C.C. Human intestinal lamina propria CD1c+ dendritic cells display an activated phenotype at steady state and produce IL-23 in response to TLR7/8 stimulation. *J. Immunol.* **2010**, *184*, 6612–6621. [CrossRef] [PubMed]

43. DeLay, M.L.; Turner, M.J.; Klenk, E.I.; Smith, J.A.; Sowders, D.P.; Colbert, R.A. HLA-B27 misfolding and the unfolded protein response augment interleukin-23 production and are associated with Th17 activation in transgenic rats. *Arthritis Rheum.* **2009**, *60*, 2633–2643. [CrossRef] [PubMed]

44. Utriainen, L.; Firmin, D.; Wright, P.; Cerovic, V.; Breban, M.; McInnes, I.; Milling, S. Expression of HLA-B27 causes loss of migratory dendritic cells in a rat model of spondyloarthritis. *Arthritis Rheum.* **2012**, *64*, 3199–3209. [CrossRef] [PubMed]

45. Sherlock, J.P.; Joyce-Shaikh, B.; Turner, S.P.; Chao, C.C.; Sathe, M.; Grein, J.; Gorman, D.M.; Bowman, E.P.; McClanahan, T.K.; Yearley, J.H.; et al. IL-23 induces spondyloarthropathy by acting on ROR-γt(+)CD3(+)CD4(-)CD8(-) entheseal resident T cells. *Nat. Med.* **2012**, *18*, 1069–1076. [CrossRef] [PubMed]

46. Nauta, A.J.; Kruisselbrink, A.B.; Lurvink, E.; Willemze, R.; Fibbe, W.E. Mesenchymal stem cells inhibit generation and function of both CD34+-derived and monocyte-derived dendritic cells. *J. Immunol.* **2006**, *177*, 2080–2087. [CrossRef] [PubMed]

47. Zhang, W.; Ge, W.; Li, C.; You, S.; Liao, L.; Han, Q.; Deng, W.; Zhao, R.C. Effects of mesenchymal stem cells on differentiation, maturation, and function of human monocyte-derived dendritic cells. *Stem Cells Dev.* **2004**, *13*, 263–271. [CrossRef] [PubMed]

48. Jiang, X.X.; Zhang, Y.; Liu, B.; Zhang, S.X.; Wu, Y.; Yu, X.D.; Mao, N. Human mesenchymal stem cells inhibit differentiation and function of monocyte-derived dendritic cells. *Blood* **2005**, *105*, 4120–4126. [CrossRef] [PubMed]

49. Spaggiari, G.M.; Abdelrazik, H.; Becchetti, F.; Moretta, L. MSCs inhibit monocyte-derived DC maturation and function by selectively interfering with the generation of immature DCs: Central role of MSC-derived prostaglandin E2. *Blood* **2009**, *113*, 6576–6583. [CrossRef] [PubMed]

50. Chiesa, S.; Morbelli, S.; Morando, S.; Massollo, M.; Marini, C.; Bertoni, A.; Frassoni, F.; Bartolomé, S.T.; Sambuceti, G.; Traggiai, E.; et al. Mesenchymal stem cells impair in vivo T-cell priming by dendritic cells. *Proc. Natl. Acad. Sci. USA* **2011**, *108*, 17384–17389. [CrossRef] [PubMed]

51. Favaro, E.; Carpanetto, A.; Caorsi, C.; Giovarelli, M.; Angelini, C.; Cavallo-Perin, P.; Tetta, C.; Camussi, G.; Zanone, M.M. Human mesenchymal stem cells and derived extracellular vesicles induce regulatory dendritic cells in type 1 diabetic patients. *Diabetologia* **2016**, *59*, 325–333. [CrossRef] [PubMed]

52. Appel, H.; Maier, R.; Wu, P.; Scheer, R.; Hempfing, A.; Kayser, R.; Thiel, A.; Radbruch, A.; Loddenkemper, C.; Sieper, J. Analysis of IL-17+ cells in facet joints of patients with spondyloarthritis suggests that the innate immune pathway might be of greater relevance than the Th17-mediated adaptive immune response. *Arthritis Res. Ther.* **2011**, *13*, R95. [CrossRef] [PubMed]

53. Maqbool, M.; Vidyadaran, S.; George, E.; Ramasamy, R. Human mesenchymal stem cells protect neutrophils from serum-deprived cell death. *Cell Biol. Int.* **2011**, *35*, 1247–1251. [CrossRef] [PubMed]

54. Raffaghello, L.; Bianchi, G.; Bertolotto, M.; Montecucco, F.; Busca, A.; Dallegri, F.; Ottonello, L.; Pistoia, V. Human mesenchymal stem cells inhibit neutrophil apoptosis: A model for neutrophil preservation in the bone marrow niche. *Stem Cells* **2008**, *26*, 151–162. [CrossRef] [PubMed]

55. Zvyagin, I.V.; Mamedov, I.Z.; Britanova, O.V.; Staroverov, D.B.; Nasonov, E.L.; Bochkova, A.G.; Chkalina, A.V.; Kotlobay, A.A.; Korostin, D.O.; Rebrikov, D.V.; et al. Contribution of functional KIR3DL1 to ankylosing spondylitis. *Cell. Mol. Immunol.* **2010**, *7*, 471–476. [CrossRef] [PubMed]

56. Sotiropoulou, P.A.; Perez, S.A.; Gritzapis, A.D.; Baxevanis, C.N.; Papamichail, M. Interactions between human mesenchymal stem cells and natural killer cells. *Stem Cells* **2006**, *24*, 74–85. [CrossRef] [PubMed]

57. Spaggiari, G.M.; Capobianco, A.; Becchetti, S.; Mingari, M.C.; Moretta, L. Mesenchymal stem cell-natural killer cell interactions: Evidence that activated NK cells are capable of killing MSCs, whereas MSCs can inhibit IL-2-induced NK-cell proliferation. *Blood* **2006**, *107*, 1484–1490. [CrossRef] [PubMed]

58. Le Blanc, K.; Mougiakakos, D. Multipotent mesenchymal stromal cells and the innate immune system. *Nat. Rev. Immunol.* **2012**, *12*, 383–396. [CrossRef] [PubMed]

59. Prigione, I.; Benvenuto, F.; Bocca, P.; Battistini, L.; Uccelli, A.; Pistoia, V. Reciprocal interactions between human mesenchymal stem cells and gammadelta T cells or invariant natural killer T cells. *Stem Cells* **2009**, *27*, 693–702. [CrossRef] [PubMed]

60. Stagg, J.; Galipeau, J. Mechanisms of immune modulation by mesenchymal stromal cells and clinical translation. *Curr. Mol. Med.* **2013**, *13*, 856–867. [CrossRef] [PubMed]

61. Aggarwal, S.; Pittenger, M.F. Human mesenchymal stem cells modulate allogeneic immune cell responses. *Blood* **2005**, *105*, 1815–1822. [CrossRef] [PubMed]

62. Francois, M.; Romieu-Mourez, R.; Li, M.; Galipeau, J. Human MSC suppression correlates with cytokine induction of indoleamine 2,3-dioxygenase and bystander M2 macrophage differentiation. *Mol. Ther.* **2012**, *20*, 187–195. [CrossRef] [PubMed]

63. Ghannam, S.; Pene, J.; Torcy-Moquet, G.; Jorgensen, C.; Yssel, H. Mesenchymal stem cells inhibit human Th17 cell differentiation and function and induce a T regulatory cell phenotype. *J. Immunol.* **2010**, *185*, 302–312. [CrossRef] [PubMed]

64. Liu, X.; Ren, S.; Qu, X.; Ge, C.; Cheng, K.; Zhao, R.C. Mesenchymal stem cells inhibit Th17 cells differentiation via IFN-γ-mediated SOCS3 activation. *Immunol. Res.* **2015**, *61*, 219–229. [CrossRef] [PubMed]

65. Rafei, M.; Campeau, P.M.; Aguilar-Mahecha, A.; Buchanan, M.; Williams, P.; Birman, E.; Yuan, S.; Young, Y.K.; Boivin, M.N.; Forner, K.; et al. Mesenchymal stromal cells ameliorate experimental autoimmune encephalomyelitis by inhibiting CD4 Th17 T cells in a CC chemokine ligand 2-dependent manner. *J. Immunol.* **2009**, *182*, 5994–6002. [CrossRef] [PubMed]

66. Huang, Z.F.; Zhu, J.; Lu, S.H.; Zhang, J.L.; Chen, X.; Du, L.X.; Yang, Z.G.; Song, Y.K.; Wu, D.Y.; Liu, B.; et al. Inhibitory effect of human umbilical cord-derived mesenchymal stem cells on interleukin-17 production in peripheral blood T cells from spondyloarthritis patients. *Zhongguo Shi Yan Xue Ye Za Zhi* **2013**, *21*, 455–459. [CrossRef]

67. Shen, H.; Goodall, J.C.; Hill Gaston, J.S. Frequency and phenotype of peripheral blood Th17 cells in ankylosing spondylitis and rheumatoid arthritis. *Arthritis Rheum.* **2009**, *60*, 1647–1656. [CrossRef] [PubMed]

68. Limón-Camacho, L.; Vargas-Rojas, M.I.; Vázquez-Mellado, J.; Casasola-Vargas, J.; Moctezuma, J.F.; Burgos-Vargas, R.; Llorente, L. In vivo peripheral blood proinflammatory T cells in patients with ankylosing spondylitis. *J. Rheumatol.* **2012**, *39*, 830–835. [CrossRef] [PubMed]

69. Luz-Crawford, P.; Kurte, M.; Bravo-Alegría, J.; Contreras, R.; Nova-Lamperti, E.; Tejedor, G.; Noël, D.; Jorgensen, C.; Figueroa, F.; Djouad, F.; et al. Mesenchymal stem cells generate a CD4$^+$CD25$^+$Foxp3$^+$ regulatory T cell population during the differentiation process of Th1 and Th17 cells. *Stem Cell Res. Ther.* **2013**, *4*, 65. [CrossRef] [PubMed]

70. Obermajer, N.; Popp, F.C.; Soeder, Y.; Haarer, J.; Geissler, E.K.; Schlitt, H.J.; Dahlke, M.H. Conversion of Th17 into IL-17A(neg) regulatory T cells: A novel mechanism in prolonged allograft survival promoted by mesenchymal stem cell-supported minimized immunosuppressive therapy. *J. Immunol.* **2014**, *193*, 4988–4999. [CrossRef] [PubMed]

71. Xueyi, L.; Lina, C.; Zhenbiao, W.; Qing, H.; Qiang, L.; Zhu, P. Levels of circulating Th17 cells and regulatory T cells in ankylosing spondylitis patients with an inadequate response to anti-TNF-alpha therapy. *J. Clin. Immunol.* **2013**, *33*, 151–161. [CrossRef] [PubMed]

72. Appel, H.; Wu, P.; Scheer, R.; Kedor, C.; Sawitzki, B.; Thiel, A.; Radbruch, A.; Sieper, J.; Syrbe, U. Synovial and peripheral blood CD4$^+$FoxP3$^+$ T cells in spondyloarthritis. *J. Rheumatol.* **2011**, *38*, 2445–2451. [CrossRef] [PubMed]

73. Guo, H.; Zheng, M.; Zhang, K.; Yang, F.; Zhang, X.; Han, Q.; Chen, Z.N.; Zhu, P. Functional defects in CD4$^+$ CD25^{high} FoxP3$^+$ regulatory cells in ankylosing spondylitis. *Sci. Rep.* **2016**, *6*, 37559. [CrossRef] [PubMed]

74. Wu, Y.; Ren, M.; Yang, R.; Liang, X.; Ma, Y.; Tang, Y.; Huang, L.; Ye, J.; Chen, K.; Wanget, P.; et al. Reduced immunomodulation potential of bone marrow-derived mesenchymal stem cells induced CCR4$^+$CCR6$^+$Th/Treg cell subset imbalance in ankylosing spondylitis. *Arthritis Res. Ther.* **2011**, *13*, R29. [CrossRef] [PubMed]

75. English, K.; Ryan, J.M.; Tobin, L.; Murphy, M.J.; Barry, F.P.; Mahon, B.P. Cell contact, prostaglandin E(2) and transforming growth factor beta 1 play non-redundant roles in human mesenchymal stem cell induction of CD4$^+$CD25^{High}forkhead box P3$^+$ regulatory T cells. *Clin. Exp. Immunol.* **2009**, *156*, 149–160. [CrossRef] [PubMed]

76. Melief, S.M.; Schrama, C.L.M.; Brugman, M.H.; Tiemessen, M.M.; Hoogduijn, M.J.; Fibbe, W.E.; Roelofs, H. Multipotent stromal cells induce human regulatory T cells through a novel pathway involving skewing of monocytes towards anti-inflammatory macrophages. *Stem Cells* **2013**, *31*, 1980–1991. [CrossRef] [PubMed]

77. LeMaoult, J.; Caumartin, J.; Daouya, M.; Favier, B.; Le Rond, S.; Gonzalez, A.; Carosella, E.D. Immune regulation by pretenders: Cell-to-cell transfers of HLA-G make effector T cells act as regulatory cells. *Blood* **2007**, *109*, 2040–2048. [CrossRef] [PubMed]

78. Selmani, Z.; Naji, A.; Zidi, I.; Favier, B.; Gaiffe, E.; Obert, L.; Borg, C.; Saas, P.; Tiberghien, P.; Rouas-Freiss, N.; et al. Human leukocyte antigen-G5 secretion by human mesenchymal stem cells is required to suppress T lymphocyte and natural killer function and to induce CD4$^+$CD25^{high}FOXP3$^+$ regulatory T cells. *Stem Cells* **2008**, *26*, 212–222. [CrossRef] [PubMed]

79. Lund, F.E.; Randall, T.D. Effector and regulatory B cells: Modulators of CD4$^+$ T cell immunity. *Nat. Rev. Immunol.* **2010**, *10*, 236–247. [CrossRef] [PubMed]

80. Nova-Lamperti, E.; Fanelli, G.; Becker, P.D.; Chana, P.; Elgueta, R.; Dodd, P.C.; Lord, G.M.; Lombardi, G.; Hernandez-Fuentesa, M.P. IL-10-produced by human transitional B-cells down-regulates CD86 expression on B-cells leading to inhibition of CD4(+)T-cell responses. *Sci. Rep.* **2016**, *6*, 20044. [CrossRef] [PubMed]

81. Cantaert, T.; Doorenspleet, M.E.; Francosalinas, G.; Paramarta, J.E.; Klarenbeek, P.L.; Tiersma, Y.; van der Loos, C.M.; De Vries, N.; Tak, P.P.; Baeten, D.L. Increased numbers of CD5+ B lymphocytes with a regulatory phenotype in spondylarthritis. *Arthritis Rheum.* **2012**, *64*, 1859–1868. [CrossRef] [PubMed]

82. Bautista-Caro, M.B.; de Miguel, E.; Peiteado, D.; Plasencia-Rodríguez, C.; Villalba, A.; Monjo-Henry, I.; Puig-Kröger, A.; Sánchez-Mateos, P.; Martín-Mola, E.; Miranda-Carús, M.E. Increased frequency of circulating CD19+CD24hiCD38hi B cells with regulatory capacity in patients with Ankylosing spondylitis (AS) naïve for biological agents. *PLoS ONE* **2017**, *12*, e0180726. [CrossRef] [PubMed]

83. Corcione, A.; Benvenuto, F.; Ferretti, E.; Giunti, D.; Cappiello, V.; Cazzanti, F.; Risso, M.; Gualandi, F.; Mancardi, G.L.; Pistoia, V.; et al. Human mesenchymal stem cells modulate B-cell functions. *Blood* **2006**, *107*, 367–372. [CrossRef] [PubMed]

84. Lee, D.S.; Yi, T.G.; Lee, H.J.; Kim, S.N.; Park, S.; Jeon, M.S.; Song, S.U. Mesenchymal stem cells infected with *Mycoplasma arginini* secrete complement C3 to regulate immunoglobulin production in b lymphocytes. *Cel Death Dis.* **2014**, *5*, e1192. [CrossRef] [PubMed]

85. Yan, H.; Wu, M.; Yuan, Y.; Wang, Z.Z.; Jiang, H.; Chen, T. Priming of Toll-like receptor 4 pathway in mesenchymal stem cells increases expression of B cell activating factor. *Biochem. Biophys. Res. Commun.* **2014**, *448*, 212–217. [CrossRef] [PubMed]

86. Ungerer, C.; Quade-Lyssy, P.; Radeke, H.H.; Henschler, R.; Konigs, C.; Kohl, U.; Seifried, E.; Schüttrumpf, J. Galectin-9 is a suppressor of T and B cells and predicts the immune modulatory potential of mesenchymal stromal cell preparations. *Stem Cells Dev.* **2014**, *23*, 755–766. [CrossRef] [PubMed]

87. Rosado, M.M.; Bernardo, M.E.; Scarsella, M.; Conforti, A.; Giorda, E.; Biagini, S.; Cascioli, S.; Rossi, F.; Guzzo, I.; Vivarelli, M.; et al. Inhibition of B-cell proliferation and antibody production by mesenchymal stromal cells is mediated by T cells. *Stem Cells Dev.* **2015**, *24*, 93–103. [CrossRef] [PubMed]

88. Ji, Y.R.; Yang, Z.X.; Han, Z.B.; Meng, L.; Liang, L.; Feng, X.M.; Yang, S.G.; Chi, Y.; Chen, D.D.; Wang, Y.W.; et al. Mesenchymal stem cells support proliferation and terminal differentiation of B cells. *Cell Physiol. Biochem.* **2012**, *30*, 1526–1537. [CrossRef] [PubMed]

89. Ding, J.; Ghali, O.; Lencel, P.; Broux, O.; Chauveau, C.; Devedjian, J.C.; Hardouin, P.; Magne, D. TNFα and IL1β inhibit RUNX2 and collagen expression but increase alkaline phosphatase activity and mineralization in human mesenchymal stem cells. *Life Sci.* **2009**, *84*, 499–504. [CrossRef] [PubMed]

90. Briolay, A.; Lencel, P.; Bessueille, L.; Caverzasio, J.; Buchet, R.; Magne, D. Autocrine stimulation of osteoblast activity by Wnt5a in response to TNF-α in human mesenchymal stem cells. *Biochem. Biophys. Res. Commun.* **2013**, *430*, 1072–1077. [CrossRef] [PubMed]

91. De Bari, C.; Kurth, T.B.; Augello, A. Mesenchymal stem cells from development to postnatal joint homeostasis, aging, and disease. *Birth Defects Res. C. Embryo Today* **2010**, *90*, 257–271. [CrossRef] [PubMed]

92. Nourissat, G.; Diop, A.; Maurel, N.; Salvat, C.; Dumont, S.; Pigenet, A.; Gosset, M.; Houard, X.; Berenbaum, F. Mesenchymal stem cell therapy regenerates the native bone-tendon junction after surgical repair in a degenerative rat model. *PLoS ONE* **2010**, *5*, e12248. [CrossRef] [PubMed]

93. Rui, Y.F.; Lui, P.P.; Ni, M.; Chan, L.S.; Lee, Y.W.; Chan, K.M. Mechanical loading increased BMP-2 expression which promoted osteogenic differentiation of tendon-derived stem cells. *J. Orthop. Res.* **2011**, *29*, 390–396. [CrossRef] [PubMed]

94. Moccia, F.; Guerra, G. Ca2+ Signalling in endothelial progenitor cells: Friend or foe? *J. Cell Physiol.* **2016**, *231*, 314–327. [CrossRef] [PubMed]

95. Ronco, V.; Potenza, D.M.; Denti, F.; Vullo, S.; Gagliano, G.; Tognolina, M.; Guerra, G.; Pinton, P.; Genazzani, A.A.; Mapelli, L.; et al. A novel Ca2+-mediated cross-talk between endoplasmic reticulum and acidic organelles: Implications for NAADP-dependent Ca2+ signaling. *Cell Calcium* **2015**, *57*, 89–100. [CrossRef] [PubMed]

96. Kim, T.J.; Sun, J.; Lu, S.; Qi, Y.X.; Wang, Y. Prolonged mechanical stretch initiates intracellular calcium oscillations in human mesenchymal stem cells. *PLoS ONE* **2014**, *9*, e109378. [CrossRef] [PubMed]

97. Kim, T.J.; Joo, C.; Seong, J.; Vafabakhsh, R.; Botvinick, E.L.; Berns, M.W.; Palmer, A.E.; Wang, N.; Ha, T.; Jakobsson, E.; et al. Distinct mechanisms regulating mechanical force-induced Ca2+ signals at the plasma membrane and the ER in human MSCs. *eLife* **2015**, *4*, e04876. [CrossRef] [PubMed]

98. Xie, Z.; Wang, P.; Li, Y.; Deng, W.; Zhang, X.; Su, H.; Li, D.; Wu, Y.; Shen, H. Imbalance between BMP2 and Noggin induces abnormal osteogenic differentiation of mesenchymal stem cells in ankylosing spondylitis. *Arthritis Rheumatol.* **2016**, *68*, 430–440. [CrossRef] [PubMed]

99. Bassi, E.J.; Moraes-Vieira, P.M.; Moreira-Sa, C.S.; Almeida, D.C.; Vieira, L.M.; Cunha, C.S.; Hiyane, M.I.; Basso, A.S.; Pacheco-Silva, A.; Câmara, N.O. Immune regulatory properties of allogeneic adipose-derived mesenchymal stem cells in the treatment of experimental autoimmune diabetes. *Diabetes* **2012**, *61*, 2534–2545. [CrossRef] [PubMed]

100. Anderson, P.; Souza-Moreira, L.; Morell, M.; Caro, M.; O'Valle, F.; Gonzalez-Rey, E.; Delgado, M. Adipose-derived mesenchymal stromal cells induce mmunomodulatory macrophages which protect from experimental colitis and sepsis. *Gut* **2013**, *62*, 1131–1141. [CrossRef] [PubMed]

101. Bartholomew, A.; Sturgeon, C.; Siatskas, M.; Ferrer, K.; McIntosh, K.; Patil, S.; Hardy, W.; Devine, S.; Ucker, D.; Deans, R.; et al. Mesenchymal stem cells suppress lymphocyte proliferation in vitro and prolong skin graft survival in vivo. *Exp. Hematol.* **2002**, *30*, 42–48. [CrossRef]

102. Oh, J.Y.; Lee, R.H.; Yu, J.M.; Ko, J.H.; Lee, H.J.; Ko, A.Y.; Roddy, G.W.; Prockop, D.J. Intravenous mesenchymal stem cells prevented rejection of allogeneic corneal transplants by aborting the early inflammatory response. *Mol. Ther.* **2012**, *20*, 2143–2152. [CrossRef] [PubMed]

103. Zappia, E.; Casazza, S.; Pedemonte, E.; Benvenuto, F.; Bonanni, I.; Gerdoni, E.; Giunti, D.; Ceravolo, A.; Cazzanti, F.; Frassoni, F.; et al. Mesenchymal stem cells ameliorate experimental autoimmune encephalomyelitis inducing T-cell anergy. *Blood* **2005**, *106*, 1755–1761. [CrossRef] [PubMed]

104. Mathias, L.J.; Khong, S.M.; Spyroglou, L.; Payne, N.L.; Siatskas, C.; Thorburn, A.N.; Boyd, R.L.; Heng, T.S. Alveolar macrophages are critical for the inhibition of allergic asthma by mesenchymal stromal cells. *J. Immunol.* **2013**, *191*, 5914–5924. [CrossRef] [PubMed]

105. Zanotti, L.; Sarukhan, A.; Dander, E.; Castor, M.; Cibella, J.; Soldani, C.; Trovato, A.E.; Ploia, C.; Luca, G.; Calvitti, M.; et al. Encapsulated mesenchymal stem cells for in vivo immunomodulation. *Leukemia* **2013**, *27*, 500–503. [CrossRef] [PubMed]

106. Swart, J.F.; Wulffraat, N.M. Mesenchymal stromal cells for treatment of arthritis. *Best Pract. Res. Clin. Rheumatol.* **2014**, *28*, 589–603. [CrossRef] [PubMed]

107. Wyles, C.C.; Houdek, M.T.; Behfar, A.; Sierra, R.S. Mesenchymal stem cell therapy for osteoarthritis: Current perspectives. *Stem Cells Cloning* **2015**, *8*, 117–124. [CrossRef] [PubMed]

108. Hinterberger, W.; Hinterberger-Fischer, M.; Marmont, A. Clinically demonstrable anti-autoimmunity mediated by allogeneic immune cells favorably affects outcome after stem cell transplantation in human autoimmune diseases. *Bone Marrow Transplant.* **2002**, *30*, 753–759. [CrossRef] [PubMed]

109. Slavin, S.; Nagler, A.; Varadi, G.; Or, R. Graft vs autoimmunity following allogeneic non-myeloablative blood stem cell transplantation in a patient with chronic myelogenous leukaemia and severe systemic psoriasis and psoriatic polyarthritis. *Exp. Hematol.* **2000**, *28*, 853–857. [CrossRef]

110. Woods, A.C.; Mant, M.J. Amelioration of severe psoriasis with psoriatic arthritis for 20 years after allogeneic haematopoietic stem cell transplantation. *Ann. Rheum. Dis.* **2006**, *65*, 697. [CrossRef] [PubMed]

111. Braiteh, F.; Hymes, S.R.; Giralt, S.A.; Jones, R. Complete remission of psoriasis after autologous hematopoietic stem-cell transplantation for multiple myeloma. *J. Clin. Oncol.* **2008**, *26*, 4511–4513. [CrossRef] [PubMed]

112. Jantumen, E.; Myllykangas-Luosujärvi, R.; Kaipiainen-Seppänen, O.; Nousiainen, T. Autologous stem cell transplantation in a lymphoma patient with a long history of ankylosing spondylitis. *Rheumatology* **2000**, *39*, 563–564. [CrossRef]

113. Yang, H.K.; Moon, S.J.; Shin, J.H.; Kwok, S.K.; Park, K.S.; Park, S.H.; Kim, H.Y.; Ju, J.H. Regression of syndesmophyte after bone marrow transplantation for acute myeloid leukemia in a patient with ankylosing spondylitis: A case report. *J. Med. Case Rep.* **2012**, *6*, 250. Available online: https://www.ncbi.nlm.nih.gov/pmc/articles/PMC3459693/ (accessed on 25 November 2017). [CrossRef] [PubMed]

114. Britanova, O.V.; Bochkova, A.G.; Staroverov, D.B.; Feforenko, D.A.; Bolotin, D.A.; Memedove, I.Z.; Turchaaninova, M.A.; Putintseva, E.V.; Kotlobay, A.A.; Lukyanov, S.; et al. First autologous hematopoietic SCT for ankylosing spondylitis: A case report and clues to understanding the therapy. *Bone Marrow Transplant.* **2012**, *47*, 1479–1481. [CrossRef] [PubMed]

115. Wang, P.; Li, Y.; Huang, L.; Yang, J.; Yang, R.; Deng, W.; Liang, B.; Dai, L.; Meng, Q.; Gao, L.; et al. Effects and safety of allogenic mesenchymal stem cells intravenous infusion in active ankylosing spondylitis patients who failed NSAIDs: A 20 week clinical trial. *Cell Transplant.* **2014**, *23*, 1293–1303. [CrossRef] [PubMed]

116. ClinicalTrials.gov. Safety and Efficacy Study of Umbilical Cord/Placenta-Derived Mesenchymal Stem Cells to Treat Ankylosing Spondylitis. ClinicalTrials.gov Identifier: NCT01420432. Available online: www.clinicaltrials.gov (accessed on 22 October 2017).

117. ClinicalTrials.gov. A Molecule Basic Study of Early Warning of New Pathogenic Risk of Ankylosing Spondylitis. ClinicalTrial.gov Identifier: NCT01709656. Available online: www.clinicaltrials.gov (accessed on 22 October 2017).
118. ClinicalTrials.gov. A Pilot Study of MSCs Infusion and Etanercept to Treat Ankylosing Spondylitis. ClinicalTrial.gov Identifier: NCT02809781. Available online: www.clinicaltrials.gov (accessed on 22 October 2017).
119. Chinese Clinical Trial Registry. Clinical Study of Mesenchymal Stem Cells Transplantation in Ankylosing Spondylitis. Registration Number: ChiCTR-TRC-11001417. Available online: http://www.chictr.org.cn/showprojen.aspx?proj=8122 (accessed on 22 October 2017).

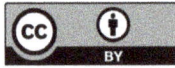

International Journal of
Molecular Sciences

MDPI

Article

The Micro-RNA Expression Profiles of Autoimmune Arthritis Reveal Novel Biomarkers of the Disease and Therapeutic Response

Steven Dudics [1,2,†], Shivaprasad H. Venkatesha [1,2,†] and Kamal D. Moudgil [1,2,3,*,‡]

1   Department of Microbiology and Immunology, University of Maryland School of Medicine, Baltimore, MD 21201, USA; sdudics1@gmail.com (S.D.); hvshivaprasad@gmail.com (S.H.V.)
2   Baltimore Veterans Affairs Medical Center, Baltimore, MD 21201, USA
3   Division of Rheumatology, Department of Medicine, University of Maryland School of Medicine, Baltimore, MD 21201, USA
*   Correspondence: kmoudgil@som.umaryland.edu; Fax: +1-410-706-2129
†   These authors contributed equally to this work.
‡   Supv. Research Health Scientist, Veterans Affairs.

Received: 16 July 2018; Accepted: 3 August 2018; Published: 5 August 2018

check for
updates

Abstract: Rheumatoid arthritis (RA) is a chronic autoimmune disease of the joints affecting about 0.3–1% of the population in different countries. About 50–60 percent of RA patients respond to presently used drugs. Moreover, the current biomarkers for RA have inherent limitations. Consequently, there is a need for additional, new biomarkers for monitoring disease activity and responsiveness to therapy of RA patients. We examined the micro-RNA (miRNA) profile of immune (lymphoid) cells of arthritic Lewis rats and arthritic rats treated with celastrol, a natural triterpenoid. Experimental and bioinformatics analyses revealed 8 miRNAs (miR-22, miR-27a, miR-96, miR-142, miR-223, miR-296, miR-298, and miR-451) and their target genes in functional pathways important for RA pathogenesis. Interestingly, 6 of them (miR-22, miR-27a, miR-96, miR-142, miR-223, and miR-296) were further modulated by celastrol treatment. Interestingly, serum levels of miR-142, miR-155, and miR-223 were higher in arthritic versus control rats, whereas miR-212 showed increased expression in celastrol-treated rats compared with arthritic rats or control rats. This is the first study on comprehensive miRNA expression profiling in the adjuvant-induced arthritis (AA) model and it also has revealed new miRNA targets for celastrol in arthritis. We suggest that subsets of the above miRNAs may serve as novel biomarkers of disease activity and therapeutic response in arthritis.

Keywords: adjuvant arthritis; arthritis; biomarkers; celastrol; inflammation; microRNA; miRNA; rat; rheumatoid arthritis; Traditional Chinese medicine; tripterine; triterpenoid

1. Introduction

Rheumatoid arthritis (RA) is a debilitating autoimmune disease characterized by chronic inflammation of the joints along with systemic manifestations [1–3]. The prevalence of RA varies from 0.3–1.0 percent globally, and it is more common in developed countries than others [4]. RA is a complex disease involving the interplay among multiple mediators and pathways of inflammation and bone damage. The expression of these mediators and their interactions in turn are controlled by a variety of regulators, including micro-RNAs (miRNAs) [5–7]. While current therapies offer a diverse choice of drugs for RA patients, only 50–60% of these patients respond to them [3,8]. Additionally, the currently used biomarkers to assess the development and progression of RA, and to monitor the patients' responsiveness to treatment, have inherent limitations. Rheumatoid factor (RF) and anti-citrullinated protein antibodies (ACPA) are the mainstay of biomarkers for arthritis, with ACPA exhibiting a similar sensitivity but better predictability of the disease course than RF [9,10]. However, RF and ACPA have also been found in other autoimmune diseases, and ACPA positivity may be limited to a subset of RA patients [11,12]. In view of the above, we proposed that certain miRNAs might serve as novel biomarkers to monitor disease activity and therapeutic response in RA.

The miRNAs are short, non-coding RNA sequences that repress gene expression. They exert their function by binding to the 3′ untranslated region (UTR) sequences of the target messenger RNAs (mRNAs), and either initiate their degradation or inhibit their translation [13,14]. The miRNAs have been studied extensively in the cancer field [15–17]. It has been shown that miRNAs can be used as biomarkers for certain cancers, such as breast cancer [18]. Interestingly, miRNAs are gaining increasing recognition for their involvement in autoimmune diseases, as well [19–26]. In RA, miR-146a and miR-155 are among the most studied miRNAs [27]. It has been reported that miR-146a is increased in RA in serum, peripheral blood, CD4+ T cells, and synovial tissue [5,27–29]. However, a reduction in miR-146a in RA fibroblast-like synoviocytes (FLS) has also been reported, implicating this miRNA in anti-inflammatory effects on FLS [6]. This miRNA is also increased in the joint tissue of osteoarthritis patients [30]. Both miR-146a and miR-155 have also been shown to be increased in IL-1β-stimulated human chondrocytes [14]. Similarly, increased levels of miR-155 in RA and its animal models have been reported [7,20,27,31,32]. However, there is a need to determine the role of additional miRNAs in the progression of RA, as well as their utility as biomarkers of disease activity and/or therapeutic response. In this context, we examined the rat adjuvant-induced arthritis (AA) model of human RA [33,34] and also tested the effect on miRNAs of celastrol, a natural triterpenoid that possesses anti-arthritic activity [35]. Celastrol is a pentacyclic triterpenoid ($C_{29}H_{38}O_4$), and it is a bioactive component of plants belonging to the Celastraceae family, such as *Tripterygium wilfordii* and *Celastrus orbiculatus* [36]. The choice of celastrol in this proof-of-concept study was based on our earlier study showing its beneficial effects against AA [35].

AA is a T cell-mediated autoimmune disease, and it has extensively been used to screen potential new drugs, as well as to define the mechanisms underlying RA pathogenesis [33]. Celastrol, derived from a traditional Chinese herb celastrus, has anti-inflammatory and anti-oxidant properties [35,37]. We have previously shown in the AA model that celastrol possesses anti-arthritic properties. These attributes include inhibition of the pro-inflammatory cytokines [35], skewing of the T helper 17 (Th17)/T regulatory (Treg) cell balance towards immune regulation [37], and modulation of bone remodeling in arthritic rats [35]. Accordingly, we hypothesized that celastrol alters specific miRNAs that are involved in the pathogenesis of AA, and that a subset of these miRNAs may serve as biomarkers for disease progression and responsiveness to therapy. Our results described below support this proposition. We observed that 8 specific miRNAs (miR-22, miR-27a, miR-96, miR-142, miR-223, miR-296, miR-298, and miR-451) have the potential to be key regulators of arthritis pathogenesis. Of these, 6 miRNAs (miR-22, miR-27a, miR-96, miR-142, miR-223, and miR-296) were further modulated following celastrol treatment. The testing of sera of control, arthritic, and celastrol-treated rats further validated the utility of some of these miRNAs as circulating biomarkers. We believe that the above-mentioned miRNAs, whether as a set or individually, could be used in conjunction with current biomarkers for improved diagnosis and/or prognosis of arthritis, as well as for monitoring a patient's responsiveness to therapeutic intervention. To the best of our knowledge, this is the first study describing a comprehensive miRNA expression profile of rats with AA as well as novel miRNAs targeted by celastrol. The latter may also lead to identification of additional therapeutic targets for arthritis.

2. Results

Using the adjuvant arthritis (AA) model in the Lewis rat, we determined the miRNA expression profile of 3 groups of rats: *M. tuberculosis* $H_{37}R_a$ (Mtb)-immunized rats in Incubation phase of AA, the vehicle-treated arthritic rats, and the celastrol-treated rats) following the experimental design laid out in Figure 1. Rats in the Incubation phase of AA served as the "baseline" control for the other two groups of rats, whereas vehicle-treated rats were compared with celastrol-treated rats (Figure 2). Lymph node cells (LNCs) of these rats were re-stimulated in the presence or absence of antigen (Mtb sonicate) for 24 h. Thereafter, total RNA isolated from these LNCs was tested using miRNA-microarray. As described under Methods, "miRNA elements" represent hybridization intensities in microarray against miRNA probes of rat, mouse, and human origin, as well as multiple probes of one species for a given miRNA. In subsequent analysis, "miRNA" refers to a given RNA sequence represented by the probes of a single species.

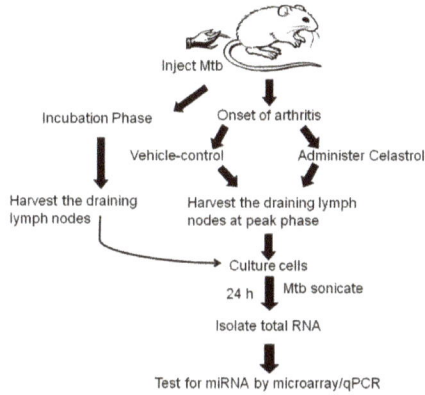

Figure 1. A flow chart showing an overview of the experimental design of the study.

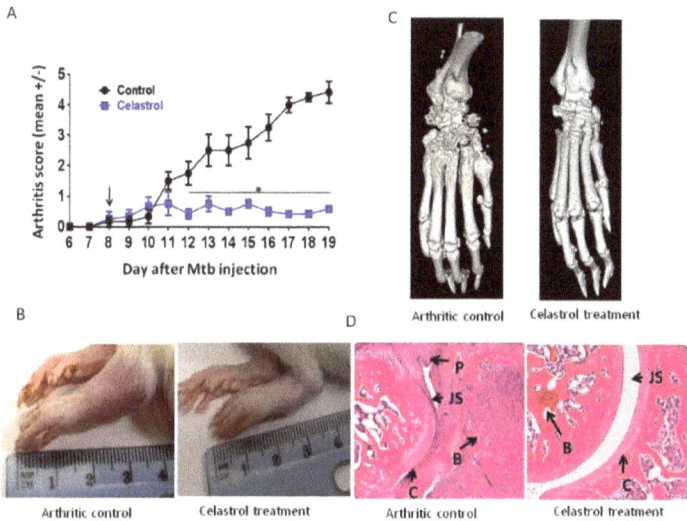

Figure 2. Celastrol inhibits the progression of adjuvant-induced arthritis (AA). (**A**) Mean scores of arthritic Lewis rats (*n* = 4 per group) treated either with celastrol or with the vehicle. Rats were administered celastrol (1 mg/kg) via intraperitoneal (i.p.) injection every day for 3 days starting at the onset of AA, followed by injections every other day until euthanization of rats on day 19 after Mtb injection. (**B**) Photographs, (**C**) computed tomographic (CT) imaging, and (**D**) histological sections of hind paws of vehicle-treated and celastrol-treated rats harvested at peak phase of the disease (day 19). The arrows point to the following: P: pannus; JS: joint space; B: bone; and C: cartilage.

2.1. LNC Micro-RNA Expression Profile of Incubation Phase Rats and Vehicle-Treated Arthritic Rats

The results of the miRNA expression of rats in the Incubation phase of AA and vehicle-treated arthritic rats are shown as a heat map (Figure 3A), principal component analysis (PCA) (Figure 3B), and Venn diagram (Figure 3C, left-titled panels). A comparison of the intensity signals of the two groups of rats revealed a total of 903 significantly altered "miRNA elements" in arthritic rats compared with Incubation phase rats (Figure 3C, left-titled panels). Of these, 748 were upregulated, which included 159 that were uniquely upregulated by antigen, meaning that celastrol treatment (described below) had no effect on these. The remaining 155 (of 903 elements) were downregulated in arthritic rats. These included 112 that were uniquely decreased by antigen, implying that these were unaffected by celastrol treatment.

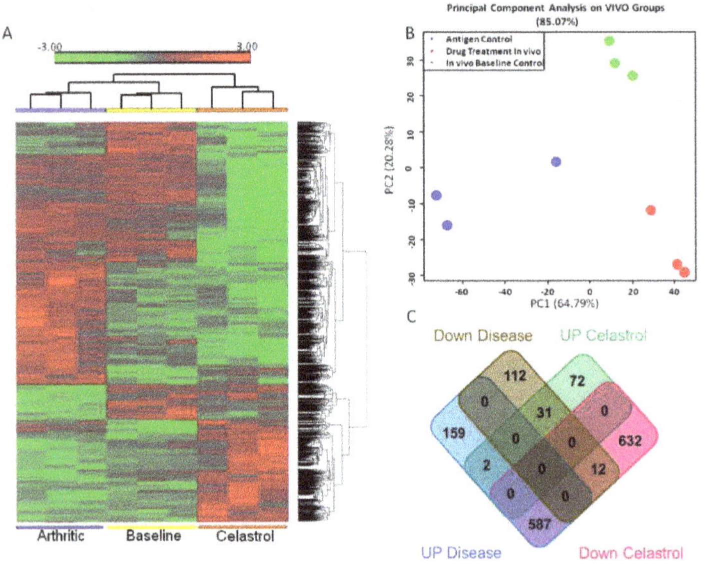

Figure 3. Microarray analysis of the miRNA expression profile of the Incubation phase (baseline) rats, control (vehicle-treated) arthritic rats, and celastrol-treated arthritic rats. (**A**) Heat map of miRNAs expressed in lymph node cells (LNCs) of the above 3 groups of rats (*n* = 3 per group) as indicated in the figure. LNCs were isolated from the draining lymph nodes of rats in the incubation phase of the disease (on day 5 after Mtb injection) and the vehicle-treated or celastrol-treated rats at peak phase of the disease (on day 19 post-Mtb immunization). Thereafter, LNCs were re-stimulated for 24 h with or without antigen (Mtb sonicate). Cells cultured in medium alone served as control for cells cultured with antigen. RNA was isolated from these samples using miRNAeasy kit (Qiagen, Germantown, MD, USA) and then subjected to hybridization using miRNA 4.0 Affymetrix gene chips (Affymetrix, Santa Clara, CA, USA). The data was then subjected to statistical and bioinformatical analyses. A heat map of statistically significant ($p \leq 0.05$; fold change ≤ -2 or ≥ 2) miRNAs was generated and samples were clustered in a hierarchical fashion. Green color indicates a decrease in intensity, whereas red color indicates an increase; (**B**) Principal component analysis (PCA) plot depicts the clustering of RNA samples of 3 groups of rats, each tested in triplicates; (**C**) Venn diagram shows the distribution of statistically significant miRNAs whose expression was altered by antigen (Left-tilted panels) versus antigen-cum-drug (Right-tilted panels) under the indicated sub-groups.

Following extensive analysis using Ingenuity Pathway Analysis (IPA) and target prediction software, we examined in detail 27 miRNAs for further consideration (Figure 4A). Out of 27, 18 showed increased expression in disease (Figure 4B), whereas 9 had reduced expression in disease (Figure 4C).

2.2. LNC Micro-RNA Expression Profile of Celastrol-Treated Arthritic Rats

The results, including the heat map (Figure 3A), PCA (Figure 3B), and Venn diagram (Figure 3C, right-tilted panels), of the miRNA testing of LNCs of celastrol-treated rats are shown. A comparison of the celastrol-treated rats and the vehicle-treated arthritic rats revealed a total of 1336 differentially expressed miRNA elements (Figure 3C, right-tilted panels). Of these, 1231 were downregulated, while 105 were upregulated in celastrol-treated rats. Of the 1231 downregulated miRNA elements, 632 were uniquely downregulated by celastrol implying that these were not affected by antigen, whereas 12 were reduced by antigen and then further downregulated by celastrol. The remaining 587 were increased by antigen, but reduced by celastrol. On the contrary, of the 105 miRNA upregulated elements in celastrol-treated rats, 72 were uniquely increased by celastrol in that antigen had no significant effect on them, whereas 31 were decreased by antigen but increased by celastrol. The remaining 2 were increased by antigen and then further upregulated by celastrol.

The relative levels of expression of select miRNAs of arthritic rats were then compared with celastrol-treated rats (Figure 4). The miRNAs affected by celastrol treatment belonged to 3 different categories (Figure 4B,C): 12 increased in disease but reduced by celastrol; 38 reduced by celastrol, but unaffected by disease; and 2 decreased in disease but upregulated by celastrol. Figure 4D shows the relative expression levels of those 38 miRNAs reduced by celastrol but not affected by the disease. These 38 miRNAs might be reduced by the direct effect of celastrol, involving mechanisms not related to the disease condition. Among these is miR-22, which has two different miRNA types, such that Figure 4A shows miR-22-5p, whereas Figure 4D shows miR-22-3p.

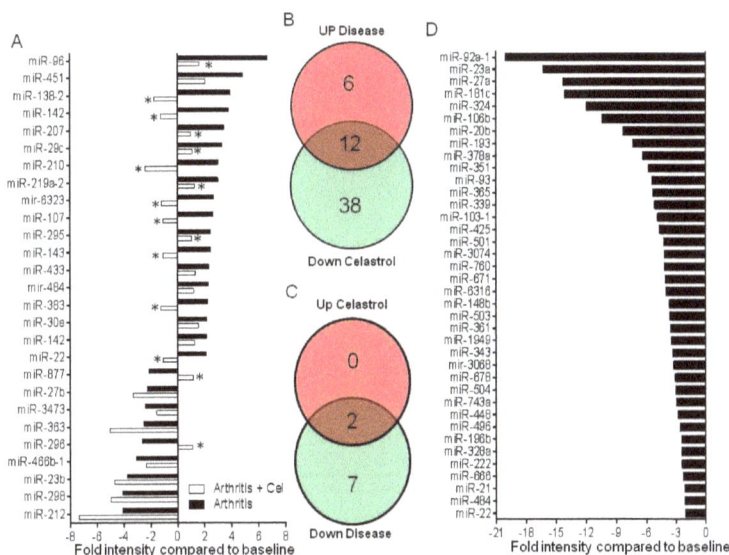

Figure 4. The differential expression of miRNAs in untreated arthritic rats versus celastrol-treated rats. (**A**) The miRNAs that are differentially expressed in arthritic rats compared to baseline control are shown in filled bars. The levels of all filled bars are statistically significant ($p < 0.05$) for at least one of 3 species' probes (mouse, human, rat) in the microarray chip. The respective miRNAs in celastrol-treated rats are shown in open bars. Here, an asterisk (*) represents significant down- or upregulated miRNAs upon celastrol treatment compared to disease controls; (**B,C**) Venn diagrams showing the number of miRNAs that are up- or down-regulated in untreated arthritic rats compared with celastrol-treated rats; (**D**) The miRNAs that are uniquely downregulated in celastrol-treated group compared to the untreated group (meaning that they are not changed upon disease development) are shown here as a Waterfall plot.

2.3. Functional Analysis of Specific Micro-RNAs Identified Following Initial Screening

To examine the potential biological functions of the select miRNAs, the data was subjected to IPA Core analysis. The selected genes were then further grouped into functional categories and plotted as a bar graph (Figure 5A). This analysis revealed several different functional categories including inflammatory disease, inflammatory response, immunological disease, cellular development, connective tissue disorder, and others (Figure 5B–F). A detailed list of these categories is given in Supplementary Materials Figure S1A,B. Additional pathways are shown in Supplementary Materials Figure S2A–C. The above analyses indicated that these pathways are quite likely to be influenced by miRNAs induced upon arthritis development.

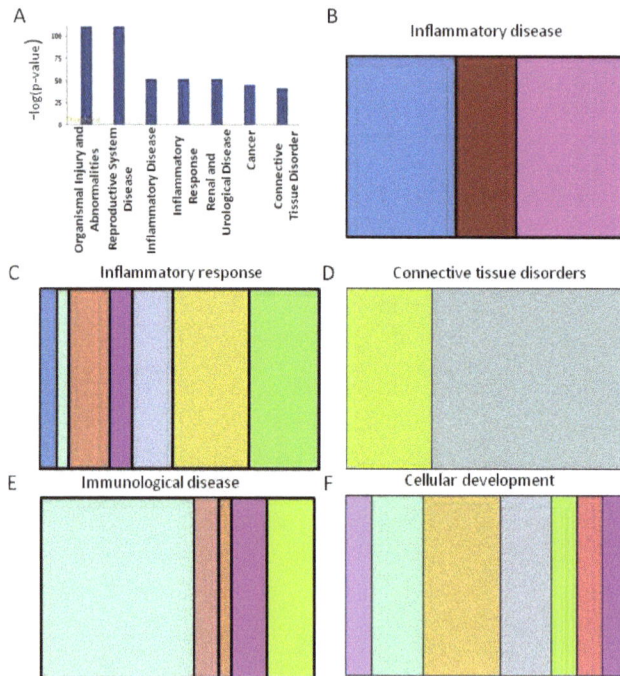

Figure 5. In silico analysis of miRNAs that are modulated following AA induction. (**A**) Bar graph indicating the number of miRNAs that are predicted to target genes in each category listed on the x-axis; (**B–F**) Vertical slice plots depict the percentage of miRNA-associated molecules and their indicated categories. The details of the distribution of miRNAs in different colored vertical slices and the categories of each plot are given in Supplementary Materials Figure S1A,B, and additional pathways in Supplementary Materials Figure S2A–C.

2.4. The Micro-RNA-Messenger RNA Interactions and Network Mapping

We also examined the key miRNA-mRNA interactions using the network mapping tool (Figures 6–8) for gaining further insight into how these miRNAs might affect different mediators and pathways in RA. The mediators that are associated with important pathways in RA were considered for further analysis. Interestingly, some of these pathways, such as IL-17 signaling and NF-κB signaling, which are known to be involved in RA, are also known to serve as targets of celastrol action [37,38].

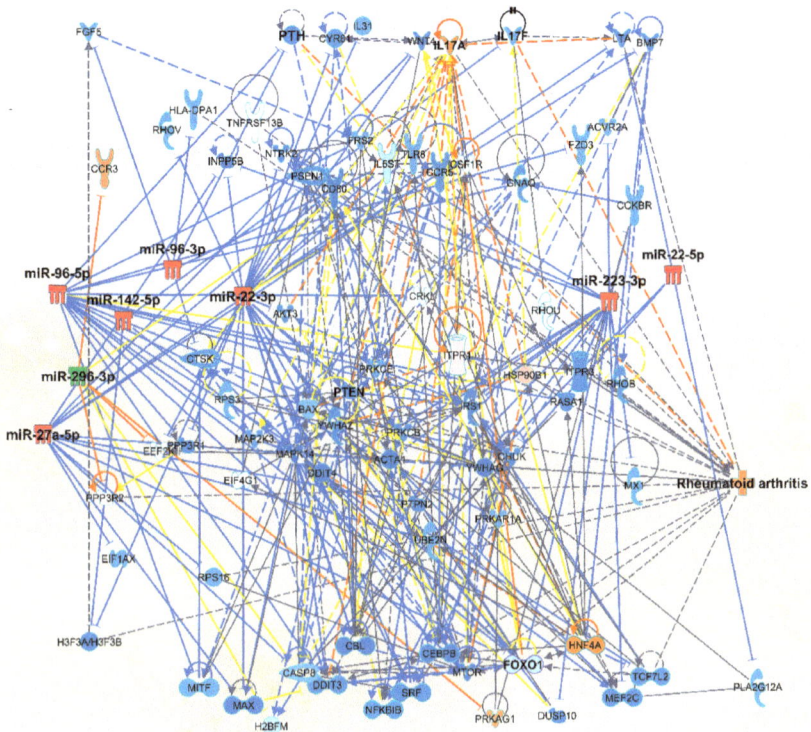

Figure 6. Network analysis of select miRNAs and the mRNAs targeted by them, as well as their impact on the progression of rheumatoid arthritis. The known interactions between the genes are represented by lines showing activation (arrow) or inhibition (blunt end). Further, solid line indicates direct interaction, whereas dashed line indicates indirect interaction. Colored lines indicate the following: orange line for activation; blue line for inhibition; yellow line for uncertain state of the downstream molecule; and gray line for effect not predicted. For the Micro-RNA symbols, red indicates increased level, whereas green indicates decreased level. For the target genes, orange indicates predicted activation, whereas blue indicates predicted inhibition.

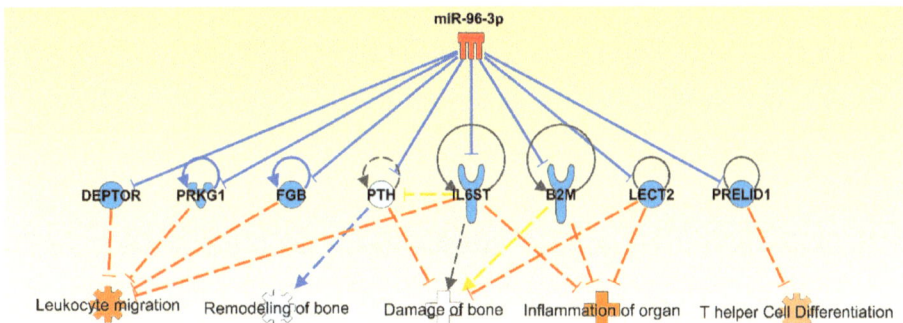

Figure 7. Network analysis showing the impact of miR-96 on various mediators and pathways involved in the pathogenesis of rheumatoid arthritis. The impact of an increase in the level of miR-96 on arthritis is also shown here. The description of lines, arrows, color, etc. is same as in the legend to Figure 6.

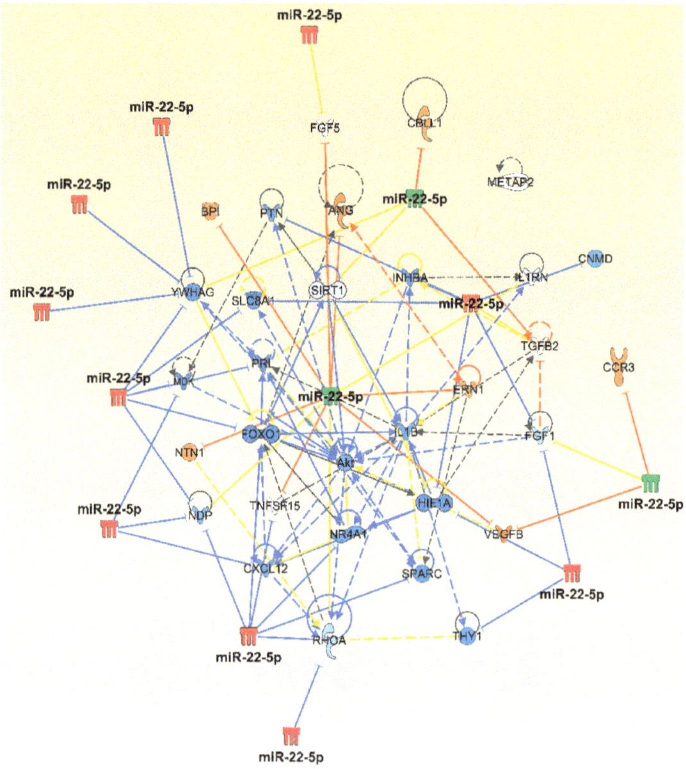

Figure 8. Network analysis of select miRNAs and the mRNAs targeted by them, as well as their impact on the proliferation of endothelial cells in inflammatory arthritis. The description of lines, arrows, color, etc. is same as in the legend to Figure 6.

2.5. Micro-RNA Expression in Endothelial Cells and Their Functional Relevance

Chronic inflammation, as in the case of human RA, is linked with endothelial dysfunction and aberrant new blood vessel formation (angiogenesis) [39–41]. In this regard, we also examined the involvement of miRNAs in endothelial activation and proliferation. Our network analysis (Figure 8) revealed that several miRNAs identified in lymphoid cells (e.g., LNCs) of arthritic rats modulate a variety of inflammatory mediators that affect endothelial cell activation/proliferation. Furthermore, some of these miRNAs are the same as those altered by celastrol in the LNCs described above. These results indicate that celastrol might also be able to modulate endothelial cell function via these miRNAs, in addition to its other anti-inflammatory effects as mentioned above.

2.6. Selection of Micro-RNAs as Biomarkers of Arthritis and Therapeutic Response

Thereafter, using multiple criteria, we selected 8 miRNAs, namely miR-22, miR-27a, miR-96, miR-142, miR-223, miR-296, miR-298, and miR-451, which have the potential to be key regulators of arthritis pathogenesis. Of these 8 miRNAs, five miRNAs (miR-22, miR-27a, miR-96, miR-142, and miR-223) were upregulated following disease development, but downregulated with celastrol treatment. However, two other miRNAs (miR-296 and miR-298) were reduced upon disease development. Of these, miR-296 was increased, but miR-298 was unaffected by celastrol treatment. Another miRNA (miR-451) was increased in disease, but not affected by celastrol treatment. We propose the above 8 miRNAs for further validation as biomarkers of disease activity in RA patients.

For the purpose of selecting biomarkers of therapeutic response, we preferred 6 of the 8 miRNAs, whose expression was changed significantly in disease and then further modulated by drug treatment. These include miR-22, miR-27a, miR-96, miR-142, miR-223, and miR-296. A representative network analysis of these is shown in Figure 6. Here, celastrol is used as a proof-of-concept drug. In this context, we propose that more than 6 miRNAs may serve as biomarkers of therapeutic response in RA patients. However, it is conceivable that another anti-arthritic drug might target a slightly different subset of miRNAs than celastrol. However, as our initial selection of miRNAs is based on the disease-related miRNAs, we anticipate that miRNAs targeted by celastrol would overlap with those affected by other anti-arthritis drugs.

2.7. Circulating Micro-RNAs in Sera of Rats

We then quantitated the levels of the above miRNAs, which were identified based on microarray miRNA expression analysis of LNC, in serum samples of control (naïve) rats, arthritic rats at peak phase of AA, and celastrol-treated rats at peak phase of AA. The levels of miR-142, miR-155, and miR-223 were higher in arthritic versus control rats, whereas miR-212 showed increased expression when comparing celastrol-treated and arthritic rats/ control rats (Figure 9). Changes in some other miRNAs had trends similar to the above 4 miRNAs, but the difference was not statistically significant. Another pattern observed with miR-96, miR-219a2, and miR-298 was a reduction in the level upon disease development, but reversal (increase) in level after celastrol treatment. However, the difference was not statistically significant.

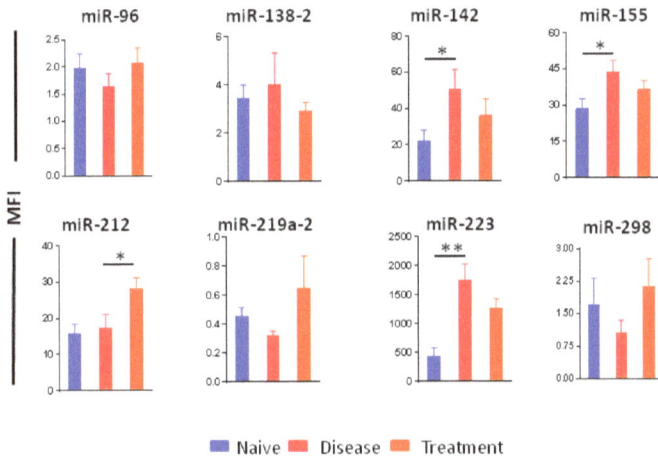

Figure 9. Testing miRNA levels in sera of rats. The levels of miRNAs were determined in serum samples obtained from normal (naïve) control, arthritic rats, and celastrol-treated arthritic rats ($n = 6$ each) using Multiplex miRNA assay. The data is presented as mean fluorescence intensity. (*, $p < 0.05$; ** <0.025).

2.8. Messenger RNA Targets of Select Micro-RNAs

Using multiple criteria, including the use of target prediction software, we identified the mRNA targets of the 8 selected miRNAs mentioned above. These targets are categorized into 3 groups (Table 1). We noted that our select miRNAs were highly predicted and/or experimentally observed to bind to the 3' UTR of the mRNAs identified by us. For example, miR-96 is predicted to bind to mRNA encoding parathyroid hormone (PTH), which would result in reduced PTH activity (Figures 6 and 7). PTH is an important hormone for mediating a homeostatic state of bone morphology, and can display anabolic or catabolic properties for bone remodeling depending on its concentration and pattern of secretion [42,43]. It has been shown that dysregulation of PTH can lead to an imbalance of critical mediators of bone remodeling. This in turn can lead to bone damage [43]. This situation can aggravate bone damage associated with inflammation of the joint in arthritis. Another interesting miRNA revealed in our analysis is miR-27a. This miRNA is predicted to target the gene Wingless-Type MMTV Integration Site Family, Member 4 (Wnt4) (Figure 6). While Wnt4 has also been associated with reproductive functions [44,45], it also plays a role in bone remodeling. For example, it has been demonstrated that Wnt4 can reduce the expression of NF-κB and subsequently inhibit bone resorption and inflammation [46]. This suggests that miR-27a could influence bone erosion and inflammation in part via Wnt4. Finally, miR-223 was predicted to target an important gene in RA, Forkhead Box O 1 (FOXO1) (Figure 6). FOXO1 has been shown to be reduced in expression in the peripheral blood of RA patients [47]. Furthermore, a reduction in FOXO1 promotes the survival of fibroblast-like synoviocytes (FLS). This implies that miRNA-induced changes in FOXO1 levels can influence FLS proliferation and joint inflammation. Our network analysis further revealed that when the expression of most of the above-mentioned miRNAs is decreased, for example, miR-96, the expression of their target mRNAs is increased, leading to the suppression of RA (Supplementary Materials Figure S3). The reverse effect is predicted when the expression of these miRNAs is increased.

Table 1. The target mRNAs of the selected top 8 miRNAs.

miRNA	High Prediction	Moderate Prediction	Experimentally Observed
miR-22	*CHUK, LTA*	*BCL2, CXCL13, IL36G, MMP1, PTK2, TGFA, VCAM1, TLR7*	*Cyr61*
miR-27a	*CASP8, CCR5, EIF1AX, GNAO1, INPP5B, RPS16, UBE2N, WNT4*	*BCL2, CD40LG, CD80, CXCL6, CXCR4, CXCR6, FLT1, TGFB1, WNT2, WNT6, LTA, FOXO1, IL10, IL1R1, IL2, IL2RA*	*FSTL1*
miR-96	*CTSB, CTSK, MTOR, PPP3R1, PRKAR1A, PRKCE, PTH, RARG, RASA1, TCF7L2*	*AHR, BCL10, BMP5, BMP8B, FGF9, FOXO3, FOXO4, HSP90AA1, IL17B, SMAD7, TGFBR1, TNFSF4, IL12A, IL22RA2, IL6ST, VEGFC*	*FOXO1, IRS1, MITF*
miR-142	*IL17F*	*FGF20, IL22, SOCS1, TNFSF13B*	*TGFBR1*
miR-223	*ACTA1, ACVR2A, CCKBR, DUSP10, FOXO1, HSP90B1, IL6ST, INPP5B, MX1, PTPN2, YWHAG*	*CCL11, CD86, DKK1, STAT1, FOXO3, IL23A, IL5*	*IRS1, RHOB, MEF2C*
miR-296	*CCR3, H2BFM, PPP3R2, PRKAG1*	*CD14, CD40LG, CXCL8, FGF1, ICAM1, IL6ST, MMP13, MMP8, VEGFB*	
miR-298	*CASP9, CHP1, EIF1, FKBP1A, IL1RN, RHOA, RHOG, VEGFB, WNT3A*	*SOCS3, TCF7L1, TLR9, ICOS, IL6R, VDR, CXCL13, CXCL5, CXCR3, DKK2, EGFR, MYD88, GATA3, IL10RA, IL12RB2, IL17F, IL2RB*	
miR-451	*ATF2, PSMB8, TSC1*	*BMP6, FGF5, IL6R, NFATC1*	*MIF, CPNE3, Rab5*

3. Discussion

The pathogenesis of RA involves complex interactions among several mediators and pathways of inflammation and bone remodeling. Micro-RNAs are known to regulate a variety of mRNAs. Information about changes in miRNA expression following the development of arthritis can provide insights into disease pathogenesis, new biomarkers of disease, and potential therapeutic targets. In this context, we examined the miRNA expression profile of arthritic rats using the AA model. This experimental model of RA has extensively been used for decades to study the pathogenesis of human RA as well as several potential therapeutics [33,34]. However, at present, there is barely any information on the expression of miRNAs and their role in AA. Our study is the first in AA that provides comprehensive insights in this regard. Furthermore, we have used celastrol as a therapeutic agent to determine the changes in the miRNA profile of arthritic rats following treatment. Although several studies by others [48–50] and us [35,37] have uncovered the biochemical and immunological aspects of the anti-inflammatory properties of celastrol, the miRNA profile of arthritic rats following celastrol treatment has not been reported previously.

Here, we have combined the miRNA-microarray technology and bioinformatics-based analysis to comprehensively determine the miRNA expression profile of untreated and celastrol-treated arthritic rats. Analysis of these miRNA profiles uncovered a set of new potential biomarkers of arthritis progression as well as response to therapy. Our results show that 8 specific miRNAs (miR-22, miR-27a, miR-96, miR-142, miR-223, miR-296, miR-298, and miR-451) have the potential to be key regulators of arthritis pathogenesis. Of these, 6 miRNAs (miR-22, miR-27a, miR-96, miR-142, miR-223, and miR-296) are significantly modulated by celastrol treatment. Importantly, the significance of some of these miRNAs is further evident from the results of serum testing, which showed that miR-142, miR-155, and miR-223 were significantly higher in the sera of arthritic rats than normal rats. Furthermore, miR-212 showed increased expression when comparing arthritic rats and celastrol-treated rats. Changes in miR-96, miR-219a-2, and miR-298 also showed an interesting trend, reduction with disease but increase with celastrol treatment. We suggest that changes in miRNAs induced by celastrol treatment might be attributable to both direct effect of celastrol on miRNA expression and indirect effect of reduced inflammation. Taken together, the above miRNAs represent circulating biomarkers of disease activity as well as therapeutic response in AA. We believe that above-mentioned miRNAs, whether as a set or individually, could be used in conjunction with current biomarkers for improved diagnosis and/or prognosis of arthritis, as well as for monitoring responsiveness to therapeutic intervention.

We tested serum samples to determine which of the miRNAs that are found to be altered in immune cells (such as LNC) might also be changed in the blood (using serum). We believe that similar to serum RF and ACPA, a serum test to check for miRNA levels can be a useful adjunct for RA diagnosis. For that reason, we preferred serum over peripheral blood mononuclear cells (PBMC) so that in subsequent comparative studies, changes in serum miRNAs can be easily compared with changes in other biomarkers of RA. Regarding serum miRNAs, it is well documented that circulating miRNAs can be detected in many disease conditions [51–54]. Such miRNAs are produced by different cells/tissues, but some of these miRNAs are then released into circulation in the form of exosomes budding from living cells [51–54]. Another interesting function aspect of exosomes is that they can also be used as therapeutic targets or delivery systems [55–58]. In the above context, we hope that our results for serum miRNAs will be of practical utility for diagnosis and prognosis of arthritis.

A brief summary of the expression of specific miRNAs and their potential targets and effects in arthritis are given below:

miR-22. This miRNA was shown to be an important regulator of FLS. It has been demonstrated that miR-22 is able to directly target Cyr61, an important mediator that promotes FLS proliferation, and that miR-22 was downregulated in the synoviocytes of RA patients [59]. In turn, this led to an increase in Cyr61 expression and subsequent FLS proliferation. Moreover, in the collagen-induced arthritic (CIA) model of RA, miR-22 had an opposite effect. The inhibition of miR-22 resulted in increased suppression of proliferation and higher apoptosis rates of FLS, as well as a decrease in pro-inflammatory cytokine production [60]. Additional studies are required to resolve its action in arthritis.

miR-27a. There are a couple of reports describing the role miR-27a in RA. For example, miR-27a targets follistatin-like protein 1 (FSTL1), an important protein that promotes FLS migration and invasion [61]. In addition, it limits the TLR4/NF-kB pathway. In RA patients, miR-27a is downregulated in the serum, synovial tissue, and FLS, suggesting that it plays a crucial role in FLS proliferation and RA pathogenesis [61]. Another study revealed that miR-27a expression is reduced in chondrocytes in osteoarthritis, and that this miRNA downregulates, albeit indirectly, two critical genes involved in the pathogenesis of osteoarthritis, namely insulin-like growth factor binding protein-5 (IGFBP-5) and matrix metalloproteinase-13 (MMP-13) [62]. A recent study in a mouse model of arthritis showed that miR-27a controls arthritis via peroxisome proliferator activated receptor gamma (PPARγ), which also involved a similar set of genes as above [63]. Also, miR-27a levels were altered in RA patients following treatment with Adalimumab and/or Methotrexate [21], suggesting that this miRNA can be used to assess the patient's responsiveness to therapy.

miR-96. To the best of our knowledge, there is no prior report yet on a direct association between arthritis and miR-96, and therefore, our study has revealed miR-96 as a promising candidate for further exploration. However, a few in vitro studies have pointed to some likely ways in which miR-96 might influence the disease process in arthritis. For example, the expression of miR-96 was found to be markedly reduced in chondrogenesis in mice when testing chondroblasts derived from mouse marrow stromal cells [64]. In another study, miR-96 was shown to facilitate osteogenic differentiation in MC3T3-E1 cells, a mouse osteoblast cell line [65]. This activity involved inhibition by miR-96 of heparin-binding EGF-like growth factor (HBEGF)-epidermal growth factor receptor (EGFR) signaling. Similarly, miR-96 was reported to regulate gene expression vital for human mesenchymal stromal cells (hMSCs) [66].

miR-142. This miRNA has been involved in signaling leading to enhanced inflammation. In regard to joint pathology, the expression level of miR-142 was found to be reduced in the cartilage in a mouse model of osteoarthritis [67]. Furthermore, over-expression of miR-451 resulted in inhibition of chondrocyte apoptosis and inflammation in these mice. This effect involved a reduction in high mobility group box 1 (HMGB1)-induced NF-κB signaling.

miR-155. Our results of serum testing showed that miR-155 is increased in arthritic rats. This observation is supported by a similar finding of increased miR-155 in sera and synovial tissue of RA patients [7,68,69]. This miRNA modulates several pro-inflammatory cytokines, chemokines, and chemokine receptors involved in arthritis pathogenesis. Furthermore, mice lacking miR-155 are resistant to CIA, further validating the role of this miRNA in arthritis [7].

miR-212. Another miRNA found to be increased in celastrol-treated rats compared with arthritic and control rats was miR-212. Thus, reduction in the severity of arthritis correlated with increase in miR-212 in serum. This finding is supported by the observation in RA sera and synovial tissue, where miR-212 is reduced in RA compared to healthy controls [70,71]. This miRNA modulates the proliferation and activity of FLS by targeting SRY-related HMG box 5 (SOX5) [71].

miR-223. It has been demonstrated that this miRNA is overexpressed in RA patients compared to healthy controls [69]. This overexpression led to a decrease in insulin growth factor-1 receptor (IGF-1R), subsequently impairing IL-10 activation in RA cells [72]. This impairment contributes to the imbalance of pro-inflammatory and anti-inflammatory cytokines, and exacerbates arthritis. Similarly, a study in a mouse model of arthritis revealed that silencing of miR-223 reduced the severity of the disease, indicating a role of this miRNA in disease progressions [73]. On the contrary, another study in RA showed increased expression of miR-223 in the synovial tissue of RA patients and its inhibitory effect on osteoclastogenesis [74]. Thus, both pro- and anti-inflammatory effects of miR-223 have been observed.

miR-296. It has been shown that TNF-α stimulation of bone marrow-derived macrophages increased the expression of miR-296, along with two other miRNAs in our list, namely miR-27a and miR-298 [25].

miR-298. As mentioned above, the expression of miR-298 has been reported to be increased following stimulation of macrophages with TNF-α [25]. While miR-298 currently has no reported role in RA, its expression has been shown to be increased in lupus patients compared to controls [75].

miR-451. As for miR-451, it has been shown to play a key role in controlling neutrophil chemotaxis, and is present in lower amounts in RA patient neutrophils compared to healthy controls [76]. This miRNA can directly target copine III (CPNE3) and Ras-related protein Rab-5A (Rab5a), thereby suppressing the p38/MAPK pathway. Furthermore, the over-expression of miR-451 in arthritic mice led to a reduction of neutrophil chemotaxis and severity of arthritis [76]. Similarly, in another study involving FLS from RA patients, it was shown that transfection of FLS with miR-451 resulted in inhibition of pro-inflammatory cytokines such as TNF-α, IL-1β, and IL-6, thereby supporting the anti-arthritic effect of this miRNA [77]. Furthermore, this effect of miR-451 involved inhibition of p38MAPK. On the contrary, another set of reports showed that miR-451 was increased in the RA sera [69] and T cells of RA patients, and that its levels correlated positively with serum IL-6 and arthritis severity [78].

In regard to arthritis therapy, with only about 60% of patients responding to the biologics [8], and the therapies taking weeks before clinical changes might be evident, there is a need for better biomarkers to monitor patient responsiveness. In this study on AA, we have shown that not only are miR-22, miR-27a, miR-96, miR-142, and miR-223 upregulated following disease development, but they are also downregulated with celastrol treatment. Furthermore, miR-296 was reduced upon disease development, but increased upon celastrol treatment. Upon serum testing, 3 miRNAs (miR-142, miR-155, and miR-223) were increased in arthritic rats, whereas one miRNA (miR-212) was increased in celastrol-treated rats compared with arthritic rats. Given that AA is a widely used model of RA and that miRNAs are highly conserved among species, our results suggest that above-mentioned miRNAs might serve as biomarkers to assess an RA patient's response to therapy, and thereby indicate the need to switch to a different medication, if necessary. This in turn would help cut down on the time with therapies that are not efficacious at remedying disease morbidity. Moreover, based on our results, we further suggest that one or more of these 8 miRNAs might serve as effective targets for therapy. For example, a miRNA mimic can be delivered via a suitable vector to increase the expression of that miRNA in vivo with the purpose of suppressing the expression of a gene encoding a pro-inflammatory mediator of arthritis. The opposite can be achieved with an antagomir, an antagonist to the select miRNA by reducing the miRNA level but increasing the expression of the corresponding target mRNA for an anti-inflammatory cytokine or other regulatory protein.

Endothelial cell activation and proliferation, leading to the formation of new blood vessels (angiogenesis), is an integral part of the pathogenic events in arthritis [41,79,80]. Pro-inflammatory cytokines (e.g., TNF-α, IL-1β, IL-6, IL-17, and IL-18) and other inflammatory mediators (e.g., C-reactive protein) cause endothelial cell activation. Continuous endothelial cell activation enhances the expression of leukocyte adhesion molecules and chemokines, which in turn cause a sustained recruitment of leukocytes to the site of inflammation—as well as enhancing the levels of intracellular reactive oxygen species (ROS) and those of matrix metalloproteinases—and enhances angiogenesis [79,80]. These changes provide increased blood flow, nutrients, and inflammatory cells to the target site, the joints. Importantly, however, endothelial dysfunction has been reported not only in RA [39], but also in the rat AA model [40], further emphasizing the significant role of endothelial cells in arthritis. Therefore, a detailed study of the factors affecting endothelial cell activation/proliferation can provide insights into the disease process, and also offer vital clues to the molecules/pathways targeted by certain anti-arthritic agents that inhibit new blood vessel formation in arthritis [41]. As described above under Results, we observed that several miRNAs can modulate a variety of inflammatory mediators that affect endothelial cell activation/proliferation. Furthermore, celastrol can target some of the mediators and pathways involving these miRNAs. It is conceivable that these endothelial cell-related miRNAs can be targeted for developing novel therapies for rectifying the endothelial dysfunction observed in RA as well as for inhibiting new blood vessel formation in this disease. Taken together, we describe the changes above in miRNAs induced following celastrol treatment of arthritic rats. Previous studies in other disease models have similarly shown the effect of other natural products on different miRNAs, for example, that of resveratrol in colitis-associated tumorigenesis model [81].

4. Materials and Methods

4.1. Induction and Evaluation of Adjuvant-induced Arthritis (AA) in Lewis Rats

Animal experiments were performed following approval from the Institutional Animal Care and Use Committee (IACUC) of the University of Maryland School of Medicine, Baltimore (UMB), protocol# 0417011 (20 April 2017) and #0817006 (17 August 2017). AA was induced in a cohort of male Lewis rats (LEW/SsNHsd (RT.1^1)) (Envigo, Madison, WI, USA), 5–6 weeks old, by subcutaneous injection at the base of the tail with heat-killed *M. tuberculosis* H$_{37}$Ra (Mtb) (Becton, Dickinson and Company, Sparks, MD, USA) (1.5 mg/rat) suspended in mineral oil (Sigma-Aldrich, St. Louis, MO, USA). (Male rats were used for consistency with previous studies by others and us using the AA model.) Thereafter, the onset and progression of arthritis in the paws was evaluated daily or on alternate days. The grading of arthritis on a scale of 0 to 4 per paw was based on redness and swelling as described previously [35]. Furthermore, the total arthritic score for a rat is derived by the addition of the arthritic scores of all 4 paws. The onset of arthritis occurs about d 8–10 after Mtb injection, and the severity of AA peaks around d 18–19. The period between Mtb injection and onset of arthritis is the "Incubation phase". The photographs, histological analysis, and computed tomographic (CT) imaging of hind paws was performed following procedures described elsewhere [35,37,82]. CT was performed at the Core for Translational Research in Imaging (C-TRIM), UMB.

4.2. Treatment of Arthritic Rats with Celastrol

Celastrol (Calbiochem, Darmstadt, Germany) was dissolved in phosphate-buffered saline (PBS) containing 0.1% dimethyl sulfoxide (DMSO) (Sigma-Aldrich, St. Louis, MO, USA) (PBS-DMSO). This celastrol solution (1.0 mg/kg) was then administered to rats via intraperitoneal (i.p.) injection beginning at the onset of the disease and then continued daily for 3 more days, followed by injection every other day until the day of euthanization. Control rats were injected with the vehicle (PBS-DMSO) on the corresponding days.

4.3. Lymph Node Cell (LNC) Culture and Total RNA Extraction

We harvested the draining LNCs from different groups of rats, cultured them in vitro, and isolated total RNA from them as described below.

4.3.1. LNC of In Vivo Vehicle/Celastrol Treatment Group:

Arthritic Lewis rats, treated either with the vehicle (PBS-DMSO) or with celastrol in PBS-DMSO (=celastrol), were euthanized at the peak phase of AA (day 19 after Mtb injection) and their draining lymph nodes (superficial inguinal and popliteal) were collected. These lymph nodes were crushed between frosted glass slides (Fischer Scientific, Bridgewater, NJ, USA) to extract LNCs, which were then filtered through a mesh and washed. These LNCs were then cultured for 24 h at 37 °C in a six-well plate (5×10^6 cells/well) in Dulbecco's modified eagle medium (DMEM) containing 10% fetal bovine serum (FBS), 1% glutamine, 1% penicillin/streptomycin, and 0.1% β-mercaptoethanol, in the presence or absence of Mtb sonicate (10 μg/mL) as the antigen. (The latter was prepared by sonicating heat-killed Mtb described above and collecting the centrifuged supernatant.) The LNCs cultured in medium alone served as controls for cells cultured with antigen. The purpose of the in vitro re-stimulation of the LNC is to increase the level of expression of various immune mediators (e.g., miRNAs), and thereby to increase the sensitivity of their detection. This change involves an increase in the generation of total RNA, including miRNAs. In vitro restimulation of LNC with antigen is a standard protocol for testing various immune mediators during the course of a disease [35,37]. However, under the conditions of antigen restimulation in vitro, the naïve T cells or B cells will not be activated and not be able to skew the results of the assay. Therefore, we do not anticipate any negative effects of antigen restimulation on the measurement of miRNAs in this regard.

4.3.2. LNC of Incubation Phase Rats:

LNCs of Mtb-immunized rats were harvested during the incubation phase of AA (day 5 after Mtb injection) and then cultured in the presence or absence of Mtb sonicate (10 μg/mL) as described above. The LNCs cultured in medium alone served as controls for cells cultured with antigen. Furthermore, the LNCs of Incubation phase rats served as the "baseline" controls for the above-mentioned LNCs of in vivo celastrol/vehicle treatment group.

4.3.3. RNA Isolation from LNC of Rats:

Total RNA was extracted from LNCs of each of the above-mentioned groups of rats using miRNeasy mini kit (Qiagen, Germantown, MD, USA) following the manufacturer's protocol. RNA concentration was determined spectrophotometrically using the NanoDrop ND-1000 (NanoDrop Technologies/Thermo Scientific, Wilmington, DE, USA), and the quality of RNA was determined by checking the ratio of 260/280 nm and 260/230 nm. RNA integrity number (RIN) was determined by the Bioanalyzer RNA 6000 Nano Kit (Agilent, Wilmington, NC, USA) following manufacturer's protocol prior to using that RNA for miRNA-microarray analysis.

4.4. Micro-RNA Hybridization and Microarray Analysis

Following the schematic plan laid out in Figure 1, the expression profile of miRNAs in LNCs of the 3 groups of rats (celastrol-/vehicle-treated arthritic rats and Incubation phase rats), each in triplicate, was determined using GeneChip™ miRNA 4.0 Array (Affymetrix, Santa Clara, CA, USA). Raw microarray data (CEL files) were first pre-processed using the Robust Multi-Array Average (RMA) technique. The RMA algorithm was used to conduct background corrections, to normalize the distribution, and to summarize probe intensities. Thereafter, principal component analysis (PCA) was performed. The PCA covered 85.07% of the variability for the 3 groups of LNCs/rats. Following RMA and PCA, ANOVA was performed. After adjusting for *p*-value (<0.05) and more than two-fold change, those miRNA elements that met the cut-off values were identified. The microarray platform had miRNA probes of multiple species (e.g., rat, mouse, and human), as well as multiple probes of each species for a single miRNA. Therefore, the hybridization intensities for all such probes were collectively recorded as "miRNA elements". In subsequent analysis, "miRNA" refers to a given RNA sequence represented by the probes of a single species.

We then employed Ingenuity Pathway Analysis (IPA) (Qiagen), as well as TargetScan, miRbase, and miRNA.org (available online: www.microRNA.org) software, to further analyze the top miRNAs and their potential gene targets. Using "Context score", a score that determines how likely it is for a miRNA to bind to a specific gene target, the highest-scoring and most relevant genes for RA targeted by select miRNA were identified. We have also included in our analysis a few miRNAs (e.g., miR-27a) that are altered under in vitro settings (i.e., LNCs of arthritic rats treated with antigen/celastrol in vitro). This testing was necessary because the in vitro exposure of LNCs and other cell types to celastrol is required to carrying out some of the subsequent validation and mechanistic studies. In the Venn diagram depiction, "uniquely" up-/downregulated refers to change in miRNA elements that are evident in response to only one entity—antigen only or celastrol only—not by both. To examine the potential biological functions of the select miRNAs, the data was subjected to IPA Core analysis. The selected genes were then further grouped into functional categories and plotted as a bar graph. We also examined the key miRNA–mRNA interactions using the network mapping tool for gaining further insight into how these miRNAs might affect different mediators and pathways in RA.

4.5. Testing Micro-RNA Levels in Sera of Rats

The levels of miRNAs in sera of control (naïve) rats, arthritic rats at peak phase of AA, and celastrol-treated rats at peak phase of AA were tested using Multiplex miRNA assays with FirePlex Particle Technology (Abcam, Cambridge, MA, USA). Briefly, blood samples were collected from rats at the peak phase of arthritis or age- and sex-matched control rats. Thereafter, serum was prepared from blood and 20 μL of each sample was subjected to multiplex miRNA assay [83]. The results obtained by Multiplex assay were analyzed using FirePlex Analysis Workbench software. The data was presented after normalizing with three endogenous normalizers selected using the geNorm algorithm: miR-146a-5p, miR-451-5p and miR-17-5p.

5. Conclusions

In summary, this is the first study in the AA model to unravel 8 miRNAs (miR-22, miR-27a, miR-96, miR-142, miR-223, miR-296, miR-298, and miR-451) that can serve as biomarkers of disease. Of these, 6 miRNAs (miR-22, miR-27a, miR-96, miR-142, miR-223, and miR-296) can also serve as biomarkers of therapeutic response in arthritis to celastrol. At present, it is not clear if these 6 biomarkers would also be applicable to monitoring therapeutic response to other anti-arthritic drugs. We believe that this information would open new avenues for better diagnosis, prognosis, and treatment of autoimmune arthritis.

Supplementary Materials: The following are available online at http://www.mdpi.com/1422-0067/19/8/2293/s1.

Declaration: The contents do not represent the views of the U.S. Department of Veterans Affairs or the United States Government.

Author Contributions: Conceptualization, S.D., S.H.V. and K.D.M.; Methodology, S.H.V., S.D., and K.D.M.; Software, S.D., S.H.V.; Validation, S.D., S.H.V.; Formal Analysis, S.D., S.H.V.; Investigation, S.D., S.H.V.; Resources, K.D.M.; Data Curation, S.D., S.H.V.; Writing–Original Draft Preparation, S.D., S.H.V.; Writing–Review & Editing, S.D., S.H.V., and K.D.M.; Funding Acquisition, K.D.M. and S.D.

Funding: This research was supported by R01 AT004321 (to K.D.M.) and F31 AT009421 (S.D.) grants from the National Institutes of Health (NIH), Bethesda, MD, and in part by Merit Review Award # 5 I01 BX002424 (to K.D.M.) from the United States (U.S.) Department of Veterans Affairs (Biomedical Laboratory Research and Development Service).

Acknowledgments: We thank Qun Zhou for his generous help in experimental design and selection of miRNAs; Tariq M. Haqqi (Northeast Ohio Medical University, OH) for helpful advice in mRNA target selection; Jing Yin, Li Tang, and Nick Ambulos for helping with the miRNA-microarray testing; Ming Tan and James Li for assistance in statistical analysis of the miRNA-microarray data; Yang Song and Anup Mahurkar for help in bioinformatics analysis of data; Rakeshchandra Meka for help with CT and data discussion; Bret Hassel, Tonya Webb, and Amit Golding for helpful discussions; and Carol Fowler and Tom Bowen for help with the VA Research Facilities. This material is the result of work supported in part with resources and the use of facilities at the VA Maryland Health Care System, Baltimore, Maryland.

Conflicts of Interest: The authors declare no conflict of interest.

References

1. Harris, E.D.J. Rheumatoid arthritis. Pathophysiology and implications for therapy. *N. Engl. J. Med.* **1990**, *322*, 1277–1289. [PubMed]
2. Birch, J.T., Jr.; Bhattacharya, S. Emerging trends in diagnosis and treatment of rheumatoid arthritis. *Prim. Care* **2010**, *37*, 779–792. [CrossRef] [PubMed]
3. *Rheumatoid Arthritis: National Clinical Guideline for Management and Treatment in Adults. National Collaborating Centre for Chronic Conditions (UK)*; Royal College of Physicians (UK): London, UK, 2009; Chapter 1; pp. 3–8.
4. Alamanos, Y.; Drosos, A.A. Epidemiology of adult rheumatoid arthritis. *Autoimmun. Rev.* **2005**, *4*, 130–136. [CrossRef] [PubMed]
5. Abou-Zeid, A.; Saad, M.; Soliman, E. MicroRNA 146a expression in rheumatoid arthritis: Association with tumor necrosis factor-α and disease activity. *Genet. Test. Mol. Biomark.* **2011**, *15*, 807–812. [CrossRef] [PubMed]
6. Saferding, V.; Puchner, A.; Goncalves-Alves, E.; Hofmann, M.; Bonelli, M.; Brunner, J.S.; Sahin, E.; Niederreiter, B.; Hayer, S.; Kiener, H.P.; et al. MicroRNA-146a governs fibroblast activation and joint pathology in arthritis. *J. Autoimmun.* **2017**, *82*, 74–84. [CrossRef] [PubMed]

7. Kurowska-Stolarska, M.; Alivernini, S.; Ballantine, L.E.; Asquith, D.L.; Millar, N.L.; Gilchrist, D.S.; Reilly, J.; Ierna, M.; Fraser, A.R.; Stolarski, B.; et al. MicroRNA-155 as a proinflammatory regulator in clinical and experimental arthritis. *Proc. Natl. Acad. Sci. USA* **2011**, *108*, 11193–11198. [CrossRef] [PubMed]
8. Yuasa, S.; Yamaguchi, H.; Nakanishi, Y.; Kawaminami, S.; Tabata, R.; Shimizu, N.; Kohno, M.; Shimizu, T.; Miyata, J.; Nakayama, M.; et al. Treatment responses and their predictors in patients with rheumatoid arthritis treated with biological agents. *J. Med. Investig.* **2013**, *60*, 77–90. [CrossRef]
9. Kastbom, A.; Strandberg, G.; Lindroos, A.; Skogh, T. Anti-CCP antibody test predicts the disease course during 3 years in early rheumatoid arthritis (the Swedish TIRA project). *Ann. Rheum. Dis.* **2004**, *63*, 1085–1089. [CrossRef] [PubMed]
10. Gavrila, B.I.; Ciofu, C.; Stoica, V. Biomarkers in Rheumatoid Arthritis, what is new? *J. Med. Life* **2016**, *9*, 144–148. [PubMed]
11. Skare, T.L.; Nisihara, R.; Barbosa, B.B.; da Luz, A.; Utiyama, S.; Picceli, V. Anti-CCP in systemic lupus erythematosus patients: A cross sectional study in Brazilian patients. *Clin. Rheumatol.* **2013**, *32*, 1065–1070. [CrossRef] [PubMed]
12. Szodoray, P.; Szabo, Z.; Kapitany, A.; Gyetvai, A.; Lakos, G.; Szanto, S.; Szucs, G.; Szekanecz, Z. Anti-citrullinated protein/peptide autoantibodies in association with genetic and environmental factors as indicators of disease outcome in rheumatoid arthritis. *Autoimmun. Rev.* **2010**, *9*, 140–143. [CrossRef] [PubMed]
13. Pillai, R.S. MicroRNA function: Multiple mechanisms for a tiny RNA? *RNA* **2005**, *11*, 1753–1761. [CrossRef] [PubMed]
14. Haseeb, A.; Makki, M.S.; Khan, N.M.; Ahmad, I.; Haqqi, T.M. Deep sequencing and analyses of miRNAs, isomiRs and miRNA induced silencing complex (miRISC)-associated miRNome in primary human chondrocytes. *Sci. Rep.* **2017**, *7*, 15178. [CrossRef] [PubMed]
15. Eades, G.; Yang, M.; Yao, Y.; Zhang, Y.; Zhou, Q. miR-200a regulates NRF2 activation by targeting Keap1 mRNA in breast cancer cells. *J. Biol. Chem.* **2011**, *286*, 40725–40733. [CrossRef] [PubMed]
16. Berindan-Neagoe, I.; Monroig Pdel, C.; Pasculli, B.; Calin, G.A. MicroRNAome genome: A treasure for cancer diagnosis and therapy. *CA Cancer J. Clin.* **2014**, *64*, 311–336. [CrossRef] [PubMed]
17. Brower, J.V.; Clark, P.A.; Lyon, W.; Kuo, J.S. MicroRNAs in cancer: Glioblastoma and glioblastoma cancer stem cells. *Neurochem. Int.* **2014**, *77*, 68–77. [CrossRef] [PubMed]
18. Parrella, P.; Barbano, R.; Pasculli, B.; Fontana, A.; Copetti, M.; Valori, V.M.; Poeta, M.L.; Perrone, G.; Righi, D.; Castelvetere, M.; et al. Evaluation of microRNA-10b prognostic significance in a prospective cohort of breast cancer patients. *Mol. Cancer* **2014**, *13*, 142. [CrossRef] [PubMed]
19. Ceribelli, A.; Nahid, M.A.; Satoh, M.; Chan, E.K. MicroRNAs in rheumatoid arthritis. *FEBS Lett.* **2011**, *585*, 3667–3674. [CrossRef] [PubMed]
20. Stanczyk, J.; Pedrioli, D.M.; Brentano, F.; Sanchez-Pernaute, O.; Kolling, C.; Gay, R.E.; Detmar, M.; Gay, S.; Kyburz, D. Altered expression of MicroRNA in synovial fibroblasts and synovial tissue in rheumatoid arthritis. *Arthritis Rheum.* **2008**, *58*, 1001–1009. [CrossRef] [PubMed]
21. Sode, J.; Krintel, S.B.; Carlsen, A.L.; Hetland, M.L.; Johansen, J.S.; Horslev-Petersen, K.; Stengaard-Pedersen, K.; Ellingsen, T.; Burton, M.; Junker, P.; et al. Plasma MicroRNA Profiles in Patients with Early Rheumatoid Arthritis Responding to Adalimumab plus Methotrexate vs Methotrexate Alone: A Placebo-controlled Clinical Trial. *J. Rheumatol.* **2018**, *45*, 53–61. [CrossRef] [PubMed]
22. Du, C.; Liu, C.; Kang, J.; Zhao, G.; Ye, Z.; Huang, S.; Li, Z.; Wu, Z.; Pei, G. MicroRNA miR-326 regulates TH-17 differentiation and is associated with the pathogenesis of multiple sclerosis. *Nat. Immunol.* **2009**, *10*, 1252–1259. [CrossRef] [PubMed]
23. Lindberg, R.L.; Hoffmann, F.; Mehling, M.; Kuhle, J.; Kappos, L. Altered expression of miR-17-5p in CD4$^+$ lymphocytes of relapsing-remitting multiple sclerosis patients. *Eur. J. Immunol.* **2010**, *40*, 888–898. [CrossRef] [PubMed]
24. Wang, H.; Peng, W.; Ouyang, X.; Li, W.; Dai, Y. Circulating microRNAs as candidate biomarkers in patients with systemic lupus erythematosus. *Transl. Res.* **2012**, *160*, 198–206. [CrossRef] [PubMed]
25. Miller, C.H.; Smith, S.M.; Elguindy, M.; Zhang, T.; Xiang, J.Z.; Hu, X.; Ivashkiv, L.B.; Zhao, B. RBP-J-Regulated miR-182 Promotes TNF-α-Induced Osteoclastogenesis. *J. Immunol.* **2016**, *196*, 4977–4986. [CrossRef] [PubMed]

26. Ma, X.; Zhou, J.; Zhong, Y.; Jiang, L.; Mu, P.; Li, Y.; Singh, N.; Nagarkatti, M.; Nagarkatti, P. Expression, regulation and function of microRNAs in multiple sclerosis. *Int. J. Med. Sci.* **2014**, *11*, 810–818. [CrossRef] [PubMed]

27. Pauley, K.M.; Satoh, M.; Chan, A.L.; Bubb, M.R.; Reeves, W.H.; Chan, E.K. Upregulated miR-146a expression in peripheral blood mononuclear cells from rheumatoid arthritis patients. *Arthritis Res. Ther.* **2008**, *10*, R101. [CrossRef] [PubMed]

28. Li, J.; Wan, Y.; Guo, Q.; Zou, L.; Zhang, J.; Fang, Y.; Zhang, J.; Zhang, J.; Fu, X.; Liu, H.; et al. Altered microRNA expression profile with miR-146a upregulation in CD4+ T cells from patients with rheumatoid arthritis. *Arthritis Res. Ther.* **2010**, *12*, R81. [CrossRef] [PubMed]

29. Nakasa, T.; Miyaki, S.; Okubo, A.; Hashimoto, M.; Nishida, K.; Ochi, M.; Asahara, H. Expression of microRNA-146 in rheumatoid arthritis synovial tissue. *Arthritis Rheum.* **2008**, *58*, 1284–1292. [CrossRef] [PubMed]

30. Kopanska, M.; Szala, D.; Czech, J.; Gablo, N.; Gargasz, K.; Trzeciak, M.; Zawlik, I.; Snela, S. MiRNA expression in the cartilage of patients with osteoarthritis. *J. Orthop. Surg. Res.* **2017**, *12*, 51. [CrossRef] [PubMed]

31. Murata, K.; Yoshitomi, H.; Tanida, S.; Ishikawa, M.; Nishitani, K.; Ito, H.; Nakamura, T. Plasma and synovial fluid microRNAs as potential biomarkers of rheumatoid arthritis and osteoarthritis. *Arthritis Res. Ther.* **2010**, *12*, R86. [CrossRef] [PubMed]

32. Mookherjee, N.; El-Gabalawy, H.S. High degree of correlation between whole blood and PBMC expression levels of miR-155 and miR-146a in healthy controls and rheumatoid arthritis patients. *J. Immunol. Methods* **2013**, *400–401*, 106–110. [CrossRef] [PubMed]

33. Van Eden, W.; Wagenaar-Hilbers, J.P.; Wauben, M.H. Adjuvant arthritis in the rat. *Curr. Protoc. Immunol.* **2001**, *19*, 15.4.1–15.4.8. [CrossRef]

34. Moudgil, K.D.; Chang, T.T.; Eradat, H.; Chen, A.M.; Gupta, R.S.; Brahn, E.; Sercarz, E.E. Diversification of T cell responses to carboxy-terminal determinants within the 65-kD heat-shock protein is involved in regulation of autoimmune arthritis. *J. Exp. Med.* **1997**, *185*, 1307–1316. [CrossRef] [PubMed]

35. Venkatesha, S.H.; Yu, H.; Rajaiah, R.; Tong, L.; Moudgil, K.D. Celastrus-derived celastrol suppresses autoimmune arthritis by modulating antigen-induced cellular and humoral effector responses. *J. Biol. Chem.* **2011**, *286*, 15138–15146. [CrossRef] [PubMed]

36. Venkatesha, S.H.; Dudics, S.; Astry, B.; Moudgil, K.D. Control of autoimmune inflammation by celastrol, a natural triterpenoid. *Pathog. Dis.* **2016**, *74*. [CrossRef] [PubMed]

37. Astry, B.; Venkatesha, S.H.; Laurence, A.; Christensen-Quick, A.; Garzino-Demo, A.; Frieman, M.B.; O'Shea, J.J.; Moudgil, K.D. Celastrol, a Chinese herbal compound, controls autoimmune inflammation by altering the balance of pathogenic and regulatory T cells in the target organ. *Clin. Immunol.* **2015**, *157*, 228–238. [CrossRef] [PubMed]

38. He, D.; Xu, Q.; Yan, M.; Zhang, P.; Zhou, X.; Zhang, Z.; Duan, W.; Zhong, L.; Ye, D.; Chen, W. The NF-κB inhibitor, celastrol, could enhance the anti-cancer effect of gambogic acid on oral squamous cell carcinoma. *BMC Cancer* **2009**, *9*, 343. [CrossRef] [PubMed]

39. Dessein, P.H.; Joffe, B.I.; Singh, S. Biomarkers of endothelial dysfunction, cardiovascular risk factors and atherosclerosis in rheumatoid arthritis. *Arthritis Res. Ther.* **2005**, *7*, R634–R643. [CrossRef] [PubMed]

40. Haruna, Y.; Morita, Y.; Komai, N.; Yada, T.; Sakuta, T.; Tomita, N.; Fox, D.A.; Kashihara, N. Endothelial dysfunction in rat adjuvant-induced arthritis: Vascular superoxide production by NAD(P)H oxidase and uncoupled endothelial nitric oxide synthase. *Arthritis Rheum.* **2006**, *54*, 1847–1855. [CrossRef] [PubMed]

41. Szekanecz, Z.; Koch, A.E. Angiogenesis and its targeting in rheumatoid arthritis. *Vascul. Pharmacol.* **2009**, *51*, 1–7. [CrossRef] [PubMed]

42. Poole, K.E.; Reeve, J. Parathyroid hormone—A bone anabolic and catabolic agent. *Curr. Opin. Pharmacol.* **2005**, *5*, 612–617. [CrossRef] [PubMed]

43. Lombardi, G.; Di Somma, C.; Rubino, M.; Faggiano, A.; Vuolo, L.; Guerra, E.; Contaldi, P.; Savastano, S.; Colao, A. The roles of parathyroid hormone in bone remodeling: Prospects for novel therapeutics. *J. Endocrinol. Investig.* **2011**, *34*, 18–22.

44. Chassot, A.A.; Bradford, S.T.; Auguste, A.; Gregoire, E.P.; Pailhoux, E.; de Rooij, D.G.; Schedl, A.; Chaboissier, M.C. WNT4 and RSPO1 together are required for cell proliferation in the early mouse gonad. *Development* **2012**, *139*, 4461–4472. [CrossRef] [PubMed]

45. Franco, H.L.; Dai, D.; Lee, K.Y.; Rubel, C.A.; Roop, D.; Boerboom, D.; Jeong, J.W.; Lydon, J.P.; Bagchi, I.C.; Bagchi, M.K.; et al. WNT4 is a key regulator of normal postnatal uterine development and progesterone signaling during embryo implantation and decidualization in the mouse. *FASEB J.* **2011**, *25*, 1176–1187. [CrossRef] [PubMed]

46. Yu, B.; Chang, J.; Liu, Y.; Li, J.; Kevork, K.; Al-Hezaimi, K.; Graves, D.T.; Park, N.H.; Wang, C.Y. Wnt4 signaling prevents skeletal aging and inflammation by inhibiting nuclear factor-κB. *Nat. Med.* **2014**, *20*, 1009–1017. [CrossRef] [PubMed]

47. Grabiec, A.M.; Angiolilli, C.; Hartkamp, L.M.; van Baarsen, L.G.; Tak, P.P.; Reedquist, K.A. JNK-dependent downregulation of FoxO1 is required to promote the survival of fibroblast-like synoviocytes in rheumatoid arthritis. *Ann. Rheum. Dis.* **2015**, *74*, 1763–1771. [CrossRef] [PubMed]

48. Yadav, V.R.; Prasad, S.; Sung, B.; Kannappan, R.; Aggarwal, B.B. Targeting inflammatory pathways by triterpenoids for prevention and treatment of cancer. *Toxins* **2010**, *2*, 2428–2466. [CrossRef] [PubMed]

49. Salminen, A.; Lehtonen, M.; Paimela, T.; Kaarniranta, K. Celastrol: Molecular targets of Thunder God Vine. *Biochem. Biophys. Res. Commun.* **2010**, *394*, 439–442. [CrossRef] [PubMed]

50. Cascao, R.; Vidal, B.; Raquel, H.; Neves-Costa, A.; Figueiredo, N.; Gupta, V.; Fonseca, J.E.; Moita, L.F. Effective treatment of rat adjuvant-induced arthritis by celastrol. *Autoimmun. Rev.* **2012**, *11*, 856–862. [CrossRef] [PubMed]

51. Fujiwara, W.; Kato, Y.; Hayashi, M.; Sugishita, Y.; Okumura, S.; Yoshinaga, M.; Ishiguro, T.; Yamada, R.; Ueda, S.; Harada, M.; et al. Serum microRNA-126 and -223 as new-generation biomarkers for sarcoidosis in patients with heart failure. *J. Cardiol.* **2018**. [CrossRef] [PubMed]

52. Guo, J.; Liu, C.; Wang, W.; Liu, Y.; He, H.; Chen, C.; Xiang, R.; Luo, Y. Identification of serum miR-1915-3p and miR-455-3p as biomarkers for breast cancer. *PLoS ONE* **2018**, *13*, e0200716. [CrossRef] [PubMed]

53. Mandourah, A.Y.; Ranganath, L.; Barraclough, R.; Vinjamuri, S.; Hof, R.V.; Hamill, S.; Czanner, G.; Dera, A.A.; Wang, D.; Barraclough, D.L. Circulating microRNAs as potential diagnostic biomarkers for osteoporosis. *Sci. Rep.* **2018**, *8*, 8421. [CrossRef] [PubMed]

54. Ouboussad, L.; Hunt, L.; Hensor, E.M.A.; Nam, J.L.; Barnes, N.A.; Emery, P.; McDermott, M.F.; Buch, M.H. Profiling microRNAs in individuals at risk of progression to rheumatoid arthritis. *Arthritis Res. Ther.* **2017**, *19*, 288. [CrossRef] [PubMed]

55. Zhang, J.; Li, S.; Li, L.; Li, M.; Guo, C.; Yao, J.; Mi, S. Exosome and exosomal microRNA: Trafficking, sorting, and function. *Genom. Proteom. Bioinform.* **2015**, *13*, 17–24. [CrossRef] [PubMed]

56. Wang, N.; Wang, L.; Yang, Y.; Gong, L.; Xiao, B.; Liu, X. A serum exosomal microRNA panel as a potential biomarker test for gastric cancer. *Biochem. Biophys. Res. Commun.* **2017**, *493*, 1322–1328. [CrossRef] [PubMed]

57. Bellavia, D.; Raimondi, L.; Costa, V.; De Luca, A.; Carina, V.; Maglio, M.; Fini, M.; Alessandro, R.; Giavaresi, G. Engineered exosomes: A new promise for the management of musculoskeletal diseases. *Biochim. Biophys. Acta* **2018**, *1862*, 1893–1901. [CrossRef] [PubMed]

58. Behera, J.; Tyagi, N. Exosomes: Mediators of bone diseases, protection, and therapeutics potential. *Oncoscience* **2018**, *5*, 181–195. [PubMed]

59. Lin, J.; Huo, R.; Xiao, L.; Zhu, X.; Xie, J.; Sun, S.; He, Y.; Zhang, J.; Sun, Y.; Zhou, Z.; et al. A novel p53/microRNA-22/Cyr61 axis in synovial cells regulates inflammation in rheumatoid arthritis. *Arthritis Rheumatol.* **2014**, *66*, 49–59. [CrossRef] [PubMed]

60. Fan, P.; He, L.; Hu, N.; Luo, J.; Zhang, J.; Mo, L.F.; Wang, Y.H.; Pu, D.; Lv, X.H.; Hao, Z.M.; et al. Effect of 1,25-(OH)2D3 on Proliferation of Fibroblast-Like Synoviocytes and Expressions of Pro-Inflammatory Cytokines through Regulating MicroRNA-22 in a Rat Model of Rheumatoid Arthritis. *Cell. Physiol. Biochem.* **2017**, *42*, 145–155. [CrossRef] [PubMed]

61. Shi, D.L.; Shi, G.R.; Xie, J.; Du, X.Z.; Yang, H. MicroRNA-27a Inhibits Cell Migration and Invasion of Fibroblast-Like Synoviocytes by Targeting Follistatin-Like Protein 1 in Rheumatoid Arthritis. *Mol. Cells* **2016**, *39*, 611–618. [CrossRef] [PubMed]

62. Tardif, G.; Hum, D.; Pelletier, J.P.; Duval, N.; Martel-Pelletier, J. Regulation of the IGFBP-5 and MMP-13 genes by the microRNAs miR-140 and miR-27a in human osteoarthritic chondrocytes. *BMC Musculoskelet. Disord.* **2009**, *10*, 148. [CrossRef] [PubMed]

63. Xiao, Y.; Li, B.; Liu, J. miRNA27a regulates arthritis via PPARgamma in vivo and in vitro. *Mol. Med. Rep.* **2018**, *17*, 5454–5462. [PubMed]

64. Suomi, S.; Taipaleenmaki, H.; Seppanen, A.; Ripatti, T.; Vaananen, K.; Hentunen, T.; Saamanen, A.M.; Laitala-Leinonen, T. MicroRNAs regulate osteogenesis and chondrogenesis of mouse bone marrow stromal cells. *Gene Regul. Syst. Biol.* **2008**, *2*, 177–191. [CrossRef]

65. Yang, M.; Pan, Y.; Zhou, Y. miR-96 promotes osteogenic differentiation by suppressing HBEGF-EGFR signaling in osteoblastic cells. *FEBS Lett.* **2014**, *588*, 4761–4768. [CrossRef] [PubMed]

66. Laine, S.K.; Alm, J.J.; Virtanen, S.P.; Aro, H.T.; Laitala-Leinonen, T.K. MicroRNAs miR-96, miR-124, and miR-199a regulate gene expression in human bone marrow-derived mesenchymal stem cells. *J. Cell. Biochem.* **2012**, *113*, 2687–2695. [CrossRef] [PubMed]

67. Wang, X.; Guo, Y.; Wang, C.; Yu, H.; Yu, X.; Yu, H. MicroRNA-142-3p Inhibits Chondrocyte Apoptosis and Inflammation in Osteoarthritis by Targeting HMGB1. *Inflammation* **2016**, *39*, 1718–1728. [CrossRef] [PubMed]

68. Elmesmari, A.; Fraser, A.R.; Wood, C.; Gilchrist, D.; Vaughan, D.; Stewart, L.; McSharry, C.; McInnes, I.B.; Kurowska-Stolarska, M. MicroRNA-155 regulates monocyte chemokine and chemokine receptor expression in Rheumatoid Arthritis. *Rheumatology* **2016**, *55*, 2056–2065. [CrossRef] [PubMed]

69. Kriegsmann, M.; Randau, T.M.; Gravius, S.; Lisenko, K.; Altmann, C.; Arens, N.; Kriegsmann, J. Expression of miR-146a, miR-155, and miR-223 in formalin-fixed paraffin-embedded synovial tissues of patients with rheumatoid arthritis and osteoarthritis. *Virchows Arch.* **2016**, *469*, 93–100. [CrossRef] [PubMed]

70. Balzano, F.; Deiana, M.; Dei Giudici, S.; Oggiano, A.; Pasella, S.; Pinna, S.; Mannu, A.; Deiana, N.; Porcu, B.; Masala, A.G.E.; et al. MicroRNA Expression Analysis of Centenarians and Rheumatoid Arthritis Patients Reveals a Common Expression Pattern. *Int. J. Med. Sci.* **2017**, *14*, 622–628. [CrossRef] [PubMed]

71. Liu, Y.; Zhang, X.L.; Li, X.F.; Tang, Y.C.; Zhao, X. miR-212-3p reduced proliferation, and promoted apoptosis of fibroblast-like synoviocytes via down-regulating SOX5 in rheumatoid arthritis. *Eur. Rev. Med. Pharmacol. Sci.* **2018**, *22*, 461–471. [PubMed]

72. Lu, M.C.; Yu, C.L.; Chen, H.C.; Yu, H.C.; Huang, H.B.; Lai, N.S. Increased miR-223 expression in T cells from patients with rheumatoid arthritis leads to decreased insulin-like growth factor-1-mediated interleukin-10 production. *Clin. Exp. Immunol.* **2014**, *177*, 641–651. [CrossRef] [PubMed]

73. Li, Y.T.; Chen, S.Y.; Wang, C.R.; Liu, M.F.; Lin, C.C.; Jou, I.M.; Shiau, A.L.; Wu, C.L. Brief report: Amelioration of collagen-induced arthritis in mice by lentivirus-mediated silencing of microRNA-223. *Arthritis Rheum.* **2012**, *64*, 3240–3245. [CrossRef] [PubMed]

74. Shibuya, H.; Nakasa, T.; Adachi, N.; Nagata, Y.; Ishikawa, M.; Deie, M.; Suzuki, O.; Ochi, M. Overexpression of microRNA-223 in rheumatoid arthritis synovium controls osteoclast differentiation. *Mod. Rheumatol.* **2013**, *23*, 674–685. [CrossRef] [PubMed]

75. Dai, Y.; Huang, Y.S.; Tang, M.; Lv, T.Y.; Hu, C.X.; Tan, Y.H.; Xu, Z.M.; Yin, Y.B. Microarray analysis of microRNA expression in peripheral blood cells of systemic lupus erythematosus patients. *Lupus* **2007**, *16*, 939–946. [CrossRef] [PubMed]

76. Murata, K.; Yoshitomi, H.; Furu, M.; Ishikawa, M.; Shibuya, H.; Ito, H.; Matsuda, S. MicroRNA-451 down-regulates neutrophil chemotaxis via p38 MAPK. *Arthritis Rheumatol.* **2014**, *66*, 549–559. [CrossRef] [PubMed]

77. Wang, Z.C.; Lu, H.; Zhou, Q.; Yu, S.M.; Mao, Y.L.; Zhang, H.J.; Zhang, P.C.; Yan, W.J. MiR-451 inhibits synovial fibroblasts proliferation and inflammatory cytokines secretion in rheumatoid arthritis through mediating p38MAPK signaling pathway. *Int. J. Clin. Exp. Pathol.* **2015**, *8*, 14562–14567. [PubMed]

78. Smigielska-Czepiel, K.; van den Berg, A.; Jellema, P.; van der Lei, R.J.; Bijzet, J.; Kluiver, J.; Boots, A.M.; Brouwer, E.; Kroesen, B.J. Comprehensive analysis of miRNA expression in T-cell subsets of rheumatoid arthritis patients reveals defined signatures of naive and memory Tregs. *Genes Immun.* **2014**, *15*, 115–125. [CrossRef] [PubMed]

79. Ezaki, T.; Baluk, P.; Thurston, G.; La Barbara, A.; Woo, C.; McDonald, D.M. Time course of endothelial cell proliferation and microvascular remodeling in chronic inflammation. *Am. J. Pathol.* **2001**, *158*, 2043–2055. [CrossRef]

80. Szmitko, P.E.; Wang, C.H.; Weisel, R.D.; de Almeida, J.R.; Anderson, T.J.; Verma, S. New markers of inflammation and endothelial cell activation: Part I. *Circulation* **2003**, *108*, 1917–1923. [CrossRef] [PubMed]

81. Altamemi, I.; Murphy, E.A.; Catroppo, J.F.; Zumbrun, E.E.; Zhang, J.; McClellan, J.L.; Singh, U.P.; Nagarkatti, P.S.; Nagarkatti, M. Role of microRNAs in resveratrol-mediated mitigation of colitis-associated tumorigenesis in Apc(Min/+) mice. *J. Pharmacol. Exp. Ther.* **2014**, *350*, 99–109. [CrossRef] [PubMed]

82. Silva, M.D.; Savinainen, A.; Kapadia, R.; Ruan, J.; Siebert, E.; Avitahl, N.; Mosher, R.; Anderson, K.; Jaffee, B.; Schopf, L.; et al. Quantitative analysis of micro-CT imaging and histopathological signatures of experimental arthritis in rats. *Mol. Imaging* **2004**, *3*, 312–318. [CrossRef] [PubMed]

83. Tackett, M.R.; Diwan, I. Using FirePlex™ Particle Technology for Multiplex MicroRNA Profiling Without RNA Purification. *Methods Mol. Biol.* **2017**, *1654*, 209–219. [PubMed]

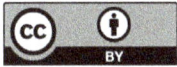

International Journal of
Molecular Sciences

MDPI

Article

Deduction of Novel Genes Potentially Involved in Osteoblasts of Rheumatoid Arthritis Using Next-Generation Sequencing and Bioinformatic Approaches

Yi-Jen Chen [1,2,3], Wei-An Chang [1,4], Ya-Ling Hsu [5], Chia-Hsin Chen [2,3,6,7,*] and Po-Lin Kuo [1,8,*]

[1]   Graduate Institute of Clinical Medicine, College of Medicine, Kaohsiung Medical University, Kaohsiung 807, Taiwan; chernkmu@gmail.com (Y.-J.C.); 960215kmuh@gmail.com (W.-A.C.)
[2]   Department of Physical Medicine and Rehabilitation, Kaohsiung Medical University Hospital, Kaohsiung 807, Taiwan
[3]   Department of Physical Medicine and Rehabilitation, Kaohsiung Municipal Ta-Tung Hospital, Kaohsiung 801, Taiwan
[4]   Division of Pulmonary and Critical Care Medicine, Kaohsiung Medical University Hospital, Kaohsiung 807, Taiwan
[5]   Graduate Institute of Medicine, College of Medicine, Kaohsiung Medical University, Kaohsiung 807, Taiwan; hsuyl326@gmail.com
[6]   Department of Physical Medicine and Rehabilitation, School of Medicine, College of Medicine, Kaohsiung Medical University, Kaohsiung 807, Taiwan
[7]   Orthopaedic Research Center, Kaohsiung Medical University, Kaohsiung 807, Taiwan
[8]   Institute of Medical Science and Technology, National Sun Yat-Sen University, Kaohsiung 804, Taiwan
*   Correspondence: chchen@kmu.edu.tw (C.-H.C.); kuopolin@seed.net.tw (P.-L.K.);
    Tel.: +886-7-312-1101 (ext. 5962) (C.-H.C.); +886-7-312-1101 (ext. 2512-33) (P.-L.K.)

Received: 15 October 2017; Accepted: 6 November 2017; Published: 11 November 2017

Abstract: The role of osteoblasts in peri-articular bone loss and bone erosion in rheumatoid arthritis (RA) has gained much attention, and microRNAs are hypothesized to play critical roles in the regulation of osteoblast function in RA. The aim of this study is to explore novel microRNAs differentially expressed in RA osteoblasts and to identify genes potentially involved in the dysregulated bone homeostasis in RA. RNAs were extracted from cultured normal and RA osteoblasts for sequencing. Using the next generation sequencing and bioinformatics approaches, we identified 35 differentially expressed microRNAs and 13 differentially expressed genes with potential microRNA–mRNA interactions in RA osteoblasts. The 13 candidate genes were involved mainly in cell–matrix adhesion, as classified by the Gene Ontology. Two genes of interest identified from RA osteoblasts, A-kinase anchoring protein 12 (*AKAP12*) and leucin rich repeat containing 15 (*LRRC15*), were found to express more consistently in the related RA synovial tissue arrays in the Gene Expression Omnibus database, with the predicted interactions with miR-183-5p and miR-146a-5p, respectively. The Ingenuity Pathway Analysis identified *AKAP12* as one of the genes involved in protein kinase A signaling and the function of chemotaxis, interconnecting with molecules related to neovascularization. The findings indicate new candidate genes as the potential indicators in evaluating therapies targeting chemotaxis and neovascularization to control joint destruction in RA.

Keywords: rheumatoid arthritis; bone erosion; osteoblasts; next-generation sequencing; bioinformatics; microRNA; messenger RNA

1. Introduction

Rheumatoid arthritis (RA) is an autoimmune disease characterized by systemic inflammation, presence of autoantibodies, and targeted synovitis, affecting approximately 0.5–1% of population [1]. Articular manifestation of inflammatory arthritis is the hallmark of RA and a major determinant of the disease activity [2]. Numerous cell types are involved in the pathophysiology of RA, including immune cells like T cell, B cells and macrophages, synoviocytes, and chondrocytes [3,4]. Synoviocytes and chondrocytes are cell types within the joint dominantly affected by RA. Activated synovial fibroblasts within the inflamed synovium have altered morphology and behavior, and attach directly to cartilage and release matrix degradation enzymes, leading to the destruction of cartilage tissue [1,5,6]. They also interact indirectly with adjacent macrophages through the release of receptor activator of nuclear factor κB ligand (RANKL) and mediate the differentiation of macrophage precursors into osteoclasts [6,7].

Bone erosion is a characteristic feature of affected joints in RA, known to be triggered mainly by synovitis, producing pro-inflammatory cytokines and RANKL [8]. Within the inflamed joint structure, the destructive process by the pannus, a structure formed by proliferative synovium containing infiltrates of immune cells, proliferative vessels, and increased osteoclasts, leads to bone erosion particularly at the synovium–bone interface where the pannus invades [9]. Through the direct contact of the invading pannus to the bone and increased angiogenesis within the pannus structure, the capacity of the synovial fibroblasts to damage structures within the joint has been widely proposed [8–11]. Together with synovial fibroblasts and immune cells, the critical role of osteoclasts in the disrupted bone homeostasis under pathological condition such as RA is being studied. The imbalance of bone homeostasis in RA leads to peri-articular bone loss, which usually precedes bone erosion and further progression of joint destruction [12].

While osteoclasts are the major cells responsible for bone loss and bone erosion in RA, the impaired differentiation and function of osteoblasts have been proposed in recent studies, and inflammatory tissue in RA may impair osteoblast activity, which respond differently from osteoblasts of osteoarthritic condition [12–15]. The precursors of immune cells are formed and maintained in the bone marrow, where osteoclasts and osteoblasts reside and act to maintain a balanced bone remodeling; therefore, research on the interplay between the immune system and the skeletal system has emerged to gain more knowledge on the novel field termed osteoimmunology [8,16,17].

MicroRNAs (miRNAs) are non-coding single strand RNAs consisting of 20–22 nucleotides, acting primarily on the 3′UTR of mRNAs to regulate gene expressions through a post-transcriptional manner [18]. These small non-coding RNAs participate in the regulation of numerous cellular processes and dysregulation of miRNAs are associated with various diseases [19]. The role of miRNA regulation in bone diseases has been reported, including osteoporosis and arthritis that are associated with altered bone homeostasis [20,21]. The study of gene associations using the next generation sequencing (NGS) technique and bioinformatics approaches has evolved, providing high-throughput genomic profiling and further understanding and analysis of functional annotations of identified genes and/or miRNAs [22,23]. In this study, we used various bioinformatics tools and databases to assist in identifying potential miRNA–mRNA interactions in osteoblasts of RA population, including miRmap [24], Gene Expression Omnibus (GEO) [25], Ingenuity® Pathway Analysis (IPA) [26], and Database for Annotation, Visualization and Integrated Discovery (DAVID) [27].

The role of osteoblasts in the development of peri-articular bone loss and limited repair of bone erosion in RA has received much attention, and miRNAs are hypothesized to play critical roles in the regulation of osteoblast function in RA. The aim of our current study is to explore novel miRNAs differentially expressed in osteoblasts of RA bone and to identify genes potentially involved in the dysregulated bone homeostasis in RA. Using the NGS for genomic profiling and various bioinformatics approaches, we expect the findings will provide novel insights into potential therapeutic targets that contribute to better control of RA disease activity.

2. Results

2.1. Identification of Differentially Expressed miRNAs and Potential miRNA–mRNA Interactions between Osteoblasts of Normal and Rheumatoid Arthritis Bones

To identify differentially expressed miRNAs and mRNAs between osteoblasts of normal and RA bones, and potential miRNA–mRNA interactions involved in the inflammatory process and bone homeostasis, we simultaneously performed RNA-seq and small RNA-seq by NGS of normal osteoblasts and RA osteoblasts. There were 35 miRNAs with >2.0-fold change and >10 reads per million (RPM) of either origin of osteoblasts identified. Sixteen up-regulated and 19 down-regulated miRNAs in RA osteoblasts compared to normal osteoblasts were identified, as listed in Table 1. Figure 1A presents the heat map analysis of the 35 differentially expressed miRNAs with z-score values. In addition, we found 434 protein-coding genes with >2.0-fold change and >0.3 fragments per kilobase of transcript per million (FPKM), where 199 genes were up-regulated and 235 genes were down-regulated in RA osteoblasts, compared to normal osteoblasts. To determine potential miRNA–mRNA interactions in normal and RA osteoblasts, we first analyzed putative targets of the 35 miRNAs by miRmap database, and selected targets with miRmap score of more than 99.0. The results yielded 435 targets (520 interactions) of 16 up-regulated miRNAs and 391 targets (477 interactions) of 19 down-regulated miRNAs. We then matched these predicted targets by up-regulated (down-regulated) miRNAs to down-regulated (up-regulated) genes from the 434 protein-coding genes selected. By Venn diagram analysis, we identified 13 genes (eight down-regulated genes and five up-regulated genes) with potential miRNA–mRNA interactions in RA osteoblast (Figure 1B).

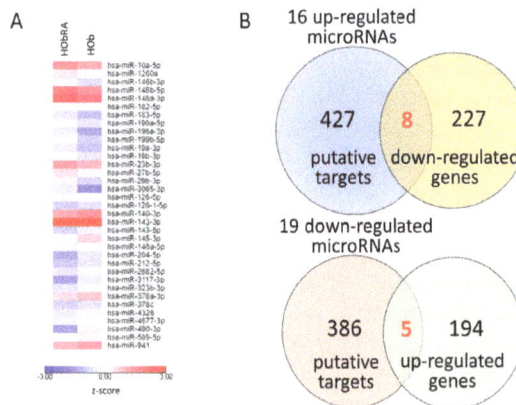

Figure 1. Identification of differentially expressed microRNAs and potential microRNA–mRNA interactions in rheumatoid arthritis primary osteoblasts. (**A**) The next generation sequencing (NGS) identified 35 differentially expressed microRNAs (thresholds of >2.0-fold change and reads per million (RPM) >10) in rheumatoid arthritis (RA) osteoblasts, compared to normal osteoblasts. The heat map analysis with z-score values is shown here. (**B**) The 16 up-regulated and 19 down-regulated microRNAs predicted 435 and 391 putative targets, respectively, using the miRmap database with selection threshold of miRmap score ≥99.0. Additionally, 434 protein-coding genes with >2.0-fold change and >0.3 fragments per kilobase of transcript per million (FPKM) were identified from the NGS, where 199 genes were up-regulated and 235 genes were down-regulated in RA osteoblasts. The putative targets of up-regulated (down-regulated) microRNAs were matched to the down-regulated (up-regulated) protein-coding genes by the Venn diagram analysis. Finally, thirteen genes (eight down-regulated and five up-regulated) with potential miRNA–mRNA interactions were identified.

Table 1. Differentially expressed miRNAs in normal and rheumatoid arthritis (RA) osteoblasts.

microRNA	Precursor	HObRA Seq (Norm)	HOb Seq (Norm)	Fold Change
hsa-miR-3065-3p	hsa-mir-3065	14.08	1.26	11.17
hsa-miR-199b-5p	hsa-mir-199b	55.42	7.36	7.53
hsa-miR-196a-3p	hsa-mir-196a-2	14.34	2.31	6.21
hsa-miR-148a-3p	hsa-mir-148a	12,452.28	4404.25	2.83
hsa-miR-19a-3p	hsa-mir-19a	13.43	4.83	2.78
hsa-miR-19b-3p	hsa-mir-19b-1	35.6	14.08	2.53
hsa-miR-29b-3p	hsa-mir-29b-1	22.17	8.83	2.51
hsa-miR-23b-3p	hsa-mir-23b	1117.61	471.84	2.37
hsa-miR-182-5p	hsa-mir-182	67.94	28.69	2.37
hsa-miR-146b-5p	hsa-mir-146b	4319.58	1843	2.34
hsa-miR-183-5p	hsa-mir-183	11.08	4.83	2.29
hsa-miR-10a-5p	hsa-mir-10a	1708.04	752.73	2.27
hsa-miR-1260a	hsa-mir-1260a	126.48	56.64	2.23
hsa-miR-190a-5p	hsa-mir-190a	28.56	13.24	2.16
hsa-miR-146b-3p	hsa-mir-146b	21.38	10.61	2.02
hsa-miR-27b-5p	hsa-mir-27b	160.78	80.29	2.00
hsa-miR-490-3p	hsa-mir-490	1.43	21.12	−14.77
hsa-miR-3117-3p	hsa-mir-3117	1.56	15.87	−10.17
hsa-miR-204-5p	hsa-mir-204	2.22	14.82	−6.68
hsa-miR-143-3p	hsa-mir-143	54,069.61	16,0924.3	−2.98
hsa-miR-143-5p	hsa-mir-143	6.39	18.92	−2.96
hsa-miR-212-5p	hsa-mir-212	4.3	12.51	−2.91
hsa-miR-323b-3p	hsa-mir-323b	10.95	31.53	−2.88
hsa-miR-2682-5p	hsa-mir-2682	10.3	29.63	−2.88
hsa-miR-146a-5p	hsa-mir-146a	22.69	64.84	−2.86
hsa-miR-145-3p	hsa-mir-145	77.45	212.17	−2.74
hsa-miR-140-3p	hsa-mir-140	814.97	1900.06	−2.33
hsa-miR-4326	hsa-mir-4326	12.65	28.69	−2.27
hsa-miR-4677-3p	hsa-mir-4677	16.69	37.1	−2.22
hsa-miR-128-1-5p	hsa-mir-128-1	5.35	11.66	−2.18
hsa-miR-378a-3p	hsa-mir-378a	174.47	376.1	−2.16
hsa-miR-126-5p	hsa-mir-126	23.47	50.02	−2.13
hsa-miR-378c	hsa-mir-378c	5.87	12.4	−2.11
hsa-miR-941	hsa-mir-941-1	516.36	1049.39	−2.03
hsa-miR-589-5p	hsa-mir-589	49.16	98.36	−2.00

2.2. The 13 Candidate Genes Were Involved in the Cell Matrix Adhesion and Related Molecular Functions

The 13 candidate genes identified from normal and RA osteoblasts were analyzed by DAVID database to determine the functional annotations of these genes. Setting the EASE threshold at 1.0, the Gene Ontology classified these genes to be involved in cell–matrix adhesion and G-protein coupled receptor signaling pathway in the domain of biological process. In the domain of molecular function, the genes were involved in the bindings of collagen, protease, heparin and protein, as shown in Figure 2A. In the domain of cellular component, the genes were mostly active in the extracellular exosome, cytoskeleton, cytoplasm, and plasma membrane (Figure 2B). The KEGG pathway identified *CREB5*, *BDKRB2* and *COL5A3* to be involved in the cGMP-PKG and PI3K-Akt signaling pathways.

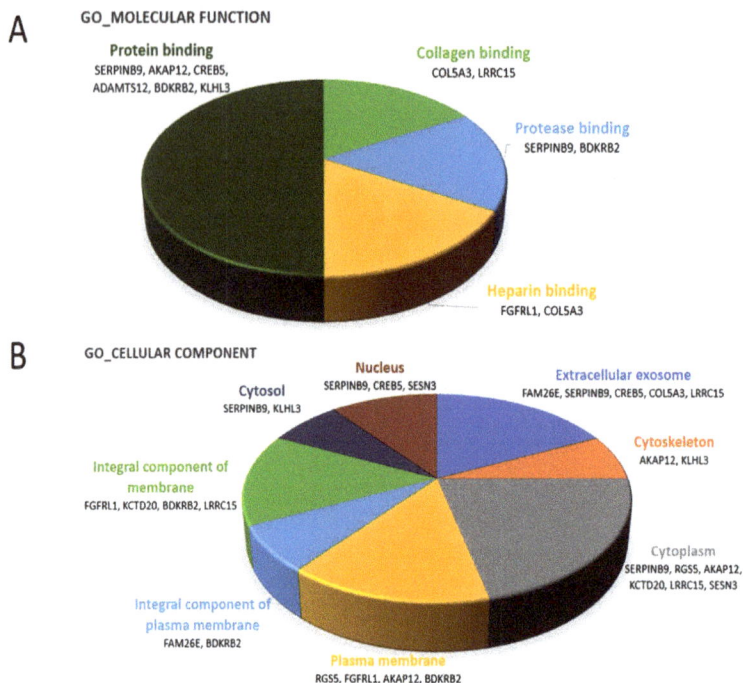

Figure 2. Gene ontology terms involved in the 13 candidate genes of rheumatoid arthritis primary osteoblasts. Using the functional annotation analysis in the DAVID database, the 13 candidate genes were classified by terms of the Gene Ontology in: the molecular function domain (**A**); and the cellular component domain (**B**). The related genes are listed below each term. The selected criteria for functional annotation analysis was EASE = 1.0.

2.3. Analysis of Candidate Genes from Normal and Rheumatoid Arthritis (RA) Osteoblasts in Gene Expression Omnibus (GEO) Database and Identification of Potential Molecular Signatures in RA Joint Microenvironment

The 13 candidate genes with potential miRNA–mRNA interactions identified from normal and RA osteoblasts are listed in Table 2. To determine the involvement of these genes in the joint microenvironment of RA patients, we searched in the GEO database for RA related arrays. There were no arrays comparing osteoblasts or bones of normal and RA patients available in the GEO database. However, we found five arrays comparing synovial tissues of normal and RA patients (GSE1919, GSE55235, GSE55475, GSE7307 and GSE77298), one array comparing synovial fibroblasts isolated from synovial tissues of normal and RA patients (GSE29746) and two arrays comparing synovial macrophages of normal and RA patients (GSE10500 and GSE97779). We analyzed the expression values of the 13 candidate genes identified from normal and RA osteoblasts in these RA related arrays and found two genes that were expressed in the same direction in RA synovial tissues more consistently. As shown in Table 3, the up-regulated *LRRC15* in RA osteoblasts was found up-regulated in four out of the five arrays of synovial tissues; the down-regulated *AKAP12* in RA osteoblasts was found down-regulated in four out of the five arrays of synovial tissues; and up-regulated in one array of synovial macrophages. Additionally, the up-regulated *CREB5* and down-regulated *KCTD20* in RA osteoblasts were observed to express in the same direction in arrays of synovial macrophages. The expression values of the 13 candidate genes in the representative array dataset (GSE77298) are shown in Figure 3.

Table 2. Candidate genes identified from putative targets of microRNAs and differentially expressed genes between normal and RA osteoblasts.

Gene Symbol	Gene Name	Fold-Change (HObRA/HOb)
BDKRB2	bradykinin receptor B2	3.20
CREB5	cAMP responsive element binding protein 5	3.11
FGFRL1	fibroblast growth factor receptor-like 1	2.76
LRRC15	leucine rich repeat containing 15	5.85
SESN3	sestrin 3	2.17
ADAMTS12	ADAM metallopeptidase with thrombospondin type 1 motif 12	0.37
AKAP12	A-kinase anchoring protein 12	0.39
COL5A3	collagen, type V, alpha 3	0.07
FAM26E	family with sequence similarity 26 member E	0.46
KCTD20	potassium channel tetramerization domain containing 20	0.32
KLHL3	kelch like family member 3	0.38
RGS5	regulator of G-protein signaling 5	0.11
SERPINB9	serpin family B member 9	0.32

Table 3. Analysis of 13 candidate genes in RA related arrays in Gene Expression Omnibus (GEO) datasets.

Accession #	GSE7307	GSE55475	GSE77298	GSE55235	GSE1919	GSE29746	GSE10500	GSE97779
Specimen			Synovial tissue			Fibroblast	Synovial macrophage	
Numbers	N/RA	N/RA	N/RA	N/RA	N/RA	N/RA	N/RA	N/RA
	5/5	10/13	7/16	10/10	5/5	11/9	3/5	5/9
Up-regulated mRNA								
BDKRB2	n.s.	n.s.	n.s.	DOWN	n.s.	n.s.	UP	n.s.
CREB5	n.s.	n.s.	n.s.	n.s.	n.s.	n.s.	UP	UP
FGFRL1	n.s.	−	n.s.	−	−	n.s.	−	n.s.
LRRC15	n.s.	UP	UP	UP	UP	n.s.	n.s.	n.s.
SESN3	UP	−	n.s.	−	−	n.s.	−	n.s.
Down-regulated mRNA								
ADAMTS12	n.s.	n.s.	n.s.	n.s.	−	n.s.	−	DOWN
AKAP12	DOWN	n.s.	DOWN	DOWN	DOWN	n.s.	UP	n.s.
COL5A3	UP	n.s.	n.s.	n.s.	−	n.s.	−	n.s.
FAM26E	n.s.	−	n.s.	−	−	n.s.	−	n.s.
KCTD20	n.s.	DOWN	n.s.	n.s.	n.s.	n.s.	DOWN	DOWN
KLHL3	DOWN	n.s.	n.s.	UP	−	n.s.	−	n.s.
RGS5	n.s.	n.s.	DOWN	n.s.	n.s.	n.s.	UP	DOWN
SERPINB9	n.s.	n.s.	n.s.	n.s.	UP	n.s.	n.s.	UP

The genes and their directions of expression marked in **bold** were those that were expressed more consistently in the same directions in RA synovial tissues from GEO datasets. N, normal population; RA, rheumatoid arthritis patients; UP, up-regulated in RA; DOWN, down-regulated in RA; n.s., non-significant between normal and RA; −, no identical probes within the array.

A

B

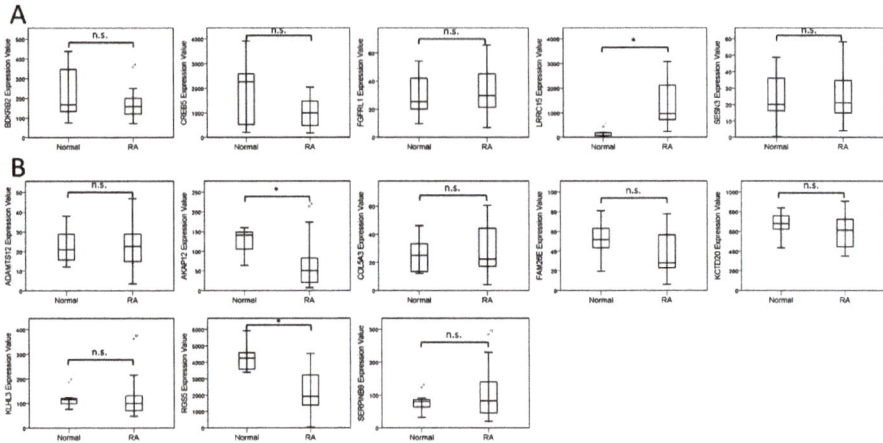

Figure 3. Analysis of 13 genes with potential microRNA–mRNA interactions in the Gene Expression Omnibus (GEO) database. The expression values of: five up-regulated genes (**A**); and eight down-regulated genes (**B**) identified from normal and rheumatoid arthritis (RA) osteoblasts were validated in a representative array (GSE77298) of normal and RA synovial tissues from the GEO database. Significant up-regulation of *LRRC15* and down-regulation of *AKAP12* and *RGS5* were observed in the synovial tissues of patients with RA, compared to the normal subjects. * indicated $p < 0.05$, and n.s. indicated no statistical significance. (Probe ID reference: *BDKRB2*, 205870_at; *CREB5*, 229228_at; *FGFRL1*, 223321_s_at; *LRRC15*, 213909_at; *SESN3*, 242899_at; *ADAMTS12*, 221421_s_at; *AKAP12*, 231067_s_at; *COL5A3*, 218975_at; *FAM26E*, 230254_at; *KCTD20*, 228299_at; *KLHL3*, 221221_s_at; *RGS5*, 209071_s_at; and *SERPINB9*, 242814_at).

2.4. Potential miRNA–mRNA Interactions of LRRC15 and AKAP12 in RA Osteoblasts

We used miRmap database to analyze potential miRNA regulations of *LRRC15* and *AKAP12*. Forty-four miRNAs with miRmap score >99.0 were potentially involved in the *LRRC15* regulation, and 11 miRNAs with miRmap score >99.0 were potentially involved in the *AKAP12* regulation. Matching to our differentially expressed miRNA database, we identified down-regulated miR-146a-5p that potentially up-regulated *LRRC15*, and up-regulated miR-183-5p that potentially down-regulated *AKAP12*, as shown in Table 4. The sequences and putative 3′UTR binding sites of representative miRNAs in *LRRC15* and *AKAP12* were then validated in miRmap, TargetScan and miRDB databases. The target binding sites of miR-146a-5p in the 3′UTR of *LRRC15* at the positions of 388–394 and 537–543 were validated in miRmap and TargetScan (Figure 4), while the target binding site of miR-183-5p in the 3′UTR of *AKAP12* at the position of 959–966 was validated in miRmap, TargetScan and miRDB (Figure 5).

Table 4. Potential miRNA regulations of corresponding predicted targets.

Down-Regulated miRNA	Precursor	Fold-Change	miRmap Score	Predicted Target Up-Regulated mRNA	Fold-Change (HObRA/HOb)
hsa-miR-146a-5p	hsa-mir-146a	−2.86	99.08	*LRRC15*	5.85
Up-Regulated miRNA	**Precursor**	**Fold-Change**	**miRmap Score**	**Predicted Target Down-Regulated mRNA**	**Fold-Change (HObRA/HOb)**
hsa-miR-183-5p	hsa-mir-183	2.29	99.56	*AKAP12*	0.39

A

B

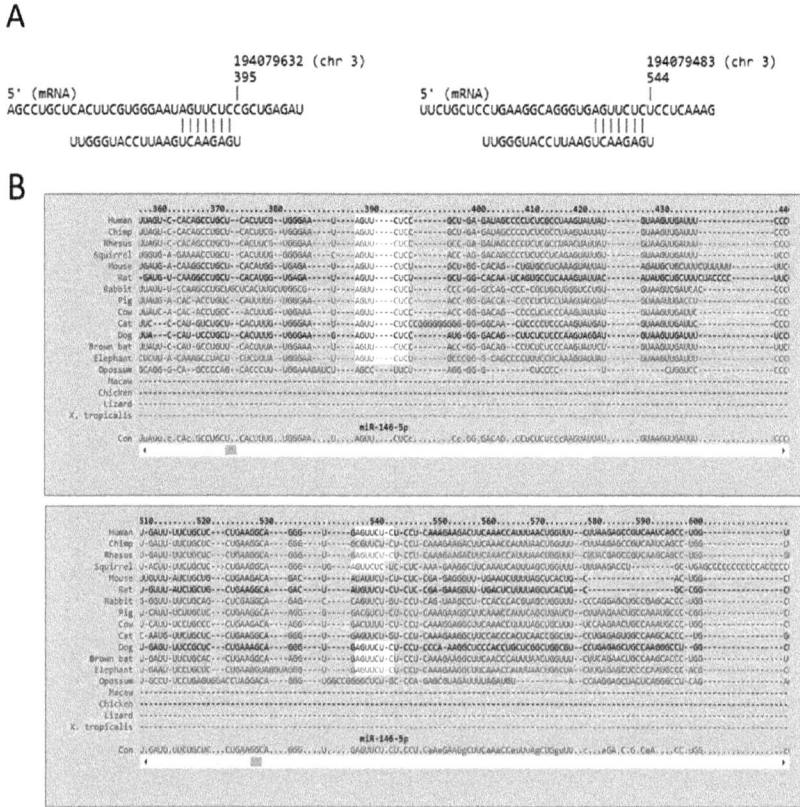

Figure 4. The putative binding sites of miR-146a-5p on *LRRC15*. The sequences and putative binding sites of miR-146a-5p on the 3′UTR of *LRRC15* at positions of 388–394 and 537–543 were validated in: miRmap (**A**); and TargetScan (**B**).

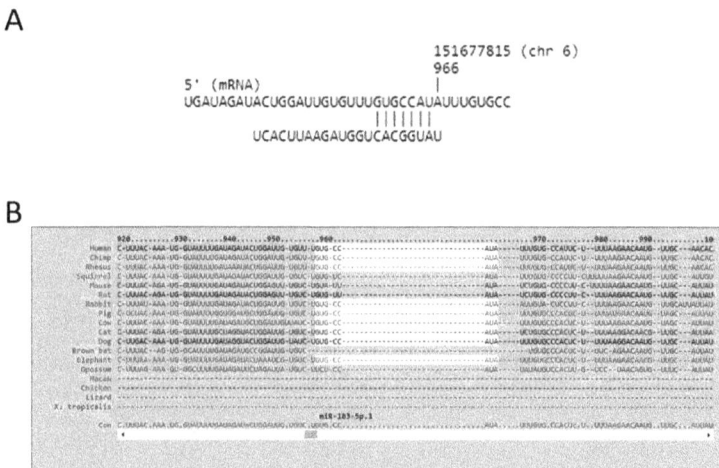

A

B

Figure 5. *Cont.*

C

3' UTR Sequence

```
   1 AACATCATGC AGTTAAACTC ATTGTCTGTT TGGAAGACCA GAATGTGAAG ACAAGTAGTA
  61 GAAGAAAATG AATGCTGCTG CTGAGACTGA AGACCAGTAT TTCAGAACTT TGAGAATTGG
 121 AGAGCAGGCA CATCAACTGA TCTCATTTCT AGAGAGCCCC TGACAATCCT GAGGCTTCAT
 181 CAGGAGCTAG AGCCATTTAA CATTTCCTCT TTCCAAGACC AACCTACAAT TTTCCCTTGA
 241 TAACCATATA AATTCTGATT TAAGGTCCTA AATTCTTAAC CTGGAACTGG AGTTGGCAAT
 301 ACCTAGTTCT GCTTCTGAAA CTGGAGTATC ATTCTTTACA TATTTATATG TATGTTTTAA
 361 GTAGTCCTCC TGTATCTATT GTATATTTTT TTCTTAATGT TTAAGGAAAT GTGCAGGATA
 421 CTACATGCTT TTTGTATCAC ACAGTATATG ATGGGGCATG TGCCATAGTG CAGGCTTGGG
 481 GAGCTTTAAG CCTCAGTTAT ATAACCCACG AAAAACAGAG CCTCCTAGAT GTAACATTCC
 541 TGATCAAGGT ACAATTCTTT AAAATTCACT AATGATTGAG GTCCATATTT AGTGGTACTC
 601 TGAAATTGGT CACTTTCCTA TTACACGGAG TGTGCTAAAA CTAAAAAGCA TTTTGAAACA
 661 TACAGAATGT TCTATTGTCA TTGGGAAATT TTTCTTTCTA ACCCAGTGGA GGTTAGAAAG
 721 AAGTTATATT CTGGTAGCAA ATTAACTTTA CATCCTTTTT CCTACTTGTT ATGGTTGTTT
 781 GGACCGATAA GTGTGCTTAA TCCTGAGGCA AAGTAGTGAA TATGTTTTAT ATGTTATGAA
 841 GAAAAGAATT GTTGTAAGTT TTTGATTCTA CTCTTATATG CTGGACTGCA TTCACACATG
 901 GCATGAAATA AGTCAGGTTC TTTACAAATG GTATTTTGAT AGATACTGGA TTGTGTTTGT
 961 GCCATATTTG TGCCATTCTT TTAAGAACAA TGTTGCAACA CATTCATTTG GATAAGTTGT
1021 GATTTGACGA CTGATTTAAA TAAAATATTT GCTTCACTTA GATTTGCTGG TTTTATTAGA
1081 TACCAGGAAG CCTGGGACAT ATGTGTACCA CATTAGAATT CTAAAGATAA TGATTGATAA
1141 GCTAGAACTT TCTGATGTAG TCATTACATG AAACCCCTTG TCACTGGTTT GTGTGTTCAG
1201 AGGAAGCCAT GGCCGAGATA GCTTTCCTGA AATAAACCAG TAGCTTTTCA GATTGACGTT
1261 CTTGCTACAA TTGTACCATC TGGTAATTCC TGAAAATGTC AATTTTTTTG TGTTAATATT
1321 TTTGGTTTCA AACAATAACA AATGTCTCTA GAAAGAAATT TTAAGAAAGC TTAATTAATA
1381 GTAAAAATGC CTTTCCTGAA ATAATCTTGG AAAATTTTTT AAATGTCAAA ATGATGAGTC
1441 ATGCTAATAC ATTGAGGGTT TGTTTTTTTG TTTGTTTGTT TGTTTGTTTT TGAGACAGAG
1501 TTTCGCTCTT GTTGCCCAGG CTGGAGTGCA ATGGCACGAT CTCAGCTCAC CGCAACCTCC
1561 ACCTCCCGGA TTCCAGCGAT TCTCCTGCCT CAGCCTACAT TAAGGGTTTT GTCAGACAAT
1621 TGTCACACGA AGAATAGTGT CACTTATCTA CTCTTGACAC ACAGAACTGG CCTGGCATAT
1681 AGCTTTCCAG ATTTTACTCA AACTTGGTAC TCCAGTTTGA AAATTTAAAT TTTGACTGCT
1741 GATTAGCTGG AAAGCCTAGT TTTAATGGAA AGAAAGTTTG CTTTTAAAAC TGAAAGTAGT
1801 TTCTTTTTGC TAACAAATCT AACTTCATAC ATAATTGGCC ATATTAGTAA AACACCTCAT
1861 GATAGCAGTG TATATATAGT CTTGTTTGTA GTTGGAAGTC ATCTTTTAGG AGTTATTCTC
1921 AAATATATAT AATAGCTACC CATGCATCAT TATTAAAATC CCCAAATTCA AAAAACCTCT
1981 GATATATATA TATAATTTTT TTTTTTTTTT TTTTTTGGCC AACTGAGATT GAAATCCAAG
2041 TGCTGGTTTC TAGTTCTGAA CATCAACTAA AGAGTTTTGG AAATGACAGC AATTTATAAC
2101 AAGTTCATAT TGACTTCCTC TCTATGGCAG GAAGACATTC TGTGCTGTTT TGAACAGATT
2161 AAAGATTTGT GTAGTTTGTG GGAAATTGAC GTTTTTGTTT AAATTCCACC CGCGTTTGTC
2221 TTTTCCTACC ACCTGTGGCC AGGTGCTCGC TGGCCATCAC AGTTGCGATT CCATGAGTAG
2281 CTGCTTTATG ACTGCTTTTT GTACTATCTG GATGTGCCCA GAGTTACTTC TGTACAAGCT
2341 CTGTATCTAT GTCCGTTGAG AACATTATTT TAACAAGAAG AACACCAACA GTAGCATGAA
2401 ATATAATACT GTTTTATAAT TCTAAAGCTG CTGTTAATTT ATGAAGTACA TAATAATCTA
2461 ATGTAAACTG CAGAAGTCAG AGCAAGTGCC TACATTTTGT TATTTTTGGC ATTACTACAG
2521 AGCCATGTAC AATAGAAAGC AATGCAAGAC TTGTAAACTC TCACCACTTC TTGTAATATC
2581 AAATGTTCCC CCTCAGGTTA TTTTGCTTAT GGTACCCATG AGTTGCCTCT CTCTGTACAT
2641 AGATAAAATTG TTCCAATATT TTCCTTTGAT GTTTGGAACT ACAGATAGTC AAGGGCTGGA
2701 AATTTTAGTT TTCAATATAA GCTTCCAGCT TAGCAATTAC CTCTAGTCGA AGACAATATT
2761 TGATTCCTAG TTCTGTTTGG GGCAAATTTT CATTTATCTA AATAAAAATGC AATCTAATTA
2821 AATGCCATGG ATTTTCTTTC TGTAAAAAAA AAAAAAAAAA A
```

Figure 5. The putative binding site of miR-183-5p on *AKAP12*. The sequence and putative binding site of miR-183-5p on the 3'UTR of *AKAP12* at the position of 959–966 was validated in: miRmap (**A**); TargetScan (**B**); and miRDB (**C**).

Using the IPA software, diseases and functions associated with the 13 candidate genes identified between normal and RA osteoblasts were further analyzed. There were two networks classified, as shown in Table 5, with 10 of the 13 candidate genes involved in network 1 (Figure 6). The previously identified *AKAP12* was involved in network 1, while *LRRC15* was involved in network 2. One of the miRNAs identified between normal and RA osteoblasts, miR-146a-5p, was also involved in network 1. Using the overlay diseases and functions tool in the IPA software, we disclosed *ADAMTS12*, *BDKRB1*, *BDKRB2*, *BMP1*, *FGF2*, *FOXO1*, *KCTD20*, *NOTCH4*, *PPARG*, *TGFB1* and miR-146a-5p to be associated with "rheumatic disease" and "inflammation of joint" in network 1, as indicated by purple frames in Figure 6.

Table 5. Networks associated with 13 candidate genes differentially expressed in RA osteoblasts.

	Top Diseases and Functions	Score	Focus Molecules	Molecules in Network
1.	Cardiovascular System Development and Function, Cellular Development, Cellular Growth and Proliferation	27	10	↓ADAMTS12, ↓AKAP12, AKT2, BDKRB1, ↑BDKRB2, BMP1, COL5A1, ↓COL5A3, collagen, Collagen type I, ↑CREB5, ERK1/2, ↓FAM26E, FGF2, Fgfr, ↑FGFRL1, FOXO1, GPC1, Hspg2, Kallikrein, ↓KCTD20, KLKB1, MAPK1, mir-25, mir-181, miR-146a-5p, MIR17HG, NOTCH2, NOTCH4, plasminogen activator, Plc beta, PPARG, ↓RGS5, ↑SESN3, TGFB1
2.	Cellular Compromise, Organismal Injury and Abnormalities, Hereditary Disorder	6	3	AKT2, COASY, DOLPP1, FOSB, FOSL2, FURIN, GBP2, H2AFB3, IGSF8, JUND, KEAP1, ↓KLHL3, ↑LRRC15, MAFG, MAPK3, MARK4, miR-3656, miR-423-5p, miR-4537, miR-6825-5p, MRPS27, NOS3, P2RY8, PLEKHM1, PRKCG, RAB11B, SELPLG, ↓SERPINB9, SLC9A1, SMARCD1, TAGLN, UNC119, USF2, WNK2, WNK4

The genes marked in **bold** were the 13 candidate genes identified in normal and RA osteoblasts.

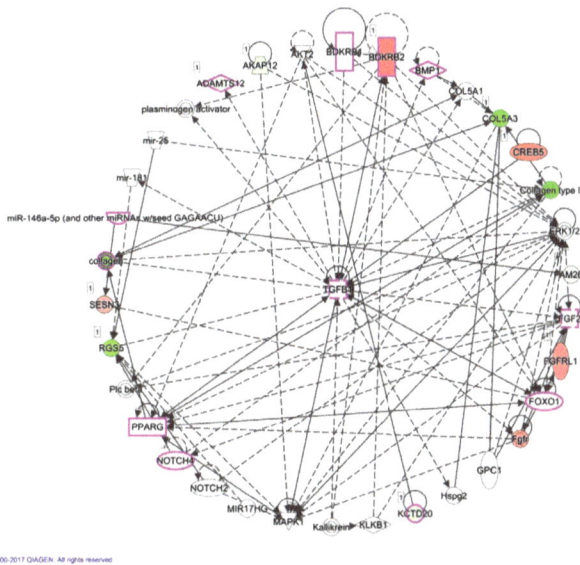

Figure 6. Network analysis by Ingenuity® Pathway Analysis (IPA) indicated molecules associated with rheumatic disease and inflammation of joint. The network analysis was performed by IPA software to indicate networks involved in the 13 candidate genes from rheumatoid arthritis (RA) osteoblasts. Ten of the 13 candidate genes were grouped in one network associated with cardiovascular system development and function, cellular development, cellular growth and proliferation. Molecules including *ADAMTS12, BDKRB1, BDKRB2, BMP1, FGF2, FOXO1, KCTD20, NOTCH4, PPARG, TGFB1* and miR-146a-5p were associated with rheumatic disease and inflammation of joint in the network, as indicated in purple frames. Molecules in green indicated down-regulated expressions, and molecules in red indicated up-regulated expressions in RA osteoblasts compared to normal osteoblasts. The green and red color scales disclosed the relative gene expression values of RA to normal osteoblasts.

In addition to network analysis, we found miR-29b-3p to be one of the significant upstream regulators (*p*-value of overlap = 3.94×10^{-4}), which was 2.51-fold up-regulated in RA osteoblasts compared to normal osteoblasts. The effectors potentially involved in the miR-29b-3p regulation were *BDKRB2, COL5A3, CREB5, KCTD20,* and *SERPINB9* (Table 6).

Table 6. Upstream regulator miR-29b-3p and potential downstream effectors of RA osteoblasts.

Analysis	Molecules in 13 Candidate Genes	p-Value of Overlap
miR-29b-3p	*BDKRB2, COL5A3, CREB5, KCTD20, SERPINB9*	3.94×10^{-4}

Analysis	Molecules in 434 Differentially Expressed Genes	p-Value of Overlap
miR-29b-3p	*RUNX1T1, PALM, PDPN, LAMA2, ITGA6, CEMIP, DPP4, HS3ST3B1, KIF26B, CACNA1A, GPR85, CELF2, HAPLN1, BDKRB2, NDN, CRYBG1, CREB5, WISP1, FAM167A, SLC12A8, COL11A1, DMKN, MEGF6, ENPP2, ID3, PDGFRB, RTL5, TRAF5, LASP1, CSPG4, HAPLN3, NEDD9, KCTD20, SERPINB9, PEG10, UACA, ADAM19, CTPS1, CCDC85A, FCRLA, TRPC6, COL5A3, CCDC81, HEYL*	1.76×10^{-5}

2.5. The Differentially Expressed Genes in RA Osteoblasts Were Associated with Chemotaxis, Neovascularization, Cell Adhesion and Extracellular Matrix Organization

To identify pathways and biological functions involved in RA osteoblasts, the 434 differentially expressed protein-coding genes (199 up-regulated genes and 235 down-regulated genes) between normal and RA osteoblasts were further analyzed by the IPA software and the functional annotation tool in the DAVID database. The results of IPA analysis identified *TGFB1*, *TNF*, *IFNG*, and *IL1B* among the top upstream regulators. miR-29b-3p was also a significant upstream regulator (p-value of overlap = 1.76×10^{-5}), with its effectors listed in Table 6. The differentially expressed genes were categorized into 25 networks. *AKAP12*, along with 24 other dysregulated genes were involved in diseases and functions related to cellular development, cellular growth and proliferation, and organ development, whereas 17 dysregulated genes, including *LRRC15*, were involved in diseases and functions related to hereditary disorder, immunological disease, and organismal injury and abnormalities (Table 7).

Table 7. Two of the networks associated with 434 candidate genes differentially expressed in RA osteoblasts.

Top Diseases and Functions	Score	Focus Molecules	Molecules in Network
Cellular Development, Cellular Growth and Proliferation, Organ Development	38	25	↓**AKAP12**, Cbp/p300, ↓**CDA**, ↑**CEMIP**, ↓**CNN1**, ↑**CRLF1**, ↓**DOCK10**, E2f, EGLN, ↑**EPHA4**, ↓**EPHA5**, ↑**FGFRL1**, ↓**FHL1**, ↓**FLT1**, GTPase, ↓**GUCY1B3**, Hedgehog, ↓**HGF**, ↑**ICA1**, Importin alpha, ↑**ITGA6**, ↑**ITGB8**, ↓**LMOD1**, ↓**MYOCD**, ↓**NOTCH1**, ↓**PDLIM3**, ↑**PHLDA1**, ↑**PLXNA2**, Proinsulin, ↓**SCUBE3**, Sfk, Smad2/3, ↑**SOX9**, Vegf, ↑**VLDLR**
Hereditary Disorder, Immunological Disease, Organismal Injury and Abnormalities	22	17	↑**ADM2**, ATP6AP1, ATP6V1F, CASP2, CDK2AP2, ↑**CMKLR1**, CTSA, ↓**CYGB**, ↑**ELFN1**, ↓**FAM46B**, FOXRED2, GPR84, GRM4, ↓**HAAO**, ↓**HEYL**, ↓**IRX2**, ↓**KCTD20**, ↑**KIF26B**, LDB1, ↑**LRRC15**, ↓**LRRC32**, ↓**LYPD1**, miR-4656, miR-504-3p, ↑**MKX**, ↓**MX1**, PLPPR2, ↓**PLPPR4**, PPP1CA, RASSF8, ↓**SERPINA9**, TBC1D22A, TRIM67, TUFT1, ZNF677

The genes marked in **bold** were the 434 differentially expressed protein-coding genes identified in normal and RA osteoblasts.

We then determined the interconnection between various diseases and functions, including inflammation of joint, chemotaxis, damage of connective tissue, migration of connective tissue cells, proliferation of osteoblasts, and neovascularization. *AKAP12* is one of the genes involved in chemotaxis, having connection with *HGF* and *ARRB1*, which are involved in damage of connective tissue and neovascularization. Using the overlay canonical pathway tool in the IPA, molecules involved in protein kinase A signaling, including *AKAP12, MAP3K1, VASP, PTK2B, TGFB2, ITPR3,* and *NFATC1*, also take part in the above selected diseases and functions, as indicated by light blue lines in Figure 7.

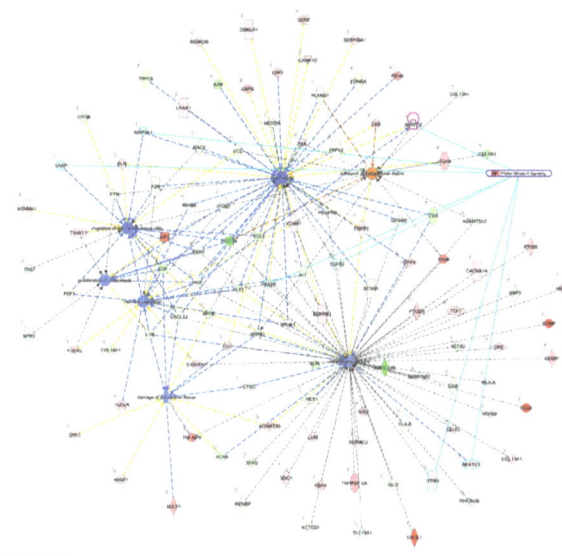

Figure 7. Analysis of the interconnection between *AKAP12* and the merged networks of related joint diseases and functions. The 434 differentially expressed genes identified in normal and rheumatoid arthritis (RA) osteoblasts were analyzed by the IPA to be categorized into 25 networks. Diseases and functions related to joint destruction in RA microenvironment, including inflammation of joint, chemotaxis, damage of connective tissue, migration of connective tissue cells, proliferation of osteoblasts, and neovascularization were selected to identify related genes. *AKAP12*, one of the genes involved in chemotaxis, was connected to *HGF* and *ARRB1*, molecules involved in damage of connective tissue and neovascularization. In addition, the overlay canonical pathway analysis indicated *AKAP12, MAP3K1, VASP, PTK2B, TGFB2, ITPR3,* and *NFATC1* (marked in light blue) to be involved in the protein kinase A signaling, and participated in various indicated networks.

Using the DAVID database for the analysis of biological functions, the top 10 biological functions involved in these differentially expressed genes of RA osteoblasts were cell adhesion (38 genes), extracellular matrix organization (23 genes), positive regulation of cell migration (21 genes), skeletal system development (18 genes), angiogenesis (22 genes), type I interferon signaling pathway (12 genes), positive regulation of cell proliferation (31 genes), response to hypoxia (18 genes), heart development (18 genes), and positive regulation of PI3K signaling (11 genes), as shown in Figure 8.

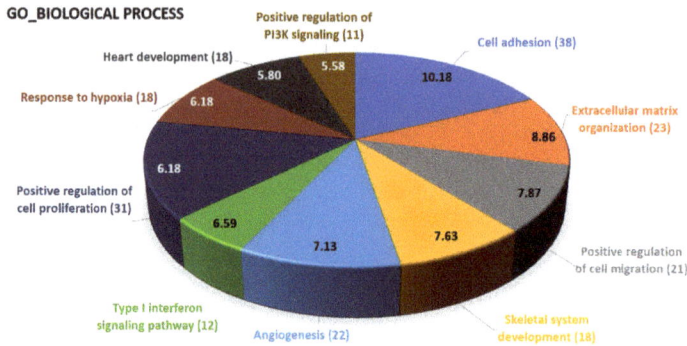

Figure 8. The biological process analysis of differentially expressed genes in rheumatoid arthritis osteoblasts. The 434 differentially expressed genes in rheumatoid arthritis osteoblasts were analyzed in the DAVID database for the identification of involved biological processes. The results indicated these genes were potentially involved in cell adhesion (38 genes), extracellular matrix organization (23 genes), positive regulation of cell migration (21 genes), skeletal system development (18 genes), angiogenesis (22 genes), type I interferon signaling pathway (12 genes), positive regulation of cell proliferation (31 genes), response to hypoxia (18 genes), heart development (18 genes), and positive regulation of PI3K signaling (11 genes). The selected criteria for functional annotation analysis were EASE = 0.1 and fold enrichment >1.3. The proportions of the pie chart were drawn according to the numbers of genes involved in each biological term, and the numbers within the pie chart indicated $-\log$ (p-value) of each biological term.

3. Discussion

The current study identified 35 differentially expressed miRNAs and 13 candidate genes potentially involved in osteoblasts of RA, using NGS and bioinformatics analysis. Two of the 13 candidate genes differentially expressed in osteoblasts of RA, *LRRC15* and *AKAP12*, were found to have consistent direction of expression in the synovial tissue of RA patients identified in four of the five RA array datasets (GSE7307, GSE55475, GSE77298, GSE55235, and GSE1919). The potential miRNA regulation on *LRRC15* was miR-146a-5p, whereas the potential miRNA regulation on *AKAP12* was miR-183-5p, predicted by miRmap, TargetScan and miRDB database. We proposed the novel findings of miR-146a-5p–*LRRC15* and miR-183-5p–*AKAP12* regulations in the altered function of osteoblasts in RA microenvironment.

The role of osteoblasts in the development of bone loss and limited capacity of repair of bone erosion in RA has received more attention recently, and miRNAs are hypothesized to play critical roles in the regulation of the function of osteoblasts in RA [13,15,28]. The results of IPA analysis identified miR-29b-3p to be a potential upstream regulator of the differentially expressed genes in RA. The regulation of the miR-29 family is proposed to participate in osteoarthritis and cartilage homeostasis [29]. In addition, the miR-29 family has been shown to promote osteoblast differentiation by targeting inhibitors of the Wnt signaling pathway, and to possess numerous distinct activities at different stages of osteoblast differentiation. In the mature osteoblasts, miR-29 targets collagen type I, reducing the rate of collagen synthesis and facilitating structural stability of the bone [30]. In a review article by Miao et al., the Wnt signaling pathway participates in the pathogenesis of RA and bone remodeling. They suggested that inhibition of the Wnt signaling pathway may contribute to impaired osteoblast function in RA, and increased expression of several inhibitors of the Wnt signaling pathway may contribute to bone resorption in RA [31]. Two of the effectors of miR-29b-3p in our candidate genes, *BDKRB2* and *SERPINB9*, were categorized into the molecular function of protease binding by gene ontology, as shown in Figure 2A and Table 6, which may support the involvement of miR-29b-3p in the regulation of bone matrix in RA.

A-kinase anchoring protein 12 (AKAP12), one of the A-kinase anchoring proteins, is a scaffold protein for protein kinase A (PKA) and protein kinase C (PKC) that control cytoskeleton dynamics, cell migration, and cell adhesion [32,33]. Studies suggested that the down-regulation of AKAP12 induces the formation of stress fibers and proliferation of adhesion complexes; increased cellular senescence was also observed in AKAP12-null mice [34]. The findings potentially link *AKAP12* to the disrupted bone homeostasis in RA, where the study by Yudoh and colleagues revealed the higher rate of cellular senescence and greater decline in the replicative capacity of peri-articular osteoblasts in RA patients, compared to osteoarthritic patients [15]. The expressions of AKAP12 in inflammatory responses were studied. The increased protein expression of AKAP12 in the fibrotic scar may restrict excessive inflammation during central nervous system repair [35], and decreased protein levels of AKAP12 were observed in the lung tissue of patients with chronic obstructive pulmonary disease [36], suggesting the participation of AKAP12 in the regulation of inflammatory response. There is not much literature discussing the role of AKAP12 in the bone homeostasis or the inflamed joint microenvironment. One study identified *Akap12* to be one of the genes possibly involved in the alternative splicing in bone following mechanical loading in rat model [37]. The altered joint structures along with inflamed peri-articular soft tissue in RA predispose the affected joint to increased mechanical loading, which may disrupt the PKA-mediated mechanotransduction.

Scaffold proteins serve as connecting hubs that modulate both upstream signaling molecules and the downstream effectors within cells. The expression and activity of AKAP12 is proposed to be affected by the hypoxic tumor microenvironment [38]. Studies also suggested *AKAP12* to be a tumor suppressor and angiogenesis suppressor gene that down-regulates vascular endothelial growth factor, potentially through epigenetic regulation [39]. The role of miRNA regulation in altered bone homeostasis has been reported [20,21]. Few studies also reported that miR-183 increased osteoclastogenesis through the binding on the 3′UTR of heme oxygenase-1 [40], and oxidative stress within the bone marrow microenvironment may alter miRNA cargo of extracellular vesicles, expressing high abundance of miR-183 cluster and miR-183-5p transfection inhibits the osteogenic differentiation of bone marrow stromal cells [41]. Altogether, with these literature reviews, the up-regulated miR-183-5p with its putative target of down-regulated *AKAP12* in our NGS result suggests the novel finding of potential miR-183-5p–*AKAP12* regulation in the changed bone homeostasis in RA joint microenvironment.

Leucine rich repeat containing 15 (*LRRC15*), also named *LIB*, is a gene encoding leucine-rich transmembrane protein that participates in the cell–matrix adhesion and cell migration, and is induced and highly expressed in various cancer types [42–44]. The role of *LRRC15* in inflammation is also proposed, as it is induced by beta-amyloid and pro-inflammatory cytokines in astrocytes of Alzheimer's disease brain [45,46] and up-regulated by pro-inflammatory stimuli during the process of dental caries [47]. There is still lack of related literature on the role of *LRRC15* in the arthritic joint microenvironment or other bone diseases.

miR-146a-5p was identified to be one of the molecules associated with the inflammation of joint in the IPA analysis, as indicated in Figure 6. miR-146 is one of the miRNAs strongly implicated in RA, regulating a group of target genes related to inflammation. The level of miR-146a is increased in synovial tissue, synovial fluid, whole blood and many other cells types such as T cells, B cells and macrophages. However, the association between the expression level of miR-146a and disease activity is still inconclusive [48]. miR-146a is also proposed to prevent joint destruction in arthritic mice by inhibiting osteoclastogenesis [49]. Our results indicated the potential regulation of miR-146a-5p on *LRRC15*. Whether the regulation of miR-146a-5p in bone is mediated by inflammatory joint microenvironment or other stimuli merits further clarification.

The interconnection between different cell types and the arthritic microenvironment is complex yet important in the understanding of the RA disease entity. The area of pannus formation is infiltrated by synoviocytes, immune cells, osteoclasts and proliferative vessels, and comes into direct contact with adjacent bone surface, where osteoblasts reside [9]. Along with immune cells and synovial fibroblasts, the role of osteoblasts in the pathogenesis of articular destruction in RA have gained much attention, with the function of osteoblasts being compromised at sites of focal erosion and reduced mineralization of the newly formed bone in the arthritic joints [50]. The activity and function of osteoblasts is also inhibited by the hypoxia within the arthritic joint microenvironment [51]. In the current study, we explored novel miRNAs and the putative targets expressed in the osteoblasts of RA origin. Several of the target genes identified in our study were also found to have consistent directions of expression in the synovial tissues of RA patients from related GEO array datasets. The schematic potential molecular mechanisms are summarized in Figure 9. These identified miRNA–mRNA regulations may provide novel perspectives into deeper understanding of the cell–cell communication between different cell types within the joint structure and the role of arthritic joint microenvironment in the altered bone homeostasis.

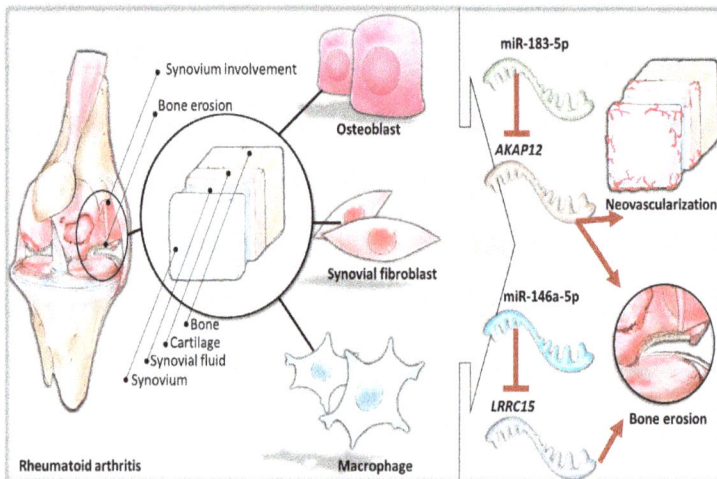

Figure 9. The proposed novel molecular signatures and microRNA regulations in rheumatoid arthritis osteoblasts.

4. Materials and Methods

4.1. Primary Cell Culture

Osteoblasts isolated from normal human bones (HOb, Catalog No. 406-05a, Lot No. 3145) and bones of patients with RA (HObRA, Catalog No. 406RA-05a, Lot No. 1796) were purchased from Cell Applications, Inc. (San Diego, CA, USA). In detail, osteoblasts of normal bone were obtained from a 66-year-old female, and osteoblasts of RA bone were obtained from a 72-year-old female with RA. Osteoblasts were grown in human osteoblast growth medium (Cell Applications, Inc.) and maintained in 37 °C incubator containing 5% CO_2 until confluence. The HOb and HObRA cells were then harvested for total RNA extraction and further mRNA and small RNA profiling.

4.2. RNA Sequencing

To prepare samples for mRNA and small RNA profiling, total RNAs from HOb and HObRA cells were extracted by Trizol® Reagent (Invitrogen, Carlsbad, CA, USA) according to the manufacturer's instructions. Before further sequencing, the quality of extracted RNAs were analyzed by OD_{260} detection using ND-1000 spectrophotometer (Nanodrop Technology, Wilmington, DE, USA) and validated by RNA integrity number (RIN) with Agilent Bioanalyzer (Agilent Technology, Santa Clara, CA, USA), where RINs for HOb and HObRA were 9.9 and 10, respectively. Total RNA sequencing analysis for RNA-seq and small RNA-seq were performed by Welgene Biotechnology Company

(Welgene, Taipei, Taiwan). We set the criteria for differentially expressed mRNAs and miRNAs at fold change >2.0, FPKM >0.3 for mRNA and RPM >10 for miRNA.

4.3. miRmap Database

miRmap is an open-source database that provides miRNA target prediction using a comprehensive approach with various computational tools, including thermodynamic, evolutionary, probabilistic and sequence-based approaches. The repression strength of a miRNA–mRNA interaction of interest is indicated by the miRmap score. The higher miRmap score indicates higher repression strength. The 35 differentially expressed miRNAs were consecutively inputted to obtain putative target genes, and those with miRmap scores higher than 99.0 were selected for further analysis [24].

4.4. Gene Expression Omnibus (GEO)

The GEO database provides public access to high-throughput array- and sequence-based data. The dataset of interest also provides link to web-based tool such as GEO2R and users can look for candidate genes and perform further analysis by obtaining raw data with expression values of specific genes in the array [25]. The arrays related to joint tissues of RA patients (GSE1919, GSE55235, GSE55475, GSE7307, GSE77298, GSE29746, GSE10500 and GSE7779) were used in this study to identify genes that expressed in consistent directions with our NGS results.

4.5. Ingenuity® Pathway Analysis (IPA)

The Ingenuity® Pathway Analysis (IPA) software (Ingenuity systems, Redwood City, CA, USA) contains large database with detailed and structured findings reviewed by experts which was derived from thousands of biological, chemical and medical researches, and provide researchers with quick searching. The IPA also enables analysis, integration, and recognition of data from gene and SNP arrays, RNA and small RNA sequencing, proteomics and many other biological experiments; in addition, deeper understanding and identification of related signaling pathways, upstream regulators, molecular interactions, disease process and candidate biomarkers are also available [26].

4.6. DAVID Database

The DAVID database is a bioinformatics resource that assists in the analysis of a list of genes derived from high-throughput genomic sequencing experiments, using different tools such as functional annotation and gene functional classification. The analysis results help researchers gain overall understanding of the involved terms of gene ontology, signaling pathways and diseases within the genes of interest [27].

4.7. Statistical Analysis

The expression values of target genes obtained from arrays of GEO database were analyzed using IBM SPSS Statistics for Windows, version 19 (IBM Corp., Armonk, NY, USA). To compare the differences of expression values between normal and RA groups, non-parametric method with Mann-Whitney U test was used. A statistically significant difference was determined by p-value < 0.05.

5. Conclusions

Our study indicates that miR-183-5p–*AKAP12* and miR-146a-5p–*LRRC15* regulations participate in the altered function of osteoblasts in RA joint microenvironment, which are partly responsible for the pathogenesis of bone erosions. The current findings suggest new candidate genes as potential indicators in evaluating therapies targeting chemotaxis and neovascularization to control joint destruction in RA.

Acknowledgments: The authors gratefully acknowledge the support of research grants from the Ministry of Science and Technology (MOST 104-2320-B-037-014-MY3 and MOST-105-2314-B-037-012), Kaohsiung Medical University Aim for the Top Universities Grants (KMU-TP104B10 and KMU-TP105B11), Kaohsiung Medical

University Hospital (KMUHS10601, KMUH105-5R66, KMUH104-4K35, and KMUH104-4M54), Kaohsiung Municipal Ta-Tung Hospital (kmtth-102-009), and the "KMU-KMUH Co-Project of Key Research" (Grant No. KMU-DK 107009) from Kaohsiung Medical University).

Author Contributions: Po-Lin Kuo, Chia-Hsin Chen, and Ya-Ling Hsu conceived and designed the experiments; Yi-Jen Chen and Wei-An Chang performed the experiments; Yi-Jen Chen, Wei-An Chang, Chia-Hsin Chen, and Po-Lin Kuo analyzed the data; Yi-Jen Chen wrote the manuscript; and all authors contributed to the editing and final approval of the manuscript.

Conflicts of Interest: The authors declare no conflict of interest.

Abbreviations

AKAP12	A-Kinase Anchoring Protein 12
DAVID	Database for Annotation, Visualization and Integrated Discovery
FPKM	Fragments per Kilobase of Transcript per Million
GEO	Gene Expression Omnibus
HOb	Osteoblasts Isolated from Normal Human Bones
HObRA	Osteoblasts Isolated from Rheumatoid Arthritis Bones
IPA	Ingenuity® Pathway Analysis
LRRC15	Leucine Rich Repeat Containing 15
miRNAs	microRNAs
NGS	Next Generation Sequencing
PKA	Protein Kinase A
RA	Rheumatoid Arthritis
RANKL	Receptor Activator of Nuclear Factor κB Ligand
RPM	Reads per Million

References

1. Scott, D.L.; Wolfe, F.; Huizinga, T.W. Rheumatoid arthritis. *Lancet* **2010**, *376*, 1094–1108. [CrossRef]
2. Grassi, W.; De Angelis, R.; Lamanna, G.; Cervini, C. The clinical features of rheumatoid arthritis. *Eur. J. Radiol.* **1998**, *27* (Suppl. 1), S18–S24. [CrossRef]
3. Choy, E. Understanding the dynamics: Pathways involved in the pathogenesis of rheumatoid arthritis. *Rheumatology* **2012**, *51* (Suppl. 5), v3–v11. [CrossRef] [PubMed]
4. Otero, M.; Goldring, M.B. Cells of the synovium in rheumatoid arthritis. Chondrocytes. *Arthritis Res. Ther.* **2007**, *9*, 220. [CrossRef] [PubMed]
5. Lipsky, P.E. Why does rheumatoid arthritis involve the joints? *N. Engl. J. Med.* **2007**, *356*, 2419–2420. [CrossRef] [PubMed]
6. Pap, T.; Meinecke, I.; Muller-Ladner, U.; Gay, S. Are fibroblasts involved in joint destruction? *Ann. Rheum. Dis.* **2005**, *64* (Suppl. 4), iv52–iv54. [CrossRef] [PubMed]
7. Lories, R. The balance of tissue repair and remodeling in chronic arthritis. *Nat. Rev. Rheumatol.* **2011**, *7*, 700–777. [CrossRef] [PubMed]
8. Schett, G.; Gravallese, E. Bone erosion in rheumatoid arthritis: Mechanisms, diagnosis and treatment. *Nat. Rev. Rheumatol.* **2012**, *8*, 656–664. [CrossRef] [PubMed]
9. Jung, S.M.; Kim, K.W.; Yang, C.W.; Park, S.H.; Ju, J.H. Cytokine-mediated bone destruction in rheumatoid arthritis. *J. Immunol. Res.* **2014**, *2014*, 263625. [CrossRef] [PubMed]
10. Elshabrawy, H.A.; Chen, Z.; Volin, M.V.; Ravella, S.; Virupannavar, S.; Shahrara, S. The pathogenic role of angiogenesis in rheumatoid arthritis. *Angiogenesis* **2015**, *18*, 433–448. [CrossRef] [PubMed]
11. Biniecka, M.; Connolly, M.; Gao, W.; Ng, C.T.; Balogh, E.; Gogarty, M.; Santos, L.; Murphy, E.; Brayden, D.; Veale, D.J.; et al. Redox-mediated angiogenesis in the hypoxic joint of inflammatory arthritis. *Arthritis Rheumatol.* **2014**, *66*, 3300–3310. [CrossRef] [PubMed]
12. Alves, C.H.; Farrell, E.; Vis, M.; Colin, E.M.; Lubberts, E. Animal models of bone loss in inflammatory arthritis: From cytokines in the bench to novel treatments for bone loss in the bedside—A comprehensive review. *Clin. Rev. Allergy Immunol.* **2016**, *51*, 27–47. [CrossRef] [PubMed]

13. Walsh, N.C.; Reinwald, S.; Manning, C.A.; Condon, K.W.; Iwata, K.; Burr, D.B.; Gravallese, E.M. Osteoblast function is compromised at sites of focal bone erosion in inflammatory arthritis. *J. Bone Miner. Res.* **2009**, *24*, 1572–1585. [CrossRef] [PubMed]

14. Abbas, S.; Zhang, Y.H.; Clohisy, J.C.; Abu-Amer, Y. Tumor necrosis factor-alpha inhibits pre-osteoblast differentiation through its type-1 receptor. *Cytokine* **2003**, *22*, 33–41. [CrossRef]

15. Yudoh, K.; Matsuno, H.; Osada, R.; Nakazawa, F.; Katayama, R.; Kimura, T. Decreased cellular activity and replicative capacity of osteoblastic cells isolated from the periarticular bone of rheumatoid arthritis patients compared with osteoarthritis patients. *Arthritis Rheum.* **2000**, *43*, 2178–2188. [CrossRef]

16. Jones, D.; Glimcher, L.H.; Aliprantis, A.O. Osteoimmunology at the nexus of arthritis, osteoporosis, cancer, and infection. *J. Clin. Investig.* **2011**, *121*, 2534–2542. [CrossRef] [PubMed]

17. Takayanagi, H. Osteoimmunology: Shared mechanisms and crosstalk between the immune and bone systems. *Nat. Rev. Immunol.* **2007**, *7*, 292–304. [CrossRef] [PubMed]

18. Tran, N.; Hutvagner, G. Biogenesis and the regulation of the maturation of miRNAs. *Essays Biochem.* **2013**, *54*, 17–28. [CrossRef] [PubMed]

19. Krol, J.; Loedige, I.; Filipowicz, W. The widespread regulation of microRNA biogenesis, function and decay. *Nat. Rev. Genet.* **2010**, *11*, 597–610. [CrossRef] [PubMed]

20. Pi, C.; Li, Y.P.; Zhou, X.; Gao, B. The expression and function of microRNAs in bone homeostasis. *Front. Biosci.* **2015**, *20*, 119–138.

21. Moore, B.T.; Xiao, P. MiRNAs in bone diseases. *Microrna* **2013**, *2*, 20–31. [CrossRef] [PubMed]

22. Zhao, M.; Liu, D.; Qu, H. Systematic review of next-generation sequencing simulators: Computational tools, features and perspectives. *Brief Funct. Genomics* **2017**, *16*, 121–128. [CrossRef] [PubMed]

23. Hao, R.; Du, H.; Guo, L.; Tian, F.; An, N.; Yang, T.; Wang, C.; Wang, B.; Zhou, Z. Identification of dysregulated genes in rheumatoid arthritis based on bioinformatics analysis. *PeerJ* **2017**, *5*, e3078. [CrossRef] [PubMed]

24. Vejnar, C.E.; Zdobnov, E.M. MiRmap: Comprehensive prediction of microRNA target repression strength. *Nucleic Acids Res.* **2012**, *40*, 11673–11683. [CrossRef] [PubMed]

25. Clough, E.; Barrett, T. The Gene Expression Omnibus Database. *Methods Mol. Biol.* **2016**, *1418*, 93–110. [CrossRef] [PubMed]

26. Thomas, S.; Bonchev, D. A survey of current software for network analysis in molecular biology. *Hum. Genomics* **2010**, *4*, 353–360. [CrossRef] [PubMed]

27. Huang da, W.; Sherman, B.T.; Lempicki, R.A. Systematic and integrative analysis of large gene lists using DAVID bioinformatics resources. *Nat. Protoc.* **2009**, *4*, 44–57. [CrossRef] [PubMed]

28. Baum, R.; Gravallese, E.M. Bone as a Target Organ in Rheumatic Disease: Impact on Osteoclasts and Osteoblasts. *Clin. Rev. Allergy Immunol.* **2016**, *51*, 1–15. [CrossRef] [PubMed]

29. Le, L.T.; Swingler, T.E.; Crowe, N.; Vincent, T.L.; Barter, M.J.; Donell, S.T.; Delany, A.M.; Dalmay, T.; Young, D.A.; Clark, I.M. The microRNA-29 family in cartilage homeostasis and osteoarthritis. *J. Mol. Med.* **2016**, *94*, 583–596. [CrossRef] [PubMed]

30. Lian, J.B.; Stein, G.S.; van Wijnen, A.J.; Stein, J.L.; Hassan, M.Q.; Gaur, T.; Zhang, Y. MicroRNA control of bone formation and homeostasis. *Nat. Rev. Endocrinol.* **2012**, *8*, 212–227. [CrossRef] [PubMed]

31. Miao, C.G.; Yang, Y.Y.; He, X.; Li, X.F.; Huang, C.; Huang, Y.; Zhang, L.; Lv, X.W.; Jin, Y.; Li, J. Wnt signaling pathway in rheumatoid arthritis, with special emphasis on the different roles in synovial inflammation and bone remodeling. *Cell Signal* **2013**, *25*, 2069–2078. [CrossRef] [PubMed]

32. Su, B.; Bu, Y.; Engelberg, D.; Gelman, I.H. SSeCKS/Gravin/AKAP12 inhibits cancer cell invasiveness and chemotaxis by suppressing a protein kinase C-Raf/MEK/ERK pathway. *J. Biol. Chem.* **2010**, *285*, 4578–4586. [CrossRef] [PubMed]

33. Wong, W.; Scott, J.D. AKAP signalling complexes: Focal points in space and time. *Nat. Rev. Mol. Cell Biol.* **2004**, *5*, 959–970. [CrossRef] [PubMed]

34. Akakura, S.; Gelman, I.H. Pivotal role of AKAP12 in the regulation of cellular adhesion dynamics: Control of cytoskeletal architecture, cell migration, and mitogenic signaling. *J. Signal Transduct.* **2012**, *2012*, 529179. [CrossRef] [PubMed]

35. Cha, J.H.; Wee, H.J.; Seo, J.H.; Ahn, B.J.; Park, J.H.; Yang, J.M.; Lee, S.W.; Kim, E.H.; Lee, O.H.; Heo, J.H.; et al. AKAP12 mediates barrier functions of fibrotic scars during CNS repair. *PLoS ONE* **2014**, *9*, e94695. [CrossRef] [PubMed]

36. Poppinga, W.J.; Heijink, I.H.; Holtzer, L.J.; Skroblin, P.; Klussmann, E.; Halayko, A.J.; Timens, W.; Maarsingh, H.; Schmidt, M. A-kinase-anchoring proteins coordinate inflammatory responses to cigarette smoke in airway smooth muscle. *Am. J. Physiol. Lung Cell. Mol. Physiol.* **2015**, *308*, L766–L775. [CrossRef] [PubMed]

37. Mantila Roosa, S.M.; Liu, Y.; Turner, C.H. Alternative splicing in bone following mechanical loading. *Bone* **2011**, *48*, 543–551. [CrossRef] [PubMed]

38. Finger, E.C.; Castellini, L.; Rankin, E.B.; Vilalta, M.; Krieg, A.J.; Jiang, D.; Banh, A.; Zundel, W.; Powell, M.B.; Giaccia, A.J. Hypoxic induction of AKAP12 variant 2 shifts PKA-mediated protein phosphorylation to enhance migration and metastasis of melanoma cells. *Proc. Natl. Acad. Sci. USA* **2015**, *112*, 4441–4446. [CrossRef] [PubMed]

39. Turtoi, A.; Mottet, D.; Matheus, N.; Dumont, B.; Peixoto, P.; Hennequiere, V.; Deroanne, C.; Colige, A.; De Pauw, E.; Bellahcene, A.; et al. The angiogenesis suppressor gene AKAP12 is under the epigenetic control of HDAC7 in endothelial cells. *Angiogenesis* **2012**, *15*, 543–554. [CrossRef] [PubMed]

40. Ke, K.; Sul, O.J.; Rajasekaran, M.; Choi, H.S. MicroRNA-183 increases osteoclastogenesis by repressing heme oxygenase-1. *Bone* **2015**, *81*, 237–246. [CrossRef] [PubMed]

41. Davis, C.; Dukes, A.; Drewry, M.; Helwa, I.; Johnson, M.H.; Isales, C.M.; Hill, W.D.; Liu, Y.; Shi, X.; Fulzele, S.; et al. MicroRNA-183-5p increases with age in bone-derived extracellular vesicles, suppresses bone marrow stromal (stem) cell proliferation, and induces stem cell senescence. *Tissue Eng. Part A* **2017**. [CrossRef] [PubMed]

42. Stanbrough, M.; Bubley, G.J.; Ross, K.; Golub, T.R.; Rubin, M.A.; Penning, T.M.; Febbo, P.G.; Balk, S.P. Increased expression of genes converting adrenal androgens to testosterone in androgen-independent prostate cancer. *Cancer Res.* **2006**, *66*, 2815–2825. [CrossRef] [PubMed]

43. Schuetz, C.S.; Bonin, M.; Clare, S.E.; Nieselt, K.; Sotlar, K.; Walter, M.; Fehm, T.; Solomayer, E.; Riess, O.; Wallwiener, D.; et al. Progression-specific genes identified by expression profiling of matched ductal carcinomas in situ and invasive breast tumors, combining laser capture microdissection and oligonucleotide microarray analysis. *Cancer Res.* **2006**, *66*, 5278–5286. [CrossRef] [PubMed]

44. Reynolds, P.A.; Smolen, G.A.; Palmer, R.E.; Sgroi, D.; Yajnik, V.; Gerald, W.L.; Haber, D.A. Identification of a DNA-binding site and transcriptional target for the EWS-WT1(+KTS) oncoprotein. *Genes Dev.* **2003**, *17*, 2094–2107. [CrossRef] [PubMed]

45. Satoh, K.; Hata, M.; Shimizu, T.; Yokota, H.; Akatsu, H.; Yamamoto, T.; Kosaka, K.; Yamada, T. Lib, transcriptionally induced in senile plaque-associated astrocytes, promotes glial migration through extracellular matrix. *Biochem. Biophys. Res. Commun.* **2005**, *335*, 631–636. [CrossRef] [PubMed]

46. Satoh, K.; Hata, M.; Yokota, H. A novel member of the leucine-rich repeat superfamily induced in rat astrocytes by beta-amyloid. *Biochem. Biophys. Res. Commun.* **2002**, *290*, 756–762. [CrossRef] [PubMed]

47. Cooper, P.R.; McLachlan, J.L.; Simon, S.; Graham, L.W.; Smith, A.J. Mediators of inflammation and regeneration. *Adv. Dent. Res.* **2011**, *23*, 290–295. [CrossRef] [PubMed]

48. Churov, A.V.; Oleinik, E.K.; Knip, M. MicroRNAs in rheumatoid arthritis: Altered expression and diagnostic potential. *Autoimmun. Rev.* **2015**, *14*, 1029–1037. [CrossRef] [PubMed]

49. Nakasa, T.; Shibuya, H.; Nagata, Y.; Niimoto, T.; Ochi, M. The inhibitory effect of microRNA-146a expression on bone destruction in collagen-induced arthritis. *Arthritis Rheum.* **2011**, *63*, 1582–1590. [CrossRef] [PubMed]

50. Corrado, A.; Maruotti, N.; Cantatore, F.P. Osteoblast role in rheumatic diseases. *Int. J. Mol. Sci.* **2017**, *18*, 1272. [CrossRef] [PubMed]

51. Chang, J.; Jackson, S.G.; Wardale, J.; Jones, S.W. Hypoxia modulates the phenotype of osteoblasts isolated from knee osteoarthritis patients, leading to undermineralized bone nodule formation. *Arthritis Rheumatol.* **2014**, *66*, 1789–1799. [CrossRef] [PubMed]

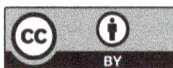

International Journal of
Molecular Sciences

MDPI

Article

Arthroprotective Effects of Cf-02 Sharing Structural Similarity with Quercetin

Feng-Cheng Liu [1], Jeng-Wei Lu [2], Chiao-Yun Chien [1], Hsu-Shan Huang [3], Chia-Chung Lee [3], Shiu-Bii Lien [4], Leou-Chyr Lin [4], Liv Weichien Chen [1], Yi-Jung Ho [5], Min-Chung Shen [6], Ling-Jun Ho [7,8] and Jenn-Haung Lai [9,*]

[1] Rheumatology/Immunology and Allergy, Department of Medicine, Tri-Service General Hospital, National Defense Medical Center, No. 161, Section 6, Minquan East Road, Taipei 114, Taiwan; lfc10399@yahoo.com.tw (F.-C.L.); epichien@gmail.com (C.-Y.C.); mslivcat@gmail.com (L.W.C.)
[2] Department of Biological Sciences, National University of Singapore, 14 Science Drive 4, Singapore 117543, Singapore; jengweilu@gmail.com
[3] Graduate Institute of Cancer Biology and Drug Discovery, College of Medical Science and Technology, Taipei Medical University, Taipei 110, Taiwan; huanghs99@tmu.edu.tw (H.-S.H.); levi0963309363@gmail.com (C.-C.L.)
[4] Department of Orthopaedics, Tri-Service General Hospital, National Defense Medical Center, No. 161, Section 6, Minquan East Road, Taipei 114, Taiwan; LSB3612@yahoo.com.tw (S.-B.L.); lchlin66@hotmail.com (L.-C.L.)
[5] School of Pharmacy, National Defense Medical Center, No. 161, Section 6, Minquan East Road, Taipei 114, Taiwan; ejung330@gmail.com
[6] Rheumatology/Immunology and Allergy, Department of Medicine, Armed Forces Taoyuan General Hospital; Taoyuan 325, Taiwan; airfly100@gmail.com
[7] Institute of Cellular and System Medicine, National Health Research Institute, No. 35, Keyan Road, Zhunan, Miaoli County 350, Taiwan; lingjunho@nhri.org.tw
[8] Graduate Institute of Microbiology and Immunology, National Defense Medical Center, No. 161, Section 6, Minquan East Road, Taipei 114, Taiwan
[9] Division of Allergy, Immunology and Rheumatology, Department of Internal Medicine, Chang Gung Memorial Hospital, Chang Gung University, No. 5, Fusing St., Gueishan Township, Tao-Yuan County 333, Taiwan
* Correspondence: laiandho@gmail.com; Tel.: +886-3-328-1200 (ext. 3333)

check for updates

Received: 20 April 2018; Accepted: 11 May 2018; Published: 14 May 2018

Abstract: In this study, we synthesized hundreds of analogues based on the structure of small-molecule inhibitors (SMIs) that were previously identified in our laboratory with the aim of identifying potent yet safe compounds for arthritis therapeutics. One of the analogues was shown to share structural similarity with quercetin, a potent anti-inflammatory flavonoid present in many different fruits and vegetables. We investigated the immunomodulatory effects of this compound, namely 6-(2,4-difluorophenyl)-3-(3-(trifluoromethyl)phenyl)-2H-benzo[e][1,3]oxazine-2,4(3H)-dione (Cf-02), in a side-by-side comparison with quercetin. Chondrocytes were isolated from pig joints or the joints of patients with osteoarthritis that had undergone total knee replacement surgery. Several measures were used to assess the immunomodulatory potency of these compounds in tumor necrosis factor (TNF-α)-stimulated chondrocytes. Characterization included the protein and mRNA levels of molecules associated with arthritis pathogenesis as well as the inducible nitric oxide synthase (iNOS)–nitric oxide (NO) system and matrix metalloproteinases (MMPs) in cultured chondrocytes and proteoglycan, and aggrecan degradation in cartilage explants. We also examined the activation of several important transcription factors, including nuclear factor-kappaB (NF-κB), interferon regulatory factor-1 (IRF-1), signal transducer and activator of transcription-3 (STAT-3), and activator protein-1 (AP-1). Our overall results indicate that the immunomodulatory potency of Cf-02 is fifty-fold more efficient than that of quercetin without any indication of cytotoxicity. When tested in vivo using the induced edema method, Cf-02 was shown to suppress inflammation and cartilage damage. The proposed method shows considerable promise for the identification of candidate disease-modifying immunomodulatory drugs and leads compounds for arthritis therapeutics.

Keywords: arthritis; osteoarthritis; rheumatoid arthritis; small-molecule inhibitor; chondrocytes; tumor necrosis factor-alpha; inflammation

1. Introduction

Arthritis is an inflammation of the joints, the most common types are rheumatoid arthritis (RA) and osteoarthritis [1,2]. Many factors such as aging, obesity, trauma, genetic predisposition, and endocrine makeup can contribute to the development of osteoarthritis [3–6]. Several catabolic factors are known to contribute to joint damage in osteoarthritis. These include molecules such as proinflammatory cytokines (e.g., interleukin-1 (IL-1) and tumor necrosis factor-alpha (TNF-α), matrix metalloproteinases (MMPs), and aggrecanases (a disintegrin and metalloproteinase with thrombospondin motifs (ADAMTS), as well as the inducible nitric oxide synthase (iNOS)–nitric oxide (NO) system [7–11]. Importantly, these factors interact closely with one another. For example, the production of MMP-13 and NO can be efficiently induced by both TNF-α and IL-1 in chondrocytes [12].

Extensive genetic analysis has led to the identification of several transcription factors which act as determinants that regulate the expression of many osteoarthritis pathogenesis-contributing factors [13,14]. A series of reports from our lab, as well as work completed by other research teams, have shown that these transcription factors include nuclear factor-kappaB (NF-κB), interferon regulatory factor-1 (IRF-1), the signal transducer and activator of transcription-3 (STAT-3), and activator protein-1 (AP-1) [15–17]. The activities of these transcription factors faithfully reflect the status of joint inflammation and are highly predictive of joint damage in a variety of arthritis models [18]. Recent research has highlighted epigenetic factors as contributing to osteoarthritis [19].

Candidate disease-modifying antiarthritis drugs should preserve immunomodulatory effects and have very limited or no toxicity [20–22]. Small molecules that target specific signaling pathways and/or mechanisms have considerable potential to meet these criteria [23,24]. Screening a mini-library containing three-hundred benzamide-linked small molecules allowed us to identify three compounds that could potentially act as disease-modifying antiarthritis drugs. The three compounds are 2-hydroxy-*N*-[3-(trifluoromethyl)phenyl]benzamide (HS-Cf) [15], *N*-(4-chloro-2-fluorophenyl) -2-hydroxybenzamide (HS-Cm) [25], and *N*-(3-chloro-4-fluorophenyl)-2-hydroxybenzamide (HS-Ck). While seeking to synthesize potent derivatives from the synthesized analogues of HS-Cf, we accidentally found a novel compound, 6-(2,4-difluorophenyl)-3-(3-(trifluoromethyl)phenyl)-2*H* -benzo[*e*][1,3]oxazine-2,4(3*H*)-dione (Cf-02), which shares many structural similarities with quercetin, a potent immunomodulatory compound that is present in many different fruits and vegetables [26]. In the present study, we characterized the immunomodulatory potencies of the new compound using a variety of methods and conducted a direct comparison with quercetin. Our results revealed that the immunomodulatory potency of Cf-02 is more than fifty-fold stronger than that of quercetin, making it a strong candidate for disease-modifying drugs against arthritis.

2. Results

2.1. Inhibiting iNOS–NO Production in TNF-α-Stimulated Porcine Chondrocytes via Cf-02

We performed experiments to compare the effectiveness of Cf-02 and quercetin (Figure 1A) in suppressing the activation of the iNOS–NO pathway in TNF-α-stimulated chondrocytes. At a concentration of 1 μM, both Cf-02 and quercetin significantly suppressed the production of NO and expression of iNOS in stimulated chondrocyte cells (Figure 1B). The IC_{50} value of Cf-02 was 0.55 µM (Figure 1C). Based on the (4,5-dimethylthiazol-2-yl)-2,5-diphenyltetrazolium bromide) (MTT) assay and lactate dehydrogenase (LDH) releasing assay, neither Cf-02 nor quercetin gave any detectable indication of cytotoxicity in porcine chondrocytes (Figure 1D,E).

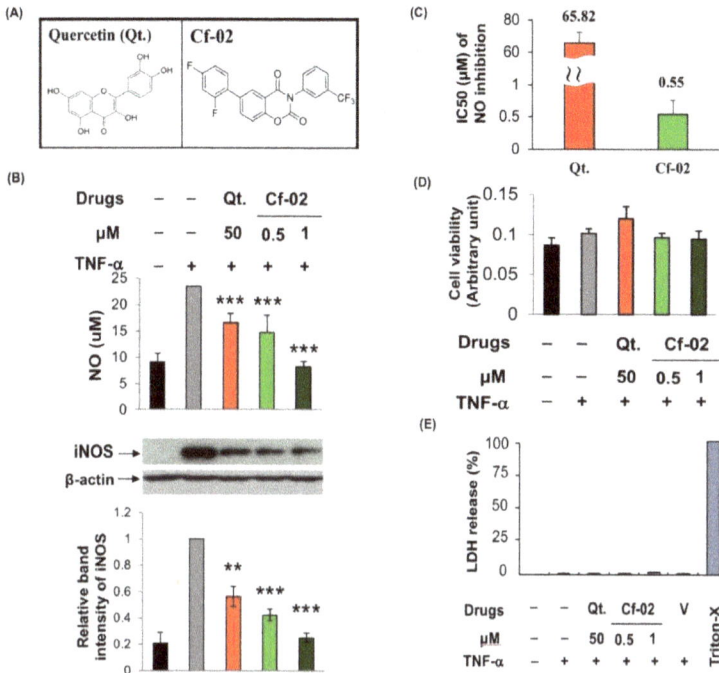

Figure 1. iNOS–NO production inhibited by Cf-02 in a dose-dependent manner in porcine chondrocytes stimulated by TNF-α. Structures of quercetin and Cf-02 (**A**); Porcine chondrocytes were pretreated with various doses of quercetin, Cf-02, or dimethyl sulfoxide (DMSO) for 2 h and then stimulated with TNF-α for 24 h. The expression of iNOS was determined by Western blotting according to the measurement of band intensities. The concentration of NO in the supernatant was determined using the Griess reaction (**B**); The IC_{50} for quercetin and Cf-02 were measured and given (**C**); Possible cytotoxic effects of Cf-02 were detected by treating porcine chondrocytes with Cf-02 at various concentrations for 48 h. Subsequently, the cell viability was analyzed by MTT assay. (**D**) and LDH release assays (**E**). Positive control: Equal numbers of cells treated with 1% Triton X-100 were used as the positive control. Representative data from no fewer than three independent experiments are presented in the figure. Data are mean ± SD from three independent experiments. ** $p < 0.01$; *** $p < 0.001$ compared to chondrocytes stimulated by TNF-α in the absence of Cf-02 treatment. V: vehicle (DMSO).

2.2. Inhibiting the Production of Chondro-Destructive Enzymes via Cf-02

MMP-13 was directly responsible for damage to the cartilage matrix; therefore, we examined the effects of Cf-02 on TNF-induced *MMP-13* mRNA and MMP-13 protein expression. The results of real-time reverse transcription polymerase chain reaction (RT-PCR) and Western blot analysis revealed that (1) TNF-induced *MMP-13* mRNA expression and (2) proMMP-13 protein levels were significantly suppressed by 1 µM of Cf-02 (Figure 2A). The zymographic analysis further revealed that a Cf-02 concentration of 1 µM significantly suppressed TNF-induced MMP-13 enzyme activity (Figure 2B). Other proteinases genes, such as *MMP-1*, *MMP-3*, and *ADAMTS4* were also inhibited by

Cf-02, although the intensity of the effects varied (Figure 2C). However, treatment with Cf-02 did not appear to have any effect on *ADAMTS5* and *TIMP-2* mRNA expression.

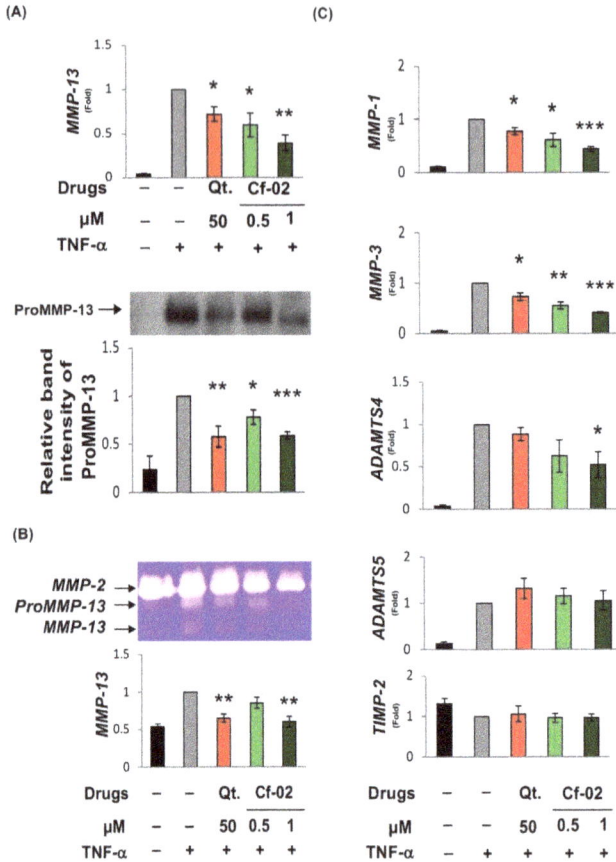

Figure 2. Cf-02 suppressed enzyme activity as well as the expression of TNF-α-induced matrix metalloproteinases (MMPs) and disintegrin and metalloproteinase with thrombospondin motifs (*ADAMTS*) genes. Chondrocytes were pretreated with quercetin, solvent, or Cf-02 (in various doses) for 2 h and then stimulated using 5 ng/mL TNF-α for another 8 or 24 h. Following treatment with TNF-α for 8 h, real-time RT-PCR was performed to measure the levels of *MMP-13* mRNA (**A**); Conversely, the activity of MMP-13 released into the culture supernatant was characterized using gelatin zymography following TNF-α stimulation for 24 h. Representative data pooled from at least three independent experiments are presented (**B**). Porcine chondrocytes that were treated for 2 h with various doses of quercetin, solvent, or various doses of Cf-02 were stimulated using TNF-α for 8 h. The cells were then collected for the preparation of total RNA in order to determine mRNA expression using real-time RT-PCR. The relative expression levels of *MMP-1*, *MMP-3*, *ADAMTS4*, *ADAMTS5*, and *TIMP-2* mRNA were normalized to glyceraldehyde 3-phopshate dehydrogenase (*GAPDH*), with subsequent normalization to the TNF-α-stimulated sample in each experiment (**C**). The significance of differences between sample groups was determined using one-way analysis of variance (ANOVA) with the Bonferroni *post-hoc* test. Results from three independent experiments are shown. Data are mean ± SD from three independent experiments. * $p < 0.05$; ** $p < 0.01$; *** $p < 0.001$ compared to TNF-α-stimulated chondrocytes that did not undergo Cf-02 treatment. V: vehicle (DMSO).

2.3. Regulating the Activity of Transcriptional Factors via Cf-02

We also compared the effects of quercetin and Cf-02 on several transcriptional factors which are important to the activation of pro-inflammatory mediators in TNF-α-activated chondrocytes. Chondrocytes are stimulated by TNF-α to trigger NF-κB in the nucleus to drive downstream gene expression, thereby indicating that TNF-α-induced NF-κB DNA-binding activity was suppressed by Cf-02 (Figure 3A). Our results also showed that Cf-02 can significantly inhibit TNF-α-induced STAT-3 and IRF-1 activation (Figure 3B,C). However, Cf-02 was ineffectual in inhibiting TNF-α-induced AP-1 DNA-binding activity in chondrocytes (Figure 3D).

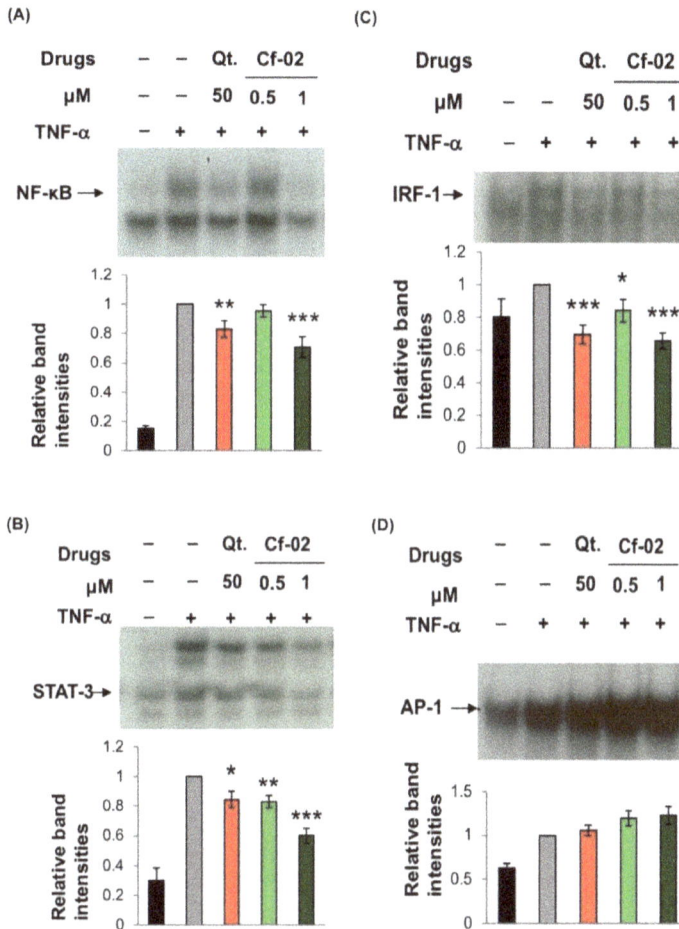

Figure 3. Cf-02 suppressed TNF-α induced DNA-binding of NF-κB, STAT-3, and IRF-1 but not AP-1. Nuclear extracts of chondrocytes treated for 2 h with 5 ng/mL TNF-α in the presence of quercetin, solvent, or various doses of Cf-02 were analyzed in order to quantify the DNA-binding activity of NF-κB (**A**), STAT-3 (**B**), IRF-1 (**C**), and AP-1 (**D**) with electrophoretic mobility shift assay (EMSA). For this, band intensity results were averaged from at least 3 independent experiments. Data are mean ± SD from three independent experiments. * $p < 0.05$; ** $p < 0.01$; *** $p < 0.001$ compared to TNF-α-stimulated chondrocytes that did not undergo Cf-02 treatment.

2.4. Effects of Cf-02 on TNF-α-Induced Proteoglycan/Aggrecan Degradation in Cartilage Explants

We also examined the chondroprotective effects of Cf-02 in order to elucidate its anti-inflammatory properties. Specifically, our objective was to determine whether Cf-02 could be used to prevent TNF-α-induced degradation of the cartilage matrix. After treating samples with TNF-α, we observed a significant reduction in Safranin-O positive proteoglycan and an increase in the cleavage products of aggrecan (NITEGE). However, these TNF-α-induced effects were prevented by pre-treatment with Cf-02 (Figure 4). Our results consistently demonstrated the effectiveness of Cf-02 in preventing the TNF-α-mediated release of proteoglycan and aggrecan into the culture supernatants of cartilage explants (Figure 4A–D). Treatment with Cf-02 was also shown to reduce the immunohistochemistry (IHC) staining associated with MMP-13 protein expression in porcine cartilage tissue blocks (Figure 4E,F).

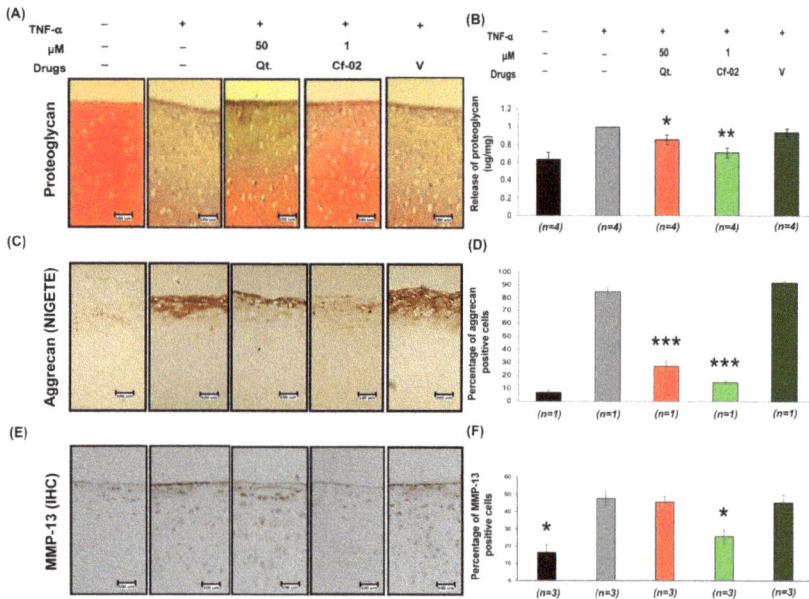

Figure 4. Effects of Cf-02 on TNF-α-induced proteoglycan/aggrecan degradation. In 24-well plates, the porcine cartilage blocks were cultured for 2 h with or without pretreatment with 1 μM Cf-02. Cartilage was then stimulated with 5 ng/mL TNF-α for another 72 h incubation. The proteoglycan retained in cartilage explants was monitored using Safranin-O staining (**A**) (100×). The release of proteoglycan into the culture medium was normalized with the weight of the cartilage (**B**). The intensity of aggrecan staining was examined in parallel (**C,D**) (100×). IHC staining of MMP-13 protein expression in porcine cartilage tissue blocks (**E,F**) (100×). Representative data from 3 independent experiments using cartilage from different donor blocks are presented. Data are mean ± SD from in each group. * $p < 0.05$; ** $p < 0.01$; *** $p < 0.001$ compared to TNF-α-stimulated chondrocytes that did not undergo Cf-02 treatment. Scale bars = 100 um.

2.5. Immunomodulatory Effects of Cf-02 on Human Chondrocytes

To enhance the clinical significance of Cf-02, we examined human chondrocytes prepared from surgical specimens of patients with osteoarthritis patients under conditions similar to those associated with porcine chondrocytes. Unlike the results from porcine chondrocytes, the results from human chondrocytes indicated that Cf-02 and quercetin significantly inhibited the production of TNF-α-induced NO (Figure 5A). Moreover, Cf-02 and quercetin also inhibited proMMP-13 production, especially at a concentration of 1 μM of Cf-02 (Figure 5B). Cf-02 also significantly suppressed the expression of *MMP-13* mRNA in TNF-α-activated human chondrocytes (Figure 5C). However, the expression of *TIMP-2* mRNA was unaffected by the tested Cf-02. Molecular approaches further demonstrated that Cf-02 can inhibit the TNF-α-induced DNA-binding activity of NF-κB (Figure 5D). Despite variations among the assays, the Cf-02 that was the focus of this study preserved immunomodulatory effects with a potency that was approximately 50-fold efficient than that of quercetin.

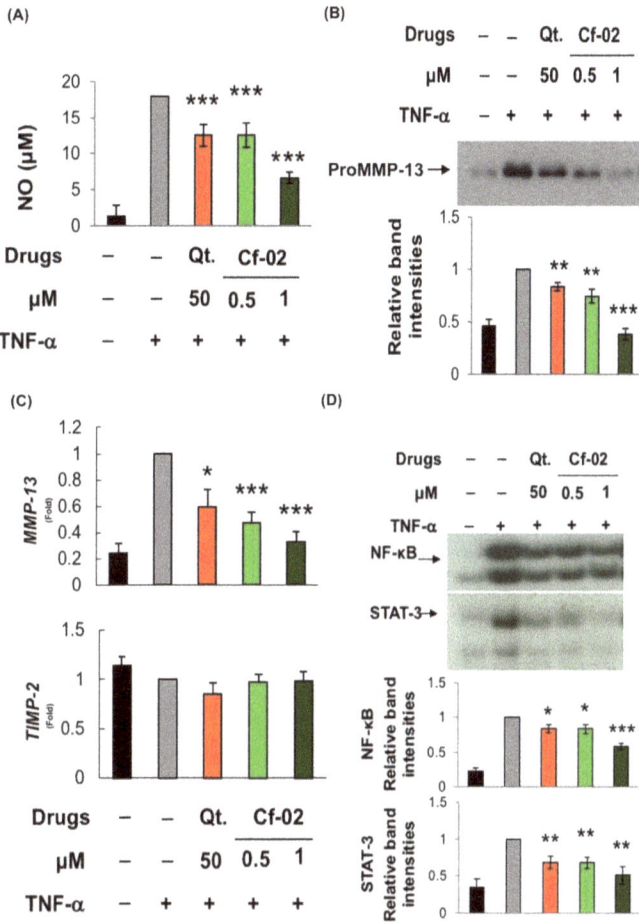

Figure 5. Effects of Cf-02 on TNF-α-stimulated human chondrocytes. Human chondrocytes (prepared from cartilage samples collected from patients who underwent total knee replacement) were first pretreated with quercetin, solvent, or Cf-02 in various doses for 2 h and then treated with 5 ng/mL TNF-α for an additional 24 h. Measurement of NO production (**A**), proMMP-13 expression (**B**), *MMP-13* mRNA expression (**C**), and NF-κB and STAT-3 DNA-binding (**D**) were performed according to the same methods as those used for porcine chondrocytes. Band intensity results were averaged from at least 3 independent experiments. Data are mean ± SD from three independent experiments. * $p < 0.05$; ** $p < 0.01$; *** $p < 0.001$ compared to TNF-α-stimulated chondrocytes that did not undergo Cf-02 treatment.

2.6. Prevention of Collagen Loss by Cf-02 in an Arthritis Animal Model

Cf-02 was shown to inhibit TNF-α-induced signaling, prevent the degradation of cartilage matrix, and inhibit inflammation. The anti-inflammatory activity Cf-02 was tested in vivo using a collagen II-induced edema method. As shown in Figure 6A, collagen-induced arthritis (CIA) rat treated with vehicle developed arthritis at the end of week 2, the severity of which increased throughout the study. However, in the Cf-02-treated CIA (Cf-02 + CIA) rat, the clinical manifestations of this effect were markedly inhibited. In our rat collagen-induced arthritis model, Cf-02 administered at a dose of 10 mg/kg/day was also shown to inhibit an increase in arthritis score (Figure 6B). Finally, hematoxylin and eosin stain (H&E) and Safranin-O staining (Figure 6C) indicated that Cf-02 suppressed inflammation and cartilage damage (Figure 6D).

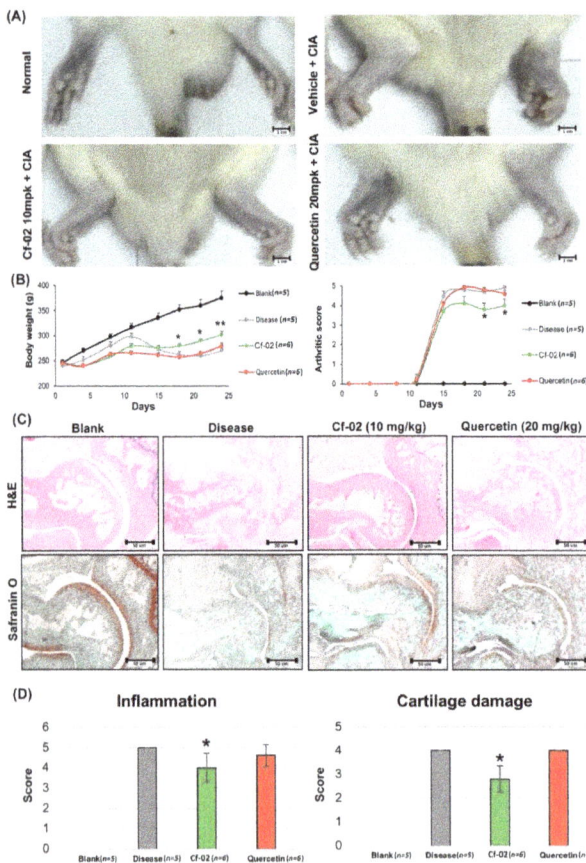

Figure 6. Cf-02 prevented collagen loss in an arthritis animal model. CIA rats were randomly divided into groups according to global assessments. The onset of arthritis occurred close to day 14 post first injection. Representative images of swelling joints (**A**) (25×). Body weight and arthritic scores were determined every 3 days (**B**). Representative joint sections from each group of rats at 24 days post-treatment. Hematoxylin and eosin (H&E) staining showing signs of inflammation. Safranin-O staining showing cartilage erosion (**C**) (200×). Frequency distribution of inflammation and cartilage damage scores from H&E staining results (**D**). Data are mean ± SD from in each group. The level of statistical significance was set at * $p < 0.05$. Scale bars = 1 cm (**A**), 50 um (**C**).

3. Discussion

Previous screening of benzamide-linked small molecules in our laboratory led to the identification of three compounds with efficient anti-inflammatory activities. Among them, 2-hydroxy-*N* -[3-(trifluoromethyl)phenyl]benzamide (HS-Cf) and *N*-(4-chloro-2-fluorophenyl)-2-hydroxybenzamide (HS-Cm) had previously been reported [15,25]. Structure-based drug design was subsequently used to synthesize additional SMIs with greater potency and lower toxicity as candidates for arthritis therapeutics. Structural modifications included the introduction of a benzyl alcohol group and a fluorine substitution. Optimization of drug-like properties led to the identification of hundreds of synthesized compounds, one of which (Cf-02) shares similarities with the anti-inflammatory flavonoid quercetin. In a side-by-side comparison, Cf-02 proved more than 50 times more effective than quercetin in suppressing (1) TNF-α-induced iNOS–NO production, (2) the mRNA expression of several *ADAMTS* and *MMPs*, and (3) the enzyme activity of MMP-13 in chondrocytes. Cf-02 was also found to be 50 times more effective than quercetin in preventing the release of proteoglycan/aggrecan in cartilage explants. Molecular examinations further revealed the potency of Cf-02 in suppressing the activation of several transcription factors, including NF-κB, STAT-3, and IRF-1, but not AP-1. Our results provide evidence that Cf-02 possess chondroprotective effects and help to elucidate the mechanisms which underlie them. We also demonstrated the potential of Cf-02 to benefit the treatment of TNF-α-induced damage to the cartilage in joints. We were also to fund that as a critical transcription factor in regulating many proinflammatory genes, the TNF-α-induced DNA-binding activity of AP-1 appeared to be resistant to all compounds examined in this study. Variations between results obtained from human chondrocyte samples and results obtained from porcine chondrocytes indicate that Cf-02 possesses a certain specificity in the targeting of signaling molecules associated with inflammatory responses in arthritis.

In terms of inflammation reduction, the potency of Cf-02 exceeded that of quercetin by 50 times. In this Cf-02, the amide motif of NH and OH were cyclized to mimic the heterocyclic pyran or pyrone ring of flavonoids, which could be used to adjust its anti-inflammatory potency. Given the success in elucidating the structure–activity relationships through several different molecular and cellular bioassays, the mechanisms observed might not fully account for the subtle different bioactivities of Cf-02. The microenvironment of arthritis is very complex. Both *ADAMTS4* and *ADAMTS5* are responsible for aggrecan degradation in a human model of arthritis. However, Cf-02 only inhibits *ADAMTS4* but does not inhibit *ADAMTS5* in porcine chondrocytes [27]. Cf-02 inhibits *MMP-1*, *MMP-3*, and *MMP-13* via signal transduction by inhibiting NF-κB, STAT-3, and IRF-1, but Cf-02 was not able to inhibit MAPK-AP1 to reduce *ADAMTS5* expression. miR-30a expression was downregulated in arthritis patients and was negatively correlated with *ADAMTS5* expression. IL-1β suppressed miR-30a expression by recruiting the AP-1 transcription factor c-jun/c-fos to the miR-30a promoter [27]. Therefore, *ADAMTS5* might be regulated by various factors which might be the reason why we cannot observe its reduction.

Nowadays, RA patients have been well treated with biological agents, and it is difficult to collect human RA fibroblasts samples from patients in a clinical setting. To make up for this deficiency, we used the collagen loss by Cf-02 in an arthritis animal model to further explore mechanisms in vivo. In vivo testing using a collagen-II induced edema method revealed that Cf-02 suppresses inflammation and cartilage damage. In our study, aside from TNF-α stimulation the primary chondrocytes from porcine and human, which is the common model to study rheumatoid arthritis disease, the collagen-II induced edema method was also used to verify the beneficial effects of Cf-02. In vivo, Cf-02 was shown to suppress inflammation and cartilage damage (Figure 6). Nevertheless, our results suggest that Cf-02 may have the potential to act as a lead compound in the subsequent identification of novel compounds. Moreover, we anticipate that our study will initiate further in vitro and in vivo research with the aim of confirming the therapeutic benefits of Cf-02 in patients with arthritis and inflammation-mediated joint disorders.

4. Materials and Methods

4.1. Reagents and Antibodies

TNF-α was supplied by an R & D commercial company (Canandaigua, NY, USA). The polyclonal antisera against iNOS (catalog number: SC-651), MMP-13 (catalog number: SC-30073), and aggrecan neoepitope (catalog number: NB100-74350) antibodies were purchased from Santa Cruz Biotechnology (Santa Cruz, CA, USA) and Novus Biologicals, (Littleton, CO, USA). Hsu-Shan Huang synthesized the small-molecule inhibitor (SMI) and provided the Cf-02 used in this study. The small molecules were reduced to concentrations that were suitable for individual experiments by diluting the stock preparation with culture medium.

4.2. Isolation and Culture of Porcine and Human Chondrocytes

Porcine cartilage specimens were taken from the hind leg joints. Chondrocytes were prepared from cartilage according to the methods outlined in a previous report [28]. Briefly, articular cartilage underwent enzymatic digestion using 2 mg/mL protease in serum-free Dulbecco's modified Eagle's medium (DMEM)/antibiotics followed by collagenase I (2 mg/mL) and hyaluronidase (0.9 mg/mL) in DMEM with fetal bovine serum (FBS) digestion overnight. Cells were collected via a cell strainer (Beckton Dickinson, Mountain View, CA, USA) and cultured in DMEM that contained 10% FBS and antibiotics for 3–4 days prior to use.

Human chondrocytes were harvested using cartilage from patients with osteoarthritis who underwent total knee replacement aseptically, human chondrocytes samples were obtained following protocols approved by the Institutional Review Board (IRB) of Tri-Service General Hospital, National Defense Medical Center Institutes Human Ethics Committee code: 1-102-05-091; Date: 02/09/2013. Chondrocytes were prepared as previously described. [29]. Briefly, articular cartilage was made into 0.5 cm^2 pieces. The protease (2 mg/mL) (EMD Millipore, Billerica, MA, USA) was for enzyme digestion at 37 °C with 5% CO$_2$ for 1 h, whereupon the specimens underwent digestion overnight using 0.25 mg/mL collagenase I and 500 U/mL hyaluronidase in DMEM medium containing 10% fetal bovine serum. Cells were collected using a cell strainer and seeded at concentrations of 6–8 × 10^6 cells in T75 flasks within DMEM containing 10% FBS and antibiotics for 3–4 days prior to use.

4.3. Cytotoxicity Analysis and Measurement of NO Concentrations

The concentration of released LDH was used as an indicator of damage to the plasma membrane according to the manufacturer's instructions (Roche, Indianapolis, IN, USA). The percentage of cytotoxicity was calculated as: ((sample value − medium control)/(high control − medium control)) × 100. Single sample values comprised the averages of absorbance values obtained in triplicate from treated culture supernatants following the subtraction of the absorbance values associated with the background control. The average absorbance values of untreated cell culture supernatants (used as control mediums) were calculated in a similar manner. Equal quantities of cells treated with 1% Triton X-100 were adopted as the high control. The amount of NO released was derived from its stable end product (nitrite) in the supernatant [28]. We performed the Griess reaction to determine the concentration of nitrite using a spectrophotometer.

4.4. Nuclear Extract Preparation and EMSA

Nuclear extract preparation and EMSA analysis were performed in accordance with methods described in our previous report [29]. Oligonucleotides containing the NF-κB, STAT-3, IRF-1, and AP-1 binding sites were used as a DNA probes. The detailed steps for the EMSA experiment were performed as described in our previous report [30].

4.5. Real-Time RT-PCR and Western Blotting

Total RNA was isolated after cells were lysed using Trizol reagent (Invitrogen; Carlsbad, CA, USA) and RNA samples were treated with DNase I (Roch, Indianapolis, IN, USA) prior to reverse transcription in accordance with the manufacturer's protocol. Total RNA (2 μg) was then reverse transcribed into cDNA using the Superscript First-Strand Synthesis System (Invitrogen, Grand Island, NY, USA). The mRNA gene expression was measured and duplicated thrice by real-time RT-PCR measurements in accordance with the manufacturer's instructions (power SYBR Green PCR Master Mix, Applied BioSystems, Foster City, CA, USA). The primer sequences for these genes were either designed by us or described by other researchers [31,32]. The primers sequences are listed in supplementary Table S1. The reactions underwent 50 cycles at 95 °C for denaturation and at 60 °C for annealing and extension. For this, the ABI Prism 7000 Sequence Detection system (Applied BioSystems) was used. After the data were collected, we calculated changes in gene expression following stimulation with TNF-α or IL-1 in the presence or absence of Cf-02 using the following formula: fold changes = $2^{-\Delta\Delta Ct}$, where $\Delta C_t = C_{t\ targeted\ gene} - C_{t\ GAPDH}$, and $\Delta(\Delta C_t) = \Delta C_{t\ stimulated} - \Delta C_{t\ control}$.

Enhanced chemiluminescence (ECL) Western blotting (Amersham-Pharmacia, Arlington Heights, IL, USA) was performed according to previous study description [29]. The protein was separated by 10% sodium dodecyl sulfate-polyacrylamide gel electrophoresis (SDS-PAGE) and then transferred to a nitrocellulose filter to analyze equal amounts of whole cellular extracts. For immunoblotting, the nitrocellulose filter was incubated in Tris-buffered saline for 1 h, and further blotting with antibodies against specific proteins for 2 h at room temperature. After being washed using milk buffer, the filter was incubated with rabbit anti-goat IgG (1:5000) or goat anti-rabbit IgG (1:5000) conjugated to horseradish peroxidase for 30 min. Finally, the filter was incubated with substrate and exposed to X-ray film (GE Healthcare, Buckinghamshire, UK).

4.6. Gelatin Zymography

Gelatin zymography was performed as previously described [22] with some modifications. Specifically, culture supernatant (16 μL) was mixed with (1) 4 μL buffer containing 4% SDS, (2) 0.15 M Tris (pH 6.8), and (3) 20% glycerol containing 0.05% bromophenol blue. A 10% polyacrylamide gel was copolymerized with 0.1% gelatin (Sigma-Aldrich, St. Louis, MO, USA); the supernatant mixture was then analyzed. After electrophoresis, gels were washed with 2.5% Triton X-100 3 times for 20 min. After incubation with the gelatinase buffer for 24 h at 37 °C, the gel was stained with 0.1% Coomassie blue. Under the background of uniform light blue staining clear bands demonstrating genatinolytic activity were found. The localization of proMMP-13 and MMP-13 was evaluated using Alpha EaseFC software (Alpha Innotech Corp, San Leandro, CA, USA) according to standard molecular weights and previous reports by other researchers [33].

4.7. Preparation of Cartilage Explants and Analysis of Cartilage Degradation

The preparation of cartilage explants was performed using the methods outlined in our previous report [28]. Briefly, articular cartilage from the femur head of the hind limb joint of pigs was excavated using a stainless steel dermal-punch that measured 3 mm in diameter (Aesculap, Tuttlingen, Germany). Following this, the extracted articular cartilage was weighed. For the dissection, each cartilage explant was cultured in DMEM and contained antibiotics and 10% FBS in a 24-well plate. Cartilage explants were then allowed to rest for 72 h in serum-free DMEM before undergoing further study. The degradation of cartilage was evaluated using a measure of proteoglycan that had been released into the cell culture medium [28]. Briefly, the 1,9-dimethylmethylene blue (DMB) solution (Sigma-Aldrich) was added to the culture medium in which the metachromatic dye was bound with sulfated glycosaminoglycan (GAG), which is a major component of proteoglycan. We then measured the quantity of the GAG-DMB complex that formed in a 96-well plate using a plate reader (TECAN

Safire, TECAN Austria GmbH, Grödig, Austria) at a wavelength of 595 nm. Finally, the loss of GAG and total GAG released per mg of cartilage were calculated.

4.8. Safranin-O Staining, IHC Staining, and Measurement of Aggrecan NITEGE Neoepitopes

Cartilage explants were placed in embedding medium (Miles Laboratories, Naperville, IL, USA) and rapidly frozen at −80 °C, continuous and discontinuous microscopic sections (7 μm) of cartilage explants were cut at −20 °C and mounted on Superfrost Plus glass slides (Menzel-Gläser, Braunschweig, Germany). These slices were used for evaluation changes in proteoglycan content by Safranin-O/fast green, countered with Weigert's iron hematoxylin staining [28]. The expression of MMP-13 and aggrecan NITEGE neoepitopes recognized was determined as described using MMP-13 and NITEGE antibodies in tissue slices [28].

4.9. Collagen-Induced Arthritis Model

Male SD rats (6–8 weeks) were housed in a 12:12-h light-dark cycle at 22 °C and allowed free access to standard rat chow and water. For the experiment, animals were first randomly divided into 3 groups. All animals then received a subcutaneous injection of 150 μg bovine collagen type II in 200 μL of 0.01 M acetic acid solution and complete Freund's adjuvant (CFA) (at a ratio of 1:1) at the base of the tail. On day 7, the rats received a booster injection of 150 μg covine collagen type II in 100 uL of 0.01 M acetic acid solution and incomplete Freund's adjuvant (CFA) at a ratio of 1:1. Clinical signs of footpad swelling and arthritic scores were monitored for 24 days. On starting, 7 days before collage II injection, and on days 1–22, rats were intraperitoneal injection treated with a dosage of Cf-02 (10 mg/kg) and Quercetin (20 mg/kg) dissolved in poly (ethylene glycol) 400. The experiment protocol was approved by the DCB institutional animal care and use committee (IACUC). Key equipment included a disperser (T 10 basic ULTRA-TURRAX®) (Sigma-Aldrich), digimatic caliper (Series No.500, Mitutoyo Corp., Tokyo, Japan), and body weight scale. The body weight of the animals was determined twice a week for three weeks. Paw thickness was measured using a caliper twice a week for three weeks. Arthritic scores ranged from 0 to 5; scoring was carried out as previously described [34].

4.10. Statistical Analysis

Wherever necessary, results were expressed as mean ± SD. Unpaired Student's *t*-tests were used to identify statistically significant differences, where $p < 0.05$ was considered significant.

Supplementary Materials: The following are available online at http://www.mdpi.com/1422-0067/19/5/1453/s1.

Author Contributions: F.-C.L. was responsible for the study design, study plan, coordination, literature collection, data management and interpretation, statistical analysis, and manuscript writing; J.-W.L. was responsible for the study plan, data management and interpretation, statistical analysis and manuscript writing; C.-Y.C., M.-C.S. and Y.-J.H. were responsible for the statistical analysis and interpretation of the statistical findings; S.-B.L., L.-C.L., H.-S.H. and C.-C.L. contributed patient samples and small-molecule inhibitors; L.W.C. and L.-J.H. performed the experiments, and J.-H.L. planned, designed, and coordinated the study over the entire period, and wrote the manuscript.

Acknowledgments: The authors' work was supported in part by grants from the National Science Council Grant (NSC 102-2314-B-016-049-MY3), the Ministry of Science and Technology (MOST 105-2314-B-016-052-MY2 and MOST 105-2314-B-182A-136-MY2), Taoyuan Armed Forces General Hospital (TAFGH-10605), Tri-Service General Hospital (TSGH-C103-070, TSGH-C104-068, TSGH-C105-063, and TSGH-C106-054), and Chang Gung Memorial Hospital (CMRPG3E2162), Taiwan. This work was supported by grants from the Core Service Platform Project for Animal Pharmacology, National Research Program, and the Ministry of Science and Technology, Taiwan.

Conflicts of Interest: The authors declare no conflicts of interest.

Abbreviations

TNF-α	tumor necrosis factor-alpha
HS-Cf	2-hydroxy-*N*-[3-(trifluoromethyl)phenyl]benzamide
Cf-02	6-(2,4-difluorophenyl)-3-(3-(trifluoromethyl)phenyl)-2*H*-benzo[*e*][1,3]oxazine-2,4(3*H*)-dione

iNOS	nitric oxide synthase
NO	nitric oxide
MMPs	matrix metalloproteinases
ADAMTS	aggrecanases like a disintegrin and metalloproteinase with thrombospondin motifs
IRF-1	interferon regulatory factor-1
NF-κB	nuclear factor-kappaB
AP-1	activator protein-1
STAT-3	signal transducer and activator of transcription-3

References

1. Pap, T.; Korb-Pap, A. Cartilage damage in osteoarthritis and rheumatoid arthritis—Two unequal siblings. *Nat. Rev. Rheumatol.* **2015**, *11*, 606–615. [CrossRef] [PubMed]
2. Robinson, W.H.; Lepus, C.M.; Wang, Q.; Raghu, H.; Mao, R.; Lindstrom, T.M.; Sokolove, J. Low-grade inflammation as a key mediator of the pathogenesis of osteoarthritis. *Nat. Rev. Rheumatol.* **2016**, *12*, 580–592. [CrossRef] [PubMed]
3. Herrero-Beaumont, G.; Roman-Blas, J.A.; Castaneda, S.; Jimenez, S.A. Primary osteoarthritis no longer primary: Three subsets with distinct etiological, clinical, and therapeutic characteristics. *Semin. Arthritis Rheum.* **2009**, *39*, 71–80. [CrossRef] [PubMed]
4. Abramson, S.B.; Attur, M. Developments in the scientific understanding of osteoarthritis. *Arthritis Res. Ther.* **2009**, *11*, 227. [CrossRef] [PubMed]
5. Toivanen, A.T.; Heliovaara, M.; Impivaara, O.; Arokoski, J.P.; Knekt, P.; Lauren, H.; Kroger, H. Obesity, physically demanding work and traumatic knee injury are major risk factors for knee osteoarthritis—A population-based study with a follow-up of 22 years. *Rheumatology* **2010**, *49*, 308–314. [CrossRef] [PubMed]
6. Peffers, M.J.; Balaskas, P.; Smagul, A. Osteoarthritis year in review 2017: Genetics and epigenetics. *Osteoarthr. Cartil.* **2018**, *26*, 304–311. [CrossRef] [PubMed]
7. Billinghurst, R.C.; Dahlberg, L.; Ionescu, M.; Reiner, A.; Bourne, R.; Rorabeck, C.; Mitchell, P.; Hambor, J.; Diekmann, O.; Tschesche, H.; et al. Enhanced cleavage of type II collagen by collagenases in osteoarthritic articular cartilage. *J. Clin. Investig.* **1997**, *99*, 1534–1545. [CrossRef] [PubMed]
8. Pelletier, J.P.; Martel-Pelletier, J. New trends in the treatment of osteoarthritis. *Semin. Arthritis Rheum.* **2005**, *34*, 13–14. [CrossRef] [PubMed]
9. Tang, B.L. ADAMTS: A novel family of extracellular matrix proteases. *Int. J. Biochem. Cell Biol.* **2001**, *33*, 33–44. [CrossRef]
10. Pelletier, J.P.; Jovanovic, D.; Fernandes, J.C.; Manning, P.; Connor, J.R.; Currie, M.G.; Di Battista, J.A.; Martel-Pelletier, J. Reduced progression of experimental osteoarthritis in vivo by selective inhibition of inducible nitric oxide synthase. *Arthritis Rheum.* **1998**, *41*, 1275–1286. [CrossRef]
11. Pelletier, J.P.; Jovanovic, D.V.; Lascau-Coman, V.; Fernandes, J.C.; Manning, P.T.; Connor, J.R.; Currie, M.G.; Martel-Pelletier, J. Selective inhibition of inducible nitric oxide synthase reduces progression of experimental osteoarthritis in vivo: Possible link with the reduction in chondrocyte apoptosis and caspase 3 level. *Arthritis Rheum.* **2000**, *43*, 1290–1299. [CrossRef]
12. Pelletier, J.P.; Martel-Pelletier, J.; Abramson, S.B. Osteoarthritis, an inflammatory disease: Potential implication for the selection of new therapeutic targets. *Arthritis Rheum.* **2001**, *44*, 1237–1247. [CrossRef]
13. Reynard, L.N.; Loughlin, J. Insights from human genetic studies into the pathways involved in osteoarthritis. *Nat. Rev. Rheumatol.* **2013**, *9*, 573–583. [CrossRef] [PubMed]
14. Gonzalez, A. Osteoarthritis year 2013 in review: Genetics and genomics. *Osteoarthr. Cartil.* **2013**, *21*, 1443–1451. [CrossRef] [PubMed]
15. Liu, F.C.; Huang, H.S.; Huang, C.Y.; Yang, R.; Chang, D.M.; Lai, J.H.; Ho, L.J. A benzamide-linked small molecule HS-Cf inhibits TNF-alpha-induced interferon regulatory factor-1 in porcine chondrocytes: A potential disease-modifying drug for osteoarthritis therapeutics. *J. Clin. Immunol.* **2011**, *31*, 1131–1142. [CrossRef] [PubMed]
16. Ho, L.J.; Hung, L.F.; Liu, F.C.; Hou, T.Y.; Lin, L.C.; Huang, C.Y.; Lai, J.H. Ginkgo biloba extract individually inhibits JNK activation and induces c-Jun degradation in human chondrocytes: Potential therapeutics for osteoarthritis. *PLoS ONE* **2013**, *8*, e82033. [CrossRef] [PubMed]

17. Rigoglou, S.; Papavassiliou, A.G. The NF-κB signalling pathway in osteoarthritis. *Int. J. Biochem. Cell Biol.* **2013**, *45*, 2580–2584. [CrossRef] [PubMed]

18. Goldring, M.B.; Otero, M. Inflammation in osteoarthritis. *Curr. Opin. Rheumatol.* **2011**, *23*, 471–478. [CrossRef] [PubMed]

19. Raman, S.; FitzGerald, U.; Murphy, J.M. Interplay of Inflammatory Mediators with Epigenetics and Cartilage Modifications in Osteoarthritis. *Front. Bioeng. Biotechnol.* **2018**, *6*, 22. [CrossRef] [PubMed]

20. Felson, D.T. Osteoarthritis in 2010: New takes on treatment and prevention. *Nat. Rev. Rheumatol.* **2011**, *7*, 75–76. [CrossRef] [PubMed]

21. Hunter, D.J. Pharmacologic therapy for osteoarthritis—The era of disease modification. *Nat. Rev. Rheumatol.* **2011**, *7*, 13–22. [CrossRef] [PubMed]

22. Liu, F.C.; Hung, L.F.; Wu, W.L.; Chang, D.M.; Huang, C.Y.; Lai, J.H.; Ho, L.J. Chondroprotective effects and mechanisms of resveratrol in advanced glycation end products-stimulated chondrocytes. *Arthritis Res. Ther.* **2010**, *12*, R167. [CrossRef] [PubMed]

23. Li, W.; Ding, S. Small molecules that modulate embryonic stem cell fate and somatic cell reprogramming. *Trends Pharmacol. Sci.* **2010**, *31*, 36–45. [CrossRef] [PubMed]

24. Ho, L.J.; Lai, J.H. Small-molecule inhibitors for autoimmune arthritis: Success, failure and the future. *Eur. J. Pharmacol.* **2014**, *747*, 200–205. [CrossRef] [PubMed]

25. Liou, J.T.; Huang, H.S.; Chiang, M.L.; Lin, C.S.; Yang, S.P.; Ho, L.J.; Lai, J.H. A salicylate-based small molecule HS-Cm exhibits immunomodulatory effects and inhibits dipeptidyl peptidase-IV activity in human T cells. *Eur. J. Pharmacol.* **2014**, *726*, 124–132. [CrossRef] [PubMed]

26. Russo, M.; Spagnuolo, C.; Tedesco, I.; Bilotto, S.; Russo, G.L. The flavonoid quercetin in disease prevention and therapy: Facts and fancies. *Biochem. Pharmacol.* **2012**, *83*, 6–15. [CrossRef] [PubMed]

27. Ji, Q.; Xu, X.; Zhang, Q.; Kang, L.; Xu, Y.; Zhang, K.; Li, L.; Liang, Y.; Hong, T.; Ye, Q.; et al. The IL-1beta/AP-1/miR-30a/ADAMTS-5 axis regulates cartilage matrix degradation in human osteoarthritis. *J. Mol. Med.* **2016**, *94*, 771–785. [CrossRef] [PubMed]

28. Huang, C.Y.; Hung, L.F.; Liang, C.C.; Ho, L.J. COX-2 and iNOS are critical in advanced glycation end product-activated chondrocytes in vitro. *Eur. J. Clin. Investig.* **2009**, *39*, 417–428. [CrossRef] [PubMed]

29. Ho, L.J.; Lin, L.C.; Hung, L.F.; Wang, S.J.; Lee, C.H.; Chang, D.M.; Lai, J.H.; Tai, T.Y. Retinoic acid blocks pro-inflammatory cytokine-induced matrix metalloproteinase production by down-regulating JNK-AP-1 signaling in human chondrocytes. *Biochem. Pharmacol.* **2005**, *70*, 200–208. [CrossRef] [PubMed]

30. Chen, L.W.; Liu, F.C.; Hung, L.F.; Huang, C.Y.; Lien, S.B.; Lin, L.C.; Lai, J.H.; Ho, L.J. Chondroprotective Effects and Mechanisms of Dextromethorphan: Repurposing Antitussive Medication for Osteoarthritis Treatment. *Int. J. Mol. Sci.* **2018**, *19*, 825. [CrossRef] [PubMed]

31. Upton, M.L.; Chen, J.; Setton, L.A. Region-specific constitutive gene expression in the adult porcine meniscus. *J. Orthop. Res.* **2006**, *24*, 1562–1570. [CrossRef] [PubMed]

32. Chou, C.H.; Cheng, W.T.; Kuo, T.F.; Sun, J.S.; Lin, F.H.; Tsai, J.C. Fibrin glue mixed with gelatin/hyaluronic acid/chondroitin-6-sulfate tri-copolymer for articular cartilage tissue engineering: The results of real-time polymerase chain reaction. *J. Biomed. Mater. Res. A* **2007**, *82*, 757–767. [CrossRef] [PubMed]

33. Schmidt-Hansen, B.; Ornas, D.; Grigorian, M.; Klingelhofer, J.; Tulchinsky, E.; Lukanidin, E.; Ambartsumian, N. Extracellular S100A4(mts1) stimulates invasive growth of mouse endothelial cells and modulates MMP-13 matrix metalloproteinase activity. *Oncogene* **2004**, *23*, 5487–5495. [CrossRef] [PubMed]

34. Jiang, H.; Hu, H.; Zhang, Y.; Yue, P.; Ning, L.; Zhou, Y.; Shi, P.; Yuan, R. Amelioration of collagen-induced arthritis using antigen-loaded dendritic cells modified with NF-kappaB decoy oligodeoxynucleotides. *Drug Des. Dev. Ther.* **2017**, *11*, 2997–3007. [CrossRef] [PubMed]

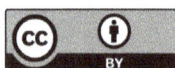

International Journal of
Molecular Sciences

MDPI

Article

Therapeutic Potential of Sclareol in Experimental Models of Rheumatoid Arthritis

Sen-Wei Tsai [1,2,†], Ming-Chia Hsieh [3,†], Shiming Li [4], Shih-Chao Lin [5,6], Shun-Ping Wang [7], Caitlin W. Lehman [5], Christopher Z. Lien [8] and Chi-Chien Lin [6,9,*]

1   Department of Physical Medicine and Rehabilitation, Taichung Tzu Chi Hospital,
     Buddhist Tzu Chi Medical Foundation, Taichung 427, Taiwan; tsaisenwei@gmail.com
2   Department of Physical Medicine and Rehabilitation, School of Medicine, Tzu Chi University,
     Hualien 970, Taiwan
3   Division of Endocrinology and Metabolism, Department of Internal Medicine, Changhua Christian Hospital,
     Changhua 500, Taiwan; mingchia570531@gmail.com
4   Hubei Key Laboratory of Processing and Application of Catalytic Materials,
     College of Chemical Engineering, Huanggang Normal University, Huanggang 438000, China;
     shiming3702@gmail.com
5   National Center for Biodefense and Infectious Diseases, School of Systems Biology,
     George Mason University, Manassas, VA 20110, USA; slin20@gmu.edu (S.-C.L.);
     cwoodso2@gmu.edu (C.W.L.)
6   Institute of Biomedical Science, National Chung-Hsing University, Taichung 40227, Taiwan
7   Department of Orthopaedics, Taichung Veterans General Hospital, Taichung 40705, Taiwan;
     wsp0120@yahoo.com.tw
8   Biodefense Program, Schar School of Policy and Government, George Mason University,
     Fairfax, VA 20110, USA; christopher.zane.lien@gmail.com
9   Department of Medical Research, China Medical University Hospital, Taichung 40402, Taiwan
*   Correspondence: lincc@dragon.nchu.edu.tw
†   These authors contributed equally to this work.

Received: 10 April 2018; Accepted: 26 April 2018; Published: 3 May 2018

check for
updates

Abstract: Previous studies have shown that the natural diterpene compound, sclareol, potentially inhibits inflammation, but it has not yet been determined whether sclareol can alleviate inflammation associated with rheumatoid arthritis (RA). Here, we utilized human synovial cell line, SW982, and an experimental murine model of rheumatoid arthritis, collagen-induced arthritis (CIA), to evaluate the therapeutic effects of sclareol in RA. Arthritic DBA/1J mice were dosed with 5 and 10 mg/kg sclareol intraperitoneally every other day over 21 days. Arthritic severity was evaluated by levels of anti-collagen II (anti-CII) antibody, inflammatory cytokines, and histopathologic examination of knee joint tissues. Our results reveal that the serum anti-CII antibody, cytokines interleukin (IL)-1β, IL-6, tumor necrosis factor (TNF)-α, and IL-17, as well as Th17 and Th1 cell population in inguinal lymph nodes, were significantly lower in sclareol-treated mice compared to the control group. Also, the sclareol treatment groups showed reduced swelling in the paws and lower histological arthritic scores, indicating that sclareol potentially mitigates collagen-induced arthritis. Furthermore, IL-1β-stimulated SW982 cells secreted less inflammatory cytokines (TNF-α and IL-6), which is associated with the downregulation of p38-mitogen-activated protein kinase (MAPK), extracellular signal-regulated kinase (ERK), and NF-κB pathways. Overall, we demonstrate that sclareol could relieve arthritic severities by modulating excessive inflammation and our study merits the pharmaceutical development of sclareol as a therapeutic treatment for inflammation associated with RA.

Keywords: sclareol; rheumatoid arthritis; synovial cell; collagen; mice; cytokines; Th17; MAPK

1. Introduction

Rheumatoid arthritis (RA) is an autoimmune disease characterized by synovial hyperplasia, chronic joint inflammation, and bone destruction, where fibroblast-like synoviocytes (FLS) appear to play a vital role in the in the pathogenesis of destructive arthritis [1]. The pathogenicity of RA exacerbated by FLS is attributed to the production of a wide range of cytokines and mediators, especially IL-6 and prostanoids, when activated by macrophage-like cells migrating from bone marrow to the synovium [2]. Specifically, RA-FLS can interact with other immune cells, including macrophages, dendritic cells, and lymphocytes, and disrupt immune homeostasis and create an inflammatory environment in the synovium, which contributes to cartilage and joint damage [3,4]. In addition, FLS can aggravate the progression of RA by secreting a number of pro-inflammatory cytokines, such as IL-6, IL-1β, TNF-α, and matrix metalloproteinases (MMPs, a matrix-degrading enzyme), and cause extracellular matrix (ECM) destruction [5,6].

Labdane diterpenes, also known as labdane-like bicyclic diterpenes, are a group of natural products sharing the same structural core and are prolific in various plants, such as Clary sage in our study. A wide variety of biological activities in labdane diterpenes have been identified, such as antimicrobial, antifungal, anti-inflammatory, and immunomodulatory functions [7–10]. Sclareol (labd-14-ene-8, 13-diol) is a member of bioactive labdane-type diterpenes, extracted from the leaves and flowers of Clary sage (*Salvia sclarea* L.) of the Lamiaceae family, one commonly cultivated for its essential oil that has been widely used as raw material for food, cosmetic products, and folk medicine. Several studies, both in vitro and in vivo, have shown that sclareol possesses immuno-modulation activities. For example, sclareol exhibits anti-inflammatory effects in lipopolysaccharide-stimulated RAW246.7 macrophages and in the λ-carrageenan-induced paw edema model via reducing expression of inducible nitric oxide synthase (iNOS) and cyclooxygenase-2 (COX-2) proteins [11]. More recently, sclareol was found to ameliorate lipopolysaccharide-induced pulmonary inflammation through the inhibition of NF-κB and MAPK and induction of heme oxygenase-1 (HO-1) signaling pathways [12]. Furthermore, sclareol exerts anti-osteoarthritic activities by regulating the balance between MMPs and TIMPs (tissue inhibitors of metalloproteinases) as well as inhibiting iNOS and COX-2 expression in interleukin-1β-induced rabbit chondrocytes and an experimental rabbit knee osteoarthritis model [13].

With its anti-inflammatory and immunomodulatory properties, sclareol is a promising candidate as an RA remedy agent. Therefore, the aims of this study were to determine and investigate the anti-arthritic activities of sclareol in a collagen-induced arthritis mouse model and SW982 human synovial cell line in order to evaluate the therapeutic potential of sclareol in treating RA.

2. Results

2.1. Amelioration of CIA by Sclareol Treatment

To determine the anti-arthritic effects of sclareol, we examined collagen-induced arthritis (CIA) progression in DBA/1J mice. On day 21 after primary immunization with CIA, when the clinical signs of arthritis first appeared, mice were intraperitoneally treated with either a daily administration of sclareol (5 and 10 mg/kg) or with a vehicle control for another 21 days. We first confirmed that the arthritic scores in CIA mice were significantly increased compared to that of the non-immunized mice throughout the experiment (Figure 1A). Mice receiving 5 and 10 mg/kg sclareol intraperitoneally displayed profound reductions in clinical scores compared to vehicle control mice. Similarly, 5 and 10 mg/kg sclareol-treated mice had reduced paw swelling compared to controls (Figure 1B,D). Histologically, the knee joints of vehicle-treated mice displayed notable synovial hyperplasia, high numbers of inflammatory cytokines, and severe cartilage damage and bone erosions. Conversely, sclareol-treated groups exhibited substantially alleviated clinical symptoms (Figure 2 and Supplementary Figure S1), suggesting that sclareol mitigates arthritic progression in our CIA mouse model, enhancing alleviation of inflammatory arthritis. Of note, sclareol treatments did not cause behavioral abnormalities or significant body changes in CIA mice (Figure 1C), whose average body weights are slightly lower than normal mice, indicating that administration of sclareol at 5 and 10 mg/kg does not induce toxicity.

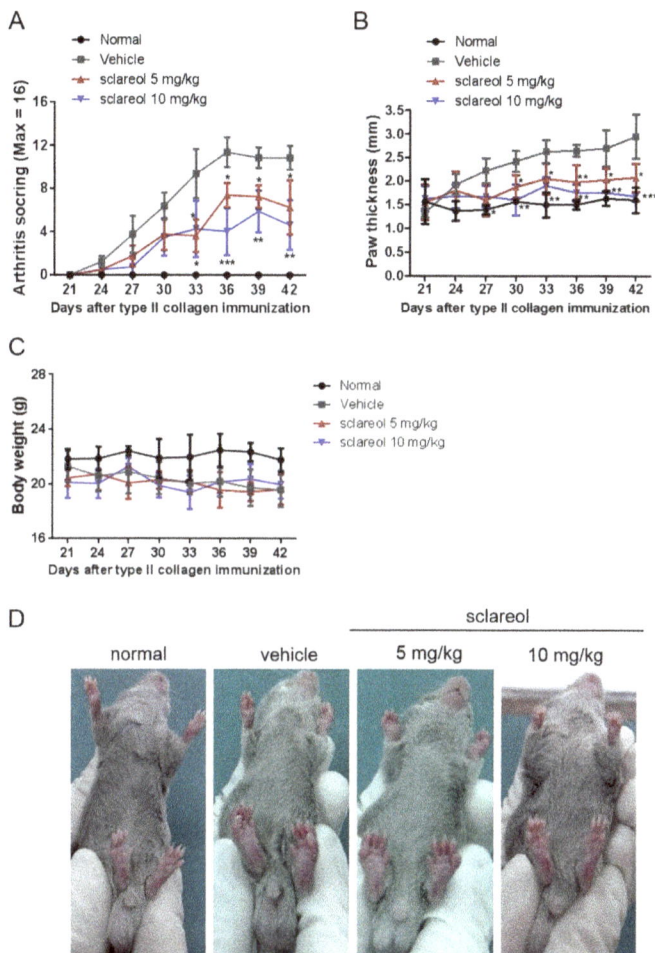

Figure 1. The effects of sclareol on the severity of collagen-induced arthritis (CIA). Mice with CIA were treated with 5 or 10 mg/kg of sclareol or vehicle every other day after arthritis onset on day 21. (**A**) The arthritis scores in each treatment group were monitored after booster immunization. (**B**) Paw swelling was measured by microcalipers, and the width of the hind paw for each mouse was averaged. Each point on the graph represents the mean ± standard deviation (SD) of six mice. (**C**) Body weight changes were monitored every 3 days after immunization with type II collagen (CII). (**D**) Photograph type (hind paw volume). The presented data are from a representative experiment that was repeated three times with similar results. * $p < 0.05$, ** $p < 0.01$, and *** $p < 0.001$ versus vehicle-treated CIA group.

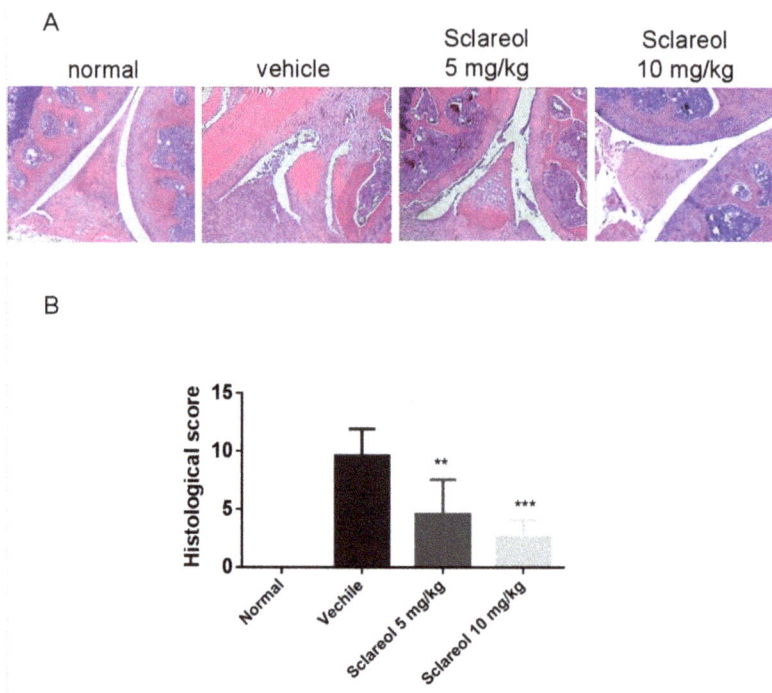

Figure 2. Histologic analysis of knee joints in mice on day 42. (**A**) Paraffin-embedded knee sections were stained with hematoxylin and eosin. Original magnification 100×. (**B**) The degrees of joint damage were scored with or without sclareol treatments. Data expressed as means ± SD of six mice in each group. The presented data are from a representative experiment that was repeated three times with similar results. ** $p < 0.01$ and *** $p < 0.001$ versus vehicle-treated CIA group.

2.2. Decreased Levels of Circulating Anti-CII Abs and Cytokines in Sclareol-Treated CIA Mice

We next explored the effect of sclareol on serum levels of anti-collagen II (anti-CII) Abs, which play an important role in the pathogenesis of CIA [14]. As shown in Figure 3A, levels of total IgG, IgG1, IgG2a, IgG2b antibodies in the serum of sclareol-treated mice were markedly reduced compared to vehicle-treated mice.

Multiple proinflammatory cytokines, such as IL-1β, IL-6, TNF-α, and IL-17, cause cartilage damage and bone destruction in aggravation of rheumatoid arthritis [15]. Thus, the regulation of these cytokines may be an appropriate approach to manage the development and progression of RA. Based on this concept, we detected the concentrations of the inflammatory cytokines in serum on day 42 by enzyme-linked immunosorbent assay (ELISA). Results (Figure 3B) reveal that compared to vehicle-treated control mice, IL-1β, IL-6, TNF-α, and IL-17 in the serum from sclareol-treated groups were markedly decreased.

Our data not only confirm that the concentrations of anti-CII antibodies and pro-inflammatory cytokines are elevated in CIA mice, which is consistent with previous works [14,15], but also imply that the humoral immune response and these pro-inflammatory cytokines could be involved in sclareol-mediated modulation of inflammation in the CIA model of inflammatory arthritis.

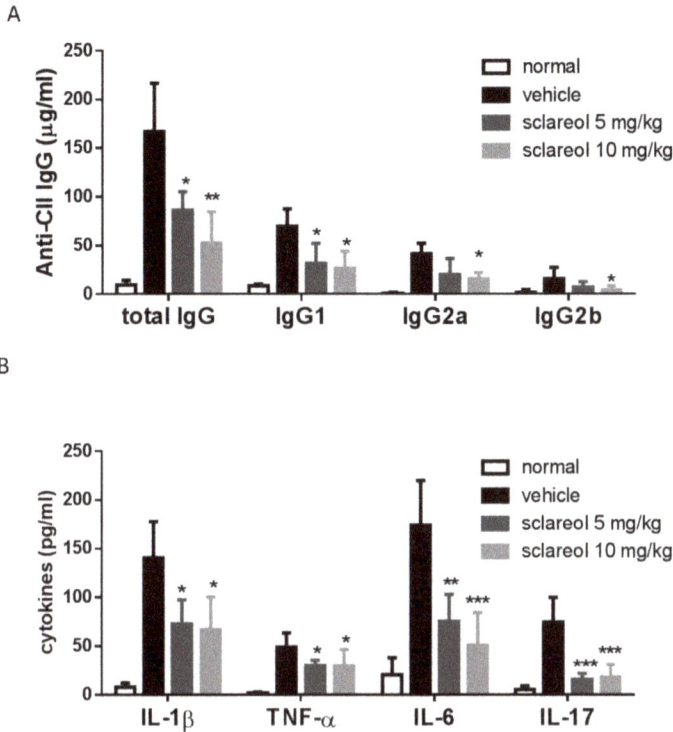

Figure 3. Effects of sclareol on anti-collagen II (anti-CII) IgG specific autoantibodies and serum cytokine levels. Serum obtained from each group on day 42 was measured for (**A**) anti-mouse collagen II IgGs and (**B**) pro-inflammatory cytokines by ELISA. Values on the graph represent the means ± SD from six mice/group. * $p < 0.05$, ** $p < 0.01$, and *** $p < 0.001$ versus vehicle-treated CIA group.

2.3. Altered Frequency of Th17 and Th1 Cells in Lymph Nodes by Sclareol Treatment

The dynamic of Th17 and regulatory (Treg) populations in peripheral blood is implicated in the pathogenesis of RA [16], and Th1 responses have also been shown to be predominant in CIA mice [17]. To elucidate whether Th17/Treg and Th1 are associated with the sclareol-mediated anti-arthritic activity, we examined the frequency of Th17, Th1, and Treg cells in draining inguinal lymph nodes (ILNs) using flow cytometry. As shown in Figure 4, the levels of CD4$^+$ IL-17$^+$ Th17 and CD4$^+$IFN-γ^+ Th1 cells, but not FOXP3$^+$ CD4$^+$ regulatory T cells, isolated from sclareol-treated CIA mice were lower than those in vehicle-treated CIA mice. This indicates that the sclareol treatment could exert its anti-arthritic effects via decreasing the Th17 and Th1 cell populations, but not increasing Treg cells, suggesting the change in Th17/Treg and the decrease of Th1 could be involved in mitigating the collagen-induced arthritis in sclareol-treated mice.

2.4. Cytotoxicity of Sclareol on Synovial Cells In Vitro

In order to have a better understanding of the effects of sclareol on RA, we next utilized a synovial cell line, SW982, as a model to investigate the interaction between FLS and sclareol. We added various doses of sclareol (from 3.125 to 100 μM) to SW982 cells for 72 h and measured cell viability by CCK-8 assay. As shown in Figure 5A, sclareol had very limited cytotoxic effects on SW982 cells in concentrations between 3.125 to 12.5 μM but not concentrations ≥25 μM. As a result, we only selected 6.25 and 12.5 μM for the following experiments. Consistent with the results from a previous study [18], treatment with IL-1β (10 ng/mL) to SW982 cells for 72 h markedly increased cell viability and proliferation, thus confirming that synovial fibroblasts, like SW982 cells, could indeed proliferate after IL-1β exposure and might play a role in the pathogenesis of RA. However, the proliferation of SW982 cells was reversed with treatment of sclareol in a dose-dependent manner (Figure 5B), indicating that sclareol significantly reduced IL-1β-induced SW982 cell viability. Notably, treatment with sclareol at the same concentrations in the absence of IL-1β did not affect cell proliferation (Figure 5A). Similarly, we also observed reversed proliferation with sclareol treatment in IL-1β-treated human primary synoviocytes (Supplementary Figure S2A).

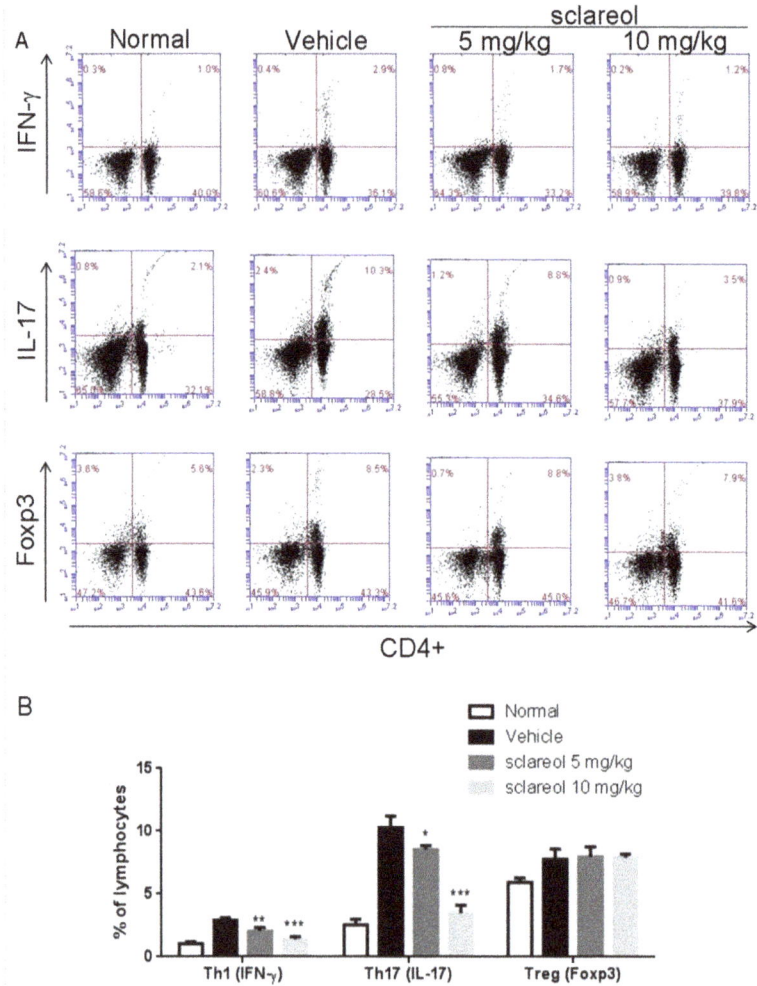

Figure 4. Sclareol reduced Th1 cells (CD4+ IFN-γ+ T cells) and Th17 cells (CD4+ IL-17+ T cells) in the inguinal lymph nodes (ILNs). (**A**) Single cell suspensions were collected from ILNs, followed by stimulation with 20 ng/mL phorbol myristate acetate (PMA) and 1 μg/mL ionomycin in the presence of 10 μg/mL brefeldin A for 4 h and then stained with anti-CD4, anti-IFN-γ, anti-IL-17A, or anti-Foxp3 Abs and analyzed by flow cytometry. Representative results in each group are shown. (**B**) Cell population results were quantified and represent as the mean ± SD with six mice per group. * $p < 0.5$, ** $p < 0.01$ and *** $p < 0.001$ versus vehicle-treated CIA group.

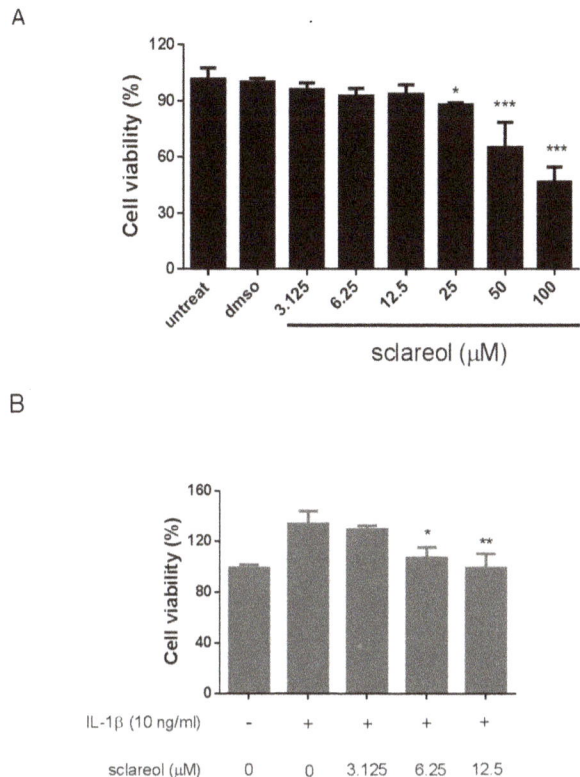

Figure 5. Effects of sclareol on SW982 cell viability. (**A**) The cytotoxicity of sclareol to SW982 cells was evaluated with the CCK-8 assay in the absence of IL-1β. (**B**) The cell viability of SW982 cells treated with IL-1β for 72 h was monitored. Each bar on the bar graph represents the mean ± SD of triplicate tests. The data are representative of three independent experiments with similar results. * $p < 0.05$, ** $p < 0.01$, and *** $p < 0.001$ versus vehicle treated dimethyl sulfoxide (DMSO) group.

2.5. Sclareol Downregulated Interleukin-1β-Induced Expression of Matrix Metalloproteinases and Proinflammatory Cytokines in Synovial Cells

IL-1β is considered one of the key cytokines involved in the pathogenesis of RA, and SW982 cells reportedly produce matrix metalloproteinase (MMP) and inflammatory cytokines in response to IL-1β, which markedly resemble the inflamed synovial tissue associated with RA [19]. Here, we stimulated SW982 cells with IL-1β (10 ng/mL) in the presence or absence of sclareol for 72 h. Western blotting assays were used to detect the expressions of MMP-1 and tissue inhibitor of metallopeptidase 1 (TIMP-1) proteins in SW982 cells. Data in Figure 6A shows that 12.5 µM of sclareol decreased the expression of IL-1β-induced MMP1, but not TIMP-1, which suggests that sclareol suppresses the degradation of extracellular matrix (ECM) caused by RA. We also investigated the effect of sclareol on the proinflammatory cytokines IL-6 and TNF-α produced by IL-1β-stimulated SW982 cells and human primary synoviocytes. The ELISA results shown in Figure 6B and Figure S2B reveal that sclareol significantly decreased IL-1β-induced TNF-α and IL-6 expression in both cells but not the anti-inflammatory cytokine IL-10 expression. Thus, our results demonstrate that sclareol can suppress inflammatory effects on IL-1β-treated synovial cells.

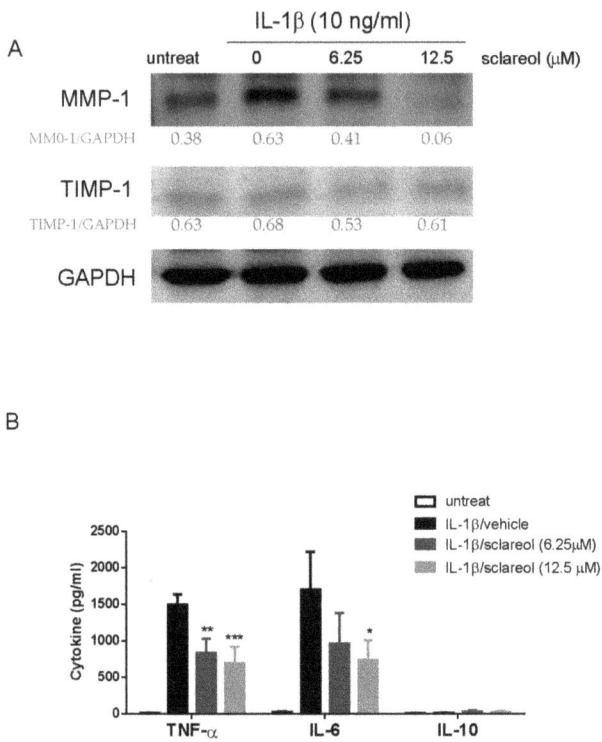

Figure 6. Effect of sclareol on IL-1β-induced production of matrix metalloproteinases (MMPs) and cytokines in SW982 cells. SW982 cells were stimulated with 10 ng/mL IL-1β with or without for sclareol for 72 h. (**A**) Expressions of MMP-1 and tissue inhibitors of metalloproteinase (TIMP)-1 in whole cell lysates were determined by Western blot with indicated antibodies. Glyceraldehyde 3-phosphate dehydrogenase (GAPDH) was used as a loading control, the normalized values (mean ± SD) compared to GAPDH were estimated by Image J software, and the normalized values were attached to each photographic band in the images. (**B**) The cytokine levels in culture supernatant were examined by ELISA. Bar graphs represent the mean ± SD of triplicate tests. * $p < 0.05$, ** $p < 0.01$, and *** $p < 0.001$ versus vehicle treated DMSO group. The data are representative of three independent experiments with similar results.

2.6. Sclareol Modulates IL-1β-Induced MAPK and NF-κB Pathways in SW982 Cells

As shown previously, the activation of MAPKs and NF-κB plays a pivotal role in the production of cytokine and MMPs by synovial fibroblasts in response to inflammatory stimuli, like IL-1β and TNF-α. To gain insight into the mechanism of inhibitory action of sclareol, we examined the protein levels of MAPKs (p38, extracellular signal-regulated kinase (ERK) -1/2, c-Jun N-terminal kinase (JNK)) and NF-κB activation in IL-1β-stimulated SW982 cells after sclareol treatments. As shown in Figure 7A, the phosphorylations of ERK and p38 induced by IL-1β were attenuated in the presence of sclareol. Furthermore, we measured the nuclear translocation of NF-κB by using the TransAM NF-κB transcription factor assay. The NF-κB binding activity was upregulated following 24 h of IL-1β stimulation, however, upon treatment with sclareol (12.5 μM), IL-1β-induced NF-κB binding activity was significantly prevented (Figure 7B). Together, these results indicate that sclareol might achieve its anti-inflammatory effects via suppressing the MAPK and NF-κB pathways in IL-1β-induced SW982 cells.

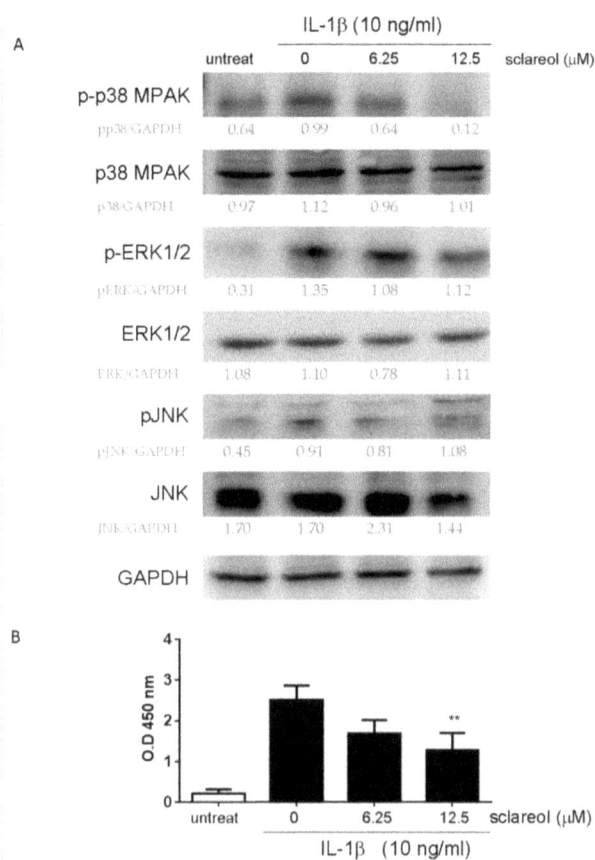

Figure 7. Effect of sclareol on MAPK and NF-κB pathways in IL-1β-stimulated SW982 cells. SW982 cells were stimulated with 10 ng/mL of IL-1β with or without sclareol and lysed after 24 h. (**A**) Expressions of c-Jun N-terminal kinase (JNK), ERK, and p38-MAPK (native and phosphorylated) in whole cell lysates were determined by Western blot with the indicated antibodies. GAPDH was used as a loading control. (**B**) The translocational activities of NF-κB with or without sclareol were determined by NF-κB activation and presented as optical density (OD) values at a wavelength of 450 nm. Bar graphs represent the mean ± SD of triplicate tests. ** $p < 0.01$ versus vehicle-treated DMSO group. The data are representative of three independent experiments with similar results.

3. Discussion

The data we show in this study have provided evidence to demonstrate that the natural diterpene, sclareol, could significantly diminish over-reactive systemic inflammation and humoral immunity in the CIA mouse model, which is characterized by lower pro-inflammatory cytokines such as IL-1β, IL-6, TNF-α, and IL-17 as well as reduced serum anti-CII antibodies. Also, sclareol treatment reduced Th17 cells from inguinal lymph nodes (ILNs) of CIA mice, contributing to the alleviation of arthritic symptoms such as reduced swelling in paws and less synovial hyperplasia in joints. We further demonstrated that sclareol treatment inhibits pro-inflammatory cytokine production from IL-1β-stimulated SW982 human synovial cells, possibly through the downregulation of MMP-1, the suppression of p38MAPK and ERK1/2 signaling pathways, and NF-κB translocation.

Sclareol is one of the main components present in the essential oil extracted from Clary sage (*Salvia sclarea* L.). Traditionally, *S. sclarea* oil has been used in herbal medicine for pain-relieving and anti-spasmodic activities [20]. More recently, sclareol was identified as an active constituent from the calyces of *S. sclarea*, contributing to the various bioactivities in *S. sclarea* [21], in particular, anti-inflammation. Sclareol has been shown to attenuate the lipopolysaccharides (LPS)-induced paw edema and pulmonary injury in mice, which justified the rationale of this study to test sclareol in arthritis [11,12]. Of note, our study is not the first report to identify the anti-arthritic function of sclareol. Zhong, Y. et al. reported that sclareol mitigated osteoarthritis in an IL-1β-stimulated rabbit model [13], but the cytokine, humoral, and cell-mediated immune responses after treatment were not investigated, whereas our study addressed this issue.

The roles of cytokines and T lymphocyte subpopulations in the pathogenesis of RA have been gradually clarified. Recent reports have implied that pathogenic Th17 cells and IL-17 mediate pannus growth [22], osteoclastogenesis [23], and synovial neoangiogenesis, explaining the severity of symptoms in RA patients [24]. Moreover, the imbalance of Th17/Treg appears to exacerbate the symptoms of RA [16]. We observed an elevated serum level of IL-17 and increased frequencies of IL-17-producing T helper (Th17) and Treg cells in the inguinal lymph nodes of CIA mice. The frequency of IL-17 and Th17 cells were decreased with the administration of sclareol, but there were no significant changes in Treg cell populations among CIA mouse groups. We reasoned that the anti-arthritic effects of sclareol could be in favor of Th17-related pathways but not Treg. However, on the contrary, an observation from a cancer study indicated that sclareol reduced the number of splenic CD4$^+$, CD25$^+$, FoxP3$^+$, and Treg cells in breast cancer mice [25]. Regardless of the differences between the two distinct disease models, it is obvious that the impact of sclareol on Treg cells needs to be further elucidated. Nevertheless, with more understanding of sclareol-inhibited Th17 and IL-17, sclareol could also be used in other immune-mediated illnesses such as systemic sclerosis or glomerular disease.

Increasing evidence shows that the activation of multiple stress signaling pathways induced by IL-1β or TNF-α (e.g., MAPKs and NF-κB) could potentially be associated with the pathogenic mechanisms of joint destruction and inflammation in RA [26,27]. Inhibitors of MAPK or NF-κB, such as bortezomib and cobimetinib, have also been shown to alleviate the synovial inflammation, bone destruction, and cartilage damage in CIA and adjuvant arthritis animal models [28,29]. Additionally, pro-inflammatory cytokines and MMP-1, which have both been verified as pathogenic factors in arthritic patients, were elevated in joint tissues in response to stimulation with transcription factor NF-κB and MAPK [30]. Therefore, the signaling cascades involving NF-κB or MAPKs are considered to be promising therapeutic targets for arthritis intervention. In the present study, sclareol appears to possess multiple facets of inhibitory function against arthritic inflammation. Sclareol not only ameliorated the histological destruction in synovial tissues but also suppressed the activation of the MAPKs and NF-κB translocation induced either by collagen or IL-1β, endowing sclareol with a new pivotal role in the combat of rheumatoid arthritis. Our results reveal that sclareol inhibits the IL-1β-induced phosphorylation and nuclear translocation of NF-κB p65 subunit, indicating the inhibiting potential of sclareol on inflammation-induced NF-κB phosphorylation in cultured FLS-like SW982 cells. Meanwhile, sclareol also significantly diminished IL-1β-triggered phosphorylation of ERK and p38, demonstrating the inhibitory effects of sclareol on MAPK activation in synoviocytes.

In this study, we present the results of the interactions between sclareol and both human FLS cell types, SW982 and primary human synoviocytes, both of which exhibit similar patterns in terms of the anti-arthritic activity when treated with sclareol (Figure 5, Figure 6, and Figure S2). When selecting cellular material for study, there are always advantages and disadvantages that must be evaluated prior to finalizing study design. For example, the stable cellular status in transformed cells is the major advantage for assessing the anti-inflammatory activities of sclareol in vitro. Contrarily, the quality of primary cells is labile due to the variable and highly dependent nature of primary cells on physiological conditions of the patient. Additionally, the sensitivity of primary cells to cultural environment conditions, such as the growth factors and the following experimental procedures, must also be considered. These variables could lead to inconsistent results, possibly jeopardizing the conclusion of a study. However, to avoid the potential abnormal growth conditions of a sarcoma cell line, it would be rational and desirable to utilize primary synovial cells for investigation of the anti-inflammatory efficacy induced by treatment with sclareol.

In summary, our study demonstrates that sclareol can decelerate the IL-1β-induced expression of MMP-1, TNF-α, and IL-6 in SW982 cells via attenuating translocation of NF-κB and phosphorylation of MAPK pathways, including p-38 and ERK. Moreover, sclareol can remarkably improve clinical symptoms, such as paw swelling and bone erosions, and reduce the number of Th17 cells in CIA mice. These findings indicate the pharmacological potential of sclareol and provide a therapeutic direction for applying sclareol towards the clinical treatments for rheumatoid arthritis and other inflammatory diseases.

4. Material and Methods

4.1. Animal Experiments

Eight-week-old male DBA/1J mice (20–22 g in weight) were purchased from Jackson Laboratory (Bar Harbor, MA, USA) and kept under specific-pathogen-free (SPF) conditions with food and water ad libitum. All animals were treated in accordance with the Institutional Animal Care and Use Committee (IACUC) of National Chung Hsing University (NCHU), and the study protocols were approved by the Committee on Animal Research and Care in NCHU (NO. 104070). The animal model of collagen type II-induced arthritis (CIA) was used as described previously [31]. Sclareol was purchased directly from Sigma Aldrich Co. (St. Louis, MO, USA) and dissolved in the corn oil/DMSO vehicles (v/v, 95/5). Male DBA/1J mice were randomly divided into four groups of equal number ($n = 6$): (1) normal/control group; (2) the CIA + vehicle group; (3) the CIA + 5 mg/kg sclareol group; and (4) the CIA + 10 mg/kg sclareol group. The mice in groups 2, 3, and 4 received either vehicle or sclareol via intraperitoneal injection every other day from day 21 to day 42, whereas group 1 was given 100 µL corn oil/DMSO as a vehicle control. Disease severities of CIA mice were scored by clinical symptoms of limbs by two investigators in a blinded manner from day 21 post-immunization. Clinical arthritis scores from 0 to 4 were recorded based on swelling levels of paws measured with microcalipers, erythema, edema, and joint rigidity. The maximal arthritis score per paw is 4, where 0 means no swelling; each limb was graded, and therefore, a maximal score was 16 for each animal. Mice were sacrificed on day 42 post-immunization for further histological examination.

4.2. Histological Analysis

The knee joints were removed at the end of the experiments. Samples were fixed in 10% formalin decalcified with 15% ethylenediaminetetraacetic acid (EDTA) and embedded in paraffin for tissue sections (5 µM thick), which in turn were stained with hematoxylin and eosin (H & E) according to standard methods. Histopathological damage was blindly scored according to previously defined parameters [32]. In brief, cell infiltration, synovial hyperplasia, and cartilage destruction were assigned scores of 0–4 by a pathologist based on the following criteria: 0, no changes; 1, mild changes; 2, moderate changes; 3, severe changes; 4, total destruction of joint architecture. A value for each knee joint was obtained and yielded the maximum possible score of 8.

4.3. ELISA for Serum Anti-Mouse Collagen II Antibodies (Anti-CII Abs)

Anti-CII Ab ELISA kits were purchased from Chondrex (Redmond, WA, USA). Sera samples were collected from each mouse at the end of the experiment and the titers of anti-CII Abs (total IgG, IgG1, IgG2a, and IgG2b) were assessed following the manufacturer's instructions. Tested sera were diluted 2500-fold and added to mouse CII-coated 96-well plates overnight at 4 °C. Bound IgG was detected by incubation with horseradish peroxidase (HRP)-conjugated anti-mouse IgG, followed by o-Phenylenediamine (OPD) substrate. Serum cytokines were measured by standard sandwich ELISA according to the manufacturer's protocol, eBioscience Co., Ltd. (San Diego, CA, USA).

4.4. Flow Cytometry

Intracellular cytokine staining and flow cytometry were modified from our previous report [30]. Briefly, on day 42, single cell suspensions from inguinal lymph nodes (ILNs) were pulsed with 20 ng/mL PMA (Sigma-Aldrich, St. Louis, MO, USA) and 1 µg/mL ionomycin (Sigma-Aldrich, St. Louis, MO, USA) for 18 h, with 10 µg/mL brefeldin A was added during the last 4 h of culture. After stimulation, the cells were surface stained with phycoerythrin- (PE-) anti-CD4 antibody (BD Biosciences, San Diego, CA, USA), permeabilized/fixed with cytofix/Cytoperm Plus (BD Biosciences), and stained with FITC-anti-IL-17A antibody and FITC-anti-IFN-γ antibody (Biolegend). To analyze regulatory T cells (Tregs), single cell suspensions from ILNs were stained with PE-anti-CD4 antibody (BD Biosciences), fixed, permeabilized, and stained with anti-Foxp3 antibody (BD Biosciences) according to the manufacturer's instructions. Flow cytometer analysis was performed in an AccuriTM C5 cytometer.

4.5. Cell Culture

The SW982 human synovial cell line was purchased from the American Type Culture Collection (ATCC; Manassas, VA, USA) and was maintained in Leibovitz-15 medium with 10% fetal bovine serum (FBS), 100 U/mL penicillin, and 100 µg/mL streptomycin. The human synovial primary cell was purchased from Celprogen (36069-02, San Pedro, CA, USA) and was cultured in human synovial fluid membrane fibroblast primary cell culture complete media with serum (M36069-03S, Celprogen). Both cell lines were maintained at 37 °C under a humidified atmosphere containing 5% CO_2 with medium changed every 3 days.

4.6. Cell Counting Kit-8 (CCK8) Assay

Cell viability was determined using the CCK8 assay (Dojindo, Kumamoto, Japan). In brief, the SW982 cells or human synovial primary cells were seeded in 96-well plates (Corning Costar, Corning, NY, USA) or extra-cellular matrix pre-coated 96 well plates (Celprogen, Torrance, CA, USA) at a density of 10^5 cells per well in 100 µL medium, incubated overnight, and then treated with sclareol (3.125–100 µM) with or without IL-1β (10 ng/mL) for 72 h. The control wells contained an equivalent amount of medium containing 0.1% DMSO. CCK8 regent was added to each well, incubated for 1 h, and absorbance (optical density, OD) was determined using a microplate reader (Tecan Sunrise, Männedorf, Switzerland) at 450 nm.

4.7. Western Blot Analysis

SW982 cells (2×10^5/well) were seeded into 6-well plates and treated with sclareol (6.25 or 12.5 µM) with or without IL-1β (10 ng/mL) for 24 h. The cells were then lysed in RIPA buffer (Sigma-Aldrich, St. Louis, MO, USA) containing 1% protease inhibitor cocktail (Sigma-Aldrich). Equal loading protein concentration was measured by using the BCA Protein Assay Kit (Thermo Fisher Scientific, Waltham, MA, USA). Proteins were separated by 10% sodium dodecyl sulfate polyacrylamide gel electrophoresis (SDS-PAGE), and then transferred to a polyvinylidene difluoride (PVDF) membrane. After blocking with 5% skim milk for 2 h at room temperature, the membranes were incubated with anti-MMP-1 (R & D systems, Minneapolis, MN, USA), anti-tissue inhibitor of metalloproteinase 1 (TIMP-1) (Sigma, St. Louis, MO, USA), anti-phospho-p38 (Thr180/Tyr182), anti-p38, anti-phospho-p42/44 (Thr202/Tyr204, 20G11), anti-total p42/44 (137F5), anti-phosphor-c-Jun N-terminal kinase (anti-phospho-JNK) (81E11), anti-JNK (all purchased from Cell Signaling, Danvers, `MA, USA) and glyceraldehyde 3-phosphate dehydrogenase (GAPDH) (Cat# ab8245, Abcam, Cambridge, MA, USA) antibodies at 4 °C overnight. The membranes were then incubated with appropriate HRP-conjugated secondary antibodies (Jackson ImmunoResearch Laboratories, West Grove, PA, USA) overnight at 4 °C. The immunoactive bands were detected with an enhanced

Int. J. Mol. Sci. **2018**, *19*, 1351

chemiluminescence (ECL) system and developed using the Hansor Luminescence Image System (Taichung, Taiwan). All bands in the blots were normalized to the level of GAPDH for each lane. The band density was measured with the ImageJ v1.47 program for Windows from the National Institute of Health (NIH) (Bethesda, Rockville, MD, USA).

4.8. NF-κB Activity Assay

The SW982 cells were harvested after 24 h treatment with sclareol, and nuclear extracts were prepared using the NE-PER Nuclear and Cytoplasmic Extraction system (Thermo Fisher Scientific, Waltham, MA, USA). For each assay, a total of 10 µg nuclear extract was used in a TransAM NF-κB p65 ELISA kit (Active Motif, Carlsbad, CA, USA) according to the manufacturer's instructions.

4.9. Measurement of the Cytokine Concentrations in Cell Culture

After washing with PBS (pH 7.4), the SW982 or human synovial fluid normal membrane fibroblast primary cells (2×10^5/well) were incubated at 37 °C with or without sclareol and IL-1β (10 ng/mL) in Leibovitz-15 medium containing 10% (v/v) FBS for 24 h. Culture supernatants were collected and stored at −80 °C. The cytokine (TNF-α and IL-6) concentrations in the medium were measured by standard sandwich ELISA according to the manufacturer's protocol (eBioscience).

4.10. Statistical Analysis

Data were expressed as the mean ± SD. All statistical analyses were performed using either one-way ANOVA or two-way ANOVA with subsequent Tukey's HSD (honest significant difference) test to compare multiple treatments using GraphPad Prism (version 5 for Windows; GraphPad Software, La Jolla, CA, USA). The significance of difference was defined as p values < 0.05.

Supplementary Materials: Supplementary materials can be found at http://www.mdpi.com/1422-0067/19/5/1351/s1.

Author Contributions: S.-C.L. and S.-P.W. carried out animal experimental work. S.L. designed the experimental work and data analysis. C.W.L. and C.Z.L. wrote the paper and data analysis. S.-W.T., M.-C.H., and C.-C.L. designed the experiments, coordinated the study, and wrote the paper.

Acknowledgments: This work was supported by grants from the Ministry of Science and Technology, China (105-2320-B-005-006).

Conflicts of Interest: The authors declare no conflict of interest.

References

1. Bustamante, M.F.; Garcia-Carbonell, R.; Whisenant, K.D.; Guma, M. Fibroblast-like synoviocyte metabolism in the pathogenesis of rheumatoid arthritis. *Arthritis Res. Ther.* **2017**, *19*, 110. [CrossRef] [PubMed]
2. Bartok, B.; Firestein, G.S. Fibroblast-like synoviocytes: Key effector cells in rheumatoid arthritis. *Immunol. Rev.* **2010**, *233*, 233–255. [CrossRef] [PubMed]
3. Bresnihan, B. Pathogenesis of joint damage in rheumatoid arthritis. *J. Rheumatol.* **1999**, *26*, 717–719. [PubMed]
4. Chang, S.K.; Gu, Z.; Brenner, M.B. Fibroblast-like synoviocytes in inflammatory arthritis pathology: The emerging role of cadherin-11. *Immunol. Rev.* **2010**, *233*, 256–266. [CrossRef] [PubMed]
5. Ganesan, R.; Rasool, M. Fibroblast-like synoviocytes-dependent effector molecules as a critical mediator for rheumatoid arthritis: Current status and future directions. *Int. Rev. Immunol.* **2017**, *36*, 20–30. [CrossRef] [PubMed]
6. Yoshida, K.; Hashimoto, T.; Sakai, Y.; Hashiramoto, A. Involvement of the circadian rhythm and inflammatory cytokines in the pathogenesis of rheumatoid arthritis. *J. Immunol. Res.* **2014**, *2014*, 282495. [CrossRef] [PubMed]
7. Kennedy, B.S.; Nielsen, M.T.; Severson, R.F. Biorationals from *Nicotiana* protect cucumbers against *Colletotrichum lagenarium* (Pass.) ell. & halst disease development. *J. Chem. Ecol.* **1995**, *21*, 221–231. [PubMed]

8. Sun, Y.J.; Gao, M.L.; Zhang, Y.L.; Wang, J.M.; Wu, Y.; Wang, Y.; Liu, T. Labdane Diterpenes from the Fruits of *Sinopodophyllum emodi. Molecules* **2016**, *21*, 434. [CrossRef] [PubMed]

9. Tran, Q.T.N.; Wong, W.S.F.; Chai, C.L.L. Labdane diterpenoids as potential anti-inflammatory agents. *Pharmacol. Res.* **2017**, *124*, 43–63. [CrossRef] [PubMed]

10. Singh, M.; Pal, M.; Sharma, R.P. Biological activity of the labdane diterpenes. *Planta Med.* **1999**, *65*, 2–8. [CrossRef] [PubMed]

11. Huang, G.J.; Pan, C.H.; Wu, C.H. Sclareol exhibits anti-inflammatory activity in both lipopolysaccharide-stimulated macrophages and the lambda-carrageenan-induced paw edema model. *J. Nat. Prod.* **2012**, *75*, 54–59. [CrossRef] [PubMed]

12. Hsieh, Y.H.; Deng, J.S.; Pan, H.P.; Liao, J.C.; Huang, S.S.; Huang, G.J. Sclareol ameliorate lipopolysaccharide-induced acute lung injury through inhibition of MAPK and induction of HO-1 signaling. *Int. Immunopharmacol.* **2017**, *44*, 16–25. [CrossRef] [PubMed]

13. Zhong, Y.; Huang, Y.; Santoso, M.B.; Wu, L.D. Sclareol exerts anti-osteoarthritic activities in interleukin-1beta-induced rabbit chondrocytes and a rabbit osteoarthritis model. *Int. J. Clin. Exp. Pathol.* **2015**, *8*, 2365–2374. [PubMed]

14. Cho, Y.G.; Cho, M.L.; Min, S.Y.; Kim, H.Y. Type II collagen autoimmunity in a mouse model of human rheumatoid arthritis. *Autoimmun. Rev.* **2007**, *7*, 65–70. [CrossRef] [PubMed]

15. McInnes, I.B.; Schett, G. Cytokines in the pathogenesis of rheumatoid arthritis. *Nat. Rev. Immunol.* **2007**, *7*, 429–442. [CrossRef] [PubMed]

16. Astry, B.; Venkatesha, S.H.; Moudgil, K.D. Involvement of the IL-23/IL-17 axis and the Th17/Treg balance in the pathogenesis and control of autoimmune arthritis. *Cytokine* **2015**, *74*, 54–61. [CrossRef] [PubMed]

17. Mauri, C.; Williams, R.O.; Walmsley, M.; Feldmann, M. Relationship between Th1/Th2 cytokine patterns and the arthritogenic response in collagen-induced arthritis. *Eur. J. Immunol.* **1996**, *26*, 1511–1518. [CrossRef] [PubMed]

18. Choi, Y.J.; Lee, W.S.; Lee, E.G.; Sung, M.S.; Yoo, W.H. Sulforaphane inhibits IL-1beta-induced proliferation of rheumatoid arthritis synovial fibroblasts and the production of MMPs, COX-2, and PGE2. *Inflammation* **2014**, *37*, 1496–1503. [CrossRef] [PubMed]

19. Yamazaki, T.; Yokoyama, T.; Akatsu, H.; Tukiyama, T.; Tokiwa, T. Phenotypic characterization of a human synovial sarcoma cell line, SW982, and its response to dexamethasone. *In Vitro Cell. Dev. Biol. Anim.* **2003**, *39*, 337–339. [CrossRef]

20. Ou, M.C.; Hsu, T.F.; Lai, A.C.; Lin, Y.T.; Lin, C.C. Pain relief assessment by aromatic essential oil massage on outpatients with primary dysmenorrhea: A randomized, double-blind clinical trial. *J. Obstet. Gynaecol. Res.* **2012**, *38*, 817–822. [CrossRef] [PubMed]

21. Caissard, J.C.; Olivier, T.; Delbecque, C.; Palle, S.; Garry, P.P.; Audran, A.; Valot, N.; Moja, S.; Nicole, F.; Magnard, J.L.; et al. Extracellular localization of the diterpene sclareol in clary sage (*Salvia sclarea* L., *Lamiaceae*). *PLoS ONE* **2012**, *7*, e48253. [CrossRef] [PubMed]

22. Kim, E.K.; Kwon, J.E.; Lee, S.Y.; Lee, E.J.; Kim, D.S.; Moon, S.J.; Lee, J.; Kwok, S.K.; Park, S.H.; Cho, M.L. IL-17-mediated mitochondrial dysfunction impairs apoptosis in rheumatoid arthritis synovial fibroblasts through activation of autophagy. *Cell Death Dis.* **2017**, *8*, e2565. [CrossRef] [PubMed]

23. Kim, K.W.; Kim, H.R.; Kim, B.M.; Cho, M.L.; Lee, S.H. Th17 cytokines regulate osteoclastogenesis in rheumatoid arthritis. *Am. J. Pathol.* **2015**, *185*, 3011–3024. [CrossRef] [PubMed]

24. Fazaa, A.; Ben Abdelghani, K.; Abdeladhim, M.; Laatar, A.; Ben Ahmed, M.; Zakraoui, L. The level of interleukin-17 in serum is linked to synovial hypervascularisation in rheumatoid arthritis. *Jt. Bone Spine* **2014**, *81*, 550–551. [CrossRef] [PubMed]

25. Noori, S.; Hassan, Z.M.; Salehian, O. Sclareol reduces CD4+ CD25+ FoxP3+ Treg cells in a breast cancer model in vivo. *Iran. J. Immunol.* **2013**, *10*, 10–21. [PubMed]

26. Jeong, J.W.; Lee, H.H.; Lee, K.W.; Kim, K.Y.; Kim, S.G.; Hong, S.H.; Kim, G.Y.; Park, C.; Kim, H.K.; Choi, Y.W.; et al. Mori folium inhibits interleukin-1beta-induced expression of matrix metalloproteinases and inflammatory mediators by suppressing the activation of NF-kappaB and p38 MAPK in SW1353 human chondrocytes. *Int. J. Mol. Med.* **2016**, *37*, 452–460. [CrossRef] [PubMed]

27. Zhang, L.; Luo, J.; Wen, H.; Zhang, T.; Zuo, X.; Li, X. MDM2 promotes rheumatoid arthritis via activation of MAPK and NF-kappaB. *Int. Immunopharmacol.* **2016**, *30*, 69–73. [CrossRef] [PubMed]

28. Herrington, F.D.; Carmody, R.J.; Goodyear, C.S. Modulation of NF-kappaB Signaling as a Therapeutic Target in Autoimmunity. *J. Biomol. Screen* **2016**, *21*, 223–242. [CrossRef] [PubMed]

29. Zhang, Q.; Lenardo, M.J.; Baltimore, D. 30 Years of NF-kappaB: A Blossoming of Relevance to Human Pathobiology. *Cell* **2017**, *168*, 37–57. [CrossRef] [PubMed]

30. Mahmoud, R.K.; El-Ansary, A.K.; El-Eishi, H.H.; Kamal, H.M.; El-Saeed, N.H. Matrix metalloproteinases MMP-3 and MMP-1 levels in sera and synovial fluids in patients with rheumatoid arthritis and osteoarthritis. *Ital. J. Biochem.* **2005**, *54*, 248–257. [PubMed]

31. Li, Y.R.; Chen, D.Y.; Chu, C.L.; Li, S.; Chen, Y.K.; Wu, C.L.; Lin, C.C. Naringenin inhibits dendritic cell maturation and has therapeutic effects in a murine model of collagen-induced arthritis. *J. Nutr. Biochem.* **2015**, *26*, 1467–1478. [CrossRef] [PubMed]

32. McCann, F.E.; Perocheau, D.P.; Ruspi, G.; Blazek, K.; Davies, M.L.; Feldmann, M.; Dean, J.L.; Stoop, A.A.; Williams, R.O. Selective tumor necrosis factor receptor I blockade is antiinflammatory and reveals immunoregulatory role of tumor necrosis factor receptor II in collagen-induced arthritis. *Arthritis Rheumatol.* **2014**, *66*, 2728–2738. [CrossRef] [PubMed]

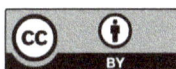

International Journal of
Molecular Sciences

MDPI

Article

Fraxinellone Attenuates Rheumatoid Inflammation in Mice

Seung Min Jung [1], Jaeseon Lee [2], Seung Ye Baek [2], Juhyun Lee [2], Se Gwang Jang [2], Seung-Min Hong [2], Jin-Sil Park [2], Mi-La Cho [2], Sung-Hwan Park [2,3] and Seung-Ki Kwok [2,3,*]

[1] Division of Rheumatology, Department of Internal Medicine, Yonsei University College of Medicine, 15-1 Yonseo-ro, Seodaemun-gu, Seoul 03722, Korea; jsmin00@yuhs.ac
[2] Rheumatism Research Center, Catholic Institutes of Medical Science, College of Medicine, The Catholic University of Korea, 222 Banpo-daero, Seocho-gu, Seoul 06591, Korea; llooo@naver.com (J.L.); syeee23@catholic.ac.kr (S.Y.B.); um26sw@hanmail.net (J.L.); yourelite@naver.com (S.G.J.); dkask0809@naver.com (S.-M.H.); wlstlf81@catholic.ac.kr (J.-S.P.); iammila@catholic.ac.kr (M.-L.C.); rapark@catholic.ac.kr (S.-H.P.)
[3] Division of Rheumatology, Department of Internal Medicine, Seoul St. Mary's Hospital, College of Medicine, The Catholic University of Korea, 222 Banpo-daero, Seocho-gu, Seoul 06591, Korea
*   Correspondence: seungki73@catholic.ac.kr; Tel.: +82-2-2258-6014; Fax: +82-2-3476-2274

Received: 31 December 2017; Accepted: 3 March 2018; Published: 13 March 2018

Abstract: This study aimed to evaluate the therapeutic effect of fraxinellone on inflammatory arthritis and identify the underlying mechanisms. Fraxinellone (7.5 mg/kg) or a vehicle control was injected into mice with collagen-induced arthritis (CIA). The severity of arthritis was evaluated clinically and histologically. The differentiation of CD4$^+$ T cells and CD19$^+$ B cells was investigated in the presence of fraxinellone. Osteoclastogenesis after fraxinellone treatment was evaluated by staining with tartrate-resistant acid phosphatase (TRAP) and by measuring the mRNA levels of osteoclastogenesis-related genes. Fraxinellone attenuated the clinical and histologic features of inflammatory arthritis in CIA mice. Fraxinellone suppressed the production of interleukin-17 and the expression of *RAR-related orphan receptor γ t* and phospho-signal transducer and activator of transcription 3 in CD4$^+$ T cells. CD19$^+$ B cells showed lower expression of *activation-induced cytidine deaminase* and *B lymphocyte-induced maturation protein-1* after treatment with fraxinellone. The formation of TRAP-positive cells and the expression of osteoclastogenesis-related markers were reduced in the presence of fraxinellone. Inhibition of interleukin-17 and osteoclastogenesis was also observed in experiments using human peripheral mononuclear cells. Fraxinellone alleviated synovial inflammation and osteoclastogenesis in mice. The therapeutic effect of fraxinellone was associated with the inhibition of cellular differentiation and activation. The data suggests that fraxinellone could be a novel treatment for inflammatory arthritis, including rheumatoid arthritis.

Keywords: fraxinellone; collagen-induced arthritis; rheumatoid arthritis; inflammatory arthritis; osteoclastogenesis

---

1. Introduction

Rheumatoid arthritis (RA) is a systemic autoimmune disease characterized by inflammatory polyarthritis that lead to joint destruction and functional disability. The pathogenesis of RA still remains to be determined, but the interplay between various immune cells would be critical in the development and progression of RA [1]. The pathologic roles of T cells have been extensively studied, and the inflammatory subset of T cells producing interleukin (IL)-17 (Th17 cells) is considered to play a key role in the pathogenesis of inflammatory arthritis [2]. IL-17 stimulates RA synoviocytes to produce IL-6, which promotes the production of proinflammatory mediators, such as IL-1β, tumor necrosis factor-alpha (TNF-α), and matrix metalloproteinase, and accelerates synovial inflammation and bone destruction. IL-6 also induces reciprocal differentiation of CD4[+] T cells into Th17 cells. IL-17 induces the expression of receptor activator of nuclear factor-κB (RANK) ligand (RANKL), and accelerates erosion of bone. In addition, B cells producing specific autoantibodies contribute to the pathogenesis of RA. Although the pathologic role of B cells is unclear, targeted-therapy-blocking B cells has long-lasting therapeutic effects in patients with RA [3,4]. Treatment of RA aims to suppress the inflammatory response provoked by these immune cells, and thus reduce the synovitis and osteoclastogenesis [5].

Recent advances in RA treatment have generated greater therapeutic opportunity, which has led to improved clinical outcomes in RA patients. Drug therapy in RA aims to reach and maintain a disease remission state via treatment with disease modifying antirheumatic drugs (DMARDs). However, some patients still show inadequate response to DMARDs, or the use of DMARDs is often limited due to comorbidities and drug complications. Thus, there are efforts to investigate novel therapeutic agents to treat RA in an effective and safe way. For development of new drugs, traditional medicine could be a promising approach.

The root bark of *Dictamnus dasycarpus*, a plant widely distributed throughout Korea and China, is a traditional herb used to treat inflammatory conditions. There have been recent efforts to identify the active components of *D. dasycarpus*, and the identified compounds have included dictamdiol, rutevin, limonoid, fraxinellone, fraxinellonone, obacunone, and dictamine [6,7]. Among these constituents, fraxinellone is suggested to have anti-inflammatory and neuroprotective effects [8–14]. Recent studies have suggested that fraxinellone has a potential therapeutic effect in animal models with inflammatory diseases. Fraxinellone demonstrated therapeutic efficacy in mice with experimental colitis, and T cell-dependent hepatitis [13,15]. In an allergy murine model, treatment with *D. dasycarpus* extract was also effective [16].

This study aimed to evaluate the therapeutic effect of fraxinellone in mice with inflammatory arthritis and identify the underlying mechanisms that contribute to alleviating inflammatory arthritis. We compared clinical arthritis between collagen-induced arthritis (CIA) mice treated with fraxinellone and a vehicle control, and investigated the inhibitory effects of fraxinellone on inflammatory immune cell functions.

2. Results

2.1. Fraxinellone Alleviates Inflammatory Arthritis in CIA Mice

Either fraxinellone (7.5 mg/kg) or a vehicle control was administered intraperitoneally into CIA mice in order to evaluate the therapeutic effects of fraxinellone on inflammatory arthritis. The arthritis score was not significantly different between fraxinellone-treated mice and control CIA mice until five weeks after primary immunization. After five weeks, fraxinellone-treated CIA mice showed a mild form of inflammatory arthritis when compared to control CIA mice (Figure 1A). The difference in arthritis severity between CIA mice treated with fraxinellone or the vehicle control was maintained during the evaluation period. The tarsal joints of control CIA mice showed destruction of articular structures and inflammatory cell infiltration, whereas the joints of fraxinellone-treated CIA mice showed retained structure (Figure 1B). The serum level of immunoglobulin G (IgG) in fraxinellone-treated mice was also decreased (Figure 1C). To evaluate the effect of fraxinellone on cytokine production, splenocytes of CIA mice treated with fraxinellone or the vehicle control were stimulated with anti-cluster of differentiation (CD) 3 antibodies. The levels of TNF-α and interferon-γ (IFN-γ) in the culture supernatant were lower in the fraxinellone-treated group as compared to the control group, although the difference was not statistically significant (Figure 1D).

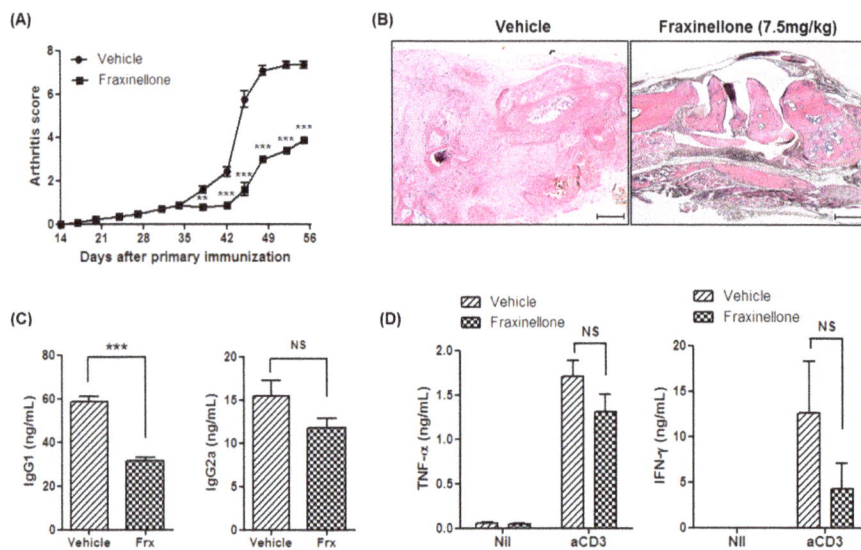

Figure 1. Fraxinellone attenuates inflammatory arthritis in mice. (**A**) Mice with collagen-induced arthritis (CIA) were treated with fraxinellone (7.5 mg/kg) or the vehicle control ($n = 10$ in each group). The arthritic score was defined as the sum of the scores of three paws (excluding the boosted paw); scores ranged from 0 to 12. (**B**) Tarsal joint tissues of CIA mice treated with fraxinellone or the control vehicle were stained with haematoxylin & eosin. The scale bars at the bottom right of the images indicate 200 μm. (**C**) Serum levels of IgG1 and IgG2a of CIA mice were determined using an enzyme-linked immunosorbent assay (ELISA). (**D**) Splenocytes of CIA mice were stimulated with or without anti-CD3 antibodies. The level of TNF-α and IFN-γ in culture media were measured by ELISA. Data are expressed as mean ± standard error of the mean (SEM). IgG1, immunoglobulin G1; IgG2a, immunoglobulin G2a; Frx, fraxinellone; TNF-α, tumor necrosis factor-α; IFN-γ, interferon-γ; Nil, no treatment; aCD3, stimulation with anti-CD3 antibodies; NS, not significant; ** $p < 0.01$; *** $p < 0.001$.

2.2. Fraxinellone Suppresses a Th17 Cell-Related Pathway

Since Th17 cells play a critical role in the pathogenesis of RA, we investigated the effect of fraxinellone on Th17 differentiation in vitro. To determine the dose of fraxinellone in a cell-based assay, an in vitro cytotoxicity assay was performed (Figure 2A). More than 80% of cells were viable until the concentration of fraxinellone was increased to 80 μM. Based on the cytotoxicity assay, CD4+ T cells isolated from murine spleens were cultured under Th17 differentiation conditions with a fraxinellone dose between 30 and 50 μM (Figure 2B). The proportion of CD4+IL-17+ cells was reduced by treatment with fraxinellone in a dose-dependent manner, however the difference was not statistically significant.

The expression of *IL-17* and *RAR-related orphan receptor gamma t* (*RORγt*) in CD4+ T cells was also evaluated in the absence or presence of 40 μM of fraxinellone. Although we did not observe a statistically significant inhibitory effect of fraxinellone on Th17 differentiation, the expression of *IL-17* and *RORγt* was markedly decreased by treatment with fraxinellone (Figure 2C). The expression of signal transducer and activator of transcription 3 (STAT3), one of the most important transcription factors in Th17 differentiation, was also investigated using Western blot analysis of T cells cultured with IL-6. The expression of phospho-STAT3 was suppressed in the presence of fraxinellone, suggesting that the signaling pathway associated with Th17 differentiation is downregulated by fraxinellone (Figure 2D).

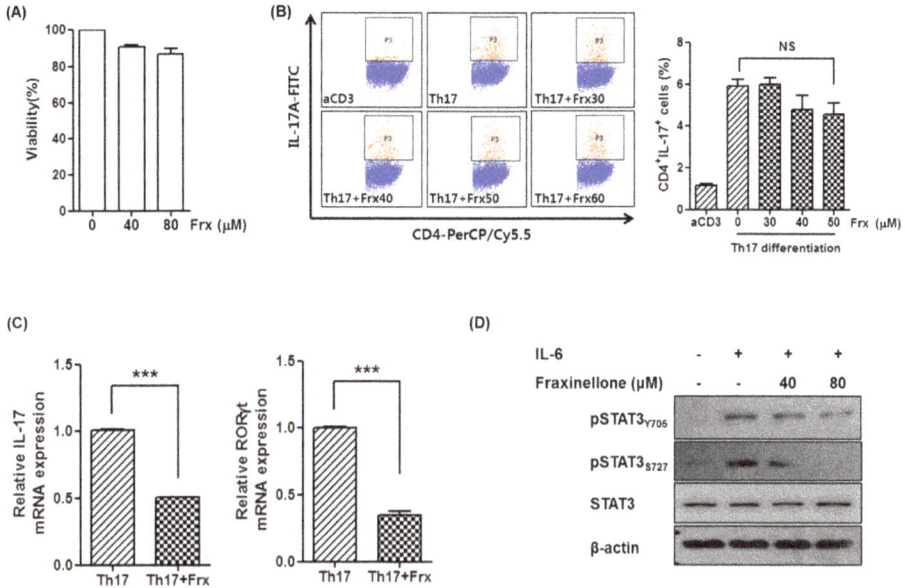

Figure 2. Fraxinellone inhibits Th17 differentiation. (**A**) Cell viability was evaluated using Cell Counting Kit-8 after treatment with 0, 40, and 80 μM of fraxinellone. Doses of fraxinellone with cell viability over 80% were considered tolerable. (**B**) CD4$^+$ T cells were differentiated into Th17 cells in the presence of various doses of fraxinellone. The proportion of CD4$^+$IL-17A$^+$ cells was measured by flow cytometry. (**C**) Relative mRNA expression of *IL-17* and *RORγt* after treatment with or without fraxinellone was determined by reverse transcriptase-polymerase chain reaction (RT-PCR). CD4$^+$ T cells were cultured with or without fraxinellone (40 μM) under Th17-favoring conditions. Data represent the mean of three independent experiments ± SEM. NS, not significant; *** $p < 0.001$. (**D**) Expression of STAT3 in CD4$^+$ T cells in the presence or absence of fraxinellone was evaluated using Western blot analysis. CD4$^+$ T cells were stimulated with IL-6, and the expression levels of STAT3 and phospho-STAT3 were determined by Western blot analysis. Frx, fraxinellone; aCD3, stimulation with anti-CD3 antibodies; RORγt, RAR-related orphan receptor γ t; STAT3, signal transducer and activator of transcription 3; pSTAT3$_{Y705}$, phosphor-STAT3 at Tyrosine 705; pSTAT3$_{S727}$, phosphor-STAT3 at Serine 727.

2.3. Fraxinellone Controls B Cell Function

Because we observed reduced production of IgG in fraxinellone-treated CIA mice, we evaluated the effect of fraxinellone on immunoglobulin production and mRNA expression of CD19$^+$ cells in vitro. The expression levels of *B lymphocyte-induced maturation protein-1* (*Blimp-1*) and *activation-induced cytidine deaminase* (*AID*), important transcription factors involved in development of germinal centers and antibody production, were upregulated after stimulation by lipopolysaccharides (LPS), but were significantly decreased by treatment with 40 μM of fraxinellone (Figure 3A,B). The production of immunoglobulin after LPS stimulation was also reduced by fraxinellone in a dose-dependent manner (Figure 3C).

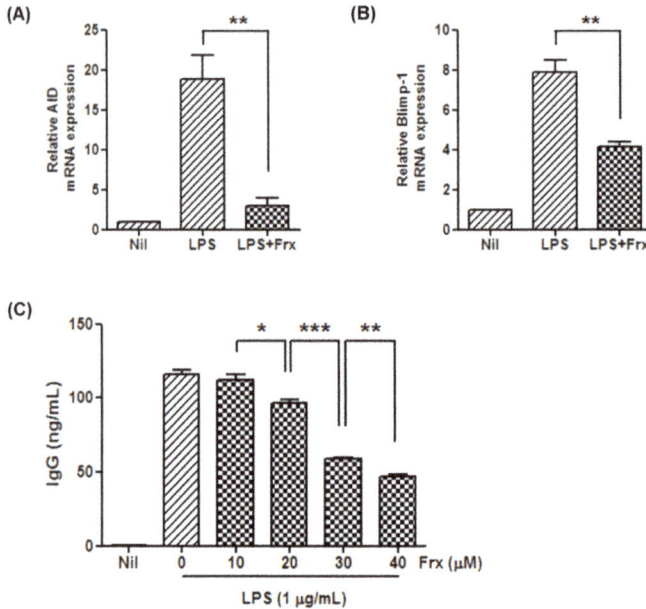

Figure 3. Fraxinellone inhibits B cell maturation. (**A,B**) CD19$^+$ B cells were activated by lipopolysaccharide. After treatment with or without fraxinellone (40 μM), the relative expression levels of *AID* and *Blimp-1* in CD19$^+$ B cells were determined with RT-PCR. (**C**) The level of immunoglobulin G in the culture supernatant was measured using ELISA in the presence of fraxinellone at doses of 0–40 μM. In all culture conditions, CD19$^+$ B cells were stimulated by lipopolysaccharide. Data represent the mean of three independent experiments ± SEM. Nil, no stimulation; LPS, stimulation with lipopolysaccharide; Frx, fraxinellone; AID, activation-induced cytidine deaminase; Blimp-1, B lymphocyte-induced maturation protein-1; IgG, immunoglobulin G; * $p < 0.05$; ** $p < 0.01$; *** $p < 0.001$.

2.4. Fraxinellone Inhibits Murine Osteoclastogenesis

CIA mice treated with fraxinellone showed a significant improvement in bone erosion as compared to control CIA mice. Because the production of IL-17, which is responsible for osteoclastogenesis, was inhibited by fraxinellone, we hypothesized that fraxinellone would inhibit osteoclastogenesis. To confirm the inhibitory effect of fraxinellone on osteoclastogenesis, murine bone marrow-derived monocytes were cultured with macrophage-colony stimulating factor (M-CSF) and RANKL, in the presence or absence of fraxinellone.

Monocyte cultures with various doses of fraxinellone between 10 to 40 μM showed a dose-dependent inhibition of osteoclast formation, which was determined by tartrate-resistant acid phosphatase (TRAP) staining (Figure 4A). The expression levels of osteoclastogenesis-related markers, such as *TRAP*, *cathepsin K*, and *matrix metalloproteinase 9* (*MMP9*), were significantly lower in the presence of 40 μM of fraxinellone (Figure 4B). The expression levels of other osteoclast markers, *osteoclast-associated immunoglobulin-like receptor* (*OSCAR*) and *calcitonin receptor*, were also reduced, although the difference was not statistically significant.

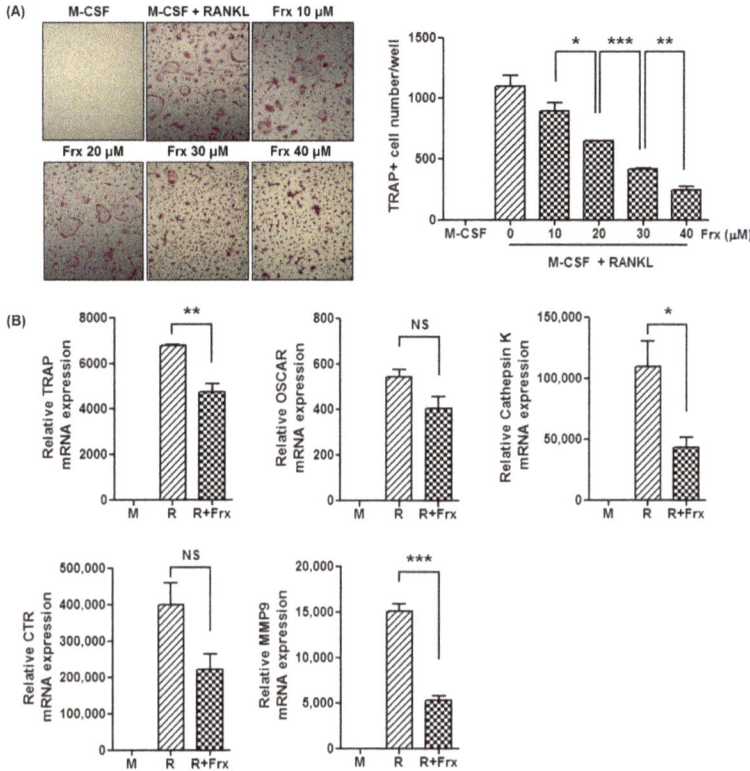

Figure 4. Fraxinellone suppresses murine osteoclastogenesis. (**A**) Murine monocytes obtained from the femur and tibia were cultured with M-CSF and RANKL to induce osteoclatogenesis. TRAP-positive multinucleated cells were counted in the culture dishes at various doses of fraxinellone (original magnification x100). (**B**) The relative mRNA levels of osteoclastogenesis-related markers, such as *TRAP, OSCAR, Cathepsin K, CTR,* and *MMP9*, were evaluated using RT-PCR. Data represent the mean of three independent experiments ± SEM. M-CSF, macrophage-colony stimulating factor; RANKL, receptor activator of nuclear factor-κB ligand; Frx, fraxinellone; TRAP, tartrate-resistant acid phosphatase; OSCAR, osteoclast-associated receptor; CTR, calcitonin receptor; MMP9, matrix metalloproteinase 9; M, culture with M-CSF; R, culture with M-CSF and RANKL; R + Frx, culture with M-CSF, RANKL, and fraxinellone; NS, not significant; * $p < 0.05$; ** $p < 0.01$; *** $p < 0.001$.

2.5. Fraxinellone Inhibits Th17 Differentiation and Osteoclastogenesis in Human

Based on the results from CIA mice, the inhibitory effects on Th17 differentiation and osteoclastogenesis were evaluated using peripheral blood mononuclear cells obtained from healthy controls.

Human CD4$^+$ T cells were cultured under Th17 differentiation condition with or without 40 μM of fraxinellone. Consistent with results from the animal experiments, the proportion of Th17 cells was not significantly different after treatment with fraxinellone, but the production of IL-17 was suppressed in the presence of fraxinellone (Figure 5A).

Fraxinellone also inhibited osteoclast differentiation from human peripheral blood mononuclear cells. Multinucleated cells stained with TRAP were significantly reduced in the presence of fraxinellone (Figure 5B). Fraxinellone also reduced the mRNA expression of osteoclastogenesis-related markers: *MMP9, RANK, cathepsin K, integrin β3*, and *nuclear factor of activated T-cells 1 (NFATc1)* (Figure 5C).

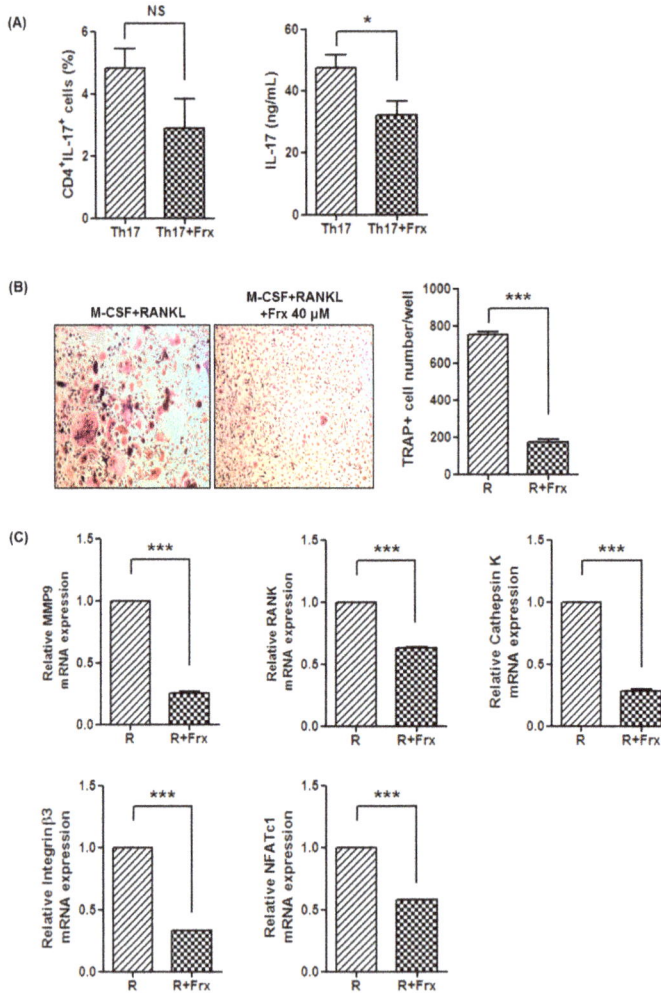

Figure 5. Fraxinellone regulates Th17 differentiation and osteoclastogenesis in human monocytes. (**A**) CD4[+] T cells isolated from human peripheral blood mononuclear cells were cultured under Th17 differentiation conditions. After treatment with or without fraxinellone, the proportion of CD4[+]IL17[+] T cells and IL-17 production were determined using flow cytometry and enzyme-linked immunosorbent assays, respectively. (**B**) Human peripheral blood mononuclear cells were cultured with M-CSF and RANKL to induce osteoclastogenesis. The number of TRAP-positive multinucleated cells was counted in the culture dishes with or without fraxinellone (40 μM) (original magnification ×100). (**C**) The expression levels of osteoclastogenesis-related markers, *MMP9*, *RANK*, *Cathepsin K*, *integrin β3*, and *NFATc1* were determined using RT-PCR in the absence or presence of fraxinellone (40 μM). Data represent the mean of three independent experiments ± SEM. Frx, fraxinellone; M-CSF, macrophage-colony stimulating factor; RANKL, receptor activator of nuclear factor-κB ligand; TRAP, tartrate-resistant acid phosphatase; MMP9, matrix metalloproteinase 9; RANK, receptor activator of nuclear factor-κB; NFATc1, nuclear factor of activated T-cells 1; R, culture with M-CSF and RANKL; R + Frx, culture with M-CSF, RANKL, and fraxinellone; NS, not significant; * $p < 0.05$; *** $p < 0.001$.

3. Discussion

Fraxinellone is a natural compound isolated from a widely distributed plant in Korea. In this study, fraxinellone showed a therapeutic effect on inflammatory arthritis. Fraxinellone alleviates synovial inflammation and osteoclast formation in CIA mice through inhibition of immune cells. This inhibitory effect was reproduced with in vitro experiments using human peripheral blood mononuclear cells. To the best of our knowledge, this is the first report that suggests an antiarthritic role of fraxinellone.

The root bark of *D. dasycarpus* has been a traditional herb used in the inflammatory conditions, such as colds, rheumatism, and jaundice. Recently, there have been efforts to delineate the underlying mechanisms of traditional medicines, and the anti-inflammatory effect of an active component of *D. dasycarpus*, fraxinellone, was evaluated in animal models with inflammatory diseases [12,13,15–17]. Previous research studies have proposed several mechanisms to explain the anti-inflammatory effects of fraxinellone.

In this study, we observed the inhibition of Th17 cell differentiation by fraxinellone. The expression levels of IL-17 and Th17 cell-related transcription factors were markedly reduced in the presence of fraxinellone. Although the proportion of Th17 cells showed no statistically significant difference between treatment with or without fraxinellone, there was a dose-dependent reduction. The critical transcription factors for Th17 differentiation, RORγt and phospho-STAT3, were downregulated by fraxinellone, which would explain inhibition of Th17 cells. A previous study had also suggested an inhibitory effect of fraxinellone on STAT1/3 expression in murine microglial cells [11]. Fraxinellone suppressed the activation of STAT1/3 signalling pathway triggered by viral components, leading to inhibition of inducible nitric oxide synthetase expression. Given that Th17 cells have a critical role in the pathogenesis of autoimmune diseases [2], fraxinellone may have a therapeutic effect in other inflammatory diseases.

However, inhibition of IL-17 does not guarantee the therapeutic effect in RA. Although the previous research provided a robust evidence for the therapeutic effect of inhibiting Th17 cell differentiation in animal studies, anti-IL-17 therapy failed to show the consistent therapeutic benefit in patients with active RA [18]. It is difficult to explain what makes this discrepancy. One study suggested that the highly variable expression of IL-17 in synovium between individual patients with RA could be responsible for inadequate response to anti-IL-17 therapy in subsets of patients [19]. Other possible explanations may be whether the drug targets Th17 cells or only IL-17. The previous research have suggested that IL-17 is not a potent inducer of inflammation by itself [20]. IL-17 accelerates the inflammatory response, in combination with other cytokines, such as TNF-α and IL-22 [21]. Th17 cells produce IL-22 as well as IL-17, and the synergistic activity of these cytokines might enhance the inflammatory reaction in RA. Given the importance of Th17 cells in the pathogenesis of RA, further investigations should be performed to elucidate the mechanisms underlying the inconsistent effect of anti-IL-17 therapy in RA patients.

Fraxinellone also inhibited the function of B cells in vivo and in vitro. Consistent with the lower serum levels of IgG in fraxinellone-treated CIA mice as compared to control CIA mice, in vitro experiments also showed fraxinellone-dependent suppression of IgG production from CD19$^+$ B cells. The expression levels of critical transcription factors for B cell maturation were markedly downregulated in the presence of fraxinellone. AID and Blimp-1 play a key role for switch recombination/hypermutation in B cells and differentiation into plasma cells, respectively [22,23]. Thus, inhibition of *AID* and *Blimp-1* in B cells would reduce the production of autoantibodies in immune-mediated diseases. To our knowledge, there have been no data on the suppression of B cells by fraxinellone. Considering that B cell-depleting therapy is effective for the treatment of RA, the inhibition of B-cell function would be a credible mechanism for the therapeutic effect of fraxinellone on inflammatory arthritis.

Previous studies have suggested that there is a fraxinellone-dependent inhibitory effect on macrophages under inflammatory conditions. Fraxinellone significantly reduced the expression of inducible nitric oxide synthetase and cyclooxygenase-2 through inhibition of nuclear factor-κB

(NF-κB) in LPS-treated RAW264.7 cells. THP-1 cells and mouse primary peritoneal cells also showed downregulated expression of NF-κB signalling after treatment with fraxinellone [13]. NF-κB is a critical transcription factor that induces osteoclastogenesis [24,25]. Consistent with those previous observations, we observed the inhibition of osteoclastogenesis in the presence of fraxinellone. Because the therapeutic goal in RA treatment is to prevent joint destruction and to preserve joint function, the anti-osteoclastogenic effect of fraxinellone would provide better clinical outcomes in RA treatment.

Interestingly, fraxinellone seems to have an anti-inflammatory effect through inhibition of cellular differentiation or activation. In an animal model with T-cell-dependent hepatitis, fraxinellone induced apoptosis of activated CD4$^+$ T cells in vivo and in vitro and inhibited the activation and infiltration of CD4$^+$ T cells to the liver [15]. In a murine allergy model, the extract of *D. dasycarpus* significantly inhibited histamine release from activated mast cells [16]. Fraxinellone also controlled the activation of macrophages in mice with experimental colitis. The production of inflammatory mediators including IL-1β and nitric oxide from macrophages was significantly reduced by fraxinellone [13]. It is unclear whether the inhibitory effect of fraxinellone is limited to proinflammatory immune cells, or fraxinellone globally suppresses cellular differentiation and activation. Because drug safety is one of the most important issues for drug development, further investigation would be required to clarify the side effects of fraxinellone on normal cells.

In conclusion, fraxinellone has an inhibitory effect on synovial inflammation and osteoclastogenesis in mice with inflammatory arthritis. Fraxinellone could have a therapeutic effect through inhibition of cellular differentiation and activation. Although the safety profile should be determined, fraxinellone could be a novel treatment in inflammatory arthritis, such as RA.

4. Materials and Methods

4.1. Induction of CIA and Treatment with Fraxinellone

Male DBA/1J mice at 7 weeks of age (purchased from Charles River Laboratories, Yokohama, Japan) were injected intradermally at the base of the tail with 100 μg of type II collagen (CII) in complete Freund's adjuvant (Chondrex, Redmond, WA, USA). Two weeks later, the mice were boosted in one hind footpad with 100 μg of CII emulsified in incomplete Freund's adjuvant (Chondrex). The mice received intraperitoneal injection with either fraxinellone (7.5 mg/kg) or vehicle control (saline) three times per week beginning on day 14 after primary immunization. All procedures involving animals were in accordance with the Laboratory Animals Welfare Act, the Guide for the Care and Use of Laboratory Animals, and the Guidelines and Policies for Rodent Experimentation provided by the Institutional Animal Care and Use Committee of the Catholic University of Korea School of Medicine (CUMC-2014-0074-02, approved on 15 May 2014).

4.2. Assessment of Arthritis

The severity of inflammation was determined on a graded scale of 0 to 4 by three independent investigators as described previously [26]: 0 = no evidence of erythema and swelling; 1 = erythema and mild swelling confined to the mid-foot (tarsal) or ankle joint; 2 = erythema and mild swelling extending from the ankle to the mid-foot; 3 = erythema and moderate swelling extending from the ankle to the metatarsal joints; 4 = erythema and severe swelling encompassing the ankle, foot, and digits. The arthritic score was expressed as the sum of the scores from three limbs, excluding the boosted paw. Thus, the highest possible score was 12 points. Clinical arthritis was evaluated three times per week for eight weeks after primary immunization in order to investigate the effects of fraxinellone on CIA.

4.3. Histological Evaluation

Joint tissues of CIA mice were fixed in 10% paraformaldehyde, decalcified in Calci-Clear Rapid bone decalcifier (National Diagnostics, Atlanta, GA, USA), and embedded in paraffin. Tissue sections with 7-μm thickness were prepared and stained with hematoxylin and eosin (H&E).

4.4. Analysis of Immunoglobulin G

Blood drawn from the orbital sinuses of mice was stored at $-20\,^{\circ}$C until use. The serum samples were diluted to 1:100,000 or 1:50,000 in Tris-buffered saline (pH 8.0) containing 1% bovine serum albumin and 0.5% Tween-20 for measurement of IgG1 or IgG2a, respectively. The concentrations of total IgG1 and IgG2a were measured using mouse IgG1 and IgG2a enzyme-linked immunosorbent assay (ELISA) Quantitation Kits (Bethyl Laboratories, Montgomery, TX, USA), respectively. Absorbance values were determined with an ELISA microplate reader operating at 450 nm.

4.5. Cytokine Measurement

Total splenocytes (1×10^6 cells/mL/well) were stimulated with plate-bound anti-CD3 monoclonal antibodies (0.5 μg/mL) for 3 days. The levels of TNF-α, IFN-γ and IL-17 were determined using the DuoSet ELISA Development System (R&D Systems, Minneapolis, MN, USA).

4.6. Cytotoxicity

Total splenocytes (2×10^5 cells/well) were seeded into 96-well flat-bottomed plates and stimulated with various doses (30, 40, 50 and 80 μM) of fraxinellone for 24 h. Two hours before termination of the culture, Cell Counting Kit-8 (Dojindo Molecular Technologies, Rockville, MD, USA) solution was added to the culture in order to evaluate the absorbance at 450 nm via a microplate reader.

4.7. Culture of CD4$^+$ T Cells and CD19$^+$ B Cells

Murine CD4$^+$ T cells and CD19$^+$ B cells were purified from spleens, and human CD4$^+$ T cells were isolated from peripheral blood using a MACS isolation kit (Miltenyi Biotec Inc., Bergisch Gladbach, Germany) according to the manufacturer's instructions. Protocols involving human samples were approved by the Institutional Review Board of Seoul St. Mary's Hospital (KC15TISI0059, Approved on 15 March 2016). Cells were cultured in RPMI1640 media (Gibco, Grand Island, NY, USA) containing 10% fetal bovine serum (FBS).

Human or murine CD4$^+$ T cells were treated with plate-bound anti-CD3 (0.5 μg/mL) and anti-CD28 (1 μg/mL) (BD PharMingen, San Diego, CA, USA). To evaluate the effect of fraxinellone on Th17 differentiation, CD4$^+$ T cells were cultured with recombinant transforming growth factor-β (2 ng/mL) (PeproTech, Rocky Hill, NJ, USA), IL-6 (20 ng/mL), anti-interferon-γ (2 μg/mL), and anti-IL-4 (2 μg/mL) (R&D Systems) in the absence or presence of fraxinellone. Three days later, RNA was extracted for evaluation of mRNA expression, and culture media was obtained for measurement of IL-17.

The effect of fraxinellone on B cells was investigated with CD19$^+$ B cells stimulated with 1 μg/mL LPS (Sigma-Aldrich, St. Louis, MO, USA) in the presence of fraxinellone. RNA and culture media were obtained for analysis after a 4-day culture.

4.8. Flow Cytometry

For intracellular detection of IL-17, CD4$^+$ T cells were incubated with 25 ng/mL phorbol 12-myristate 13-acetate (PMA), 250 ng/mL ionomycin (Sigma-Aldrich), and monensin-containing GolgiStop (BD Biosciences, San Jose, CA, USA) for 4 h. The harvested cells were stained with PerCP-conjugated anti-CD4 antibodies (Biolegend, San Diego, CA, USA). After fixation with fixation/permeabilization solution, the cells were stained with 0.125 μg FITC-conjugated anti-IL-17 antibodies (eBioscience, San Diego, CA, USA) to determine the population of Th17 cells.

All analyses were performed using a BD LSRII fortessa (BD Biosciences) and FACS DIVA version 10.0 (BD Biosciences).

4.9. Real-Time Reverse Transcription Polymerase Chain Reaction (RT-PCR)

Total RNA was extracted using Trizol (Invitrogen, Carlsbad, CA, USA). PCR amplification and analyses were performed with a LightCycler 480 II instrument (Roche Life Science, Penzberg, Germany) according to the manufacturer's instructions. LightCycler 480 SYBR Green I Master Mix (Roche Life Science) was used to develop all reactions. The primers for RT-PCR are given in Table 1. All mRNA expression levels were normalized to β-actin mRNA levels.

Table 1. Primer sequences for real-time RT-PCR.

Gene		Sense (5′–3′)	Anti-Sense (5′–3′)
Mouse	IL-17	CCTCAAAGCTCAGCGTGTCC	GAGCTCACTTTTGCGCCAAG
	RORγt	TGTCCTGGGCTACCCTACTG	GTGCAGGAGTAGGCCACATT
	Blimp-1	CTGTCAGAACGGGATGAACA	TGGGGACACTCTTTGGGTAG
	AID	CGTGGTGAAGAGGAGAGATAGTG	CAGTCTGAGATGTAGCGTAGGAA
	TRAP	TCCTGGCTCAAAAAGCAGTT	ACATAGCCCACACCGTTCTC
	OSCAR	CCTAGCCTCATACCCCCAG	CAAACCGCCAGGCAGATTG
	Cathepsin K	CAGCAGAGGTGTGTACTATG	GCGTTGTTCTTACTTCGAGC
	CTR	CGGACTTTGACACAGCAGAA	AGCAGCAATCGACAAGGAGT
	MMP9	CTGTCCAGACCAAGGGTACAGCCT	GAGGTATAGTGGGACACATAGTGG
	β-Actin	GAAATCGTGCGTGACATCAAAG	TGTAGTTTCATGGATGCCACAG
Human	MMP9	TGGGGGGCAACTCGGC	GGAATGATCTAAGCCCAG
	Cathepsin K	TGAGGCTTCTCTTGGTGTCCATAC	AAAGGGTGTCATTACTGCGGG
	Integrin β3	GCAATGGGACCTTTGAGTGT	GTGGCAGACACATTGACCAC
	RANK	GCTCTAACAAATGTGAACCA	GCCTTGCCTGTATCACAAAC
	NFATc1	GCATCACAGGGAAGACCGTGTC	GAAGTTCAATGTCGGAGTTTCTGAG
	β-actin	GGACTTCGAGCAAGAGATGG	TGTGTTGGGGTACAGGTCTTTG

IL-17, interleukin-17; RORγt, RAR-related orphan receptor γ t; Blimp-1, B lymphocyte-induced maturation protein-1; AID, activation-induced cytidine deaminase; TRAP, tartrate resistant acid phosphatase; OSCAR, osteoclast-associated immunoglobulin-like receptor; CTR, calcitonin receptor; MMP9, matrix metalloproteinase 9; RANK, receptor activator of nuclear factor-κB; NFATc1, nuclear factor of activated T-cells 1.

4.10. Western Blot Analysis

Murine splenocytes were treated with IL-6 (20 ng/mL), with or without fraxinellone for 30 min. At the given time, total cellular proteins from cells were extracted using RIPA buffer containing Halt Protease and Phosphatase Inhibitor Cocktail (Thermo scientific, Waltham, MA, USA). Polyacrylamide gel electrophoresis was performed at 100 V for 1.5 h, and proteins were transferred to polyvynilidene fluoride membrane (Bio-Rad, Hercules, CA, USA). To evaluate protein expression, membranes were incubated with the following antibodies: anti-STAT3, anti-phospho-STAT3$_{Y705}$ (pSTAT3$_{Y705}$), anti-pSTAT3$_{S727}$ (Cell Signaling Technology, Danvers, MA, USA), and anti-β-actin antibodies (Sigma-Aldrich). Subsequently, the membranes were incubated with horseradish peroxidase-conjugated goat anti-rabbit IgG (Thermo Scientific) or goat anti-mouse IgG (Santa Cruz Biotechnology, Dallas, TX, USA). Reactive signals were evaluated using SuperSignal® West Pico Chemiluminescent substrate (Thermo Scientific), and the membranes were then exposed to an Amersham Imager 600 (GE Healthcare Bioscience, Pittsburgh, PA, USA).

4.11. Osteoclastogenesis Assay

Bone marrow cells from mouse femurs and tibias and mononuclear cells isolated from peripheral blood of healthy humans were cultured in α-minimal essential medium (α-MEM; Invitrogen) containing antibiotics and 10% heat-inactivated FBS. To induce osteoclastogenesis, the floating murine monocytes and adherent human monocytes were harvested and cultured with 100 ng/mL recombinant M-CSF (R&D Systems) for 3 days. The monocytes were further stimulated with 25 ng/mL of M-CSF and 50 ng/mL of RANKL in the absence or presence of fraxinellone. On day 2, the culture media was replaced with fresh medium containing the same components. After a 4-day culture, monocytes were harvested for isolation of RNA or fixation with paraformaldehyde. The fixed cells were stained with TRAP using a commercial kit (Sigma-Aldrich) according to the manufacturer's instructions, omitting the counterstaining with hematoxylin. TRAP-positive cells containing three or more nuclei were counted under a light microscope.

4.12. Statistical Analysis

The experimental data are presented as the mean and standard error. Statistical significance was determined using the Student's *t*-test, and *p*-values < 0.05 were considered significant. All data were analyzed using SAS software (v. 9.1; SAS Institute, Cary, NC, USA) and GraphPad Prism software (v. 5.01; GraphPad, San Diego, CA, USA).

Acknowledgments: This research was supported by the Catholic Medical Center Research Foundation made in the program year of 2014.

Author Contributions: Seung Min Jung and Seung-Ki Kwok conceived and designed the experiments; Seung Min Jung, Jaeseon Lee, Seung Ye Baek, Juhyun Lee, Se Gwang Jang, Seung Ye Baek, and Seung-Min Hong performed the experiments; Seung Min Jung, Jaeseon Lee, and Seung-Ki Kwok analyzed the data; Seung Min Jung, Jin-Sil Park, Mi-La Cho, Sung-Hwan Park, and Seung-Ki Kwok contributed reagents/materials/analysis tools; Seung Min Jung, Jaeseon Lee and Seung-Ki Kwok wrote the paper.

Conflicts of Interest: The authors declare no conflicts of interest.

Abbreviations

RA	Rhematoid arthritis
IL	Interleukin
Th17	T helper cell producing IL-17
TNF-α	Tumor necrosis factor-alpha
RANK	Receptor activator of nuclear factor-κB
RANKL	Receptor activator of nuclear factor-κB ligand
DMARD	Disease modifying anti-rheumatic drug
CIA	Collagen-induced arthritis
Ig	Immunoglobulin
IFN-γ	Interferon-gamma
ELISA	Enzyme-linked immunosorbent assay
SEM	Standard error of the mean
RORγt	RAR-related orphan receptor γ t
STAT3	Signal transducer and activator of transcription 3
pSTAT3	Phospho-signal transducer and activator of transcription 3
RT-PCR	Reverse transcriptase-polymerase chain reaction
Blimp-1	B lymphocyte-induced maturation protein-1
AID	Activation-induced cytidine deaminase
LPS	Lipopolysaccharide
M-CSF	Macrophage-colony stimulating factor
TRAP	Tartrate resistant acid phosphatase
MMP9	Matrix metalloproteinase 9
OSCAR	Osteoclast-associated immunoglobulin-like receptor
CTR	Calcitonin receptor
NFATc1	Nuclear factor of activated T-cells 1.
NF-κB	Nuclear factor-κB

References

1. McInnes, I.B.; Schett, G. The pathogenesis of rheumatoid arthritis. *N. Engl. J. Med.* **2011**, *365*, 2205–2219. [CrossRef] [PubMed]
2. Miossec, P.; Korn, T.; Kuchroo, V.K. Interleukin-17 and type 17 helper T cells. *N. Engl. J. Med.* **2009**, *361*, 888–898. [CrossRef] [PubMed]
3. Cohen, S.B.; Emery, P.; Greenwald, M.W.; Dougados, M.; Furie, R.A.; Genovese, M.C.; Keystone, E.C.; Loveless, J.E.; Burmester, G.R.; Cravets, M.W.; et al. Rituximab for rheumatoid arthritis refractory to anti-tumor necrosis factor therapy: Results of a multicenter, randomized, double-blind, placebo-controlled, phase III trial evaluating primary efficacy and safety at twenty-four weeks. *Arthritis Rheum.* **2006**, *54*, 2793–2806. [CrossRef] [PubMed]
4. Emery, P.; Fleischmann, R.; Filipowicz-Sosnowska, A.; Schechtman, J.; Szczepanski, L.; Kavanaugh, A.; Racewicz, A.J.; van Vollenhoven, R.F.; Li, N.F.; Agarwal, S.; et al. The efficacy and safety of rituximab in patients with active rheumatoid arthritis despite methotrexate treatment: Results of a phase IIB randomized, double-blind, placebo-controlled, dose-ranging trial. *Arthritis Rheum.* **2006**, *54*, 1390–1400. [CrossRef] [PubMed]
5. Scott, D.L.; Wolfe, F.; Huizinga, T.W. Rheumatoid arthritis. *Lancet* **2010**, *376*, 1094–1108. [CrossRef]
6. Jiang, Y.; Li, S.P.; Chang, H.T.; Wang, Y.T.; Tu, P.F. Pressurized liquid extraction followed by high-performance liquid chromatography for determination of seven active compounds in Cortex Dictamni. *J. Chromatogr. A* **2006**, *1108*, 268–272. [CrossRef] [PubMed]
7. Sun, J.; Wang, X.; Wang, P.; Li, L.; Qu, W.; Liang, J. Antimicrobial, antioxidant and cytotoxic properties of essential oil from *Dictamnus angustifolius*. *J. Ethnopharmacol.* **2015**, *159*, 296–300. [CrossRef] [PubMed]
8. Jeong, G.S.; Byun, E.; Li, B.; Lee, D.S.; Kim, Y.C.; An, R.B. Neuroprotective effects of constituents of the root bark of *Dictamnus dasycarpus* in mouse hippocampal cells. *Arch. Pharm. Res.* **2010**, *33*, 1269–1275. [CrossRef] [PubMed]
9. Yoon, J.S.; Yang, H.; Kim, S.H.; Sung, S.H.; Kim, Y.C. Limonoids from *Dictamnus dasycarpus* protect against glutamate-induced toxicity in primary cultured rat cortical cells. *J. Mol. Neurosci.* **2010**, *42*, 9–16. [CrossRef] [PubMed]
10. Kim, J.H.; Park, Y.M.; Shin, J.S.; Park, S.J.; Choi, J.H.; Jung, H.J.; Park, H.J.; Lee, K.T. Fraxinellone inhibits lipopolysaccharide-induced inducible nitric oxide synthase and cyclooxygenase-2 expression by negatively regulating nuclear factor-κB in RAW 264.7 macrophages cells. *Biol. Pharm. Bull.* **2009**, *32*, 1062–1068. [CrossRef] [PubMed]
11. Lee, C.S.; Won, C.; Yoo, H.; Yi, E.H.; Cho, Y.; Maeng, J.W.; Sung, S.H.; Ye, S.K.; Chung, M.H. Inhibition of double-stranded RNA-induced inducible nitric oxide synthase expression by fraxinellone and sauchinone in murine microglia. *Biol. Pharm. Bull.* **2009**, *32*, 1870–1874. [CrossRef] [PubMed]
12. Kim, H.; Kim, M.; Kim, H.; Lee, G.S.; An, W.G.; Cho, S.I. Anti-inflammatory activities of *Dictamnus dasycarpus* Turcz., root bark on allergic contact dermatitis induced by dinitrofluorobenzene in mice. *J. Ethnopharmacol.* **2013**, *149*, 471–477. [CrossRef] [PubMed]
13. Wu, X.F.; Ouyang, Z.J.; Feng, L.L.; Chen, G.; Guo, W.J.; Shen, Y.; Wu, X.D.; Sun, Y.; Xu, Q. Suppression of NF-κB signaling and NLRP3 inflammasome activation in macrophages is responsible for the amelioration of experimental murine colitis by the natural compound fraxinellone. *Toxicol. Appl. Pharmacol.* **2014**, *281*, 146–156. [CrossRef] [PubMed]
14. Han, X.; Chen, H.; Zhou, J.; Tai, H.; Gong, H.; Wang, X.; Huang, N.; Qin, J.; Fang, T.; Wang, F.; et al. The inhibitory effect in Fraxinellone on oxidative stress-induced senescence correlates with AMP-activated protein kinase-dependent autophagy restoration. *J. Cell. Physiol.* **2017**, *233*, 3945–3954. [CrossRef] [PubMed]
15. Sun, Y.; Qin, Y.; Gong, F.Y.; Wu, X.F.; Hua, Z.C.; Chen, T.; Xu, Q. Selective triggering of apoptosis of concanavalin A-activated T cells by fraxinellone for the treatment of T-cell-dependent hepatitis in mice. *Biochem. Pharmacol.* **2009**, *77*, 1717–1724. [CrossRef] [PubMed]
16. Jiang, S.; Nakano, Y.; Rahman, M.A.; Yatsuzuka, R.; Kamei, C. Effects of a *Dictamnus dasycarpus* T. extract on allergic models in mice. *Biosci. Biotechnol. Biochem.* **2008**, *72*, 660–665. [CrossRef] [PubMed]
17. Yang, B.; Lee, H.B.; Kim, S.; Park, Y.C.; Kim, K.; Kim, H. Decoction of *Dictamnus Dasycarpus* Turcz. Root Bark Ameliorates Skin Lesions and Inhibits Inflammatory Reactions in Mice with Contact Dermatitis. *Pharmacogn. Mag.* **2017**, *13*, 483–487. [PubMed]

18. Kunwar, S.; Dahal, K.; Sharma, S. Anti-IL-17 therapy in treatment of rheumatoid arthritis: A systematic literature review and meta-analysis of randomized controlled trials. *Rheumatol. Int.* **2016**, *36*, 1065–1075. [CrossRef] [PubMed]

19. Van Baarsen, L.G.; Lebre, M.C.; van der Coelen, D.; Aarrass, S.; Tang, M.W.; Ramwadhdoebe, T.H.; Gerlag, D.M.; Tak, P.P. Heterogeneous expression pattern of interleukin 17A (IL-17A), IL-17F and their receptors in synovium of rheumatoid arthritis, psoriatic arthritis and osteoarthritis: Possible explanation for nonresponse to anti-IL-17 therapy? *Arthritis Res. Ther.* **2014**, *16*, 426. [CrossRef] [PubMed]

20. Gaffen, S.L. Structure and signalling in the IL-17 receptor family. *Nat. Rev. Immunol.* **2009**, *9*, 556–567. [CrossRef] [PubMed]

21. Veldhoen, M. Interleukin 17 is a chief orchestrator of immunity. *Nat. Immunol.* **2017**, *18*, 612–621. [CrossRef] [PubMed]

22. Muramatsu, M.; Kinoshita, K.; Fagarasan, S.; Yamada, S.; Shinkai, Y.; Honjo, T. Class switch recombination and hypermutation require activation-induced cytidine deaminase (AID), a potential RNA editing enzyme. *Cell* **2000**, *102*, 553–563. [CrossRef]

23. Turner, C.A., Jr.; Mack, D.H.; Davis, M.M. Blimp-1, a novel zinc finger-containing protein that can drive the maturation of B lymphocytes into immunoglobulin-secreting cells. *Cell* **1994**, *77*, 297–306. [CrossRef]

24. Lee, Z.H.; Kim, H.H. Signal transduction by receptor activator of nuclear factor κB in osteoclasts. *Biochem. Biophys. Res. Commun.* **2003**, *305*, 211–214. [CrossRef]

25. Jimi, E.; Ghosh, S. Role of nuclear factor-κB in the immune system and bone. *Immunol. Rev.* **2005**, *208*, 80–87. [CrossRef] [PubMed]

26. Brand, D.D.; Latham, K.A.; Rosloniec, E.F. Collagen-induced arthritis. *Nat. Protoc.* **2007**, *2*, 1269–1275. [CrossRef] [PubMed]

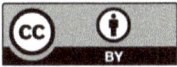

International Journal of
Molecular Sciences

MDPI

Article

Clodronate as a Therapeutic Strategy against Osteoarthritis

Maria Teresa Valenti [1,*], Monica Mottes [2], Alessandro Biotti [1], Massimiliano Perduca [3], Arianna Pisani [3], Michele Bovi [3], Michela Deiana [1,2], Samuele Cheri [1,2] and Luca Dalle Carbonare [1]

[1] Internal Medicine, Section D, Department of Medicine, University of Verona, 37134 Verona, Italy; ale.biotti89@gmail.com (A.B.); michela.deiana@univr.it (M.D.); samuele.cheri@univr.it (S.C.); luca.dallecarbonare@univr.it (L.D.C.)
[2] Department of Neurosciences, Biomedicine and Movement Sciences, University of Verona, 37134 Verona, Italy; monica.mottes@univr.it
[3] Biocrystallography Lab, Department of Biotechnology, University of Verona, 37134 Verona, Italy; massimiliano.perduca@univr.it (M.P.); ariannapisani92@gmail.com (A.P.); michele.bovi@univr.it (M.B.)
* Correspondence: mariateresa.valenti@univr.it; Tel.: +39-045-8128450; Fax: +39-045-8027496

Received: 16 November 2017; Accepted: 8 December 2017; Published: 13 December 2017

Abstract: Osteoarthritis (OA), the most prevalent musculoskeletal pathology, is mainly characterized by the progressive degradation of articular cartilage due to an imbalance between anabolic and catabolic processes. Consequently, OA has been associated with defects in the chondrocitic differentiation of progenitor stem cells (PSCs). In addition, SOX9 is the transcription factor responsible for PSCs chondrogenic commitment. To evaluate the effects of the non-amino bisphosphonate clodronate in OA patients we investigated *SOX9* gene expression in circulating progenitor cells (CPCs) and in an in vitro OA model. We evaluated pain intensity, mental and physical performance in OA patients, as well as serum biomarkers related to bone metabolism. In addition, in order to improve therapeutic strategies, we assayed nanoparticle-embedded clodronate (NPs-clo) in an in vitro model of chondrogenic differentiation. Our data showed upregulation of *SOX9* gene expression upon treatment, suggesting an increase in chondrocytic commitment. Clodronate also reduced osteoarticular pain and improved mental and physical performance in patients. Furthermore, NPs-clo stimulated *SOX9* expression more efficaciously than clodronate alone. Clodronate may therefore be considered a good therapeutic tool against OA; its formulation in nanoparticles may represent a promising challenge to counteract cartilage degeneration.

Keywords: clodronate; gene expression; osteoarthritis; progenitor cells; SOX9

1. Introduction

Osteoarthritis is a very common condition, covering 80% of all rheumatic disease, and being the main cause of population morbidity in the elderly [1]. Its prevalence increases with age, affecting especially females [2]. Its pathogenesis is related to environmental and genetic factors, some of which are still unknown [3]. Recently, osteoarthritis has been identified as a condition affecting the entire joint, not only the cartilage district [4]. Moreover, subchondral bone alterations, included osteoporosis areas, are connected to cartilage damage and caused by pro inflammatory cytokines (such as TNFα, IL6 and IL1β) and metalloproteinase (MMP) release by macrophages. Pro inflammatory molecules can bind receptors on chondrocytes surface and alter their metabolism, but they can also reduce mesenchymal stem cells (MSCs) chondrogenic differentiation [5]. All these aspects alter cartilage regeneration and subchondral bone metabolism, leading to high remodelling areas, sclerosis, microfractures, cysts and periarticular osteophytes [6,7]. Considering that both osteoarthritis and osteoporosis share these pathological changes, we tested the efficacy of clodronate as a new promising drug capable of modifying OA (osteoarthritis) natural history.

Bisphosphonates are synthetic, non-hydrolyzable analogs of pyrophosphate that contain a P-C-P core and two side chains, named R1 and R2, bound to the central carbon. According to R2 chain characteristics, they can be distinguished into two major groups: nitrogen (N-BF) and non-nitrogen (NN-BF) bisphosphonates [8,9]. Both categories inhibit osteoclast's bone resorptive action, although in different ways. N-BFs mode of action has been identified recently. Once incorporated into cells, these compounds inhibit farnesyl diphosphonate synthase (FPPS) in osteoclasts, thereby preventing the formation of isoprenoid lipids required for the prenylation of small GTPases, such as Rac, Rho and Ras. The loss of prenylated proteins accounts for osteoclastic drawbacks regarding citoskeletal rearrangement and ruffled border formation. N-BFs show a higher antiresorptive efficacy compared to NN-BFs; however, they also have a pro-inflammatory activity ascribable to isopentyl pyrophosphate backlog in Tγδ limphocytes citosol, due to FPPS inhibition [10–13]. This may be the cause of flu-like symptoms, observed especially upon intravenous administration [14]. Conversely, NN-BFs show anti-inflammatory effects due to their inhibition of macrophagic release of NO and pro- inflammatory mediators and their proapoptotic action [15–17]. For these reasons, NN-BFs have been tested for their ability to reduce inflammatory osteoarthritis and also, in animal models, to prevent acute phase reaction after N-BFs injection [18–21]. Clodronate (dichloromethylene-1,1-bisphosphonate) is a halogenated NN-BF, with proven antiresorptive efficacy in a variety of diseases associated with excessive bone resorption, including hypercalcemia of malignancy, osteolytic bone metastases, primary hyperparathyroidism and Paget's disease. As for other bisphosphonates, its affinity for bone matrix is not relevant, so patients need a long-term therapy with short intervals between doses, in order to obtain clinical benefits. Recently, clodronate efficacy has been tested upon intra-articular (erosive osteoarthritis) and intra-dermic administration [20]. Furthermore, its anti-inflammatory and analgesic efficacy, possibly related to its pro-apoptotic action on macrophages, may be beneficial for chondrogenesis. In fact, release of NO and pro-inflammatory cytokines (such as TNFα and IL1β) [15–17] may promote cartilage erosion, subchondral bone alterations, and inhibit progenitors' maturation into chondrocytes in OA early stages. Clodronate could therefore stimulate cellular differentiation by regulating inflammatory pathways [22].

MSCs feature promising sources for cell-based therapeutic strategies. They are generally defined as self-renewable, multipotent progenitor cells with the ability to differentiate into several mesenchymal lineages, including bone, cartilage, adipose and muscle tissues. SOX9 is the master transcription factor for MSC differentiation into chondrocytes, exerting its role along the whole pathway [22]. SOX9 expression is regulated by BMPs and it activates many extracellular matrix (ECM) genes such as *COL2A1*, *COL9A1*, *COL11A2* and *ACAN* (aggrecan) [23–25].

2. Results

2.1. Patients

Average age, height, weight, BMI and menopause age were 71.8 ± 7 years, 153 ± 5.8 cm, 64.2 ± 8.6 kg, 27.4 ± 3.5 kg/m^2 and 46.5 ± 7 years, respectively. Among bone metabolism parameters, only CTX values showed a significant reduction at the end of the study (0.25 ± 0.08 ng/mL at M6 vs. 0.39 ± 0.19 ng/mL at M0; $p < 0.05$). Moreover, 25 hydroxyvitamin D levels did not manifest relevant variations during therapy, and they maintained average values over insufficiency cut-off (20 ng/mL) (Table 1).

Table 1. Biochemical data.

Parameters	Basal	Treatment	*p*	Normal Range
Serum Calcium (mg/dL)	9.28 ± 0.33	9.60 ± 0.40	NS	8.41–10.42 mg/dL
PTH (pg/mL)	42.00 ± 19.20	41.23 ± 21.38	NS	10–65 pg/mL
Vit D (ng/mL)	31.45 ± 14.40	38.89 ± 9.31	NS	<30 ng/mL insufficiency <20 ng/mL depletion
CTX (ng/mL)	0.39 ± 0.19	0.25 ± 0.08	$p < 0.05$ vs. CTX M0	0.1–0.7 ng/mL
Creatinin (mg/dL)	0.74 ± 0.12	0.77 ± 0.13	NS	0.49–1.19 mg/dL
Urinary Calcium Excretion Rate (mmol/mmol creatinine)	0.42 ± 0.23	0.42 ± 0.22	NS	<0.57 mmol/mmol creatinin

NS: not significant; PTH: parathyroid hormone; Vit D: vitamin D; CTX: C-terminal telopeptide.

Moreover, visual analogue pain scale (VAS) showed relevantly decreased scores at the end of treatment in older women. Numerical rating pain scale (NRS) showed a significant decrease of symptoms after three months in the same group ($p < 0.05$ for both). A decrease in pain intensity likely warranted patients a better quality of life. This point is confirmed by significant increases of ISM and ISF scores at the end of treatment, compared to basal values. VAS and NRS average pain scores decreased rapidly; however, only NRS pain score reached a significant improvement after drug assumption (4.27 ± 2.06 at M6 vs. 6.00 ± 2.34 at M0; $p = 0.01$). ISF and ISM indexes of SF36 survey both reached relevant improvement after 6 months (ISF score: 43.04 ± 6.73 at M6 vs. 36.89 ± 12.21 at M0; $p < 0.05$; ISM score: 45.75 ± 3.86 at M6 vs. 42.54 ± 4.87 at M0; $p < 0.05$) (Table 2).

Table 2. VAS (visual analogue pain scale) and NRS (numerical rating pain scale pain scales) during the study.

VAS M0	VAS M3	VAS M6	NRS M0	NRS M3	NRS M6
5.30 (±2.7)	4.2 (±2.1) $p < 0.05$ vs. VAS M0	3.9 (±2.2) $p < 0.01$ vs. VAS M0	5.7 (±2.2)	4.9 (±2.0) p = NS	4.9 (±2.2) $p < 0.01$ vs. NRS M0
ISF MO	ISF M3	ISF M6	ISM M0	ISM M3	ISM M6
36.8 (±12.9)	39.6 (±8.9) p = NS	428 (±6.5) $p < 0.01$ vs. ISF M0	43.2 (±4.7)	45.2 (±6.4) p = NS	45.6 (±37) $p < 0.05$ vs. ISM M0

2.2. Gene Expression in OA Patients' CPCs

CPC cluster differentiation (CD) expression patterns were similar in normal donors (NDs) and Patients (Table 3). Therefore, SOX9 expression was analyzed in CPCs from patients and NDs at M0, M3 and M6, respectively. Gene expression levels were monitored in all samples. *SOX9* average expression in patients increased constantly during the study, matching (M3) and then exceeding (M6) control levels (Figure 1A). Interestingly, COL2A1 expression in patients also increased during the study (Figure 1B).

Table 3. Cell phenotype of CPCs (Circulating Progenitor Cells) after depletion.

Cluster Differentiation	NDs	M0	M3	M6
CD3	Undetectable level	Undetectable level	Undetectable level	Undetectable level
CD14	0.34 ± 0.05%	0.4% (±0.02)	0.34% (±0.4)	0.37% (±0.05)
CD19	Undetectable level	Undetectable level	Undetectable level	Undetectable level
CD45	2.35 ± 0.37%	1.51% (±0.6)	2.16% (±0.3)	1.6% (± 0.8)
CD34	Undetectable level	Undetectable level	Undetectable level	Undetectable level

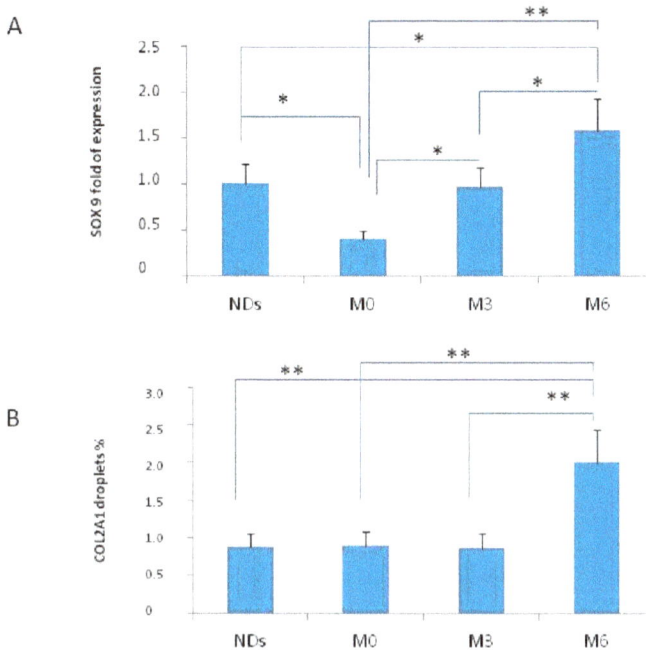

Figure 1. *SOX9* (**A**) and *COL2A1* (**B**) fold of expression in CPCs of Normal Donors (NDs) and patients at baseline (M0), after 3 (M3) and 6 (M6) months. * $p < 0.05$; ** $p < 0.001$.

2.3. Chitosan-Hyaluronic Acid-Clodronate Embedded Nanoparticles

Synthesized clodronate nanoparticles were analyzed by dynamic light scattering and showed a single peak at 135.4 nm with a polydispersity index (pdI) of 0.922 and a surface charge of 25.5 mV.

The encapsulation efficiency (EE%) was estimated to be 64.9%. It was calculated from a clodronate calibration curve. These nanoparticles were used for all further experiments.

2.4. Gene Expression in the In Vitro OA Model

As we did in vivo, we studied clodronate effects in vitro, in cultured MSCs. *SOX9* expression was surveyed in order to evaluate chondrogenic differentiation. All results were reported as normalized values compared to their expression at the end of the differentiation process (in specific mediums) without IL1β and/or clodronate addition to cultures. The in vitro experiments confirmed IL1β inhibition of chondrogenic maturation. This pro-inflammatory cytokine halved MSCs ability to differentiate. On the other hand, clodronate increased MSCs' potential to undergo chondrogenic differentiation in a dose dependent way. We then added two different combinations of IL1β + clodronate (50 nM and 100 nM) to the cultures. At the lower dose, the drug inhibited cytokine pro-inflammatory action only partially; but at the higher dose, clodronate action exceeded IL1β inhibition, stimulating MSCs maturation (Figure 2A). In order to improve the therapeutic effect against OA, we tested customized nanoparticles produced with molecules which are employed in cartilage tissue engineering, as chitosan and hyaluronic acid [26]. Nanoparticles embedded-clodronate exhibited a stronger effect in counteracting IL1β inhibition of *SOX9* (Figure 2B) and *COL2A1* (Figure 2C) expression. Notably, MSCs cultured with chondrogenic differentiation medium in the presence of clodronate alone or embedded in nanoparticles, exhibited a strong positive staining with alcian-blue indicating the production of glycosaminoglycan (GAG) and therefore the chondrogenic maturation (Figure 3).

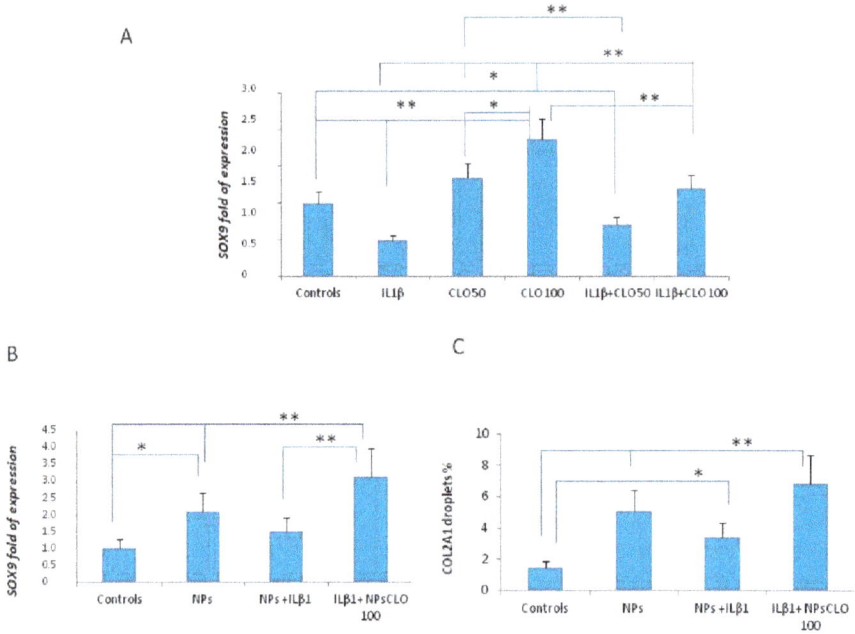

Figure 2. Effects of clodronate in mesenchymal stem cells (MSCs). *SOX9* fold of expression in MSCs treated with and w/o clodronate in chondrogenic medium in the presence or absence of ILβ1 (**A**). *SOX9* (**B**) and *COL2A1* (**C**) fold of expression in chitosan and hyaluronic acid empty nano particles (NPs) or clodronate embedded nanoparticles in chindrogenic medium with or w/o ILβ1. The synergistic action of NPs and clodronate is noteworthy. * $p < 0.05$; ** $p < 0.01$.

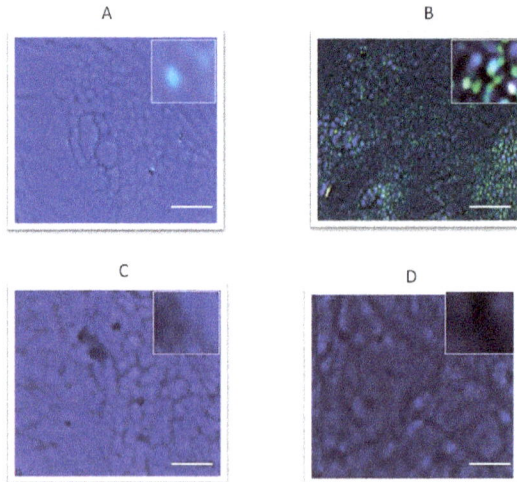

Figure 3. Alcian blue staining. After 21 days of culture, cells were fixed and stained with alcian blue in order to evaluate GAGs production. Control (**A**), cells treated with GFP nanoparticles alone (**B**); in the presence of ILβ1 (**C**); clodronate embedded NPs in the presence of ILβ1 (**D**). Scale bar 150 μm; insert 80×.

3. Discussion

Recent hypotheses regarding the pathogenesis of osteoarthritis have confirmed that subchondral bone alterations, including osteoporosis areas, appear at an early stage of the disease, influence its evolution, and are also associated to cartilage damage [1]. Moreover, these signs also occur in other bone diseases characterized by an excessive bone resorption. Pro-inflammatory cytokines, such as TNFα and IL1β, aggravate cartilage erosion due to the secretion of MMPs and other factors which destroy articular tissues and to the inhibition of progenitor cells differentiation into mature chondrocytes [27]. Articular pain depends on sinovitis which is related to macrophage inflammatory activity and bone marrow lesions, consequent to excessive bone resorption [15]. Clodronate (as other NN-BFs), with its antiresorptive and anti-inflammatory action, appears therefore an ideal candidate for osteoarthritis therapy, possibly capable of influencing the natural history of this disease. Clodronate also exerts, through its interaction with purinergic receptors on chondrocyte surface, an anabolic function on this cellular type, enhancing ECM components secretion [28].

Thus, in our study, we evaluated for the first time the in vivo and in vitro effects of clodronate on peripheral blood MSCs differentiation. We also evaluated its influence on bone metabolism, osteoarticular pain, mental and physical performance.

Our outcomes demonstrated, for the first time, that intramuscular 200 mg clodronate weekly assumption stimulates in vivo MSCs maturation toward the chondrogenic lineage. Clodronate strongly increased SOX9 expression after three and six months treatment, compared to patients' basal value. In addition, after six months of treatment, patients' *SOX9* and *COL2A1* expression exceeded NDs'. Transcription factor *SOX9* induces mesenchymal cells differentiation into chondrocytes, upregulating specific chondrogenic genes such as *COL2A1* [29]. Clodronate also exerts analgesic effects. NRS pain scale showed a significant decrease at the end of treatment in both groups. Bivariate correlations also evidenced direct concordance between mean ISF scores and mean 25 hydroxyvitamin D levels, suggesting that the hormone influences physical performance. Several studies have demonstrated that higher hormone levels enhance physical performance and strength in the elderly [30].

Clodronate, as other bisphosphonates, inhibits bone resorption since the first months of assumption: this is confirmed by the significant decrease in CTX values after six months, compared to basal values. We also recall that 25 hydroxyvitamin D mean levels did not change noticeably during our study, and constantly remained above the insufficiency cut-off (20 ng/mL): we can therefore state that SF36, VAS and NRS outcomes are not influenced by the hormone blood levels. Our results also confirmed that short-term clodronate therapy does not affect renal function: serum creatinin did not increase significantly after six months of drug assumption.

In order to analyze the molecular effects of clodronate in an OA in vitro model, we cultured a human MSC line with IL1β, an inflammatory cytokine involved in OA pathogenesis [31]. Interestingly, our data confirmed the chondrogenic differentiation induced by clodronate observed in CPCs obtained from treated patients. In fact, *SOX9* gene expression increased significantly in a dose-dependent manner in cells treated with clodronate. This effect was observed even in co-occurrence with IL1β. Clodronate, alone or embedded in nanoparticles, was able to stimulate the condrogenic maturation, proven by the alcian blue staining data.

These outcomes strengthen the idea that clodronate stimulates chondrogenic differentiation of precursors and may hinder effectively the pathogenesis and progression mechanisms of OA.

In addition, our finding that clodronate embedded in NPs may increase further SOX9 expression stimulates the search for new therapeutical strategies against osteoarthritis. Due to its multiple mechanisms of action over all the different pathways involved in OA pathogenesis, clodronate appears an ideal candidate for new therapies against this condition. However, additional studies are necessary in order to verify whether clodronate is able to influence osteoarthritis natural history.

4. Patients, Materials and Methods

4.1. Subjects

Written informed consent was obtained from all participants and the study was approved by the Ethical Committee of Azienda Ospedaliera Universitaria Integrata of Verona, Italy (number 1538, 3 December 2012).

We selected 23 female patients, (age: 60–83 years), recruited through the Veneto's Specialistic Regional Center for Skeletal and Degenerative Diseases. Patients were treated with clodronate I.M. 200 mg weekly. All subjects were affected by spondiloarthritis evaluated by dorso-lumbar X-rays. All patients at entry were administered Dibase 100,000 UI, once a month.

Exclusion criteria were: any cause of secondary osteoporosis, antiresorptive therapy (e.g., bisphosphonates, strontium ranelate, denosumab), in the previous 12 months, bone metabolism modifying drugs, (e.g., statins or tiazidics), vitamin D insufficiency (<20 ng/mL), NSAIDs, hormonal replacement therapy, smoking, alcoholism, vertebral fractures (defined with Genant criterias at the morphometric evaluation of spine).

The Control group consisted of 5 healthy females (age: 25–30 years, height 154 ± 3.2 cm, weight 63.4 ± 4.2 kg, BMI 26.7 kg/m^2). All subjects were in the bone mass peak age. Exclusion criterias were: any cause of primary or secondary osteoporosis and osteoarthritis.

Three blood samples were obtained by venipuncture from each patient at three different time points named M0 (before treatment), M3 and M6 (after 3 and 6 months, respectively, of treatment). circulating progenitor cells (CPCs) were isolated from each blood sample. At the same time, VAS, NRS and SF36 surveys were completed by each participant. Two additional blood samples were obtained from each subject at the beginning (M0) and at the end of the study (M6) for bone metabolism parameters evaluation. We quantified serum blood calcium, PTH, 25 hydroxyvitamin D, CTX (C-terminal peptide of collagen type I) serum creatinin and urinary calcium excretion rate levels in order to exclude secondary osteoporosis causes and to evaluate therapy influences on their expression at the end of study. M0 and M6 average scores were calculated for each bone metabolism index. Outcomes are expressed as mean $\pm$ standard deviation.

Control group subjects, upon written consent, were submitted to a single venipuncture in basal conditions (M0) for the isolation of CPCs. Results were calculated both for the entire study population and for patients aged ≥ 70 alone (6 subjects). We considered this subgroup as electively representative of OA affected people, since the disease incidence peak falls after age 70.

4.2. VAS, NRS, SF36 Surveys

Each patient completed anonymously the three surveys at each time point (M0, M3, M6). VAS and NRS surveys evidenced osteoarticular pain scores: in VAS, we asked patients to position a cross sign-according to the gravity of their symptoms, within a line spanning from no pain to high intensity pain. In NRS, patients were asked to associate a number to their pain, in a 0–10 points scale. SF36 survey instead consisted of a list of questions about life quality. We obtained also scores about mental and physical performance (ISM and ISF, respectively). At the end of treatment, we calculated M0, M3 and M6 average scores for VAS and NRS pain scales, ISM and ISF indexes. All results were expressed as mean $\pm$ standard deviation.

4.3. Circulating Progenitor Cells (CPCs)

CPCs were isolated from 50 mL of heparinized blood using two Ficoll procedures to deplete hematopoietic cells by antibodies cocktail, as previously reported [32,33]. The enriched cells obtained were washed in phosphate-buffered saline (PBS) and phenotype analysis was performed as previously described [33]. Then, CPCs were analyzed for gene expression.

4.4. Chondrogenic Differentiation of Mesenchymal Stem Cells

We used hMSCs (PromoCell) to analyze the effects of clodronate, alone or embedded in nanoparticles, on chondrogenic differentiation. We chose commercial MSCs in order to avoid confounding effects of different circulating growth factors as well as cytokines. Cells were plated at a density of 5×10^4 cells per well into 48-well plates in chondrogenic differentiation medium (DMEM, with 100 nM dexamethasone, 200 umol ascorbic acid and 10 ng/mL TGF β), for 21 days at 37 °C in humidified atmosphere with 5% CO_2. Medium was changed every 2 days.

4.5. Nanoparticles Synthesis

Bisphosphonate nanoparticles were prepared using chitosan and hyaluronic acid applying the ionotropic gelation method. 600 µg of clodronate were dissolved in 0.6 ml of distilled water and added to 100 mL of chitosan solution (100 µg/mL in acetic acid 1% pH 5) under magnetic stirring for 20 min. 30 mL of hyaluronic acid solution (115.2 µg/mL in 100 mM acetic acid pH 5) were added dropwise to the emulsion under stirring for 1 hour to enable complete stabilization of the system.

Green fluorescent protein (GFP) embedded nanoparticles, were prepared with the same protocol substituting clodronate with 1 mg of GFP. Finally, all nanoparticles (NPs) were divided into aliquots and lyophilized.

The nanoparticles mean size and zeta potential were estimated using the dynamic light scattering (DLS) technique (Nano ZetaSizer ZS, ZEN3600, Malvern Instruments, Malvern, Worcestershire, UK), re-suspending the synthesized NPs in PBS buffer (137 mM NaCl, 2.7 mM KCl, 10 mM Na_2HPO_4 and 1.8 mM KH_2PO_4) at the final concentration of 5 mg/mL with the sample cell temperature fixed at 25 °C.

The encapsulation efficiency was calculated from a clodronate UV absorbance calibration curve prepared with different amounts of the drug dissolved in an aqueous solution containing 1.5 mM $CuSO_4$ and 1.5 mM HNO_3 at pH 3. Absorbance was recorded at 261 nm using empty nanoparticles absorbance as basic correction [34].

4.6. In Vitro Treatments

Six different combinations of supplements were added to the cell cultures during chondrogenic differentiation. In detail: IL1β alone, NPs alone, Clodronate 50 nM, NPs + IL1β, Clodronate 100 nM, IL1β + Clodronate 50 nM, IL1β + Clodronate 100 nM, IL1β + Clodronate-embedded nanoparticles 100 nM. Noteworthy, IL1β, an inflammatory cytokine, was added in order to mimic OA conditions as previously reported [31]. Cultures without supplements were taken as controls. Three independent experiments were performed for each condition.

4.7. Total RNA Extraction

Total RNA was extracted from each cell pellet using the RNA assay Minikit (Quiagen, Hilden, Germany) with DNAse I treatment. The amount of extracted RNA was quantified by measuring the absorbance at 260 nm. The purity of RNA was checked by measuring the ratio of the absorbance at 260 and 280 nm, where a ratio ranging from 1.8 to 2.0 was taken to be pure.

4.8. Reverse Transcription

First-strand cDNA was generated, according to the manufacturer's protocol, using the First Strand cDNA Synthesis Kit (GE Healthcare, Little Chalfont, UK), with random hexamers, reverse transcriptase and 4 dNTPs. 1 µg RNA was employed in each reaction.

4.9. Real Time RT-PCR

PCR was performed in a total volume of 50 µL containing $1\times$ Taqman Universal PCR Master Mix, no AmpErase UNG and 5 µL of cDNA from each sample; pre-designed *SOX9*-specific primers and probe set was obtained from Assay-on-Demand Gene Expression (Thermofisher Corporation,

Waltham, MA, USA). Real Time RT-PCR reactions were carried out in multiplex. The real-time amplifications included 10 min at 95 °C, followed by 40 cycles at 95 °C for 15 s and at 60 °C for 1 min. Thermocycling and signal detection were performed with ABI Prism 7300 Sequence Detector. Signals were detected according to the manufacturer's instructions. *SOX9* gene expression levels during chondrogenic differentiation were calculated in triplicate for each sample after normalization against the housekeeping genes (β_2 microglobulin and GADPH), using the relative fold expression differences. Average C_t value was used to calculate the relative mRNA expression levels of the PCR targets, using the comparative C_t method with the equation: relative expression = $2^{-[Ct\,(target)\,-\,Ct\,(reference\,gene)]} \times 100$.

4.10. Ct DATA

C_t values for each reaction were determined using TaqMan SDS analysis software. For each amount of RNA tested triplicate C_t values were averaged. Since C_t values vary linearly with the logarithm of the amount of RNA, this average represents a geometric mean.

4.11. ddPCR

In order to analyze the expression of COL2A1, which is scarcely expressed in CPCs, we performed the digital droplet PCR (ddPCR). 5 µL of RNA samples (0.2 ng/µL) were added to 10 µL of ddPCR supermix for no UTP probes, and to 1 µL of COL2A1 TaqMan probe (Applied Biosystems). The mix was applied to QX200 droplet generator (BioRad, Hercules, CA, USA) with 70 µL of oil. Droplets were transferred into a 96 well plate and heat-sealed with tinfoil sheet. Thermocycling conditions were as follows: pre-incubation at 95 °C for 10 min, amplification at 95 °C for 30 s, annealing at 60 °C for 1 min, for 40 cycles, heat inactivation at 98 °C for 10 min. Plates containing droplets were placed in a QX200 droplet reader, which analyses droplets individually, through a two color detection system (FAM and VIC). Results were processed by QuantaSoft (BioRad) according to the manufacturer's instructions.

4.12. Alcian Blue Staining

Alcian blue staining was performed as previously reported [35]. Briefly, after 21 days of culture, the cell slides were fixed with 95% methanol and then stained with 1% Alcian blue 8GX HCl overnight. Subsequently, cell slides were gently washed and observed under microscope.

4.13. Statistic Analysis

Statistical analyses were performed using SPSS 21.0 for Windows operative system. For multiple comparisons, statistical analysis was assessed by one-way ANOVA. Results were expressed as mean ± standard deviation.

5. Conclusions

We conclude that clodronate assumption, over a six-month period, stimulated significantly in vivo MSCs differentiation toward the chondrogenic lineage. This drug also reduced osteoarticular pain, improved mental and physical performance and, according to other studies, also diminished bone resorption after the first months of assumption. Finally, clodronate stimulated, in a dose dependent manner, chondrogenic differentiation of MSCs also in vitro and we demonstrated that it can counteract the inflammatory inhibition of chondrogenic differentiation.

Acknowledgments: We thank Abiogen Pharma and Chiesi Farmaceutici for supporting the study.

Author Contributions: Luca Dalle Carbonare and Maria Teresa Valenti conceived and designed the experiments; Alessandro Biotti, Samuele Cheri and Michela Deiana performed the experiments; Massimiliano Perduca conceived and supervised the nanoparticles synthesis; Michele Bovi and Arianna Pisani conceived and performed the nanoparticle synthesis and characterization; Monica Mottes and Luca Dalle Carbonare analyzed the data; Monica Mottes and Maria Teresa Valenti wrote the paper.

Conflicts of Interest: The authors declare no conflict of interest.

References

1. Kirwan, J.R.; Silman, A.J. Epidemiological, sociological and environmental aspects of rheumatoid arthritis and osteoarthrosis. *Bailliere's Clin. Rheumatol.* **1987**, *1*, 467–489. [CrossRef]
2. Buchanan, W.W.; Kean, W.F.; Kean, R. History and current status of osteoarthritis in the population. *Inflammopharmacology* **2003**, *11*, 301–316. [CrossRef] [PubMed]
3. Rai, M.F.; Sandell, L.J. Inflammatory mediators: Tracing links between obesity and osteoarthritis. *Crit. Rev. Eukaryot. Gene Expr.* **2011**, *21*, 131–142. [CrossRef] [PubMed]
4. Ding, C.; Martel-Pelletier, J.; Pelletier, J.P.; Abram, F.; Raynauld, J.P.; Cicuttini, F.; Jones, G. Meniscal tear as an osteoarthritis risk factor in a largely non-osteoarthritic cohort: A cross-sectional study. *J. Rheumatol.* **2007**, *34*, 776–784. [PubMed]
5. Wang, M.; Ketheesan, N.; Peng, Z. Investigations of wear particles and selected cytokines in human osteoarthritic knee joints. *Proc. Inst. Mech. Eng. Part H J. Eng. Med.* **2014**, *228*, 1176–1182. [CrossRef] [PubMed]
6. Tanamas, S.K.; Wluka, A.E.; Pelletier, J.P.; Martel-Pelletier, J.; Abram, F.; Wang, Y.; Cicuttini, F.M. The association between subchondral bone cysts and tibial cartilage volume and risk of joint replacement in people with knee osteoarthritis: A longitudinal study. *Arthritis Res. Ther.* **2010**, *12*, R58. [CrossRef] [PubMed]
7. Zanetti, M.; Bruder, E.; Romero, J.; Hodler, J. Bone marrow edema pattern in osteoarthritic knees: Correlation between MR imaging and histologic findings. *Radiology* **2000**, *215*, 835–840. [CrossRef] [PubMed]
8. Lin, J.H. Bisphosphonates: A review of their pharmacokinetic properties. *Bone* **1996**, *18*, 75–85. [CrossRef]
9. Rogers, M.J.; Crockett, J.C.; Coxon, F.P.; Monkkonen, J. Biochemical and molecular mechanisms of action of bisphosphonates. *Bone* **2011**, *49*, 34–41. [CrossRef] [PubMed]
10. Ghinoi, V.; Brandi, M.L. Clodronate: Mechanisms of action on bone remodelling and clinical use in osteometabolic disorders. *Expert Opin. Pharmacother.* **2002**, *3*, 1643–1656. [CrossRef] [PubMed]
11. Reszka, A.A.; Rodan, G.A. Mechanism of action of bisphosphonates. *Curr. Osteoporos. Rep.* **2003**, *1*, 45–52. [CrossRef] [PubMed]
12. Luckman, S.P.; Hughes, D.E.; Coxon, F.P.; Graham, R.; Russell, G.; Rogers, M.J. Nitrogen-containing bisphosphonates inhibit the mevalonate pathway and prevent post-translational prenylation of GTP-binding proteins, including Ras. *J. Bone Miner. Res.* **1998**, *13*, 581–589. [CrossRef] [PubMed]
13. Hewitt, R.E.; Lissina, A.; Green, A.E.; Slay, E.S.; Price, D.A.; Sewell, A.K. The bisphosphonate acute phase response: Rapid and copious production of proinflammatory cytokines by peripheral blood γδ T cells in response to aminobisphosphonates is inhibited by statins. *Clin. Exp. Immunol.* **2005**, *139*, 101–111. [CrossRef] [PubMed]
14. Rogers, M.J. New insights into the molecular mechanisms of action of bisphosphonates. *Curr. Pharm. Des.* **2003**, *9*, 2643–2658. [CrossRef] [PubMed]
15. Frith, J.C.; Monkkonen, J.; Auriola, S.; Monkkonen, H.; Rogers, M.J. The molecular mechanism of action of the antiresorptive and antiinflammatory drug clodronate: Evidence for the formation in vivo of a metabolite that inhibits bone resorption and causes osteoclast and macrophage apoptosis. *Arthritis Rheumatol.* **2001**, *44*, 2201–2210. [CrossRef]
16. Dombrecht, E.J.; Schuerwegh, A.J.; Bridts, C.H.; Ebo, D.G.; Offel, J.V.; Stevens, W.J.; Clerck, L.D. Effect of bisphosphonates on nitric oxide production by inflammatory activated chondrocytes. *Clin. Exp. Rheumatol.* **2007**, *25*, 817–822. [PubMed]
17. Makkonen, N.; Salminen, A.; Rogers, M.J.; Frith, J.C.; Urtti, A.; Azhayeva, E.; Mönkkönen, J. Contrasting effects of alendronate and clodronate on RAW 264 macrophages: The role of a bisphosphonate metabolite. *Eur. J. Pharm. Sci.* **1999**, *8*, 109–118. [CrossRef]
18. Matsuo, A.; Shuto, T.; Hirata, G.; Satoh, H.; Matsumoto, Y.; Zhao, H.; Iwamoto, Y. Antiinflammatory and chondroprotective effects of the aminobisphosphonate incadronate (YM175) in adjuvant induced arthritis. *J. Rheumatol.* **2003**, *30*, 1280–1290. [PubMed]
19. Barrera, P.; Blom, A.; van Lent, P.L.; Van Bloois, L.; Beijnen, J.H.; Van Rooijen, N.; De Waal Malefijt, M.C.; Van De Putte, L.; Storm, G.; Van Den Berg, W.B. Synovial macrophage depletion with clodronate-containing liposomes in rheumatoid arthritis. *Arthritis Rheumatol.* **2000**, *43*, 1951–1959. [CrossRef]

20. Rossini, M.; Viapiana, O.; Ramonda, R.; Bianchi, G.; Olivieri, I.; Lapadula, G.; Adami, S. Intra-articular clodronate for the treatment of knee osteoarthritis: Dose ranging study vs. hyaluronic acid. *Rheumatology* **2009**, *48*, 773–778. [CrossRef] [PubMed]
21. Oizumi, T.; Yamaguchi, K.; Funayama, H.; Kuroishi, T.; Kawamura, H.; Sugawara, S.; Endo, Y. Necrotic actions of nitrogen-containing bisphosphonates and their inhibition by clodronate, a non-nitrogen-containing bisphosphonate in mice: Potential for utilization of clodronate as a combination drug with a nitrogen-containing bisphosphonate. *Basic Clin. Pharmacol. Toxicol.* **2009**, *104*, 384–392. [CrossRef] [PubMed]
22. Bi, W.; Deng, J.M.; Zhang, Z.; Behringer, R.R.; de Crombrugghe, B. SOX9 is required for cartilage formation. *Nat. Genet.* **1999**, *22*, 85–89. [PubMed]
23. Ng, L.J.; Wheatley, S.; Muscat, G.E.; Conway-Campbell, J.; Bowles, J.; Wright, E.; Bell, D.M.; Tam, P.P.; Cheah, K.S.; Koopman, P. SOX9 binds DNA, activates transcription, and coexpresses with type II collagen during chondrogenesis in the mouse. *Dev. Biol.* **1997**, *183*, 108–121. [CrossRef] [PubMed]
24. Yoon, B.S.; Ovchinnikov, D.A.; Yoshii, I.; Mishina, Y.; Behringer, R.R.; Lyons, K.M. Bmpr1a and Bmpr1b have overlapping functions and are essential for chondrogenesis in vivo. *Proc. Natl. Acad. Sci. USA* **2005**, *102*, 5062–5067. [CrossRef] [PubMed]
25. Leung, V.Y.; Gao, B.; Leung, K.K.; Melhado, I.G.; Wynn, S.L.; Au, T.Y.; Dung, N.W.; Lau, J.Y.; Mak, A.C.; Chan, D.; et al. *SOX9* governs differentiation stage-specific gene expression in growth plate chondrocytes via direct concomitant transactivation and repression. *PLoS Genet.* **2011**, *7*, e1002356. [CrossRef] [PubMed]
26. Remya, N.S.; Nair, P.D. Engineering cartilage tissue interfaces using a natural glycosaminoglycan hydrogel matrix—An in vitro study. *Mater. Sci. Eng. C Mater. Biol. Appl.* **2013**, *33*, 575–582. [CrossRef] [PubMed]
27. Stannus, O.; Jones, G.; Cicuttini, F.; Parameswaran, V.; Quinn, S.; Burgess, J.; Ding, C. Circulating levels of IL-6 and TNF-alpha are associated with knee radiographic osteoarthritis and knee cartilage loss in older adults. *Osteoarthr. Cartil.* **2010**, *18*, 1441–1447. [CrossRef] [PubMed]
28. Pingguan-Murphy, B.; El-Azzeh, M.; Bader, D.L.; Knight, M.M. Cyclic compression of chondrocytes modulates a purinergic calcium signalling pathway in a strain rate- and frequency-dependent manner. *J. Cell. Physiol.* **2006**, *209*, 389–397. [CrossRef] [PubMed]
29. Takigawa, Y.; Hata, K.; Muramatsu, S.; Amano, K.; Ono, K.; Wakabayashi, M.; Matsuda, A.; Takada, K.; Nishimura, R.; Yoneda, T. The transcription factor Znf219 regulates chondrocyte differentiation by assembling a transcription factory with Sox9. *J. Cell Sci.* **2010**, *123*, 3780–3788. [CrossRef] [PubMed]
30. Ceglia, L.; Harris, S.S. Vitamin D and its role in skeletal muscle. *Calcif. Tissue Int.* **2013**, *92*, 151–162. [CrossRef] [PubMed]
31. Kapoor, M.; Martel-Pelletier, J.; Lajeunesse, D.; Pelletier, J.P.; Fahmi, H. Role of proinflammatory cytokines in the pathophysiology of osteoarthritis. *Nat. Rev. Rheumatol.* **2011**, *7*, 33–42. [CrossRef] [PubMed]
32. Carbonare, L.D.; Valenti, M.T.; Zanatta, M.; Donatelli, L.; Lo Cascio, V. Circulating mesenchymal stem cells with abnormal osteogenic differentiation in patients with osteoporosis. *Arthritis Rheumatol.* **2009**, *60*, 3356–3365. [CrossRef] [PubMed]
33. Dalle Carbonare, L.; Mottes, M.; Malerba, G.; Mori, A.; Zaninotto, M.; Plebani, M.; Dellantonio, A.; Valenti, M.T. Enhanced osteogenic differentiation in zoledronate-treated osteoporotic patients. *Int. J. Mol. Sci.* **2017**, *18*, 1261. [CrossRef] [PubMed]
34. Koba, M.; Koba, K.; Przyborowski, L. Application of UV-derivative spectrophotometry for determination of some bisphosphonates drugs in pharmaceutical formulations. *Acta Pol. Pharm.* **2008**, *65*, 289–294. [PubMed]
35. Newton, P.T.; Staines, K.A.; Spevak, L.; Boskey, A.L.; Teixeira, C.C.; Macrae, V.E.; Canfield, A.E.; Farquharson, C. Chondrogenic ATDC5 cells: An optimised model for rapid and physiological matrix mineralisation. *Int. J. Mol. Med.* **2012**, *30*, 1187–1193. [CrossRef] [PubMed]

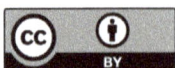

International Journal of
Molecular Sciences

MDPI

Article

Visfatin Promotes IL-6 and TNF-α Production in Human Synovial Fibroblasts by Repressing miR-199a-5p through ERK, p38 and JNK Signaling Pathways

Min-Huan Wu [1,2], Chun-Hao Tsai [3,4], Yuan-Li Huang [5], Yi-Chin Fong [6,7] and Chih-Hsin Tang [3,5,8,*]

1   Physical Education Office, Tunghai University, Taichung 40704, Taiwan; mhwu@thu.edu.tw
2   Sports Recreation and Health Management Continuing Studies, Tunghai University, Taichung 40704, Taiwan
3   School of Medicine, China Medical University, Taichung 40402, Taiwan; ritsai8615@gmail.com
4   Department of Orthopedic Surgery, China Medical University Hospital, Taichung 40402, Taiwan
5   Department of Biotechnology, College of Health Science, Asia University, Taichung 41354, Taiwan; yuanli@asia.edu.tw
6   Department of Sports Medicine, College of Health Care, China Medical University, Taichung 40402, Taiwan; yichin.fong@msa.hinet.net
7   Department of Orthopaedic Surgery, China Medical University Beigang Hospital, Yun-Lin County 65152, Taiwan
8   Graduate Institute of Basic Medical Science, China Medical University, Taichung 40402, Taiwan
*   Correspondence: chtang@mail.cmu.edu.tw; Tel.: +886-2205-2121 (ext. 7726)

Received: 15 December 2017; Accepted: 4 January 2018; Published: 8 January 2018

Abstract: Osteoarthritis (OA), an inflammatory form of arthritis, is characterized by synovial inflammation and cartilage destruction largely influenced by two key proinflammatory cytokines—interleukin-6 (IL-6) and tumor necrosis factor α (TNF-α). Notably, levels of visfatin (a proinflammatory adipokine) are elevated in patients with OA, although the relationship of visfatin to IL-6 and TNF-α expression in OA pathogenesis has been unclear. In this study, visfatin enhanced the expression of IL-6 and TNF-α in human OA synovial fibroblasts (OASFs) in a concentration-dependent manner and stimulation of OASFs with visfatin promoted phosphorylation of extracellular-signal-regulated kinase (ERK), p38, and c-Jun N-terminal kinase (JNK), while ERK, p38, and JNK inhibitors or siRNAs all abolished visfatin-induced increases in IL-6 and TNF-α production. Moreover, transfection with miR-199a-5p mimics reversed visfatin-induced increases in IL-6 and TNF-α production. Furthermore, we also found that visfatin-promoted IL-6 and TNF-α production is mediated via the inhibition of miR-199a-5p expression through the ERK, p38, and JNK signaling pathways. Visfatin may therefore be an appropriate target for drug intervention in OA treatment.

Keywords: visfatin; IL-6; TNF-α; osteoarthritis; miR-199a-5p

---

1. Introduction

Osteoarthritis (OA), a common chronic inflammatory disorder of the synovial joint, is characterized by articular cartilage degradation, cartilage remodeling/degeneration, subchondral sclerosis and osteophyte formation [1–3]. OA patients typically complain of stiffness, muscle weakness and joint pain; the etiology underlying these symptoms remains unclear [4,5]. It is known that an inflammatory reaction promotes the overexpression of macrophage-derived proinflammatory cytokines interleukin 1 β (IL-1β), IL-6 and tumor necrosis factor α (TNF-α) in the synovial membrane, which induces neovascularization and inflammation as well as the production of matrix-degrading enzymes such as matrix metalloproteinases (MMPs) that lead to cartilage degradation [6,7].

IL-6 involves several biological functions and plays a key role in hematopoiesis formation [8], the innate immune response, inflammation and promotes osteoclastogenesis which is recognized as being a critical proinflammatory cytokine in the pathophysiology of OA [9]. Another key proinflammatory cytokine, TNF-α is a potent stimulus of inflammatory responses through the up-regulation of several genes, including those responsible for cytokines, chemokines, proteinases, cyclooxygenase, and adhesion molecules [10,11]. Notably, elevated TNF-α levels are found in human OA synovial fluid [12,13].

Visfatin, a growth factor for B lymphocyte precursors, is a pro-inflammatory adipokine found in the liver, skeletal muscles and bone marrow and produced by visceral white adipose tissue, which mimics the effects of insulin [14]. Serum visfatin levels are increased in patients with OA [15,16]. Reports have highlighted the significant role played by adipocytokines, including visfatin, in mediating joint damage [17,18]. However, the role of visfatin in IL-6 and TNF-α production in osteoarthritis synovial fibroblasts (OASFs) has not been extensively studied. We therefore sought to elucidate the intracellular signaling underlying visfatin-induced IL-6 and TNF-α production in human OASF cells. Our findings show that visfatin promotes IL-6 and TNF-α production by repressing miR-199a-5p expression via the extracellular-signal-regulated kinase (ERK), p38 and c-Jun N-terminal kinase (JNK) signaling pathways. Thus, we suggest that visfatin could be an appropriate target for therapeutic intervention in OA.

2. Results

2.1. Visfatin Promotes IL-6 and TNF-α Expression in Human Osteoarthritis Synovial Fibroblasts (OASFs)

Visfatin levels are significantly higher in synovial fluid from patients with OA compared with healthy controls [17,18]. OA pathology is associated with chronically inflamed synovium, increased levels of inflammatory cells and synovial hyperplasia, as well as fibroblast-like synoviocytes [19]. We therefore used human synovial fibroblasts to investigate which signaling pathways involve visfatin in the production of IL-6 and TNF-α. Treatment of OASFs with visfatin (1–30 ng/mg) for 24 h induced *IL-6* and *TNF-α* mRNA expression in a concentration-dependent manner (Figure 1A). Visfatin also enhanced the protein expression of IL-6 and TNF-α according to Western blot and ELISA analysis (Figure 1B,C). These results indicate that visfatin enhances IL-6 and TNF-α expression in human OASFs.

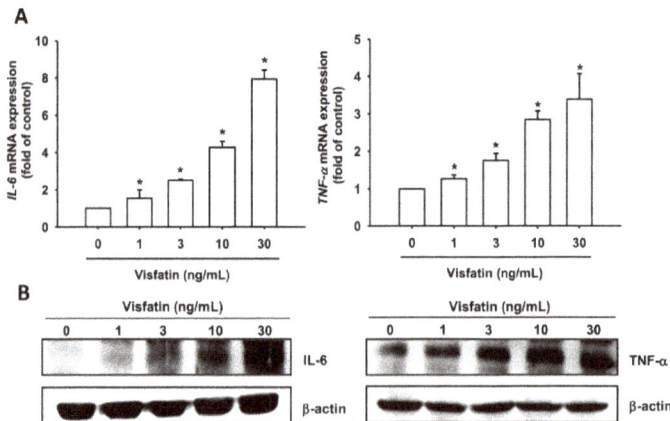

Figure 1. *Cont.*

C

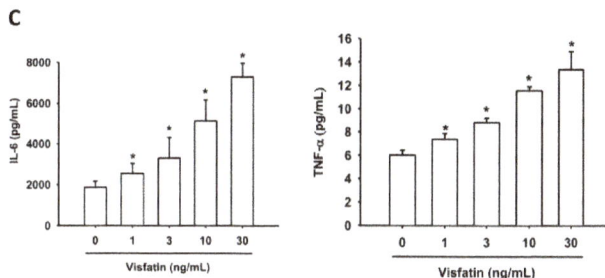

Figure 1. Visfatin induces IL-6 and TNF-α expression in human synovial fibroblasts. Osteoarthritis synovial fibroblasts (OASFs) were incubated with various concentrations of visfatin for 24 h. (**A–C**) IL-6 and TNF-α expression was examined by qPCR, Western blot and ELISA assay. Results are expressed as the mean ± SEM. * $p < 0.05$ as compared with baseline.

2.2. Visfatin Increases IL-6 and TNF-α Expression via the MAPK Signaling Pathway

Previous studies have shown that the mitogen-activated protein kinases (MAPKs), ERK, p38 MAPK and JNK are involved in the regulation of inflammatory cytokine expression [20,21]. We therefore investigated the role of MAPKs in mediating visfatin-induced IL-6 and TNF-α expression, using the specific ERK inhibitor FR180214, p38 inhibitor SB203580, and JNK inhibitor SP600125. Pretreatment of OASFs with these agents blocked visfatin-induced increases in mRNA expression of *IL-6* and *TNF-α* levels (Figure 2A–C, Figure 3A–C and Figure 4A–C). In addition, transfection of OASFs with ERK, p38 and JNK siRNAs markedly inhibited visfatin-enhanced IL-6 and TNF-α production (Figure 2A–C, Figure 3A–C and Figure 4A–C), whereas incubation of OASFs with visfatin promoted ERK, p38 and JNK phosphorylation in a time-dependent manner (Figures 2D, 3D and 4D). Thus, visfatin appears to act through the MAPK signaling pathway to promote IL-6 and TNF-α expression in OASFs.

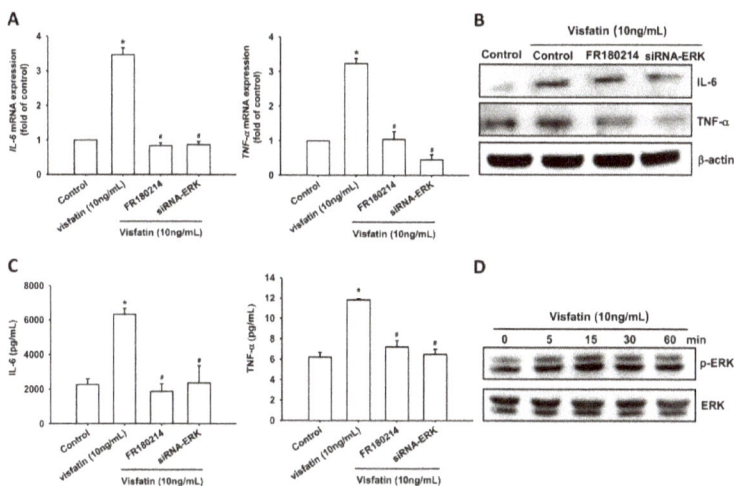

Figure 2. Visfatin induces increases in IL-6 and TNF-α expression through the ERK pathway. (**A–C**) OASFs were pretreated with FR180214 (10 μM) for 30 min or transfected with ERK siRNA for 24 h followed by stimulation with visfatin (30 ng/mL) for 24 h; IL-6 and TNF-α expression was examined by qPCR, Western blot and ELISA assay; (**D**) OASFs were incubated with visfatin for indicated time intervals; ERK phosphorylation was examined by Western blot. Results are expressed as the mean ± SEM. * $p < 0.05$ as compared with baseline. # $p < 0.05$ as compared with the visfatin-treated group.

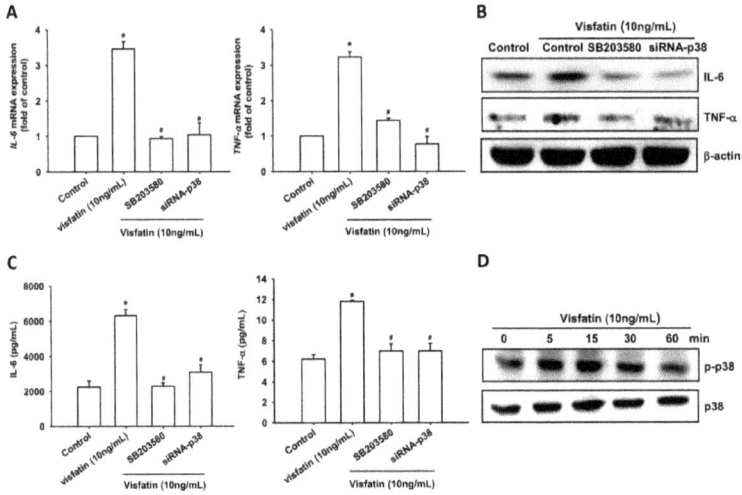

Figure 3. Visfatin induces increases in IL-6 and TNF-α expression through the p38 pathway. (**A–C**) OASFs were pretreated with SB203580 (10 μM) for 30 min or transfected with p38 siRNA for 24 h followed by stimulation with visfatin (30 ng/mL) for 24 h; IL-6 and TNF-α expression was examined by qPCR, Western blot and ELISA assay; (**D**) OASFs were incubated with visfatin for indicated time intervals; p38 phosphorylation was examined by Western blot. Results are expressed as the mean ± S.E.M. * $p < 0.05$ as compared with baseline. # $p < 0.05$ as compared with the visfatin-treated group.

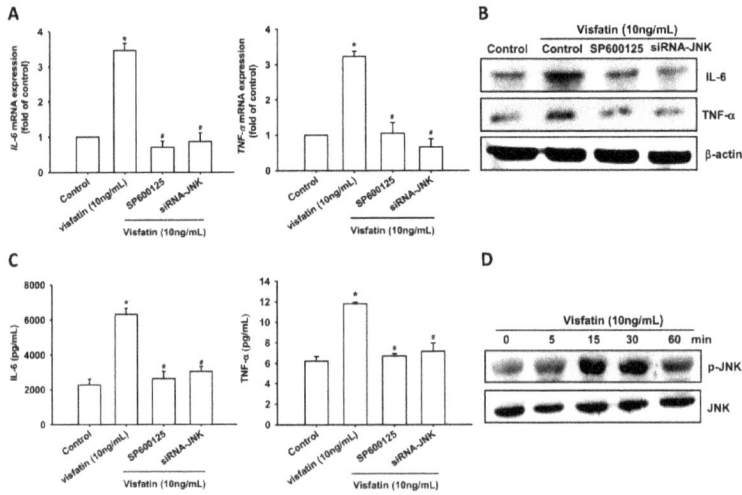

Figure 4. Visfatin induces increases in IL-6 and TNF-α expression through the JNK pathway. (**A–C**) OASFs were pretreated with SP600125 (10 μM) for 30 min or transfected with JNK siRNA for 24 h followed by stimulation with visfatin (30 ng/mL) for 24 h; IL-6 and TNF-α expression was examined by qPCR, Western blot and ELISA assay; (**D**) OASFs were incubated with visfatin for indicated time intervals; JNK phosphorylation was examined by Western blot. Results are expressed as the mean ± SEM. * $p < 0.05$ as compared with baseline. # $p < 0.05$ as compared with the visfatin-treated group.

2.3. Visfatin Increases IL-6 and TNF-α Production in OASFs by Inhibiting miR-199a-5p Expression

miRNAs are important regulators of inflammatory cytokine production [22,23] and have recently been implicated in the control of OA pathogenesis [24–26]. We therefore hypothesized that miRNAs may regulate visfatin-mediated IL-6 and TNF-α expression. Using miRNA target prediction software, we found that the 3′-UTRs of *IL-6* and *TNF-α* mRNAs harbor potential binding sites for miR-199a-5p (Figure 5A). Stimulation of OASFs with visfatin lowered miR-199a-5p expression in a concentration-dependent manner (Figure 5B). Further investigations confirmed the involvement of miR-199a-5p in visfatin-induced increases in IL-6 and TNF-α mRNA and protein expression; miR-199a-5p mimic reversed these increases (Figure 5C–E). Our data suggest that visfatin increases IL-6 and TNF-α production by inhibiting miR-199a-5p expression.

To learn whether miR-199a-5p regulates the 3′-UTRs of *IL-6* and *TNF-α*, we constructed luciferase reporter vectors harboring the wild-type 3′-UTRs of *IL-6* and *TNF-α* mRNAs (IL-6-3′-UTR-wt and TNF-α-3′-UTR-wt) and a vector containing mismatches in the predicted miR-199a-5p binding sites (IL-6-3′-UTR-mut and TNF-α-3′-UTR-mut) (Figure 5F). We found that transfection with the miR-199a-5p mimic antagonized visfatin-induced increases in luciferase activity in the IL-6-3′-UTR-wt and TNF-α-3′-UTR-wt but not in the IL-6-3′-UTR-mut and TNF-α-3′-UTR-mut plasmids (Figure 5G). In addition, treatment with ERK, p38 and JNK inhibitors reversed visfatin-mediated miR-199a-5p expression (Figure 5H). Collectively, these data suggest that miR-199a-5p directly represses IL-6 and TNF-α expression via binding to the 3′-UTR region of the human *IL-6* and *TNF-α* genes through the ERK, p38 and JNK pathways.

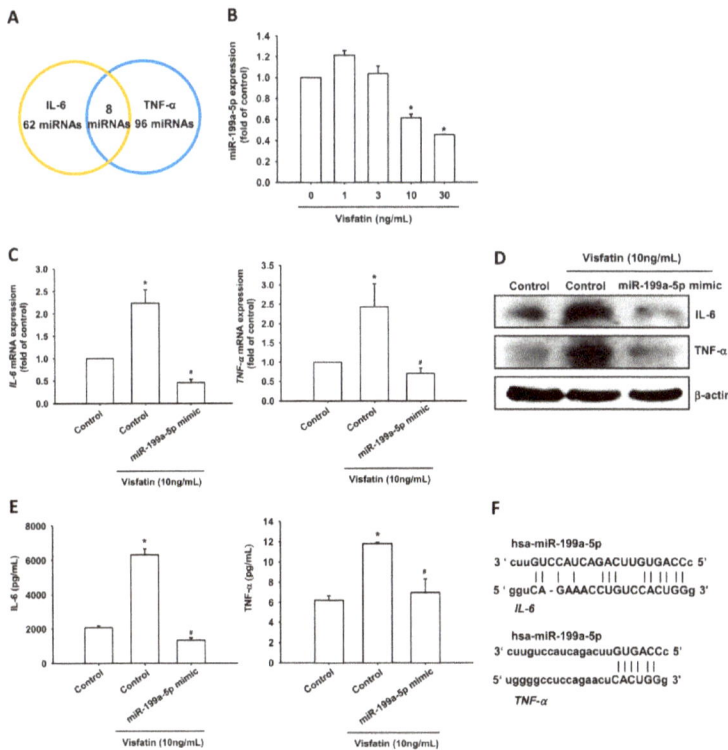

Figure 5. *Cont.*

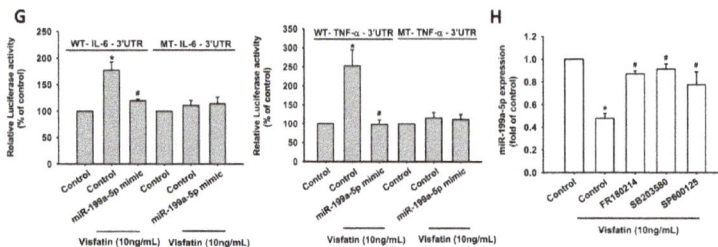

Figure 5. Visfatin increases IL-6 and TNF-α expression via inhibition of miR-199a-5p through the ERK, p38 and JNK signaling pathways. (**A**) Searches of three online computational algorithms (TargetScan, miRWalk and miRanda) for candidate miRNAs that target the IL-6 and TNF-α regions revealed the involvement of miR-199a-5p; (**B**) OASFs were incubated with visfatin for 24 h; miR-199a-5p expression was assessed by qPCR; (**C–E**) OASFs were transfected with miR-199a-5p mimic for 24 h, followed by stimulation with visfatin for 24 h; IL-6 and TNF-α expression was examined by qPCR, Western blot and ELISA assay; (**F**) Schematic 3′-UTR representation of human *IL-6* and *TNF-α* containing the miR-199a-5p binding site; (**G**) OASFs were transfected with indicated luciferase plasmids before incubation with visfatin for 24 h; Luciferase activity was assessed; (**H**) OASFs were pretreated with ERK, p38, and JNK inhibitors for 30 min followed by stimulation with visfatin (30 ng/mL) for 24 h; miR-199a-5p expression was examined by qPCR. Results are expressed as the mean ± SEM. * $p < 0.05$ as compared with baseline. # $p < 0.05$ as compared with the visfatin-treated group.

3. Discussion

It is well established that a complex cytokine network contributes to chronic inflammation of the synovial membrane and the development of disease and cartilage degradation in OA [27]. However, we lack a complete understanding of what factors are responsible for initiating the degradation and loss of articular tissue. While elevated levels of the proinflammatory adipokine, visfatin, are observed in inflammatory diseases, such as OA and rheumatoid arthritis (RA) [28], the molecular mechanisms regulating this inflammatory response are unclear. In this study, we demonstrated that IL-6 and TNF-α are target proteins for the visfatin signaling pathway regulating the cell inflammatory response. Furthermore, we found that visfatin enhances IL-6 and TNF-α production by inhibiting miR-199a-5p via the ERK, p38 and JNK signaling pathways in OASFs. These findings suggest that visfatin enhances proinflammatory cytokines, such as IL-6 and TNF-α, and the inflammatory response. IL-1β is another key proinflammatory cytokine that enhances the production of MMPs leading to cartilage degradation [6,7]. However, we did not examine the role of visfatin in IL-1β and MMPs production in OASFs; this aspect needs further analysis. It is well established that OA chondrocytes produce higher levels of MMP-1, -3 and -13 in comparison with normal chondrocytes [17,29]. Therefore, chondrocyte activity is also an important factor for progression of OA. However, our study did not investigate the role of visfatin in chondrocyte cells; this is another research area that requires further clarification.

The MAPK signaling pathway helps to regulate gene expression levels [30]. Here, we report that the ERK inhibitor FR180214, p38 inhibitor SB203580, and JNK inhibitor SP600125 all antagonized visfatin-induced increases in IL-6 and TNF-α expression. Similar results were seen after OASFs were transfected with ERK, p38 and JNK siRNAs, while stimulation of OASFs with visfatin promoted ERK, p38, and JNK phosphorylation. These results indicate that ERK, p38, and JNK activation mediates visfatin-promoted IL-6 and TNF-α production in OASFs.

miRNAs have been investigated for their role in gene regulation [31]. By binding to mRNA 3′-UTRs, miRNAs can affect many protein-encoding genes at the post-transcriptional level [32]. We therefore sought to determine whether miRNAs are implicated in IL-6 and TNF-α expression following visfatin stimulation. We found that visfatin markedly inhibits miR-199a-5p expression in OASFs. Co-transfection of cells with miR-199a-5p mimic abolished visfatin-induced increases in IL-6 and TNF-α expression. Strikingly, we found that miR-199a-5p directly inhibited IL-6 and TNF-α protein expression through binding to the 3′-UTRs of the human *IL-6* and *TNF-α* genes, thereby negatively regulating visfatin-mediated IL-6 and TNF-α expression. These findings provide insight into potential miRNA-based strategies for visfatin-mediated IL-6 and TNF-α production.

In conclusion, our investigations into the signaling pathway involved in visfatin-induced increases in IL-6 and TNF-α expression in human synovial fibroblasts reveal that visfatin inhibits miR-199a-5p expression through the ERK, p38 and JNK signaling pathways (Figure 6). These findings may provide a better understanding of the mechanisms of OA pathogenesis.

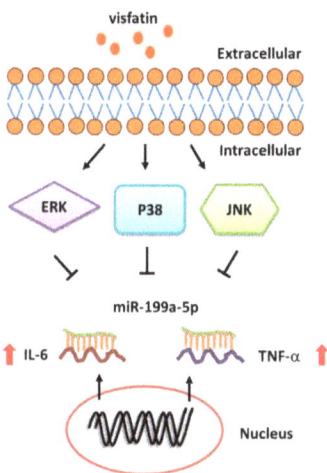

Figure 6. Schema of signaling pathways involved in visfatin-induced increases in IL-6 and TNF-α expression in synovial fibroblasts. Visfatin promotes IL-6 and TNF-α production (red arrows) in human synovial fibroblasts by inhibiting miR-199a-5p expression (T bars) via the ERK, p38 and JNK signaling pathways (black arrows).

4. Materials and Methods

4.1. Materials

We obtained control miRNA, miR-199a-5p mimic and Lipofectamine 2000 from Life Technologies (Carlsbad, CA, USA), rabbit polyclonal antibodies for P-ERK, ERK, P-p38, p38, P-JNK, JNK, TNF-α, IL-6 and β-actin; ERK, p38, JNK and control siRNA were purchased from Santa Cruz Biotechnology (Santa Cruz, CA, USA), recombinant human visfatin was purchased from PeproTech (Rocky Hill, NJ, USA). All other chemicals were purchased from Sigma-Aldrich (St. Louis, MO, USA).

4.2. Cell Culture

Human synovial fibroblasts were obtained from synovial tissue collected from generally healthy OA patients aged 50–75 years undergoing knee replacement surgery. Written approval (CMUH103-REC2-023, 6 May 2014) was obtained from the Institutional Review Board of China Medical University Hospital, Taichung, Taiwan, and also from the patients, prior to sample collection. OASFs were isolated, cultured, and characterized as previously described [33,34]. In vitro experiments were performed using cells from passages 3–6.

Int. J. Mol. Sci. **2018**, *19*, 190

4.3. Measurement of IL-6 and TNF-α

We pretreated human OASFs with various inhibitors for 30 min or transfected the OASFs for 24 h with miRNA mimic or siRNAs prior to visfatin administration. IL-6 and TNF-α in the medium was assayed using IL-6 and TNF-α enzyme immunoassay kits (R&D Systems, Minneapolis, MN, USA), as according to the manufacturer's procedure.

4.4. Real-Time Quantitative PCR of mRNA and miRNA

Total RNA was extracted from OASFs using a TRIzol kit (MDBio, Taipei, Taiwan). Reverse transcription was performed using oligo(dT) primer [35,36]. We used the Taqman® one-step PCR Master Mix (Applied Biosystems, Foster City, CA, USA) to perform real-time quantitative PCR (RT qPCR) analysis; we added 100 ng of total cDNA per 25 μL reaction with sequence-specific primers and Taqman® probes. We purchased sequences for target gene primers and probes from Applied Biosystems (GAPDH was used as the internal control); qPCR assays were carried out in triplicate using the StepOnePlus sequence detection system (Applied Biosystems, Foster City, CA, USA) [37].

For the miRNA assay, we used the TaqMan MicroRNA Reverse Transcription Kit (Applied Biosystems) to synthesize cDNA; reactions were incubated at 16 °C for 30 min, then at 42 °C for 30 min, followed by inactivation at 85 °C for 5 min. All reactions were run using the StepOnePlus sequence detection system. Relative quantification analysis of gene expression was performed with the *U6* gene as an endogenous control. The relative gene expression level was calculated using the comparative C_T method.

4.5. Western Blot Analysis

The cell lysates were resolved by SDS-PAGE [7,38] and transferred to Immobilon polyvinylidene fluoride membranes. We initially blocked blots for 1 h with 4% bovine serum albumin at room temperature, then probed the blots with rabbit anti-human antibodies against P-ERK, ERK, P-p38, p38, P-JNK or JNK (1:1000) for 1 h at room temperature (Santa Cruz Biotechnology, Santa Cruz, CA, USA). After undergoing three washes, blots were incubated secondary antibody (1:1000) visualized using LAS-4000 image reader (FujiFILM, Tokyo, Japan) [39].

4.6. Plasmid Construction and Luciferase Assay

The three prime untranslated region (3′-UTR) of human *IL-6* and *TNF-α* contains a miR-199a-5p binding site. DNA fragments containing wild-type (wt)-IL-6-3′-UTR, mutant-type (mut)-IL-6-3′-UTR, wt-TNF-α-3′-UTR and mut-TNF-α-3′-UTR were purchased from Invitrogen (Carlsbad, CA, USA). The fragments were subcloned into the luciferase reporter vector pmirGLO-control (Promega, Madison, WI, USA), upstream of the vector's promoter. These plasmids were transfected into cells using Lipofectamine 2000. Cell extracts were prepared and used to measure luciferase and β-galactosidase activity.

4.7. Statistical Analysis

The data are expressed as the mean ± SEM. Statistical analysis was performed using GraphPad Prism 4 software (GraphPad Software, La Jolla, CA, USA). One-way analysis of variance (ANOVA) and the unpaired two-tailed Student's *t*-test were used to test for any significant difference in the means. The difference was denoted significant when the *p*-value was less than 0.05.

Acknowledgments: This study was supported by grants from the Ministry of Science and Technology of Taiwan (MOST106-2320-B-029-002-; MOST106-2632-B-029-001-) and China Medical University (CMU106-ASIA-03).

Author Contributions: Min-Huan Wu and Chih-Hsin Tang conceived and designed the experiments; Min-Huan Wu, Chun-Hao Tsai, Yuan-Li Huang and Yi-Chin Fong performed the experiments; Min-Huan Wu, Chun-Hao Tsai, Yuan-Li Huang and Yi-Chin Fong analyzed the data; Chun-Hao Tsai, Yuan-Li Huang and Yi-Chin Fong contributed reagents/materials/analysis tools; Chih-Hsin Tang wrote the paper.

Conflicts of Interest: The authors declare no conflict of interest.

References

1. Bresnihan, B. Pathogenesis of joint damage in rheumatoid arthritis. *J. Rheumatol.* **1999**, *26*, 717–719. [PubMed]
2. Grossman, J.M.; Brahn, E. Rheumatoid arthritis: Current clinical and research directions. *J. Women Health* **1997**, *6*, 627–638. [CrossRef]
3. Altman, R.; Asch, E.; Bloch, D.; Bole, G.; Borenstein, D.; Brandt, K.; Christy, W.; Cooke, T.D.; Greenwald, R.; Hochberg, M.; et al. Development of criteria for the classification and reporting of osteoarthritis. Classification of osteoarthritis of the knee. Diagnostic and therapeutic criteria committee of the american rheumatism association. *Arthritis Rheumatol.* **1986**, *29*, 1039–1049.
4. Bai, T.; Chen, C.C.; Lau, L.F. Matricellular protein CCN1 activates a proinflammatory genetic program in murine macrophages. *J. Immunol.* **2010**, *184*, 3223–3232. [CrossRef] [PubMed]
5. Barksby, H.E.; Hui, W.; Wappler, I.; Peters, H.H.; Milner, J.M.; Richards, C.D.; Cawston, T.E.; Rowan, A.D. Interleukin-1 in combination with oncostatin M up-regulates multiple genes in chondrocytes: Implications for cartilage destruction and repair. *Arthritis Rheumatol.* **2006**, *54*, 540–550. [CrossRef] [PubMed]
6. Goldring, S.R.; Goldring, M.B. The role of cytokines in cartilage matrix degeneration in osteoarthritis. *Clin. Orthop. Relat. Res.* **2004**, S27–S36. [CrossRef]
7. Tang, C.H.; Hsu, C.J.; Fong, Y.C. The CCL5/CCR5 axis promotes interleukin-6 production in human synovial fibroblasts. *Arthritis Rheumatol.* **2010**, *62*, 3615–3624. [CrossRef] [PubMed]
8. Livshits, G.; Zhai, G.; Hart, D.J.; Kato, B.S.; Wang, H.; Williams, F.M.; Spector, T.D. Interleukin-6 is a significant predictor of radiographic knee osteoarthritis: The chingford study. *Arthritis Rheumatol.* **2009**, *60*, 2037–2045. [CrossRef] [PubMed]
9. Honsawek, S.; Deepaisarnsakul, B.; Tanavalee, A.; Yuktanandana, P.; Bumrungpanichthaworn, P.; Malila, S.; Saetan, N. Association of the IL-6 −174G/C gene polymorphism with knee osteoarthritis in a thai population. *Genet. Mol. Res.* **2011**, *10*, 1674–1680. [CrossRef] [PubMed]
10. Tracey, K.J.; Cerami, A. Tumor necrosis factor, other cytokines and disease. *Annu. Rev. Cell Biol.* **1993**, *9*, 317–343. [CrossRef] [PubMed]
11. Liang, C.J.; Wang, S.H.; Chen, Y.H.; Chang, S.S.; Hwang, T.L.; Leu, Y.L.; Tseng, Y.C.; Li, C.Y.; Chen, Y.L. Viscolin reduces vcam-1 expression in TNF-α-treated endothelial cells via the JNK/NF-κB and ROS pathway. *Free Radic. Biol. Med.* **2011**, *51*, 1337–1346. [CrossRef] [PubMed]
12. Di Giovine, F.S.; Nuki, G.; Duff, G.W. Tumour necrosis factor in synovial exudates. *Ann. Rheumatol. Dis.* **1988**, *47*, 768–772. [CrossRef]
13. Saxne, T.; Palladino, M.A., Jr.; Heinegard, D.; Talal, N.; Wollheim, F.A. Detection of tumor necrosis factor α but not tumor necrosis factor β in rheumatoid arthritis synovial fluid and serum. *Arthritis Rheumatol.* **1988**, *31*, 1041–1045. [CrossRef]
14. Tilg, H.; Moschen, A.R. Adipocytokines: Mediators linking adipose tissue, inflammation and immunity. *Nat. Rev. Immunol.* **2006**, *6*, 772–783. [CrossRef] [PubMed]
15. Liao, L.; Chen, Y.; Wang, W. The current progress in understanding the molecular functions and mechanisms of visfatin in osteoarthritis. *J. Bone Miner. Metab.* **2016**, *34*, 485–490. [CrossRef] [PubMed]
16. Fioravanti, A.; Giannitti, C.; Cheleschi, S.; Simpatico, A.; Pascarelli, N.A.; Galeazzi, M. Circulating levels of adiponectin, resistin, and visfatin after mud-bath therapy in patients with bilateral knee osteoarthritis. *Int. J. Biometeorol.* **2015**, *59*, 1691–1700. [CrossRef] [PubMed]
17. Tong, K.M.; Chen, C.P.; Huang, K.C.; Shieh, D.C.; Cheng, H.C.; Tzeng, C.Y.; Chen, K.H.; Chiu, Y.C.; Tang, C.H. Adiponectin increases MMP-3 expression in human chondrocytes through adipor1 signaling pathway. *J. Cell. Biochem.* **2011**, *112*, 1431–1440. [CrossRef] [PubMed]
18. Su, C.M.; Lee, W.L.; Hsu, C.J.; Lu, T.T.; Wang, L.H.; Xu, G.H.; Tang, C.H. Adiponectin induces oncostatin M expression in osteoblasts through the PI3K/AKT signaling pathway. *Int. J. Mol. Sci.* **2016**, *17*, 29. [CrossRef] [PubMed]
19. Sokolove, J.; Lepus, C.M. Role of inflammation in the pathogenesis of osteoarthritis: Latest findings and interpretations. *Ther. Adv. Musculoskelet. Dis.* **2013**, *5*, 77–94. [CrossRef] [PubMed]
20. Chen, C.Y.; Fuh, L.J.; Huang, C.C.; Hsu, C.J.; Su, C.M.; Liu, S.C.; Lin, Y.M.; Tang, C.H. Enhancement of CCL2 expression and monocyte migration by CCN1 in osteoblasts through inhibiting miR-518a-5p: Implication of rheumatoid arthritis therapy. *Sci. Rep.* **2017**, *7*, 421. [CrossRef] [PubMed]

21. Hsiao, Y.C.; Yeh, M.H.; Chen, Y.J.; Liu, J.F.; Tang, C.H.; Huang, W.C. Lapatinib increases motility of triple-negative breast cancer cells by decreasing miRNA-7 and inducing RAF-1/MAPK-dependent interleukin-6. *Oncotarget* **2015**, *6*, 37965–37978. [CrossRef] [PubMed]

22. He, X.; Jing, Z.; Cheng, G. MicroRNAs: New regulators of Toll-like receptor signalling pathways. *BioMed Res. Int.* **2014**, *2014*, 945169. [CrossRef] [PubMed]

23. Xiao, L.; Liu, Y.; Wang, N. New paradigms in inflammatory signaling in vascular endothelial cells. *Am. J. Physiol. Heart Circ. Physiol.* **2014**, *306*, H317–H325. [CrossRef] [PubMed]

24. Santini, P.; Politi, L.; Vedova, P.D.; Scandurra, R.; Scotto d'Abusco, A. The inflammatory circuitry of miR-149 as a pathological mechanism in osteoarthritis. *Rheumatol. Int.* **2014**, *34*, 711–716. [CrossRef] [PubMed]

25. Budd, E.; Waddell, S.; de Andres, M.C.; Oreffo, R.O.C. The potential of microRNAs for stem cell-based therapy for degenerative skeletal diseases. *Curr. Mol. Biol. Rep.* **2017**, *3*, 263–275. [CrossRef] [PubMed]

26. McAlinden, A.; Im, G.I. Micrornas in orthopaedic research: Disease associations, potential therapeutic applications, and perspectives. *J. Orthop. Res. Soc.* **2017**. [CrossRef] [PubMed]

27. Liu, J.F.; Hou, S.M.; Tsai, C.H.; Huang, C.Y.; Yang, W.H.; Tang, C.H. Thrombin induces heme oxygenase-1 expression in human synovial fibroblasts through protease-activated receptor signaling pathways. *Arthritis Res. Ther.* **2012**, *14*, R91. [CrossRef] [PubMed]

28. Otero, M.; Lago, R.; Gomez, R.; Lago, F.; Dieguez, C.; Gomez-Reino, J.J.; Gualillo, O. Changes in plasma levels of fat-derived hormones adiponectin, leptin, resistin and visfatin in patients with rheumatoid arthritis. *Ann. Rheumatol. Dis.* **2006**, *65*, 1198–1201. [CrossRef] [PubMed]

29. Huang, C.Y.; Lin, H.J.; Chen, H.S.; Cheng, S.Y.; Hsu, H.C.; Tang, C.H. Thrombin promotes matrix metalloproteinase-13 expression through the PKCδ/c-Src/EGFR/PI3K/Akt/AP-1 signaling pathway in human chondrocytes. *Mediat. Inflamm.* **2013**, *2013*, 326041. [CrossRef] [PubMed]

30. Latimer, H.R.; Veal, E.A. Peroxiredoxins in regulation of MAPK signalling pathways; sensors and barriers to signal transduction. *Mol. Cells* **2016**, *39*, 40–45. [PubMed]

31. Bayoumi, A.S.; Sayed, A.; Broskova, Z.; Teoh, J.P.; Wilson, J.; Su, H.; Tang, Y.L.; Kim, I.M. Crosstalk between long noncoding RNAs and microRNAs in health and disease. *Int. J. Mol. Sci.* **2016**, *17*, 356. [CrossRef] [PubMed]

32. He, L.; Hannon, G.J. Micrornas: Small RNAs with a big role in gene regulation. *Nat. Rev. Genet.* **2004**, *5*, 522–531. [CrossRef] [PubMed]

33. Kuo, S.J.; Yang, W.H.; Liu, S.C.; Tsai, C.H.; Hsu, H.C.; Tang, C.H. Transforming growth factor β1 enhances heme oxygenase 1 expression in human synovial fibroblasts by inhibiting microRNA 519b synthesis. *PLoS ONE* **2017**, *12*, e0176052. [CrossRef] [PubMed]

34. Liu, S.C.; Chiu, C.P.; Tsai, C.H.; Hung, C.Y.; Li, T.M.; Wu, Y.C.; Tang, C.H. Soya-cerebroside, an extract of cordyceps militaris, suppresses monocyte migration and prevents cartilage degradation in inflammatory animal models. *Sci. Rep.* **2017**, *7*, 43205. [CrossRef] [PubMed]

35. Tzeng, H.E.; Tsai, C.H.; Chang, Z.L.; Su, C.M.; Wang, S.W.; Hwang, W.L.; Tang, C.H. Interleukin-6 induces vascular endothelial growth factor expression and promotes angiogenesis through apoptosis signal-regulating kinase 1 in human osteosarcoma. *Biochem. Pharmacol.* **2013**, *85*, 531–540. [CrossRef] [PubMed]

36. Wang, C.Q.; Li, Y.; Huang, B.F.; Zhao, Y.M.; Yuan, H.; Guo, D.; Su, C.M.; Hu, G.N.; Wang, Q.; Long, T.; et al. EGFR conjunct FSCN1 as a novel therapeutic strategy in triple-negative breast cancer. *Sci. Rep.* **2017**, *7*, 15654. [CrossRef] [PubMed]

37. Lerner, I.; Baraz, L.; Pikarsky, E.; Meirovitz, A.; Edovitsky, E.; Peretz, T.; Vlodavsky, I.; Elkin, M. Function of heparanase in prostate tumorigenesis: Potential for therapy. *Clin. Cancer Res.* **2008**, *14*, 668–676. [CrossRef] [PubMed]

38. Huang, C.Y.; Chen, S.Y.; Tsai, H.C.; Hsu, H.C.; Tang, C.H. Thrombin induces epidermal growth factor receptor transactivation and CCL2 expression in human osteoblasts. *Arthritis Rheumatol.* **2012**, *64*, 3344–3354. [CrossRef] [PubMed]

39. Lee, M.R.; Lin, C.; Lu, C.C.; Kuo, S.C.; Tsao, J.W.; Juan, Y.N.; Chiu, H.Y.; Lee, F.Y.; Yang, J.S.; Tsai, F.J. YC-1 induces G0/G1 phase arrest and mitochondria-dependent apoptosis in cisplatin-resistant human oral cancer CAR cells. *Biomedicine* **2017**, *7*, 12. [CrossRef] [PubMed]

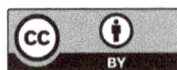

International Journal of
Molecular Sciences

MDPI

Article

Nitric Oxide Mediates Crosstalk between Interleukin 1β and WNT Signaling in Primary Human Chondrocytes by Reducing DKK1 and FRZB Expression

Leilei Zhong [1,2], Stefano Schivo [1,3], Xiaobin Huang [1], Jeroen Leijten [1], Marcel Karperien [1] and Janine N. Post [1,*]

[1] Developmental BioEngineering, MIRA Institute for Biomedical Technology and Technical Medicine, University of Twente, 7522 NB Enschede, The Netherlands; zhongleilei8@gmail.com (L.Z.); s.schivo@utwente.nl (S.S.); x.huang-1@utwente.nl (X.H.); j.c.h.leijten@utwente.nl (J.L.); h.b.j.karperien@utwente.nl (M.K.)
[2] Department of Orthopaedic Surgery, University of Pennsylvania, Philadelphia, PA 19104, USA
[3] Formal Methods and Tools, CTIT, University of Twente, 7522 NB Enschede, The Netherlands
* Correspondence: j.n.post@utwente.nl; Tel.: +31-6-53-489-4205

Received: 2 November 2017; Accepted: 17 November 2017; Published: 22 November 2017

Abstract: Interleukin 1 beta (IL1β) and Wingless-Type MMTV Integration Site Family (WNT) signaling are major players in Osteoarthritis (OA) pathogenesis. Despite having a large functional overlap in OA onset and development, the mechanism of IL1β and WNT crosstalk has remained largely unknown. In this study, we have used a combination of computational modeling and molecular biology to reveal direct or indirect crosstalk between these pathways. Specifically, we revealed a mechanism by which IL1β upregulates WNT signaling via downregulating WNT antagonists, DKK1 and FRZB. In human chondrocytes, IL1β decreased the expression of Dickkopf-1 (DKK1) and Frizzled related protein (FRZB) through upregulation of nitric oxide synthase (iNOS), thereby activating the transcription of WNT target genes. This effect could be reversed by iNOS inhibitor 1400W, which restored DKK1 and FRZB expression and their inhibitory effect on WNT signaling. In addition, 1400W also inhibited both the matrix metalloproteinase (MMP) expression and cytokine-induced apoptosis. We concluded that iNOS/NO play a pivotal role in the inflammatory response of human OA through indirect upregulation of WNT signaling. Blocking NO production may inhibit the loss of the articular phenotype in OA by preventing downregulation of the expression of DKK1 and FRZB.

Keywords: osteoarthritis; cell signaling; IL1β; WNT; antagonists; computational modeling; nitric oxide

1. Introduction

Osteoarthritis (OA) is the most common joint disorder with the knee being the most affected joint. Knee OA affects >10% of the western population over 60 years of age, and this number is likely to increase due to the aging and obesity of the population [1]. OA affects the whole joint and as yet there is no cure. OA is characterized by progressive degeneration of articular cartilage, mild signs of inflammation, and typical bone changes [2,3]. The mechanisms underlying OA pathogenesis are still largely unknown.

Accumulating evidence has strongly linked WNT activity to the onset and development of OA. Indeed, alterations of WNTs and WNT-related proteins, such as the WNT antagonists Dickkopf-1 (DKK1) and Frizzled related protein (FRZB) have been found in human OA. Multiple whole genome studies indicated that loss-of-function single nucleotide polymorphisms (SNPs) in the WNT antagonist

FRZB are related with hip OA [4,5]. In addition, FRZB-knockout mice have more severe OA cartilage deterioration in response to instability, enzymatic injury, or inflammation [6]. Moreover, FRZB$^{-/-}$ mice are shown to have increased MMP expression after load or interleukin 1β (IL1β) treatment [7]. It was shown that high levels of DKK1 have a protective function against cartilage degeneration and that lower levels of DKK1 are associated with OA development [8–10]. We have previously shown that the exogenous addition of high concentrations of DKK1 and FRZB prevented the hypertrophic differentiation of chondrogenically differentiating mesenchymal stem cells [11]. In addition, we reported the loss of DKK1 and FRZB expression in OA [12], and showed that the expression of these antagonists are negatively correlated with grading of knee OA [13].

Interleukin 1β (IL1β) is a key pro-inflammatory cytokine that drives OA progression by inducing the expression of cartilage degrading enzymes, such as matrix metalloproteinases (MMPs) [14,15]. Pro-inflammatory cytokines stimulate iNOS (nitric oxide synthase) expression resulting in the synthesis and release of nitric oxide (NO), which contributes to the joint pathology [16,17]. NO is highly expressed in OA chondrocytes [18–20] and cartilage [21]. NO inhibits both the synthesis of proteoglycan and collagen [22], activates MMPs, mediates chondrocyte apoptosis [23], and promotes inflammatory responses. All of these effects contribute to the catabolic activities of NO in cartilage [24].

Despite the important roles of WNT and IL1β signaling in OA, it remains largely unknown how these pathways cross communicate and thereby affect OA onset and development. We have shown that WNT/β-catenin inhibits IL1β induced MMP expression in human articular cartilage. Addition of IL1β to human chondrocytes increased expression of WNT7b, while decreasing the expression of the WNT antagonists DKK1 and FRZB. This correlated with an increase in β-catenin accumulation [25]. In addition, the WNT/β-catenin regulated transcription factor TCF4 (Transcription Factor 4) binds to NF-κB (Nuclear Factor κB) thereby enhancing NF-κB activity [26].

It was recently shown that IL1β induced NO production in cancer cells was responsible for a strong decrease in DKK1 expression, which in turn resulted in the upregulation of WNT/β-catenin signaling [27]. However, the mechanism by which IL1β downregulates DKK1 and FRZB in chondrocytes is as yet unknown and the subject of this manuscript.

Since OA is a complex disease, involving integration of many factors leading to a unique response in cell fate, a thorough understanding of the integration of signals in cells and disease pathologies is necessary for the development of effective therapies [28]. In the past, attempted clinical trials relied on the correlation of a single pathway. However, as yet there are no successful treatment strategies that successfully treat OA and prevent cartilage degeneration (reviewed in [29]). Static diagrams of signal transduction pathways prevent insight into the dynamic behavior of these systems. Pathways are often studied in isolation, largely deprived of the context of interaction with other pathways. To investigate the dynamic interplay of signal transduction pathways, we developed ANIMO (Analysis of Networks with Interactive Modeling) [30–33]. We have previously used ANIMO to identify a new level of crosstalk between the TNFα and EGF pathways in human colon carcinoma cells [31].

Here, we tested our hypothesis that IL-1β plays a role in initiating OA by increasing WNT/β-catenin activity via iNOS by reducing DKK1 and FRZB expression in human chondrocytes. We first tested our hypothesis computationally, and validated our hypothesis experimentally in primary human chondrocytes. Using the model, we revealed a novel cross-talk between IL1β and WNT signaling in OA, which provided novel mechanistic insights in OA and for the development of novel therapeutics.

2. Results

2.1. Expression of DKK1 and FRZB Is Decreased While IL1β, NOS2/iNOS, and AXIN2 Are Increased in Human OA

We investigated the differences in gene and protein expression levels of IL1β, NOS2/iNOS, AXIN2, and FASL, and the WNT antagonists DKK1 and FRZB in human OA cartilage as compared to those that are found in macroscopically healthy looking (preserved) cartilage. In OA cartilage,

DKK1 and FRZB mRNA expression was significantly decreased accompanied by overexpression of the pro-inflammatory factor *IL1B*, the gene encoding inflammatory mediator *iNOS*, the apoptotic factor FASL, and the WNT target gene *AXIN2* (axis inhibition protein 2) (Figure 1A). DKK1, FRZB, and β-catenin protein expression was detected with immunohistochemistry in paired preserved and OA cartilage specimens from ten patients. Preserved cartilage consistently demonstrated the high expression of cytosolic DKK1 and FRZB, especially in the superficial layer. In contrast, the matching OA cartilage from the same patient showed significantly decreased DKK1 and FRZB expression and increased nuclear localization of β-catenin. β-catenin was hardly detected in preserved cartilage in which high expression of DKK1 and FRZB was observed (Figure 1B, quantification of expression Figure 1C, data of each patient is shown in Figure S1). Interestingly, positive staining of DKK1 was also detected in cell clusters of some OA cartilage samples.

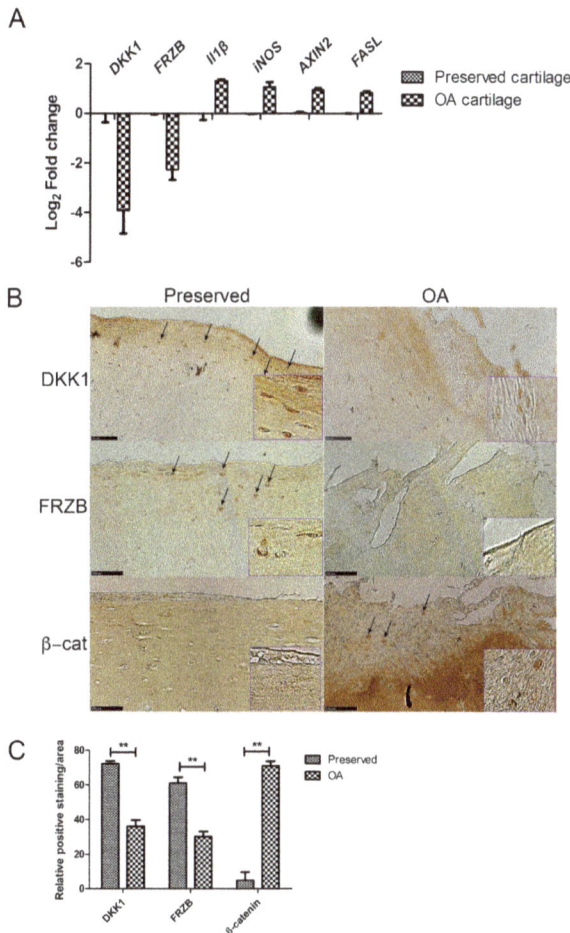

Figure 1. Gene and protein expression in preserved and Osteoarthritis (OA) cartilage. (**A**) RT-qPCR was performed to assess gene expression; (**B**) Immunohistochemistry (IHC) was used to visualize protein expression (arrows indicate positively stained areas). Representative pictures from one donor are shown. Images were taken using the Nanozoomer (scale bar 100 μm), magnified pictures were indicated in inserts; (**C**) Quantification of positive staining was performed by ImageJ software. ** $p < 0.01$: significant correlation.

2.2. ANIMO Model Predicts That IL1β Upregulates WNT Signaling via iNOS/NO by Downregulating Expression of DKK1 and FRZB

To obtain insight into the possible mechanism by which IL1β influences WNT signaling, we generated a simplified network diagram of the WNT and IL1β signaling pathway, which was composed of key proteins. The different steps that were taken to build the model are described in the supplementary information/Figure S4. We used IL1β, IL1Receptor (IL1R), NFκB, IκB, *MMP13*, and iNOS for the IL1β pathway, and WNT, β-catenin, TCF/LEF and the antagonists DKK1 and FRZB, both as mRNA and protein, for the WNT pathway. The regulation of DKK1 and FRZB expression is summarized in a node called 'ANAbolic Regulator', or ANAR. The network diagram was then formalized in ANIMO, which allows us to analyze activity-based computational models. Nodes in an ANIMO network can represent proteins or mRNAs [33], while a change in node activity can describe protein phosphorylation or mRNA expression, depending on the node type. Nodes are connected by interactions (edges), which have the effect of changing the activity level of the target node if the source node is active. The speed at which an interaction occurs was abstractly modelled as either "fast" (for reactions such as phosphorylations) or "slow" (when gene transcription is involved) [30,31].

It has been described for a human cancer that nitric oxide (NO) indirectly upregulates WNT/β-catenin signaling by inhibiting DKK1 [27]. We also identified that in chondrocytes IL1β treatment resulted in downregulation of both FRZB and DKK1 [25]. We therefore added a reaction from iNOS to inhibit both DKK1 mRNA and FRZB mRNA. This resulted in a small network that described additional cross-talk between ILβ and WNT signaling, model 1 (Figure 2 and Figure S5A,B). As expected, in model 1, the addition of IL1β activated WNT/β-catenin signaling via iNOS induced loss of DKK1 and FRZB.

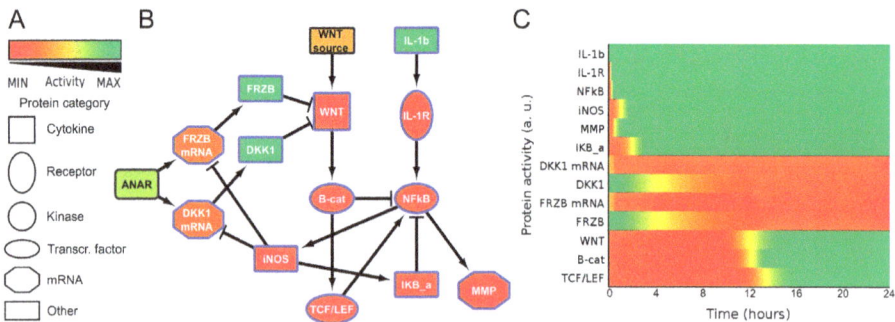

Figure 2. Network diagram ((**B**), model 1) and corresponding activity heatmap (**C**) of the interleukin 1β and Wingless-Type MMTV Integration Site Family (WNT) signaling pathway, in which nitric oxide synthase (iNOS) inhibits DKK1 and FRZB expression, resulting in WNT activity. (**A**) Activities are color coded from red = inactive, via yellow to green = fully active. The shape of the nodes indicate the type of protein or gene/mRNA; (**B**) Simplified network. Il-1b= IL1β, IKB-a = IκBα. For simplicity, the self-inactivating edges that formalize mRNA/protein activity life-time are not shown. The complete model, including self-inactivating edges can be found in the supplemental Figure S5A,B (interaction parameters are in Table S2, initial activities of all models are shown in Table S3).The colors of the nodes indicate their initial activity, and these colors correspond to the activity heatmap in (**C**); (**C**) activity heatmap of the network in (**B**).

It is often suggested that the WNT antagonists FRZB and DKK1 are functionally redundant. To visualize this, we removed the inhibition of iNOS on FRZB in our model. If DKK1 and FRZB are indeed functionally redundant, then the inhibition of only one of these factors should prevent WNT activation. Since in osteoarthritis development we found that FRZB was lost starting in grade 2, while DKK1 started to decrease in grade 1 [13], we decided to test in our model if FRZB was able to prevent WNT activity when DKK1 expression was lost. We therefore removed the inhibitory edge from iNOS to FRZB and activated only IL1β in this model, which is model 2 (Figure S5C,D). However, reduction of DKK1 expression alone did not alleviate the inhibition on WNT signaling, due to the presence of FRZB. This prediction thus suggested that IL1β would only activate WNT signaling by simultaneously downregulating both DKK1 and FRZB expression via iNOS, which we subsequently tested in the wet-lab.

2.3. IL1β Decreased DKK1 and FRZB Expression in a Time- but Not Dose-Dependent Manner

To validate that IL1β indeed regulates both mRNA and protein expression of DKK1 and FRZB in human chondrocytes (hChs), we measured the effect of IL1β on *DKK1* and *FRZB* mRNA expression by qPCR and the DKK1 and FRZB protein levels by ELISA. IL1β significantly decreased the expression of DKK1 and FRZB (Figure 3A–C).

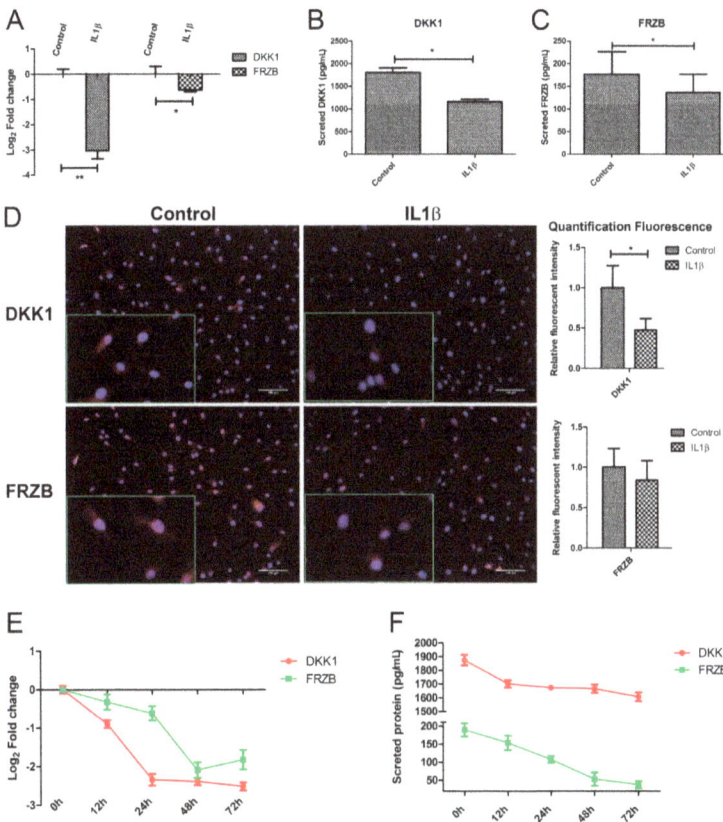

Figure 3. IL1β decreased expression of Dickkopf-1 (DKK1) and Frizzled related protein (FRZB) at mRNA and at the protein level. Human primary chondrocytes were treated with IL1β for 24 h. (**A**); (**B,C**). DKK1 and FRZB gene and protein expression were measured by qPCR and Enzyme-Linked Immunosorbent Assay (ELISA), respectively; (**D**) The expression of DKK1 and FRZB was measured by IF. DKK1 and FRZB are illustrated in red and nuclei are in blue (scale bar 100 μm), magnified pictures were indicated in inserts. Quantification of immunofluorescence intensity was performed using CellProfiler software; (**E,F**). IL1β decreased DKK1 and FRZB expression is time-dependent. Time-course evaluation of DKK1 and FRZB expression after IL1β stimulation. * $p < 0.05$, ** $p < 0.01$: significant correlation.

Immunofluorescence was used to examine the localization and expression of DKK1 and FRZB in human chondrocytes. Chondrocytes in the control group demonstrated constitutive expression of DKK1 and FRZB in the cytoplasm and also in the nucleus. IL1β exposure significantly decreased DKK1 and FRZB expression, especially in the cytoplasm (Figure 3D and Figure S2A,B). IL1β exposure had a widespread effect on the expression of WNT related genes by increasing *FZD10*, *LEF1*, and *TCF4*, while downregulating the expression of the *WNT4* and the WNT inhibitor *WIF1* (Figure S2C). In addition, the effect of IL1β treatment on expression of cartilage markers, catabolic markers, and an apoptotic factor was measured by qPCR. IL1β treatment decreased *ACAN* and *COL2A1* expression, while it increased *MMP3*, *BMP2*, and FASL expression (Figure S2D).

We explored if the IL1β regulation of DKK1 and FRZB was time-dependent by performing a time-course experiment to examine the effects of IL1β treatment for up to 72 h. To ensure the efficacy of the stimulation, we measured *IL16*, *IL1B*, and *MMP3* expression, well-established target genes of IL1β. IL1β strongly induced the mRNA levels of all of these target genes, which progressively increased until at least 72 h after treatment (Figure S2E). The expression of DKK1 and FRZB in response to IL1β was time-dependent. *DKK1* and *FRZB* mRNA expression started to decrease from 12 h after stimulation and reached the lowest expression levels at 72 and 48 h, respectively (Figure 3E). The decrease in *FRZB* mRNA level occurred more slowly. In line with the qPCR results, the secreted protein levels of DKK1 and FRZB were downregulated after IL1β stimulation (Figure 3F).

Measuring the dose-dependent effects of IL1β on *DKK1* and *FRZB* mRNA expression level after 12 h using a range of 0.4 ng/mL to 50 ng/mL, revealed that IL1β treatment was already effective at the lowest concentration of 0.4 ng/mL. There was an increase of IL1β and IL6 expression with an increased concentration (Figure S2F). Exposure to IL1β at any concentration significantly downregulated DKK1 and FRZB expression both at the mRNA as well as the protein level. However, no significant difference was observed between the different IL1β concentrations (Figure S2G).

2.4. IL1β Decreased DKK1 and FRZB Expression through Upregulation of iNOS

To determine if IL1β decreased DKK1 and FRZB by upregulating iNOS, as predicted by our ANIMO model in Figure 2, we measured *NOS2*/iNOS expression and NO production 24 h after IL1β treatment. *NOS2*/iNOS expression at mRNA level was significantly induced by IL1β (Figure 4A). The concentration of the end product of iNOS, nitrite, was increased in cell medium, as determined by a Griess assay (Figure 4B). iNOS protein was hardly detected in relatively healthy human chondrocytes while iNOS protein was strongly increased after IL1β stimulation, as determined by western blot (Figure 4C). IL1β almost linearly (R^2 = 0.9875) increased *NOS2*/iNOS expression over 48 h of stimulation (Figure 4D). Immunofluorescence staining confirmed the increase in iNOS production after exposure to IL1β for 24 h (Figure 4E). These results correspond to the data in our model, where we predicted that both DKK1 and FRZB mRNA and protein expression were affected by IL1β treatment through increase of iNOS activity.

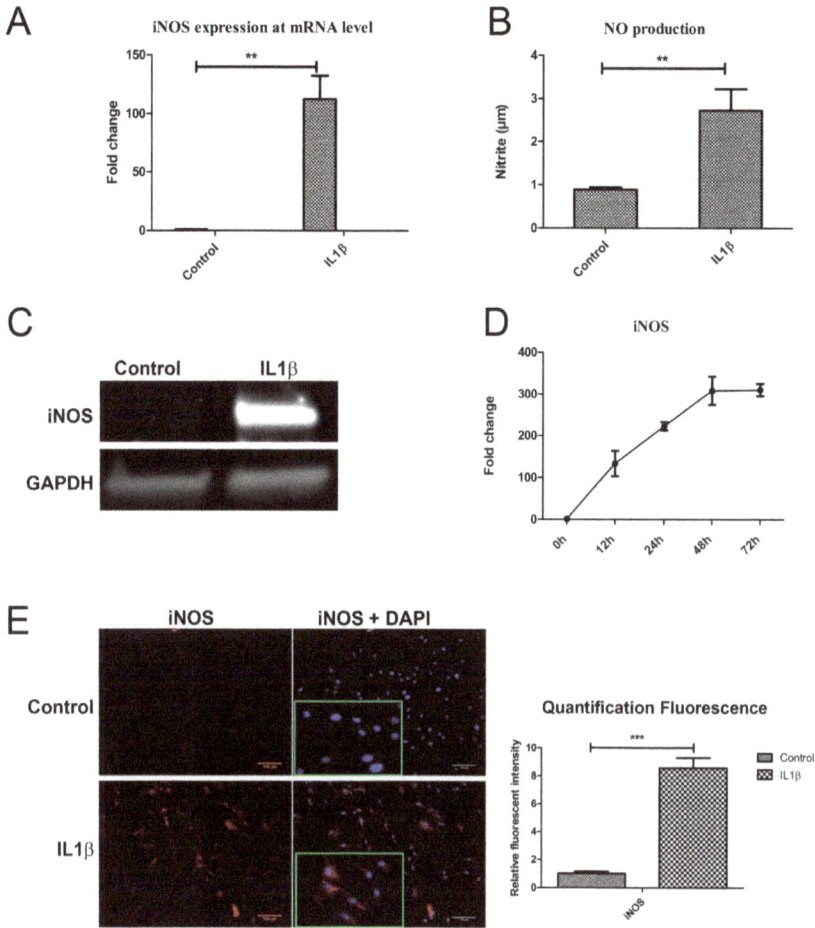

Figure 4. IL1β induced iNOS expression at both mRNA and protein level. (**A,B**) Human chondrocytes were treated with IL1β for 24 h. iNOS mRNA expression was detected by qPCR and nitric oxide (NO) production was measured by Griess assay. (**C**) Western blot was used detect iNOS protein expression. (**D**) Time course evaluation of iNOS mRNA expression after IL1β treatment. (**E**) IF was used to measure iNOS expression, magnified pictures were indicated in inserts. Scale bars 100 μm. Quantification of immunofluorescence intensity was performed by CellProfiler software. ** $p < 0.05$, *** $p < 0.01$: significant correlation.

2.5. Addition of 1400W Relieves the Break on DKK1 and FRZB Inhibition

iNOS activity can be blocked using a small molecule inhibitor 1400W [34]. To in silico confirm the hypothesis that inhibiting iNOS would be sufficient to regain expression of DKK1 and FRZB, we further extended our ANIMO model. Specifically, we added the node '1400W' to inhibit iNOS activity and started the model using the final activities of the model in Figure 2 (where DKK1 and FRZB expression were suppressed and the WNT pathway was active) as input settings. In this model, model 3, we observed that the addition of 1400W is sufficient to release the inhibition of DKK1 and FRZB, resulting in the inhibition of the WNT signaling pathway (Figure 5A and Figure S5E,F and Supplemental Table S2).

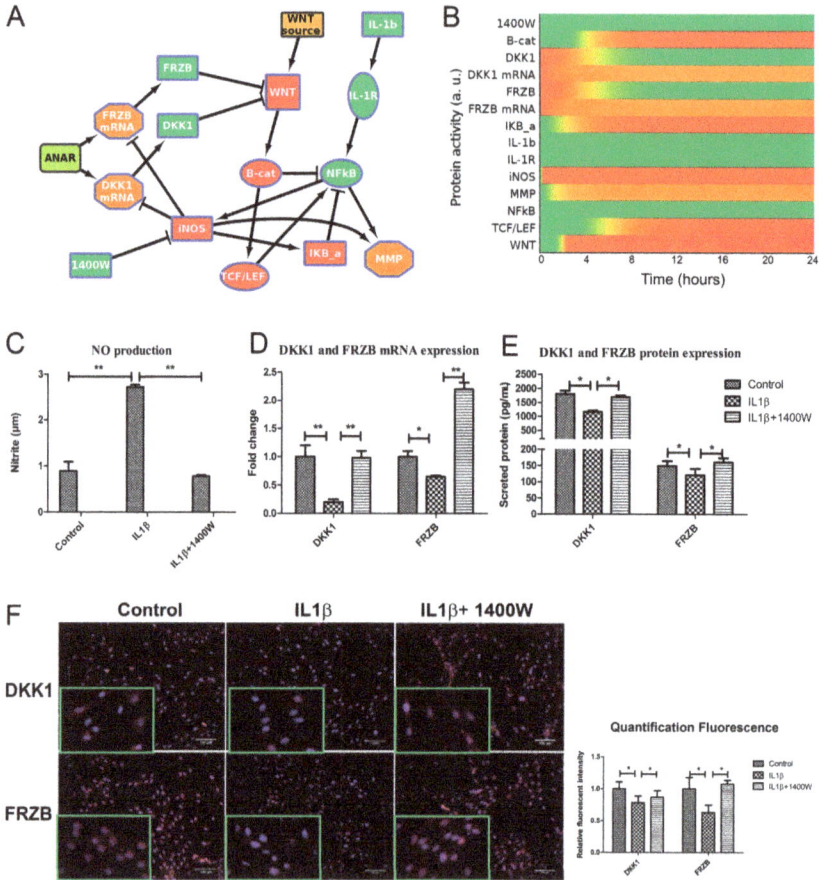

Figure 5. iNOS inhibitor 1400W blocked NO production and rescued the expression of DKK1 and FRZB both in the computational model and in cells. (**A,B**). Addition of 1400W to model 2, creating model 3, shows WNT inactivation by relieving the brake on DKK1 and FRZB expression. Activity levels at 24 h are shown. As shown in Figure 2A, Green is active, red inactive. IL-1b = IL1β, B-cat = β-catenin (protein), IKb-a = IκBα. The model with auto-inhibition edges is shown in Figure S5. (**C**) Human chondrocytes were treated with either IL1β or 1400W or both for 24 h. 1400W inhibited IL1β induced NO production, as measured by Griess assay. (**D,E**). The mRNA and protein expression of DKK1 and FRZB was rescued after addition of iNOS inhibitor, measured by qPCR and ELISA (**F**). The protein expression of DKK1 and FRZB was also measured by immunofluorescence (scale bar 100 μm), magnified pictures were indicated in inserts. Quantification of immunofluorescence intensity was performed by CellProfiler software. * $p < 0.05$, ** $p < 0.01$: significant correlation.

We experimentally tested our hypothesis that blocking iNOS using 1400W is sufficient to block WNT signaling by recovery of DKK1 and FRZB expression in human primary chondrocytes. We validated that 1400W blocked iNOS-generated nitric oxide (Figure 5C). As predicted by the model, blocking iNOS simultaneously rescued DKK1 and FRZB expression at mRNA and protein level, as was determined by qPCR (Figure 5D) and ELISA (Figure 5E), and corroborated by semi-quantified immunofluorescence microphotographs (Figure 5F and Figure S3A,B).

2.6. Blocking IL1β-Induced iNOS Decreased β-Catenin Expression

In our models, we assumed that there was crosstalk between iNOS and the WNT signaling pathway based on the observation that IL1β treatment resulted in changes of both IL1β and WNT related genes, such as *MMP1, MMP3* and *MMP13, FRZD10, LEF1, TCF4, WIF1,* and *WNT4.* To determine the relationship between IL1β, iNOS, and WNT/β-catenin signaling, we measured β-catenin expression by Western blot and IF following exposure to IL1β in the presence and absence of 1400W (Figure 6A). The control group showed low level expression of membrane bound cytosolic β-catenin. IL1β highly increased cytosolic expression and nuclear localization of β-catenin and blocking IL1β-induced iNOS by 1400W decreased β-catenin expression (Figure 6B,C, and Figure S3C). In addition, we found that 1400W inhibited IL1β-induced *MMP-1, -3* and *-13* expression and chondrocyte apoptosis (Figure 6D,E).

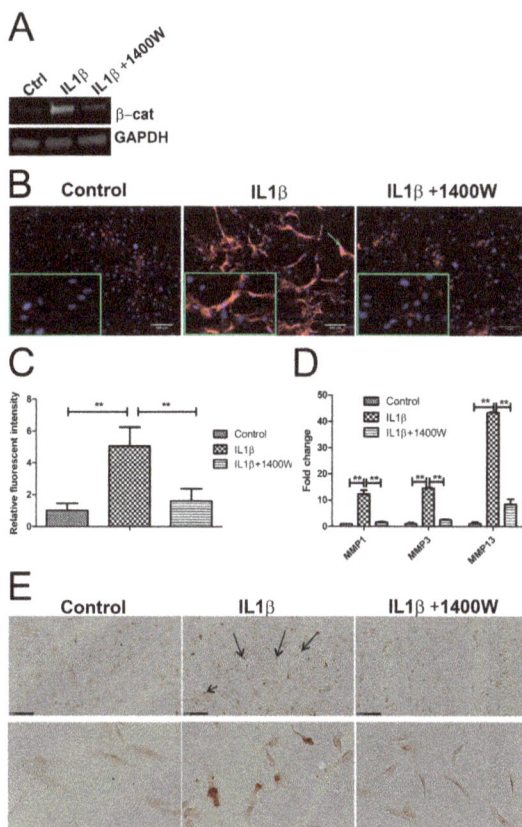

Figure 6. Blocking iNOS decreased β-catenin, matrix metalloproteinases (MMPs) expression, and inhibited apoptosis. (**A,B**) Chondrocytes were treated with 10 ng/mL recombinant human IL-1β or 100 uM iNOS inhibitor 1400W for 24 h. The protein expression of β-catenin was detected by Western blot and IF, green arrow indicated nuclear positive staining of β-catenin, magnified pictures were indicated in inserts. (**C**) Quantification of immunofluorescence intensity was performed by CellProfiler software. (**D**) MMP mRNA expression was measured by qPCR. (**E**) Apoptosis of human chondrocytes was detected using the DeadEnd colorimetric TUNEL assay. Apoptotic nuclei were stained dark brown (dark arrow). Images were taken using Hamamatsu Nanozoomer. Scale bar = 250 μm, top panel indicate overview of cell apoptosis, below panel indicates enlarged picture. ** $p < 0.01$: significant correlation.

2.7. Computational Model Highlights Role of iNOS in Regulating MMP Expression

In our computational model, *MMP* is downstream of NFκB (nuclear factor kappa-light-chain-enhancer of activated B cells) and there is no interaction between iNOS and *MMP*. Therefore, in the model, the expression of *MMP* is unaltered after 1400W addition (Figure 5B and Figure S5F). However, our wet-lab data could be explained if IL1β induced *MMP* expression is also regulated by iNOS. We therefore adapted our model by adding *MMP* downstream of iNOS and lowering the k-value for the edge from NFκB to *MMP*, resulting in the downregulation of *MMP* expression in the presence of 1400W (model 4: Figure S5G,H).

Our model explains the mechanism that iNOS is a mediator regulating both DKK1 and FRZB, as well as *MMP* expression. Combined, these are new findings in chondrocytes.

3. Discussion

The major and novel findings in this study are: (i) Facile computational activity-based models of signal transduction pathway crosstalk can be used to predict, visualize, and explain a cellular response; (ii) In paired samples of the same donor we showed that DKK1 and FRZB protein is highly expressed in the superficial layer of preserved cartilage, while it is lost in OA cartilage; and, (iii) IL1β induced iNOS expression in chondrocytes, which, with NO as a mediator, activated WNT signaling in primary human chondrocytes by simultaneously decreasing endogenous DKK1 and FRZB expression, while increasing *MMP* expression.

Making small activity-based computational models to describe cellular signaling pathways is an efficient and insightful way to visualize the effects of perturbation of the networks. Here, we showed that we can build relatively simple activity based networks in a facile manner and test hypotheses in silico to render visual and comprehensive results. This is particularly advantageous when discussing signaling crosstalk with people that are new to the field. While there are many more precise modeling tools (reviewed in [31]), we adopted relatively simple dynamics to mimic the interactions between only a few proteins in the networks. Using these simple dynamics, we are able to describe the timing of the interactions quite precisely when compared to our data and previous data [33].

We used ANIMO models of the IL1β/WNT signaling crosstalk to show that both DKK1 and FRZB need to be inhibited for IL1β to regulate β-catenin expression, through the re-activation of the WNT signaling pathway. In addition, because of the use of the activity-based model, we identified a link between iNOS/NO and MMP expression that would otherwise have been ignored.

It has been shown that nitric oxide influences the binding of specific transcription factors to DNA. In the case of c-MYB, c-MYB DNA binding was reduced in the presence of NO [35]. In addition, NO has been shown to reduce the binding of the transcriptional repressor Yin-Yang-1 at the Fas promotor [36]. In contrast, NO positively influenced IL8 expression in a process that was dependent on the activity of the transcription factors that normally regulated IL8 expression [37]. It is, therefore, possible that NO also influences the binding of NFκB to the promotor site of *MMP1*, -3, and -13, so that *MMP1*, -3 and -13 expression is higher in the presence of NO, which is what we observe. Inhibiting the NO production by 1400W would then result in a lower binding efficiency of NFκB binding to its target genes, thereby decreasing the expression of *MMP1*, -3, and -13.

In this manuscript, we chose to make the model as small as possible was based on the principle of Occam's razor: we built a model that involves a minimal amount of players and can still describe the effects that we observed thereafter in experimental data. One has to keep in mind that some edges in the model, such as the one connecting WNT and β-Catenin, do not necessarily represent actual interactions. What those edges represent is the "net effect" of the activation of some significant players. In the example, the edge represents the fact that β-Catenin concentration increases when WNT is available. We avoided the inclusion of all the intermediate steps in that process, as their presence would have increased the number of nodes in the network without increasing the capability of the model to explain our hypothesis. However, for other applications, for example when precise information on protein interactions is investigated, more detailed modeling may be necessary ([38], and reviewed in [31]).

In previous work, we found that simultaneous inhibition of endogenous DKK1 and FRZB using neutralizing VHH llama antibodies, inhibited redifferentiation of human chondrocytes and induced hypertrophic differentiation in co-cultures of human mesenchymal stem cells and human chondrocytes, indicating that the simultaneous expression of DKK1 and FRZB is important for chondrocyte development and the prevention of hypertrophic differentiation [39]. Both DKK1 and FRZB are antagonists of WNT signaling, but they antagonize WNT signaling through different mechanisms. DKK1 inhibits the canonical pathway [40,41] and FRZB antagonizes WNT signaling of both canonical and noncanonical pathways [42–45]. The canonical pathway regulates proliferation and the noncanonical pathway regulates differentiation [46]. In OA cartilage, chondrocytes not only show abnormal proliferation but also hypertrophic differentiation and dedifferentiation, suggesting that both canonical and noncanonical WNT pathways can be activated due to the inhibition of DKK1 and FRZB expression.

We find that the expression of *DKK1* and *FRZB* decreased while *IL1B*, *NOS2*/iNOS, and *AXIN2* was increased in OA cartilage. In addition, we found that DKK1 and FRZB protein is highly present in relatively healthy cartilage but is lost in the paired OA cartilage. Both of these findings are in line with previous work of our group and others [12,16,47]. In contrast, β-catenin showed high expression in OA and low expression in the paired preserved samples. This indicates that diminished DKK1 and FRZB expression favors the activation of canonical WNT signaling and consequently contributes to OA. Interestingly, in some patients, DKK1 positive staining was also observed in some of the cell clusters in the middle layer of OA cartilage. It has been reported that the overexpression of cartilage markers, such as *SOX9*, *ACAN*, and COLII is observed in cell clusters in OA [48]. Given the anabolic role of DKK1 in cartilage homeostasis, it is not surprising that some repopulated cells produce DKK1 to antagonize WNT signaling in OA cartilage.

IL1β is known as a non-specific activator of WNT signaling [49,50]. We previously showed that the expression of *DKK1* and *FRZB* mRNA decreased after exposure to IL1β, and that IL1β induces β-catenin accumulation, which may be through inhibition of WNT inhibitors in human chondrocytes [25]. We showed here that in human chondrocytes, IL1β significantly downregulated DKK1 and FRZB, and that this regulation is time dependent, but not dose dependent. In addition, IL1β induced expression of several WNT related gene such as *FRZD10*, *LEF1*, and *TCF4*, while expression of the WNT inhibitor *WIF1* was reduced. This matches with findings in a cancer cell line [27]. It has been shown that inflammatory factors reduce cartilage proteoglycan synthesis [22] and induce chondrocyte hypertrophy [51–54]. Indeed, we show that IL1β inhibited the expression of the cartilage markers *ACAN* and *COL2A1*, while it induced the expression of the hypertrophic markers *COL10A1*, *MMP13*, and *BMP2*. It thus appears that IL1β induces chondrocytes to switch their stable articular phenotype to a hypertrophic state by decreasing DKK1 and FRZB expression via iNOS.

In cancer cells, IL1β induced nitric oxide production and that this upregulated WNT/β-catenin signaling by inhibiting DKK1 expression [27]. We found that blocking iNOS rescued the expression of both of DKK1 and FRZB, and also inhibited IL1β-induced MMP expression and chondrocyte apoptosis. This matches with work by Pelletier et al., in which another iNOS inhibitor, L-NIL, was shown to reduce *MMP1* and *MMP3* expression [55] and inhibits chondrocyte apoptosis in OA dogs [56]. It is of note that other mechanisms might contribute to the inhibition of DKK1 and FRZB. For example, our group has previously shown that abnormal mechanical loading and tonicity decreased DKK1 and FRZB expression in human chondrocytes [12].

4. Materials and Methods

4.1. ANIMO

ANIMO is a software tool that is designed to be used in biological research and operates as an application in Cytoscape [57]. The supplementary methods describe the use of ANIMO. ANIMO networks can include activations (→) and inhibitions (⊣), which will increase (resp. decrease) the activity level of the target node if the source node is active. For example, A → B will increase the activity level of B if A is active. The speed at which an interaction occurs is defined by its k parameter, which can be estimated qualitatively by choosing among a pre-defined set of options (very slow, slow, medium, fast, very fast), or by directly inputting a numerical value. We initially used only the qualitative interaction speeds 'very slow, slow, medium, fast, very fast', and successively adapted some k-values to obtain more realistic behaviour from the network. In particular, we lowered the speed of some self-inhibitions to values below the 'very slow' speed. We use these interactions to represent the processes of degradation/deactivation of proteins that constantly happen in the cell, but at a rate that is normally (much) lower than the production/activation of their targets.

In all of the models, the colors of the nodes represent its activity level at a certain time-point, and correspond to the colors/activities at that time point in the heat-map. In most images, the activities at the beginning of simulation is shown, unless otherwise stated. The colors thus represent the starting activities of the nodes in the network. Instructions on how to install and use ANIMO can be found on our web site [58]. Also, all of the published models are freely available on this site.

4.2. Human Cartilage

The collection and use of human cartilage was approved by a medical ethical committee (METC) of Zorggroep Twente, The Netherlands. Cartilage was obtained from 10 patients with OA undergoing total knee replacement surgery (seven female, 1one male, two unknown, median age 62 ± 12). Preserved cartilage samples were isolated from macroscopically intact areas and OA cartilage specimens were isolated from areas that were affected by OA, as described in supplemental methods and in [13].

Cartilage samples were collected into 10 mL tubes and were washed twice with PBS. For RNA isolation, subchondral bone was removed from the cartilage, and samples were cut into small pieces (1–2 mm) and quickly snap frozen into liquid nitrogen. Samples were stored at −80 °C. For histology, cartilage samples were fixed using 10% phosphate buffered formalin (pH = 7, Sigma Aldrich, St. Louis, MO, USA) overnight at 4 °C, decalcified for four weeks in 12.5% (w/v) EDTA solution containing 0.5% phosphate buffered formalin (pH 8.0), dehydrated using graded ethanol, and embedded in paraffin.

4.3. RNA Isolation and qPCR Analysis

Total RNA was isolated using TRIzol (ThermoFisher Scientific, Waltham, MA, USA, for details see supplementary methods and [13]). mRNA was isolated from cells using the NucleoSpin RNA II kit (Macherey-Nagel, Dueren, Germany), according to the manufacturers protocol. For cartilage samples: Cartilage pieces were transferred into a pre-cooled Cryo-Cup Grinder for crushing. The obtained cartilage powder was collected into 50 mL tubes and samples were weighed. One mL TRIzol reagent per 50–100 mg sample was added.

The isolated RNA was treated with RNase-free DNase I (Invitrogen Life Technologies, ThermoFisher Scientific, MA, USA). cDNA was obtained from 1 µg of RNA with a cDNA synthesis kit (BIO-RAD, Hercules, CA, USA). QPCR was performed using SYBR Green sensimix (Bioline, London, UK) in the Bio-Rad CFX96 (Bio-Rad, Hercules, CA, USA). For each reaction, a melting curve was generated to test for primer dimer formation and non-specific priming. *GAPDH* was used for gene expression normalization. Mean fold change of gene expression was transformed to $\log_2$, which was plotted. Primer sequences are listed in Supplemental Table S1.

4.4. Immunohistochemistry (IHC) and Immunofluorescence

Immunohistochemical staining of DKK1, FRZB, and β-catenin was performed on 5 μm tissue sections, as previously described [13]. Rabbit polyclonal DKK1 (sc-25516), rabbit polyclonal FRZB (from sc-13941), rabbit polyclonal iNOS (sc-651), all from Santa Cruz Biotechnology, Dallas, TX, USA, and rabbit polyclonal β-catenin (LS-C203657, LifeSpan Biosciences, Seattle, WA, USA) were diluted 1:500 in 5% BSA in PBS and incubated overnight at 4 °C. Non-immune controls were performed without primary antibody. A biotinylated secondary antibody was diluted 1:500 and HRP-Streptavidin was added. For visualization, DAB substrate kit was used (ab64238, Abcam, Cambridge, UK). Quantification was performed using ImageJ software (FIJI) [59].

For immunofluorescence, hChs were seeded at a density of 10^4 cells/cm^2 on coverslips and cultured for 24 h in the presence or absence of 10 ng/mL of IL1β. Samples were washed three times with PBS, fixed with 10% formalin for 30 min, and permeablized with 0.5% triton X-100 in PBS for 15 min at RT. Samples were blocked in 1.5% of BSA in PBST for 1 h, then incubated with specific primary antibody against DKK1, FRZB, iNOS, or β-catenin (Cat.# and supplier, see above) overnight at 4 °C. Cells were rinsed with PBS for three times, 5 min/time. Then, Alexa® Fluor 546-labelled goat anti-rabbit or anti-mouse antibody in 1.5% BSA in PBST was added for 2 h at RT. Cells were rinsed with PBS and mounted in mounting medium with DAPI. Slides were imaged using a BD pathway confocal microscope.

4.5. Human Primary Chondrocyte Isolation and Cell Culture

Human primary articular chondrocytes (hChs) were isolated from macroscopically healthy looking areas of OA cartilage from patients undergoing total knee replacement and were cultured in DMEM (Gibco) supplemented with 10% Fetal Bovine Serum (FBS), 100 U/mL Penicillin, 100 mg/mL Streptomycin, 0.4 mM proline, 0.2 mM ascorbic acid diphosphate, and 1% nonessential amino acids. Passage two cells were used for all experiments.

4.6. Recombinant Proteins and Reagents

Recombinant human IL-1β was obtained from R&D Systems. The inhibitor of nitric oxide, 1400W, was purchased from Cayman Chemical (Ann Arbor, MI, USA).

4.7. Enzyme-Linked Immunosorbent Assay (ELISA)

Cell culture medium was collected. Secreted DKK1 and FRZB protein concentrations were determined by ELISA following the manufacturer's instructions (Cat.#: DY1906 for DKK1; DY192 for FRZB, R&D systems).

4.8. Western Blotting

Total cell proteins were collected in RIPA buffer (Cell Signaling Technology, Danvers, MA) supplemented with Halt protease and phosphatase inhibitor cocktail (ThermoFisher Scientific, MA, USA). The specific antibodies used for Western blot analysis including: Anti-iNOS (sc-651, Santa Cruz Biotechnology, TX, USA), anti-GAPDH (G8795, Sigma-Aldrich, St. Louis, MO, USA), and anti-β-catenin (LS-C203657, LifeSpan Biosciences, Seattle, WA, USA).

4.9. NO Production Assay

Cell supernatant was collected and quantified for nitrite using the Griess reaction as previously described [60].

4.10. Immunofluorescent Staining

hChs were seeded at a density of 10^4 cells/cm^2 on coverslips and cultured for 24 h in the presence or absence of 10 ng/mL of IL1β. Samples were fixed with 10% formalin. For the detection of DKK1,

FRZB, iNOS, or β-catenin, specific antibodies were used (Cat.# and supplier, see above) As a secondary antibody, Alexa® Fluor 546-labelled goat anti-rabbit or anti-mouse antibody was added. Cells were mounted in mounting medium with DAPI and imaged using a BD pathway confocal microscope.

Quantification was performed using CellProfiler 2.2.0 software. The fluorescence intensity of each cell was measured and the mean intensity of all cells was calculated as pixels/cell. The intensity of fluorescence of each experimental group was normalized to the control group. Graphs represent relative fluorescent intensities.

4.11. Apoptosis Assay

Human chondrocytes were exposed to 10 ng/mL of recombinant human IL-1β and/or 100 uM of iNOS inhibitor 1400W for 48 h. Apoptosis of human chondrocytes was detected using the DeadEnd colorimetric TUNEL assay (Promega, Madison, WI, USA) following the manufacturer's procedure. Apoptotic nuclei were stained dark brown.

4.12. Statistical Analysis

Three donors were used as biological triplicates, with at least three technical replicates per experiment. Statistical analysis between groups was performed using student's t-test. The difference between multiple groups was tested using one-way ANOVA and Tukey post hoc analysis. $p < 0.05$ was considered statistically significant.

5. Conclusions

Our data suggest a pivotal role of iNOS/NO in the inflammatory response of human OA through indirect upregulation of WNT signaling. Blocking NO production immediately after trauma using pharmacological methods may inhibit the loss of the articular phenotype in OA by preventing downregulation of the expression of DKK1 and FRZB.

Supplementary Materials: Supplemental information can be found at www.mdpi.com/1422-0067/18/11/2491/s1.

Acknowledgments: Leilei Zhong is funded by the Dutch Arthritis Foundation (Reumafonds) grant number 11-1-408 to Janine N. Post and Marcel Karperien. The Dutch Arthritis Foundation had no role in designing, collecting data, analysis, and interpreting of the work. We thank the patients, surgeons and staff of the Orthopedisch Centrum Oost Nederland (OCON), Hengelo, The Netherlands for providing patient samples.

Author Contributions: Leilei Zhong, Jeroen Leijten, Marcel Karperien and Janine N. Post designed experiments. Leilei Zhong and Xiaobin Huang performed all wet-lab experiments. Stefano Schivo and Janine N. Post performed all ANIMO modeling. Leilei Zhong, Xiaobin Huang, Stefano Schivo, Jeroen Leijten, Marcel Karperien and Janine N. Post wrote the manuscript. All authors have read and approved the final submitted manuscript.

Conflicts of Interest: The authors declare no conflict of interest.

Abbreviations

ACAN	Aggrecan
ANAR	ANAbolic regulator
ANIMO	Analysis of networks with interactive modeling
AXIN2	Axis inhibition protein 2, mRNA
COL2A1	Collagen 2 variant a1
DKK1	Dickkopf-1
EGF	Epidermal growth factor
FASL	Fas ligand/CD95L-mRNA
FRZB	Frizzled related protein
FZD10	Frizzled-10-mRNA
hCh	Human chondrocyte
IHC	Immunohistochemistry
IL	Interleukin
IL1R	IL1Receptor

iNOS/*NOS2*	nitric oxide synthase
IκB	Inhibitor of κB
LEF	Lymphoid enhancer-binding factor
MMP3	Matrix metalloproteinase 3- mRNA
NF-κB	nuclear factor kappa-light-chain-enhancer of activated B cells/nuclear factor kappa B
NO	Nitric oxide
OA	Osteoarthritis
SNP	Single nucleotide polymorphisms
TCF4	Transcription factor 4
TNFa	Tumor necrosis factor α
WIF1	Wnt inhibitory factor 1-mRNA
WNT	Wingless-type MMTV integration site family

References

1. Allen, K.D.; Golightly, Y.M. State of the evidence. *Curr. Opin. Rheumatol.* **2015**, *27*, 276–283. [CrossRef] [PubMed]
2. Issa, S.N.; Sharma, L. Epidemiology of osteoarthritis: An update. *Curr. Rheumatol. Rep.* **2006**, *8*, 7–15. [CrossRef] [PubMed]
3. Goldring, M.B.; Goldring, S.R. Osteoarthritis. *J. Cell. Physiol.* **2007**, *213*, 626–634. [CrossRef] [PubMed]
4. Loughlin, J.; Dowling, B.; Chapman, K.; Marcelline, L.; Mustafa, Z.; Southam, L.; Ferreira, A.; Ciesielski, C.; Carson, D.A.; Corr, M. Functional variants within the secreted frizzled-related protein 3 gene are associated with hip osteoarthritis in females. *Proc. Natl. Acad. Sci. USA* **2004**, *101*, 9757–9762. [CrossRef] [PubMed]
5. Min, J.L.; Meulenbelt, I.; Riyazi, N.; Kloppenburg, M.; Houwing-Duistermaat, J.J.; Seymour, A.B.; Pols, H.A.; van Duijn, C.M.; Slagboom, P.E. Association of the frizzled-related protein gene with symptomatic osteoarthritis at multiple sites. *Arthritis Rheum.* **2005**, *52*, 1077–1080. [CrossRef] [PubMed]
6. Lories, R.J.U.; Peeters, J.; Bakker, A.; Tylzanowski, P.; Derese, I.; Schrooten, J.; Thomas, J.T.; Luyten, F.P. Articular cartilage and biomechanical properties of the long bones inFrzb-knockout mice. *Arthritis Rheum.* **2007**, *56*, 4095–4103. [CrossRef] [PubMed]
7. Bougault, C.; Priam, S.; Houard, X.; Pigenet, A.; Sudre, L.; Lories, R.J.; Jacques, C.; Berenbaum, F. Protective role of frizzled-related protein B on matrix metalloproteinase induction in mouse chondrocytes. *Arthritis Res. Ther.* **2014**, *16*, R137. [CrossRef] [PubMed]
8. Lane, N.E.; Nevitt, M.C.; Lui, L.-Y.; de Leon, P.; Corr, M. Wnt signaling antagonists are potential prognostic biomarkers for the progression of radiographic hip osteoarthritis in elderly Caucasian women. *Arthritis Rheum.* **2007**, *56*, 3319–3325. [CrossRef] [PubMed]
9. Voorzanger-Rousselot, N.; Ben-Tabassi, N.C.; Garnero, P. Opposite relationships between circulating Dkk-1 and cartilage breakdown in patients with rheumatoid arthritis and knee osteoarthritis. *Ann. Rheum. Dis.* **2009**, *68*, 1513–1514. [CrossRef] [PubMed]
10. Honsawek, S.; Tanavalee, A.; Yuktanandana, P.; Ngarmukos, S.; Saetan, N.; Tantavisut, S. Dickkopf-1 (Dkk-1) in plasma and synovial fluid is inversely correlated with radiographic severity of knee osteoarthritis patients. *BMC Musculoskelet. Disord.* **2010**, *11*. [CrossRef] [PubMed]
11. Leijten, J.C.H.; Emons, J.; Sticht, C.; van Gool, S.; Decker, E.; Uitterlinden, A.; Rappold, G.; Hofman, A.; Rivadeneira, F.; Scherjon, S.; et al. Gremlin 1, Frizzled-related protein, and Dkk-1 are key regulators of human articular cartilage homeostasis. *Arthritis Rheum.* **2012**, *64*, 3302–3312. [CrossRef] [PubMed]
12. Leijten, J.C.; Bos, S.D.; Landman, E.B.; Georgi, N.; Jahr, H.; Meulenbelt, I.; Post, J.N.; van Blitterswijk, C.A.; Karperien, M. GREM1, FRZB and DKK1 mRNA levels correlate with osteoarthritis and are regulated by osteoarthritis-associated factors. *Arthritis Res. Ther.* **2013**, *15*, R126. [CrossRef] [PubMed]
13. Zhong, L.; Huang, X.; Karperien, M.; Post, J. Correlation between Gene Expression and Osteoarthritis Progression in Human. *Int. J. Mol. Sci.* **2016**, *17*, 1126. [CrossRef] [PubMed]
14. Kobayashi, M.; Squires, G.R.; Mousa, A.; Tanzer, M.; Zukor, D.J.; Antoniou, J.; Feige, U.; Poole, A.R. Role of interleukin-1 and tumor necrosis factor α in matrix degradation of human osteoarthritic cartilage. *Arthritis Rheum.* **2005**, *52*, 128–135. [CrossRef] [PubMed]
15. Wojdasiewicz, P.; Poniatowski, Ł.A.; Szukiewicz, D. The Role of Inflammatory and Anti-Inflammatory Cytokines in the Pathogenesis of Osteoarthritis. *Mediat. Inflamm.* **2014**, *2014*, 561459. [CrossRef] [PubMed]

16. Goldring, M.B.; Otero, M. Inflammation in osteoarthritis. *Curr. Opin. Rheumatol.* **2011**, *23*, 471–478. [CrossRef] [PubMed]

17. Heinegård, D.; Saxne, T. The role of the cartilage matrix in osteoarthritis. *Nat. Rev. Rheumatol.* **2010**, *7*, 50–56. [CrossRef] [PubMed]

18. Pelletier, J.-P.; Martel-Pelletier, J.; Abramson, S.B. Osteoarthritis, an inflammatory disease: Potential implication for the selection of new therapeutic targets. *Arthritis Rheum.* **2001**, *44*, 1237–1247. [CrossRef]

19. Abramson, S.B.; Attur, M.; Yazici, Y. Prospects for disease modification in osteoarthritis. *Nat. Clin. Pract. Rheumatol.* **2006**, *2*, 304–312. [CrossRef] [PubMed]

20. Amin, A.R. The expression and regulation of nitric oxide synthase in human osteoarthritis-affected chondrocytes: Evidence for up-regulated neuronal nitric oxide synthase. *J. Exp. Med.* **1995**, *182*, 2097–2102. [CrossRef] [PubMed]

21. Loeser, R.F.; Carlson, C.S.; Carlo, M.D.; Cole, A. Detection of nitrotyrosine in aging and osteoarthritic cartilage: Correlation of oxidative damage with the presence of interleukin-1β and with chondrocyte resistance to insulin-like growth factor 1. *Arthritis Rheum.* **2002**, *46*, 2349–2357. [CrossRef] [PubMed]

22. Taskiran, D.; Stefanovicracic, M.; Georgescu, H.; Evans, C. Nitric-Oxide Mediates Suppression of Cartilage Proteoglycan Synthesis by Interleukin-1. *Biochem. Biophys. Res. Commun.* **1994**, *200*, 142–148. [CrossRef] [PubMed]

23. Blanco, F.J.; Ochs, R.L.; Schwarz, H.; Lotz, M. Chondrocyte apoptosis induced by nitric oxide. *Am. J. Pathol.* **1995**, *146*, 75–85. [PubMed]

24. Abramson, S.B. Osteoarthritis and nitric oxide. *Osteoarthr. Cartil.* **2008**, *16*, S15–S20. [CrossRef]

25. Ma, B.; van Blitterswijk, C.A.; Karperien, M. A Wnt/β-catenin negative feedback loop inhibits interleukin-1-induced matrix metalloproteinase expression in human articular chondrocytes. *Arthritis Rheum.* **2012**, *64*, 2589–2600. [CrossRef] [PubMed]

26. Ma, B.; Zhong, L.; van Blitterswijk, C.A.; Post, J.N.; Karperien, M. T Cell Factor 4 Is a Pro-catabolic and Apoptotic Factor in Human Articular Chondrocytes by Potentiating Nuclear Factor κB Signaling. *J. Biol. Chem.* **2013**, *288*, 17552–17558. [CrossRef] [PubMed]

27. Du, Q.; Zhang, X.; Liu, Q.; Zhang, X.; Bartels, C.E.; Geller, D.A. Nitric Oxide Production Upregulates Wnt/-Catenin Signaling by Inhibiting Dickkopf-1. *Cancer Res.* **2013**, *73*, 6526–6537. [CrossRef] [PubMed]

28. Lenas, P.; Moos, M.; Luyten, F.P. Developmental Engineering: A New Paradigm for the Design and Manufacturing of Cell-Based Products. Part II. From Genes to Networks: Tissue Engineering from the Viewpoint of Systems Biology and Network Science. *Tissue Eng. Part B Rev.* **2009**, *15*, 395–422. [CrossRef] [PubMed]

29. Zhang, W.; Ouyang, H.; Dass, C.R.; Xu, J. Current research on pharmacologic and regenerative therapies for osteoarthritis. *Bone Res.* **2016**, *4*, 15040. [CrossRef] [PubMed]

30. Schivo, S.; Scholma, J.; Karperien, M.; Post, J.N.; van de Pol, J.; Langerak, R. Setting Parameters for Biological Models with ANIMO. *Electron. Proc. Theor. Comput. Sci.* **2014**, *145*, 35–47. [CrossRef]

31. Schivo, S.; Scholma, J.; van der Vet, P.E.; Karperien, M.; Post, J.N.; van de Pol, J.; Langerak, R. Modelling with ANIMO: Between fuzzy logic and differential equations. *BMC Syst. Biol.* **2016**, *10*. [CrossRef] [PubMed]

32. Schivo, S.; Scholma, J.; Wanders, B.; Camacho, R.A.U.; van der Vet, P.E.; Karperien, M.; Langerak, R.; van de Pol, J.; Post, J.N. Modeling Biological Pathway Dynamics With Timed Automata. *IEEE J. Biomed. Health Inf.* **2014**, *18*, 832–839. [CrossRef] [PubMed]

33. Scholma, J.; Schivo, S.; Urquidi Camacho, R.A.; van de Pol, J.; Karperien, M.; Post, J.N. Biological networks 101: Computational modeling for molecular biologists. *Gene* **2014**, *533*, 379–384. [CrossRef] [PubMed]

34. Jarvinen, K.; Vuolteenaho, K.; Nieminen, R.; Moilanen, T.; Knowles, R.G.; Moilanen, E. Selective iNOS inhibitor 1400W enhances anti-catabolic IL-10 and reduces destructive MMP-10 in OA cartilage. Survey of the effects of 1400W on inflammatory mediators produced by OA cartilage as detected by protein antibody array. *Clin. Exp. Rheumatol.* **2008**, *26*, 275–282. [PubMed]

35. Brendeford, E.M.; Andersson, K.B.; Gabrielsen, O.S. Nitric oxide (NO) disrupts specific DNA binding of the transcription factor c-Myb in vitro. *FEBS Lett.* **1998**, *425*, 52–56. [CrossRef]

36. Garban, H.J.; Bonavida, B. Nitric Oxide Inhibits the Transcription Repressor Yin-Yang 1 Binding Activity at the Silencer Region of the Fas Promoter: A Pivotal Role for Nitric Oxide in the Up-Regulation of Fas Gene Expression in Human Tumor Cells. *J. Immunol.* **2001**, *167*, 75–81. [CrossRef] [PubMed]

37. Sparkman, L. Nitric oxide increases IL-8 gene transcription and mRNA stability to enhance IL-8 gene expression in lung epithelial cells. *Am. J. Physiol. Lung Cell. Mol. Physiol.* **2004**, *287*, L764–L773. [CrossRef] [PubMed]

38. Hartung, N.; Benary, U.; Wolf, J.; Kofahl, B. Paracrine and autocrine regulation of gene expression by wnt-inhibitor dickkopf in wild-type and mutant hepatocytes. *BMC Syst. Biol.* **2017**, *11*, 98. [CrossRef] [PubMed]

39. Zhong, L.; Huang, X.; Rodrigues, E.D.; Leijten, J.C.; Verrips, T.; El Khattabi, M.; Karperien, M.; Post, J.N. Endogenous dkk1 and frzb regulate chondrogenesis and hypertrophy in three-dimensional cultures of human chondrocytes and human mesenchymal stem cells. *Stem Cells Dev.* **2016**, *25*, 1808–1817. [CrossRef] [PubMed]

40. Semënov, M.V.; Tamai, K.; Brott, B.K.; Kühl, M.; Sokol, S.; He, X. Head inducer Dickkopf-1 is a ligand for Wnt coreceptor LRP6. *Curr. Biol.* **2001**, *11*, 951–961. [CrossRef]

41. Bafico, A.; Liu, G.; Yaniv, A.; Gazit, A.; Aaronson, S.A. Novel mechanism of wnt signalling inhibition mediated by Dickkopf-1 interaction with LRP6/Arrow. *Nat. Cell Biol.* **2001**, *3*, 683–686. [CrossRef] [PubMed]

42. Lin, K.; Wang, S.; Julius, M.A.; Kitajewski, J.; Moos, M.; Luyten, F.P. The cysteine-rich frizzled domain of Frzb-1 is required and sufficient for modulation of Wnt signaling. *Proc. Natl. Acad. Sci. USA* **1997**, *94*, 11196–11200. [CrossRef] [PubMed]

43. Leyns, L.; Bouwmeester, T.; Kim, S.H.; Piccolo, S.; De Robertis, E.M. Frzb-1 is a secreted antagonist of wnt signaling expressed in the spemann organizer. *Cell* **1997**, *88*, 747–756. [CrossRef]

44. Bafico, A.; Gazit, A.; Pramila, T.; Finch, P.W.; Yaniv, A.; Aaronson, S.A. Interaction of Frizzled Related Protein (FRP) with Wnt Ligands and the Frizzled Receptor Suggests Alternative Mechanisms for FRP Inhibition of Wnt Signaling. *J. Biol. Chem.* **1999**, *274*, 16180–16187. [CrossRef] [PubMed]

45. Kawano, Y. Secreted antagonists of the Wnt signalling pathway. *J. Cell Sci.* **2003**, *116*, 2627–2634. [CrossRef] [PubMed]

46. Gough, N.R. Understanding Wnt's Role in Osteoarthritis. *Sci. Signal.* **2011**, *4*, ec134. [CrossRef]

47. Blom, A.B.; van Lent, P.L.; van der Kraan, P.M.; van den Berg, W.B. To seek shelter from the wnt in osteoarthritis? Wnt-signaling as a target for osteoarthritis therapy. *Curr. Drug Targets* **2010**, *11*, 620–629. [CrossRef] [PubMed]

48. Lotz, M.K.; Otsuki, S.; Grogan, S.P.; Sah, R.; Terkeltaub, R.; D'Lima, D. Cartilage cell clusters. *Arthritis Rheum.* **2010**, *62*, 2206–2218. [CrossRef] [PubMed]

49. Hwang, S.-G.; Yu, S.-S.; Ryu, J.-H.; Jeon, H.-B.; Yoo, Y.-J.; Eom, S.-H.; Chun, J.-S. Regulation of beta-catenin signaling and maintenance of chondrocyte differentiation by ubiquitin-independent proteasomal degradation of alpha-catenin. *J. Biol. Chem.* **2005**, *280*, 12758–12765. [CrossRef] [PubMed]

50. Sandell, L.J.; Aigner, T. Articular cartilage and changes in arthritis. An introduction: Cell biology of osteoarthritis. *Arthritis Res.* **2001**, *3*, 107–113. [CrossRef] [PubMed]

51. Cecil, D.L.; Johnson, K.; Rediske, J.; Lotz, M.; Schmidt, A.M.; Terkeltaub, R. Inflammation-Induced Chondrocyte Hypertrophy Is Driven by Receptor for Advanced Glycation End Products. *J. Immunol.* **2005**, *175*, 8296–8302. [CrossRef] [PubMed]

52. Cecil, D.L.; Rose, D.M.; Terkeltaub, R.; Liu-Bryan, R. Role of interleukin-8 in PiT-1 expression and CXCR1-mediated inorganic phosphate uptake in chondrocytes. *Arthritis Rheum.* **2005**, *52*, 144–154. [CrossRef] [PubMed]

53. Cecil, D.L.; Appleton, C.T.G.; Polewski, M.D.; Mort, J.S.; Schmidt, A.M.; Bendele, A.; Beier, F.; Terkeltaub, R. The Pattern Recognition Receptor CD36 Is a Chondrocyte Hypertrophy Marker Associated with Suppression of Catabolic Responses and Promotion of Repair Responses to Inflammatory Stimuli. *J. Immunol.* **2009**, *182*, 5024–5031. [CrossRef] [PubMed]

54. Olivotto, E.; Borzi, R.M.; Vitellozzi, R.; Pagani, S.; Facchini, A.; Battistelli, M.; Penzo, M.; Li, X.; Flamigni, F.; Li, J.; et al. Differential requirements for ikkalpha and ikkbeta in the differentiation of primary human osteoarthritic chondrocytes. *Arthritis Rheum.* **2007**, *58*, 227–239. [CrossRef] [PubMed]

55. Pelletier, J.P.; Lascau-Coman, V.; Jovanovic, D.; Fernandes, J.C.; Manning, P.; Connor, J.R.; Currie, M.G.; Martel-Pelletier, J. Selective inhibition of inducible nitric oxide synthase in experimental osteoarthritis is associated with reduction in tissue levels of catabolic factors. *J. Rheumatol.* **1999**, *26*, 2002–2014. [PubMed]

56. Pelletier, J.P.; Jovanovic, D.V.; Lascau-Coman, V.; Fernandes, J.C.; Manning, P.T.; Connor, J.R.; Currie, M.G.; Martel-Pelletier, J. Selective inhibition of inducible nitric oxide synthase reduces progression of experimental osteoarthritis in vivo: Possible link with the reduction in chondrocyte apoptosis and caspase 3 level. *Arthritis Rheum.* **2000**, *43*, 1290–1299. [CrossRef]

Int. J. Mol. Sci. **2017**, *18*, 2491

57. Shannon, P.; Markiel, A.; Ozier, O.; Baliga, N.S.; Wang, J.T.; Ramage, D.; Amin, N.; Schwikowski, B.; Ideker, T. Cytoscape: A software environment for integrated models of biomolecular interaction networks. *Genome Res.* **2003**, *13*, 2498–2504. [CrossRef] [PubMed]

58. Schivo, S.; Scholma, J.; Wanders, B.; Camacho, R.A.U.; van der Vet, P.E.; Karperien, M.; Langerak, R.; van de Pol, J.; Post, J.N. Animo. Available online: http://fmt.cs.utwente.nl/tools/animo/ (accessed on 31 October 2017).

59. Schneider, C.A.; Rasband, W.S.; Eliceiri, K.W. Nih image to imagej: 25 years of image analysis. *Nat. Methods* **2012**, *9*, 671–675. [CrossRef] [PubMed]

60. Du, Q.; Park, K.S.; Guo, Z.; He, P.; Nagashima, M.; Shao, L.; Sahai, R.; Geller, D.A.; Hussain, S.P. Regulation of human nitric oxide synthase 2 expression by wnt beta-catenin signaling. *Cancer Res.* **2006**, *66*, 7024–7031. [CrossRef] [PubMed]

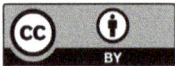

International Journal of
Molecular Sciences

MDPI

Article

The Immunogenicity of Branded and Biosimilar Infliximab in Rheumatoid Arthritis According to Th9-Related Responses

Rossella Talotta [1,*,†], Angela Berzi [2,†], Andrea Doria [3], Alberto Batticciotto [1], Maria Chiara Ditto [1], Fabiola Atzeni [1], Piercarlo Sarzi-Puttini [1] and Daria Trabattoni [2]

[1] Department of Rheumatology, Azienda Ospedaliera-Polo Universitario Luigi Sacco, Milan 20157, Italy; alberto.batticciotto@hsacco.it (A.B.); mariachiara.ditto@hsacco.it (M.C.D.); atzenifabiola@gmail.com (F.A.); sarzi@tiscali.it (P.S.-P.)
[2] Department of Biomedical and Clinical Sciences, Azienda Ospedaliera-Polo Universitario Luigi Sacco, Milan 20157, Italy; angyberzi@gmail.com (A.B.); daria.trabattoni@unimi.it (D.T.)
[3] Department of Rheumatology, University of Padua, Padua 35100, Italy; adoria@unipd.it
* Correspondence: rossella.talotta@asst-fbf-sacco.it; Tel.: +39-023-9042906; Fax +39-023-9042941
† These authors contributed equally to this work.

Received: 15 September 2017; Accepted: 6 October 2017; Published: 12 October 2017

Abstract: Our objective was to evaluate the immunogenicity of branded and biosimilar infliximab by detecting changes in T-helper-9 (Th9) percentages induced by an in vitro stimulation test. Methods: Peripheral blood mononuclear cells collected from 55 consecutive rheumatoid arthritis (RA) outpatients (15 drug free, 20 successfully treated with branded infliximab, 20 branded infliximab inadequate responders) and 10 healthy controls were cultured, with or without 50 µg/mL of infliximab originator (Remicade®) or 50 µg/mL of infliximab biosimilar (Remsima®) for 18 h. Th9 lymphocytes were identified by means of flow cytometry as PU.1 and IRF4-expressing, IL-9-secreting CD4$^+$ T cells. Furthermore, the markers CCR7 and CD45RA were used to distinguish naïve from memory IL-9 producer cells. Results: Under unstimulated conditions, the drug-free RA patients had the highest percentages of Th9 lymphocytes. Following stimulation with branded infliximab, the percentages of PU.1 and IRF4-expressing Th9 cells, CCR7$^+$, CD45RA$^-$ (central memory) and CCR7$^-$, CD45RA$^-$ (effector memory) cells significantly increased in the group of inadequate responders, but no significant variation was observed after exposure to the biosimilar of infliximab. Conclusions: Th9 cells seem to be involved in the immune response to the epitopes of branded, but not biosimilar, infliximab, and this may depend on the recall and stimulation of both central and effector memory cells.

Keywords: biosimilars; Th9 lymphocytes; rheumatoid arthritis; infliximab

1. Introduction

Rheumatoid arthritis (RA) is an autoimmune chronic disease characterized by inflammation of peripheral joints, with a varying degree of systemic involvement. The pathogenesis is partly understood and relies on the activation of cells belonging either to innate and adaptive immunity, with the subsequent production of cytokines and chemokines contributing to final synovitis and systemic inflammation. The treatment of RA has been remarkably implemented in recent decades. Several conventional and biological drugs have been developed in order to counteract the activation of the immune system by acting at different steps of the inflammatory cascade. Particularly, biological agents currently approved for RA include: anti-Tumor Necrosis Factor-α (TNF) drugs (infliximab, etanercept, adalimumab, certolizumab pegol, golimumab), an anti-CD20 drug (rituximab), a receptor antagonist of interleukin-1 (anakinra), an antagonist of the receptor of interleukin-6 (tocilizumab) and a fusion protein containing the Cytotoxic T Lymphocyte Antigen-4 domain activity (abatacept). All these drugs are characterized by high specificity that allows the recognition of a specific molecule, thus preventing further repercussions on other cells or organs. In addition, biosimilar drugs of infliximab, etanercept and rituximab have been recently commercialised, and their use has been spread due to their non-negligible cost-sparing effects and comparable profiles, in terms of efficacy and safety, with the reference products.

The use of biological drugs to treat RA has led to considerable improvements in inflammation control and the prevention of structural damage. However, there are patients who develop adverse events or experience the progressive loss of treatment efficacy. The unsuccessful outcome of biological therapy may be due to immunogenicity (i.e., the capacity of a drug to induce an immune-mediated response against its own epitopes), which may depend on a number of drug- and patient-related factors. Biological monoclonal antibodies (MoAbs) are synthesised in murine cells and contain some foreign amino acid sequences that are potentially highly antigenic. The 25% murine structure of infliximab and its biosimilar compounds make them more immunogenic than other anti-rheumatic biological agents, despite comparable immunogenicity profiles, as assessed by the production of anti-drug antibodies (ADAs) between originators and biosimilars.

RA is characterized by an aberrant activation of adaptive immunity that is mirrored by the interplay of many sub-sets of T helper (Th) lymphocytes. In an altered cytokine background, such as that of RA patients, the administration of biological drugs that are potentially highly antigenic may induce the aberrant activation of specific T and B effector responses against drug epitopes. There is considerable evidence that the production of ADAs mainly depends on the activation of a Th2 cell pathway; however, as suggested by a few reports, the paradoxical activation of Th1 and Th17 responses following the administration of infliximab may also occur in non-responding RA patients.

The levels of Th9 cells, which are specialised for producing IL-9, but can also produce IL-10, IL-17, IL-21 and IL-22, are increased in the bloodstream and synovial membranes of RA patients, where they are directly related to the degree of lymphoid organisation and the production of autoantibodies, such as anti-citrullinated peptide antibodies (ACPAs). However, no study has yet investigated the role of Th9 lymphocytes in the immunogenicity of biological agents by comparing originator and biosimilar compounds.

The aim of this study was to evaluate if Th-9 cells can mediate drug immunogenicity and to compare the Th9-related immunogenicity of the infliximab originator (Remicade®) and its biosimilar compound (Remsima®) in a cohort of infliximab-responder and inadequate responder (IR) RA patients by means of an in vitro stimulation assay, taking into account the demographic and clinimetric features of the patients, the use of concomitant drugs, and the reason for discontinuing infliximab.

2. Results

2.1. Baseline Demographic and Clinical Assessment

At the time of enrolment, five of the 15 drug-naïve RA patients (14 Caucasians and one Chinese; 12 females; mean age 54.8 ± 16.2 years; mean disease duration 2.3 ± 3.9 years) had ACPAs, seven had rheumatoid factor (RF), and two had anti-nuclear antibodies (ANAs); their mean C-reactive protein/28-joint disease activity score (CRP-DAS28) was 4.6 ± 1.0. All were taking anti-inflammatory and analgesic drugs as needed.

Fifteen of the 20 good responders to infliximab (19 Caucasians and one Hispanic; 16 females, mean age 61.3 ± 12.2 years; mean disease duration 13.4 ± 7.2 years) had ACPAs, 12 had ANAs, 11 had RF, three had anti-double stranded DNA antibodies (anti-dsDNA), one had anticardiolipin antibodies (ACLAs), and one had anti-extractable nuclear antigen antibodies (ENAs). Their RA had been well controlled by infliximab (Remicade®) for a mean of 8.3 ± 3.9 years (mean CRP-DAS28 at the time of blood sampling 2.5 ± 1.0). The concomitant medications were prednisone (2.5–10 mg/day) in eight patients, methotrexate (5–15 mg/week) in 20, and hydroxychloroquine (200–400 mg/day) in three.

Seventeen of the 20 non-responders to infliximab (19 Caucasians and one Indian; 15 females; mean age 57.0 ± 12.2 years; mean disease duration 18.1 ± 9.5 years) had ANAs, 15 had ACPAs, 15 had RF, three had ACLAs, two had anti-dsDNA, and two had anti-ENAs. Thirteen were being treated with intravenous (i.v.) abatacept (10 mg/kg every four weeks), five were being treated with i.v. tocilizumab (8 mg/kg every four weeks), one was being treated with subcutaneous (s.c.) etanercept (50 mg once a week), and one was being treated with s.c. certolizumab pegol (200 mg every other week); these treatments were the second (8 patients), third (8 patients) or fourth biological line (4 patients). The patients had been treated with infliximab (Remicade®) for a mean of 2.4 ± 1.9 years, and had discontinued the drug for a mean of 8.0 ± 2.5 years due to inefficacy (11 cases) or adverse events (mainly allergic or infusion reactions, 9 cases). Their concomitant conventional drugs were prednisone (2.5–10 mg/day) in 14 cases, methotrexate (5–15 mg/week) in nine cases and hydroxychloroquine (200–400 mg/day) in five cases. Their mean CRP-DAS28 was 2.9 ± 0.8 at the time of blood sampling. Demographic and clinical characteristics are displayed in Table 1.

Treated patients and untreated patients were matched for gender and age, and significantly differed for disease duration ($p < 0.001$, Student's *t* Test for unpaired samples); ANAs and ACPAs were more frequently detected in longstanding RA treated patients than in untreated ones ($p < 0.001$ and $p = 0.006$, respectively; Pearson's Chi squared test).

Good responders and non-responders to infliximab were matched for gender, age, disease duration, autoantibody subsets (Student's *t* Test for unpaired samples and Pearson's Chi squared test); whereas they significantly differed for methotrexate and prednisone medium dose intake, (respectively $p = 0.003$ and 0.030; Student's *t* Test for unpaired samples).

Table 1. Demographic characteristics of the population included in the study. RA: rheumatoid arthritis; IFX: infliximab; SD: standard deviation; F: females; M: males; ACPAs: anti-citrullinated-protein antibodies; RF: rheumatoid factor; ANAs: anti-nuclear antibodies; anti-dsDNA: anti-double stranded DNA antibodies; anti-ENAs: anti-extractable nuclear antigen antibodies; ACLAs: anticardiolipin antibodies; LAC: lupus anticoagulant; CRP-DAS28: C-reactive protein/28-joint disease activity score; NSAIDs: non-steroidal anti-inflammatory drugs.

Variables	Healthy Controls	Treatment-Naïve RA Patients	RA Patients Responding to IFX	RA Patients Non-Responding to IFX
Number of subjects	10	15	20	20
Mean age ± SD, years	43.9 ± 8.3	54.8 ± 16.2	61.3 ± 12.2	57.0 ± 12.2
Mean disease duration ± SD, years	/	2.3 ± 3.9	13.4 ± 7.2	18.1 ± 9.5
Gender, F/M (number)	4/6	12/3	16/4	15/5
ACPAs+, (number)	/	5	15	15
RF+, (number)	/	7	11	15
ANAs+, (number)	/	2	12	17
Anti-dsDNA Ab, (number)	/	0	3	2
Anti-ENAs Ab+, (number)	/	0	1	3
ACLAs/LAC+, (number)	/	0	1	2
Mean CRP-DAS28 ± SD	/	4.6 ± 1.0	2.5 ± 1.0	2.9 ± 0.8
Prednisone (2.5–10 mg/day), (number)	/	/	8	14
Methotrexate (5–15 mg/week), (number)	/	/	20	9
Hydroxychloroquine (200–400 mg/day), (number)	/	/	3	5
NSAIDs, (number)	/	14	as needed	as needed

2.2. T helper 9 Cells at Baseline

The baseline percentage of PU.1$^+$, IRF4$^+$ Th9 cells was higher in the drug-naïve patients than in the healthy controls and treated patients ($p < 0.01$) (Figure 1). There was no significant difference in the percentage of OX40-expressing, IL-9-producing, CD4$^+$ T cells between the healthy controls and any of the patient groups (Figure 2), possibly because of the involvement of different pathways in the differentiation of Th9 cells [1]; however, the percentage of OX40-expressing CD4$^+$ T cells was higher in the patient groups than in the controls. The greater frequency of Th9 cells among the RA patients was not associated with higher ANA or other autoantibody levels, disease duration, baseline

CRP-DAS28, nor was it associated with the reason for discontinuing infliximab or the number of previous biological drugs administered to the non-responders. Moreover, a multivariate analysis did not reveal any significant influence of concomitant conventional or biological treatments, although the heterogeneity of the biological therapies and the limited number of cases may have biased the statistical evaluation.

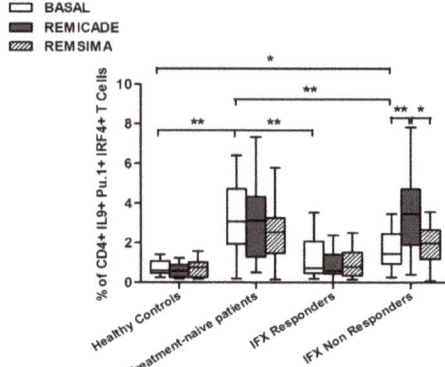

Figure 1. Percentages of PU.1[+], IRF4[+], IL-9[+] CD4[+] T cells at baseline and after exposure to branded and biosimilar infliximab. * $p < 0.05$, ** $p < 0.01$.

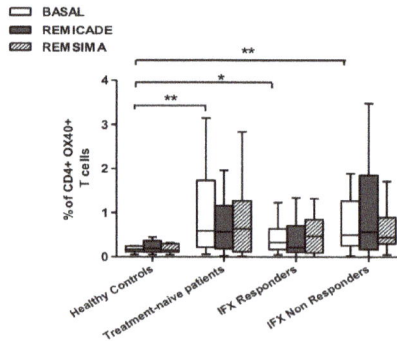

Figure 2. Percentages of OX40[+], IL-9[+] CD4[+] T cells at baseline and after exposure to branded and biosimilar infliximab. * $p < 0.05$, ** $p < 0.01$.

In brief, at baseline the difference in the percentage of Th9 cells between the healthy controls and the RA patients was observed in the group of untreated patients. This finding indicates that the activation of Th9 cells is a distinctive characteristic of RA and can be restored by concomitant efficacious conventional or biological treatments.

2.3. Effects of Infliximab (Remicade®) on T Helper 9 Cells

Stimulation with branded infliximab increased the percentage of PU.1[+] and IRF4[+] Th9 cells only in the IR group of patients (Figure 1). There were no differences in OX40-expressing, IL-9-producing CD4[+] T cells or OX40-expressing CD4[+] T cells, before and after infliximab exposure (Figure 2), possibly because of the widespread expression of OX40 in the Th cell pool [2].

We also investigated whether Th9 lymphocytes may be activated by means of a specific stimulus on Th memory cells from patients who had discontinued infliximab because of inefficacy or adverse events. Antigen stimulation can induce central memory (CCR7[+], CD45RA[−]) T cells to migrate from lymph nodes to peripheral tissues, lose CCR7, and differentiate into (CCR7$^-$, CD45RA$^-$) effector memory T cells with immediate activation. Furthermore, in the case of protracted low-dose antigen stimulation, they may be able to re-express the molecule CD45RA (terminally differentiated effector memory, TEMRA) and acquire surveillance functions with less pronounced effector properties [3,4]. We therefore subdivided IL-9-secreting CD4$^+$ T cells on the basis of the expression of CCR7 and CD45RA, which makes it possible to distinguish among naïve, central memory, effector memory and TEMRA cells. All of these cell pools were increased in the untreated RA patients in comparison with the other groups. Following the addition of infliximab, IL-9$^+$, CCR7$^+$, CD45RA$^-$ central memory cells and IL-9$^+$, CCR7$^-$, CD45RA$^-$ effector memory cells (but not naïve Th9 cells) were increased in the infliximab IR group, thus indicating that these cell pools may account for the change in the percentage in PU.1 and IRF4-expressing, IL-9-secreting CD4$^+$ T cells (Figures 3–5). On the contrary, the percentage of TEMRA lymphocytes did not vary, presumably because of the limited proliferative activity of this cell pool (Figure 6).

The gating strategy for the identification of naïve, central memory, effector memory and TEMRA CD4$^+$ T lymphocytes is shown in Figure 7.

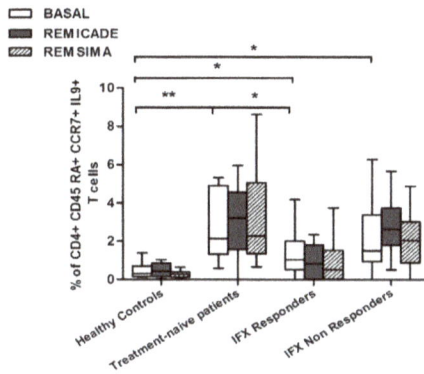

Figure 3. Percentages of CD45RA$^+$, CCR7$^+$, IL-9$^+$ CD4$^+$ (naïve) T cells at baseline and after exposure to branded and biosimilar infliximab. * $p < 0.05$, ** $p < 0.01$.

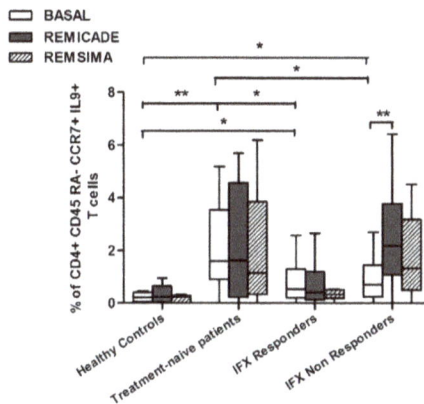

Figure 4. Percentages of CD45RA$^-$, CCR7$^+$, IL-9$^+$ CD4$^+$ (central memory) T cells at baseline and after exposure to branded and biosimilar infliximab. * $p < 0.05$, ** $p < 0.01$.

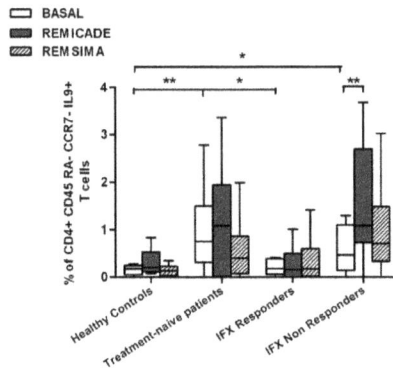

Figure 5. Percentages of CD45RA$^-$, CCR7$^-$, IL-9$^+$ CD4$^+$ (effector memory) T cells at baseline and after exposure to branded and biosimilar infliximab. * $p < 0.05$, ** $p < 0.01$.

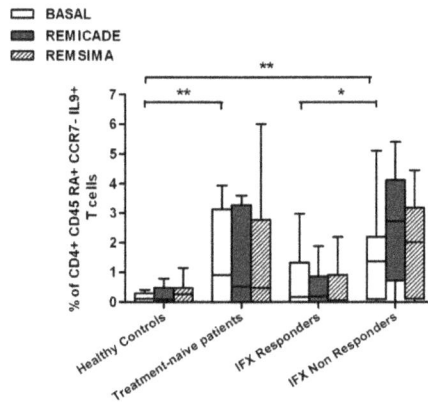

Figure 6. Percentages of CD45RA$^+$, CCR7$^-$, IL-9$^+$ CD4$^+$ (terminally differentiated effector memory, TEMRA) T cells at baseline and after exposure to branded and biosimilar infliximab. * $p < 0.05$, ** $p < 0.01$.

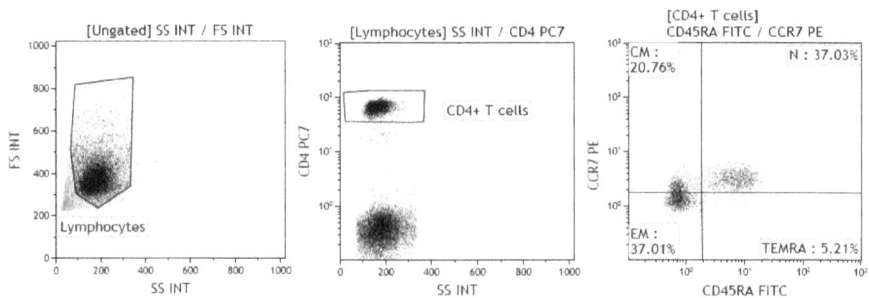

Figure 7. Gating strategy for the identification of naïve CD4$^+$ T lymphocytes (N), central memory CD4$^+$ T lymphocytes (CM), effector memory CD4$^+$ T lymphocytes (EM) and terminally differentiated effector memory (TEMRA) CD4$^+$ T lymphocytes. The lymphocyte population was gated on forward and side scatter properties, and further gated for CD4, CCR7, CD45RA expression; at least 20,000 events were acquired within the CD4 gate. The samples were acquired using a Gallios flow cytometer, and the data were analysed using Kaluza software (both Beckman Coulter).

2.4. Comparison of the Effects of Remicade® and Remsima® on T Helper 9 Cells

We repeated the previous experiment using the biosimilar compound CT-P13 (Remsima®). As in the experiment with the original infliximab, there were no significant variations in the percentages of PU.1[+], IRF4[+] Th9 cells, under basal or stimulated conditions, in the healthy controls and the untreated or responding RA patients, but the addition of the biosimilar did not significantly increase the percentage of PU.1 and IRF4-expressing, IL-9-secreting CD4[+] T cells or IL-9-secreting central and effector memory CD4[+] T cells in the infliximab IR group, as was observed after the addition of branded infliximab (Figures 1, 4 and 5). Furthermore, as in the case of branded infliximab, exposure to biosimilar CT-P13 did not induce a significant change in the percentages of IL-9-secreting naïve and TEMRA CD4[+] T lymphocytes (Figures 3 and 6), OX40-expressing, IL-9-producing CD4[+] T cells or OX40-expressing CD4[+] T cells in any of the patient groups (Figure 2).

3. Discussion

The aims of this study were to investigate the possible relationship between Th9 cells and the outcome of infliximab biological therapy, and to demonstrate that the immunogenic profiles of branded and biosimilar infliximab are comparable in terms of Th9-driven immune responses. The immunogenicity of a drug depends on the presence of the specific B and T epitopes contained in the primary amino acid sequence, or developing during post-translational modifications [5–7]. The most widely accepted hypothesis is that the production of ADAs is the mechanism underlying a drug-induced immune response [8–12], although it may also be responsible for the development of adverse events or a progressive loss of efficacy. The immunogenicity of biological drugs (especially chimeric molecules such as infliximab) may be partly due to the induction of ADAs, but we and other authors have shown that other immune pathways, such as the antigen-specific activation of Th1 or Th17 cells may be an alternative explanation for the rejection of biological treatments [13,14]. Th9 cells are a sub-set of T helper cells that develop from naïve or primed Th2 lymphocytes in the presence of IL-4 and TGFβ, and are characterised by transcriptional factors—PU-1 and IRF4. Furthermore, co-stimulatory molecules (including OX40 and Notch) and other cytokines (such as IL-1β, IL-25, IL-33, type I interferons, and thymic stromal lymphopoietin) are involved in promoting Th9 differentiation and IL-9 production [1]. These cells represent the main source of IL-9, although other cells such as Th2, Th17 and Treg cells may also make a contribution [15,16]. IL-9 is capable of activating various cells, including Th17 and Treg lymphocytes [17], and therefore, depending on the local microenvironment, Th9 lymphocytes may direct the immune response towards autoimmunity/inflammation or tolerance. IL-9 and Th9 cells are increased in subjects with inflammatory arthritis, connective tissue diseases, autoimmune colitis, and autoimmune encephalomyelitis [18–24]. In a previous experiment, we found an increased prevalence of IFNγ-, IL-4-, IL-17-, IL-9-secreting CD4[+] T cells in RA patients, although there was no significant association with therapeutic outcomes [25]; this unusual behaviour may be related to the heterogeneity and plasticity of IL-9-producing CD4[+] T cells, which may also include regulatory cells [26].

In line with these data, our results showed a higher percentage of Th9 cells in the peripheral blood of RA patients than in that of healthy controls; the levels were particularly high in untreated patients, whereas treatment with conventional or biological drugs seemed to reduce the difference. Following stimulation with original infliximab, the percentage of PU.1[+], IRF4[+] Th9 cells increased in the infliximab IR group and this finding was confirmed when the experiment was repeated with central and effector memory IL-9[+], CD4[+] T cells, but not with naïve or TEMRA IL-9 producer CD4[+] T cells.

PU1[+], IRF4[+] Th9 cells may increase following antigenic stimulation with infliximab in patients who have discontinued treatment, possibly because of the recall and activation of central and effector memory Th9 cells, but when we assessed the response of PU.1 and IRF4-expressing, IL-9-secreting CD4[+] T lymphocytes to biosimilar infliximab, we did not find any significant variation from baseline in any of the four groups, although there was a trend in the case of central and effector memory cells. A possible inhibitory effect on memory Th cells related to IL-10, produced in vitro upon reverse signaling on mTNF-α-bearing dendritic cells (DCs), or by memory T cells producing IL-10—particularly expanded in tolerant patients—cannot be excluded. Effector memory Th cells were reported to be consistently blocked by the IL-10, induced in vitro by the drug in tolerant patients and, to a lesser extent, in patients who interrupted therapy [27]. In our previous study [13], we reported an increase in the percentage of Treg cells in IFX-responders, compared to IFX naïve and IFX non-responders, even though we did not detected differences in the frequency of IL-10-producing Tregs among the groups of patients.

The discrepancy between branded and biosimilar infliximab may be due to various reasons. There was a trend towards an increase in the overall percentage of central and effector memory Th9 lymphocytes after exposure to biosimilar infliximab, but the difference was not significant, possibly because of the small number of patients. Furthermore, our experiments were carried using single batches of Remicade® and Remsima®, but it is known that there may be structural differences between one batch and another of the same drug. The epitopes recognised by Th9 cells upon exposure to branded infliximab may not be the same as those recognised upon exposure to the biosimilar, due to differences in charge, amount of aggregates and unassembled forms, and post-translational motifs such as the pattern of glycosylation [28,29]. The greater fucosylation in the crystallisable fragment (Fc) of biosimilar infliximab may prevent interaction with the FcγR (especially FCγ RIIIa and FCγ RIIIb) of mononuclear cells [30,31]. This has been related to reduced antibody-dependent cell cytotoxicity (ADCC) and may also affect immunogenicity, by reducing the internalisation of the drug–receptor complex in antigen-presenting cells. It has also been demonstrated that the infliximab originator has at least two B cell epitopes in the Fc with a glycosylated pattern [32], and this may give it a different immunogenic profile from that of its biosimilar compound. Finally, although current randomised controlled trials and spontaneous reports have indicated comparable immunogenicity profiles between biosimilar and reference infliximab [33–38], these have all been based on the production of ADAs, which may depend on different immunogenic properties and biological pathways.

One of the main limitations of this study was that none of the biologically-treated patients (enrolled prior of the commercialization of biosimilar drugs) received a treatment with biosimilar infliximab, being all treated with Remicade®. Consequently, data on the association between the efficacy/safety profile of Remsima® in vivo and Th9 cell percentages in vitro were not available. Moreover, differences in methotrexate and steroid intakes between the two groups (infliximab responders and non-responders) may have affected Th9 cell responses in vitro, despite no influence on Th9 cell percentages at baseline being reported and a lack of current scientific evidence.

4. Materials and Methods

4.1. Population

The study involved 55 outpatients with RA, diagnosed according to the ACR/EULAR 2010 criteria [39] who had participated in a previous study designed to explore the Th1/Th17-driven immunogenicity of infliximab (Remicade®) [13]: Fifteen subjects free of immunosuppressive drugs, 20 patients successfully treated with branded infliximab, and 20 patients who had switched or swapped from branded infliximab to other biological drugs because of adverse events or inefficacy.

The patients and a matched control group of 10 healthy subjects were consecutively enrolled between June 2013 and December 2013.

The exclusion criteria were concurrent infections, atopic dermatitis, hematological disorders, concomitant or recent treatment with leflunomide or cyclosporine, or vaccinations in the previous two months, because these drugs or medical conditions can variously affect the Th cell pool [40–44].

The protocol was approved by the local Ethics Committee of the University Hospital Luigi Sacco, Milan, on 27 June 2013, registered with the number 364/2013 38AP (Resolution No. 484), and conduced in accordance with the Declaration of Helsinki. Written informed consent was obtained from all participants.

4.2. Immunological Analyses

Peripheral blood mononuclear cells (PBMCs) were isolated from 18 mL blood samples collected into EDTA-containing Vacutainer tubes (Becton Dickinson, Rutherford, NJ, USA) by means of centrifugation on lymphocyte separation medium (Cedarlane Laboratories, Burlington, NC, USA), and their number and viability were determined using an ADAM-MC automatic cell counter (Digital-Bio, NanoEnTek Inc., Seoul, South Korea). The cells were cultured in RPMI 1640 plus penicillin, streptomycin, L-glutamine and 10% pooled human AB serum (all from Euroclone, Siziano, Italy) at a concentration of 1×106/mL, and were incubated for 18 h with culture medium alone, branded infliximab 50 µg/mL (Remicade®, Janssen Biologics, Leiden, The Netherlands), or its biosimilar (Remsima®, Celltrion Healthcare, Budapest, Hungary); pokeweed mitogen (PWM) (1 µg/mL of lectin from Phytolacca Americana, Sigma-Aldrich, Saint Louis, MO, USA) was used as a positive control to evaluate the cells' responsiveness [13]. The infliximab concentration of 50 µg/mL was chosen after titration testing—increasing drug concentrations and measuring median serum infliximab concentrations one hour after infusion (peak serum concentration: 39.9–219.1 µg) [45]. In order to facilitate co-stimulation, 1 µg/mL of anti-human CD28 (R&D Systems, Minneapolis, MN, USA) was added to the cell cultures. Brefeldin A 10 µg/mL (Sigma-Aldrich) was added after the first three h, in order to inhibit cytokine secretion.

The percentage of Th9 lymphocytes was determined by flow cytometric analysis. Th9 lymphocytes were identified as PU.1 and IRF4-expressing, IL-9-secreting CD4$^+$ T cells, although the percentage of OX40-expressing, IL-9-secreting CD4$^+$ T cells was also measured, as the co-stimulatory molecule may selectively drive Th differentiation toward a Th9 phenotype, while repressing both Treg and Th17 cell development [2]. IL-9 production by naïve CD4$^+$ T lymphocytes (CCR7$^+$, CD45RA$^+$), central memory CD4$^+$ T lymphocytes (CCR7$^+$, CD45RA$^-$), effector memory CD4$^+$ T lymphocytes (CCR7$^-$, CD45RA$^-$), and terminally differentiated effector memory (TEMRA) CD4$^+$ T lymphocytes (CCR7$^-$, CD45RA$^+$) was also evaluated.

The following human monoclonal antibodies (mAbs) were used: CD4 PE-Cy7, CD45RA FITC (Beckman Coulter, Milan, Italy); IRF4 PerCP-eFluor® and CD134 (OX40) FITC (eBioscience, Diego, CA, USA); IL-9 allophycocyanin (APC), CCR7 R-phycoerythrin (PE) and PU.1 PE (R&D Systems). To evaluate the percentage of IL-9-secreting PU.1- and IRF4-expressing CD4$^+$ T lymphocytes, the PBMCs were incubated with the mAbs for detecting cell surface antigens for 15 min, permeabilised with fixation/permeabilisation buffer (eBiosciences) for 30 min at 4 °C, and then stained with the antibodies for detecting intracellular transcription factors and IL-9 for a further 30 min at 4 °C. To evaluate IL-9 production by naïve and memory CD4$^+$ T cells, the PBMCs were incubated with the mAbs for detecting cell surface antigens for 15 min at room temperature (RT), fixed with 1% paraformaldehyde (PFA) for 15 min at 4 °C, permeabilised with saponin (Sigma-Aldrich), and stained with the antibodies for detecting intracellular cytokines. Following 45 min of incubation in ice, the cells were fixed with 1% PFA.

The lymphocyte population was gated on the basis of its forward and side scatter properties, and further gated for CD4, CCR7 and CD45RA expression; at least 20,000 events were acquired within the CD4 gate. The samples were acquired using a Gallios flow cytometer, and the data were analysed using Kaluza software (both Beckman Coulter).

4.3. Statistical Analysis

The data were analysed parametrically, as they were normally distributed. The groups were compared using an unpaired Student's *t* test for unequal variances, with a two-tailed *p* value and Pearson's Chi squared test. A multivariate analysis was used to detect whether the subjects' demographic characteristics or therapeutic regimens affected the Th9 percentages. A *p* value of <0.05 was considered statistically significant. The analyses were made using GraphPad Prism Software (GraphPad Software, San Diego, CA, USA) and SPSS, version 24.0 (International Business Machines Corporation, New York, NY, USA).

5. Conclusions

In conclusion, the prevalence of Th9 cells is higher in RA patients than in healthy subjects, and may be restored by concomitant conventional and biological treatments. Based on our findings, PU.1[+], IRF4[+] Th9 cells may be involved in orchestrating immune responses against epitopes of branded infliximab in patients failing the treatment; and this may be due to the recall and stimulation of both central and effector memory cells. On the other hand, despite a comparable profile in terms of immunogenicity emerged from other studies, biosimilar infliximab does not seem to activate these cell pools.

This study provides new insights into the immunogenicity of anti-TNF agents, which is routinely based on the detection of ADAs. The paradoxical activation of Th9 cells following exposure to infliximab may contribute to underlying inflammation, and thus explain the progressive loss of efficacy.

Nevertheless, the discrepancy between the Th9-driven immunogenicity of branded and biosimilar infliximab observed in our experiments may be attributable to our methodology rather than the real presence of dissimilar epitopes, and therefore deserves further investigation.

Author Contributions: Rossella Talotta conceived and designed the experiments; Rossella Talotta, Maria Chiara Ditto and Alberto Batticciotto recruited the patients; Angela Berzi and Daria Trabattoni performed the experiments; Angela Berzi and Rossella Talotta analyzed the data and performed statistical analysis; Angela Berzi and Daria Trabattoni contributed to reagents, materials and analysis tools; Rossella Talotta wrote the paper; Fabiola Atzeni, Andrea Doria and Piercarlo Sarzi-Puttini critically reviewed the manuscript.

Conflicts of Interest: The authors declare no conflict of interest.

References

1. Kaplan, M.H.; Hufford, M.M.; Olson, M.R. The development and in vivo function of T helper 9 cells. *Nat. Rev. Immunol.* **2015**, *15*, 295–307. [CrossRef] [PubMed]
2. Xiao, X.; Balasubramanian, S.; Liu, W.; Chu, X.; Wang, H.; Taparowsky, E.J.; Fu, Y.X.; Choi, Y.; Walsh, M.C.; Li, X.C. OX40 signaling favors the induction of Th 9 cells and airway inflammation. *Nat. Immunol.* **2012**, *13*, 981–990. [CrossRef] [PubMed]
3. Zielinski, C.E.; Corti, D.; Mele, F.; Pinto, D.; Lanzavecchia, A.; Sallusto, F. Dissecting the human immunologic memory for pathogens. *Immunol. Rev.* **2011**, *240*, 40–51. [CrossRef] [PubMed]
4. Harari, A.; Vallelian, F.; Pantaleo, G. Phenotypic heterogeneity of antigen-specific CD4 T cells under different conditions of antigen persistence and antigen load. *Eur. J. Immunol.* **2004**, *34*, 3525–3533. [CrossRef] [PubMed]
5. Jahn, E.M.; Schneider, C.K. How to systematically evaluate immunogenicity of therapeutic proteins—Regulatory considerations. *New Biotecnhol.* **2009**, *25*, 280–286. [CrossRef] [PubMed]
6. Spinelli, F.R.; Valesini, G. Immunogenicity of anti-tumor necrosis factor drugs in rheumatic diseases. *Clin. Exp. Rheumatol.* **2013**, *31*, 954–963. [PubMed]
7. Harding, F.A.; Stickler, M.M.; Razo, J.; DuBridge, R.B. The immunogenicity of humanised and fully human antibodies. Residual immunogenicity resides in the CDR regions. *mAbs* **2010**, *2*, 256–265. [CrossRef] [PubMed]
8. Atzeni, F.; Talotta, R.; Salaffi, F.; Cassinotti, A.; Varisco, V.; Battellino, M.; Ardizzone, S.; Pace, F.; Sarzi-Puttini, P. Immunogenicity and autoimmunity during anti-TNF therapy. *Autoimmun. Rev.* **2013**, *12*, 703–708. [CrossRef] [PubMed]
9. Aikawa, N.E.; de Carvalho, J.F.; Silva, C.A.; Bonfà, E. Immunogenicity of anti-TNF-α agents in autoimmune diseases. *Clinic Rev. Allerg. Immunol.* **2010**, *38*, 82–89. [CrossRef] [PubMed]
10. Vultaggio, A.; Matucci, A.; Nencini, F.; Pratesi, S.; Parronchi, P.; Rossi, O.; Romagnani, S.; Maggi, E. Anti-infliximab IgE and non-IgE antibodies and induction of infusion-related severe anaphylactic reactions. *Allergy* **2010**, *65*, 657–661. [CrossRef] [PubMed]

11. Baert, F.; Noman, M.; Vermeire, S.; Van Assche, G.; D'Haens, G.; Carbonez, A.; Rutgeerts, P. Influence of immunogenicity on the long-term efficacy of infliximab in Crohn's disease. *N. Engl. J. Med.* **2003**, *348*, 601–608. [CrossRef] [PubMed]

12. Vermeire, S.; Noman, M.; Van Assche, G.; Baert, F.; D'Haens, G.; Rutgeerts, P. Effectiveness of concomitant immunosuppressive therapy in suppressing the formation of antibodies to infliximab in Crohn's disease. *Gut* **2007**, *56*, 1226–1231. [CrossRef] [PubMed]

13. Talotta, R.; Berzi, A.; Atzeni, F.; Batticciotto, A.; Clerici, M.; Sarzi-Puttini, P.; Trabattoni, D. Paradoxical Expansion of Th1 and Th17 Lymphocytes in Rheumatoid Arthritis Following Infliximab Treatment: A Possible Explanation for a Lack of Clinical Response. *J. Clin. Immunol.* **2015**, *35*, 550–557. [CrossRef] [PubMed]

14. Torres, M.J.; Chaves, P.; Doña, I.; Blanca-López, N.; Canto, G.; Mayorga, C.; Blanca, M. T-cell involvement in delayed-type hypersensitivity reactions to infliximab. *J. Allergy Clin. Immunol.* **2011**, *128*, 1365–1367. [CrossRef] [PubMed]

15. Dardalhon, V.; Awasthi, A.; Kwon, H.; Galileos, G.; Gao, W.; Sobel, R.A.; Mitsdoerffer, M.; Strom, T.B.; Elyaman, W.; Ho, I.C.; et al. IL-4 inhibits TGF-beta-induced Foxp3+ T cells and, together with TGF-β, generates IL-9+ IL-10+ Foxp3− effector T cells. *Nat. Immunol.* **2008**, *9*, 1347–1355. [CrossRef] [PubMed]

16. Schmitt, E.; Klein, M.; Bopp, T. Th9 cells, new players in adaptive immunity. *Trends Immunol.* **2014**, *35*, 61–68. [CrossRef] [PubMed]

17. Elyaman, W.; Bradshaw, E.M.; Uyttenhove, C.; Dardalhon, V.; Awasthi, A.; Imitola, J.; Bettelli, E.; Oukka, M.; van Snick, J.; Renauld, J.C.; et al. IL-9 induces differentiation of TH17 cells and enhances function of FoxP3+ natural regulatory T cells. *Proc. Natl. Acad. Sci. USA.* **2009**, *106*, 12885–12890. [CrossRef] [PubMed]

18. Leng, R.X.; Pan, H.F.; Ye, D.Q.; Xu, Y. Potential role of IL-9 in the pathogenesis of systemic lupus erythematosus. *Am. J. Clin. Exp. Immunol.* **2012**, *1*, 28–32. [PubMed]

19. Nalleweg, N.; Chiriac, M.T.; Podstawa, E.; Lehmann, C.; Rau, T.T.; Atreya, R.; Krauss, E.; Hundorfean, G.; Fichtner-Feigl, S.; Hartmann, A.; et al. IL-9 and its receptor are predominantly involved in the pathogenesis of UC. *Gut* **2015**, *64*, 743–755. [CrossRef] [PubMed]

20. Yanaba, K.; Yoshizaki, A.; Asano, Y.; Kadono, T.; Sato, S. Serum interleukin-9 levels are increased in patients with systemic sclerosis: Association with lower frequency and severity of pulmonary fibrosis. *J. Rheumatol.* **2011**, *38*, 2193–2197. [CrossRef] [PubMed]

21. Khan, I.H.; Krishnan, V.V.; Ziman, M.; Janatpour, K.; Wun, T.; Luciw, P.A.; Tuscano, J. Comparison of multiplex suspension array large-panel kits for profiling cytokines and chemokines in rheumatoid arthritis patients. *Clin. Cytometry* **2009**, *76*, 159–168. [CrossRef] [PubMed]

22. Hughes-Austin, J.M.; Deane, K.D.; Derber, L.A.; Kolfenbach, J.R.; Zerbe, G.O.; Sokolove, J.; Lahey, L.J.; Weisman, M.H.; Buckner, J.H.; Mikuls, T.R.; et al. Multiple cytokines and chemokines are associated with rheumatoid arthritis-related autoimmunity in first-degree relatives without rheumatoid arthritis: Studies of the Aetiology of Rheumatoid Arthritis (SERA). *Ann. Rheum. Dis.* **2013**, *72*, 901–907. [CrossRef] [PubMed]

23. Ciccia, F.; Guggino, G.; Rizzo, A.; Manzo, A.; Vitolo, B.; La Manna, M.P.; Giardina, G.; Sireci, G.; Dieli, F.; Montecucco, C.M.; et al. Potential involvement of IL-9 and Th9 cells in the pathogenesis of rheumatoid arthritis. *Rheumatology (Oxford)* **2015**, *54*, 2264–2272. [CrossRef] [PubMed]

24. Kundu-Raychaudhuri, S.; Abria, C.; Raychaudhuri, S.P. IL-9, a local growth factor for synovial T cells in inflammatory arthritis. *Cytokine* **2016**, *79*, 45–51. [CrossRef] [PubMed]

25. Talotta, R.; Berzi, A.; Atzeni, F.; Dell'Acqua, D.; Sarzi Puttini, P.; Trabattoni, D. Evaluation of Th9 lymphocytes in peripheral blood of rheumatoid arthritis patients and correlation with anti-tumor necrosis factor therapy: Results from an in vitro pivotal study. *Reumatismo* **2016**, *68*, 83–89. [CrossRef] [PubMed]

26. Zhu, J.; Paul, W.E. Heterogeneity and plasticity of T helper cells. *Cell Res.* **2010**, *20*, 4–12. [CrossRef] [PubMed]

27. Vultaggio, A.; Petroni, G.; Pratesi, S.; Nencini, F.; Cammelli, D.; Milla, M.; Prignano, F.; Annese, V.; Romagnani, S.; Maggi, E.; et al. ABIRISK Consortium. Circulating T cells to infliximab are detectable mainly in treated patients developing anti-drug antibodies and hypersensitivity reactions. *Clin. Exp. Immunol.* **2016**, *186*, 364–372. [CrossRef] [PubMed]

28. Remsima Assessment Report. EMA/CHMP/589317/2013. Available online: http://www.ema.europa.eu/docs/en_GB/document_library/EPAR_-_Public_assessment_report/human/002576/WC500151486.pdf (accessed on 27 June 2013).

29. Jung, S.K.; Lee, K.H.; Jeon, J.W.; Lee, J.W.; Kwon, B.O.; Kim, Y.J.; Bae, J.S.; Kim, D.I.; Lee, S.Y.; Chang, S.J. Physicochemical characterization of Remsima. *mAbs* **2014**, *6*, 1163–1177. [CrossRef] [PubMed]

30. Pierri, C.L.; Bossis, F.; Punzi, G.; De Grassi, A.; Cetrone, M.; Parisi, G.; Tricarico, D. Molecular modeling of antibodies for the treatment of TNFα-related immunological diseases. *Pharmacol. Res. Perspect.* **2016**, *4*, e00197. [CrossRef] [PubMed]

31. Yamane-Ohnuki, N.; Satoh, M. Production of therapeutic antibodies with controlled fucosylation. *mAbs* **2009**, *1*, 230–236. [CrossRef] [PubMed]

32. Homann, A.; Röckendorf, N.; Kromminga, A.; Frey, A.; Jappe, U. B cell epitopes on infliximab identified by oligopeptide microarray with unprocessed patient sera. *J. Transl. Med.* **2015**, *13*, 339. [CrossRef] [PubMed]

33. Yoo, D.H.; Hrycaj, P.; Miranda, P.; Ramiterre, E.; Piotrowski, M.; Shevchuk, S.; Kovalenko, V.; Prodanovic, N.; Abello-Banfi, M.; Gutierrez-Ureña, S.; et al. A randomised, double-blind, parallel-group study to demonstrate equivalence in efficacy and safety of CT-P13 compared with innovator infliximab when coadministered with methotrexate in patients with active rheumatoid arthritis: The PLANETRA study. *Ann Rheum. Dis.* **2013**, *72*, 1613–1620. [CrossRef] [PubMed]

34. Park, W.; Hrycaj, P.; Jeka, S.; Kovalenko, V.; Lysenko, G.; Miranda, P.; Mikazane, H.; Gutierrez-Ureña, S.; Lim, M.; Lee, Y.A.; et al. A randomised, double-blind, multicentre, parallel-group, prospective study comparing the pharmacokinetics, safety, and efficacy of CT-P13 and innovator infliximab in patients with ankylosing spondylitis: The PLANETAS study. *Ann Rheum. Dis.* **2013**, *72*, 1605–1612. [CrossRef] [PubMed]

35. Ben-Horin, S.; Yavzori, M.; Benhar, I.; Fudim, E.; Picard, O.; Ungar, B.; Lee, S.; Kim, S.; Eliakim, R.; Chowers, Y. Cross-immunogenicity: Antibodies to infliximab in Remicade-treated patients with IBD similarly recognise the biosimilar Remsima. *Gut* **2016**, *65*, 1132–1138. [CrossRef] [PubMed]

36. Smits, L.J.; Derikx, L.A.; de Jong, D.J.; Boshuizen, R.S.; van Esch, A.A.; Drenth, J.P.; Hoentjen, F. Clinical Outcomes Following a Switch from Remicade® to the Biosimilar CT-P13 in Inflammatory Bowel Disease Patients: A Prospective Observational Cohort Study. *J. Crohns Colitis* **2016**, *10*, 1287–1293. [CrossRef] [PubMed]

37. Buer, L.C.; Moum, B.A.; Cvancarova, M.; Warren, D.J.; Medhus, A.W.; Høivik, M.L. Switching from Remicade® to Remsima® is safe and feasible: A prospective, open-label study. *J. Crohns Colitis* **2016**, *11*, 297–304.

38. Benucci, M.; Gobbi, F.L.; Bandinelli, F.; Damiani, A.; Infantino, M.; Grossi, V.; Manfredi, M.; Parisi, S.; Fusaro, E.; Batticciotto, A.; et al. Safety, efficacy and immunogenicity of switching from innovator to biosimilar infliximab in patients with spondyloarthritis: A 6-month real-life observational study. *Immunol. Res.* **2016**, *65*, 419–422. [CrossRef] [PubMed]

39. Aletaha, D.; Neogi, T.; Silman, A.J.; Funovits, J.; Felson, D.T.; Bingham, C.O., 3rd; Birnbaum, N.S.; Burmester, G.R.; Bykerk, V.P.; Cohen, M.D.; et al. 2010 Rheumatoid arthritis classification criteria: An American College of Rheumatology/European League Against Rheumatism collaborative initiative. *Arthritis Rheum.* **2010**, *62*, 2569–2581. [CrossRef] [PubMed]

40. García-Piñeres, A.; Hildesheim, A.; Dodd, L.; Kemp, T.J.; Williams, M.; Harro, C.; Lowy, D.R.; Schiller, J.T.; Pinto, L.A. Cytokine and chemokine profiles following vaccination with human papillomavirus type 16L1 virus-like particles. *Clin. Vaccine Immunol.* **2007**, *14*, 984–989. [CrossRef] [PubMed]

41. Purvis, S.; Asaad, R.; Valerio, I.; Sha, B.E.; Landay, A.L.; Lederman, M.M. Levels of proinflammatory cytokines in plasma after pneumoccoccal immunization in human immunodeficiency virus type 1-infected patients. *Clin. Diagn. Lab. Immunol.* **1999**, *6*, 427–428.

42. Weigmann, B.; Jarman, E.R.; Sudowe, S.; Bros, M.; Knop, J.; Reske-Kunz, A.B. Induction of regulatory T cells by leflunomide in a murine model of contact allergen sensitivity. *J. Investig. Dermatol.* **2006**, *126*, 1524–1533. [CrossRef] [PubMed]

43. Chong, A.S.; Ma, L.L.; Shen, J.; Blinder, L.; Yin, D.P.; Williams, J.W. Modification of humoral responses by the combination of leflunomide and cyclosporine in Lewis rats transplanted with hamster hearts. *Transplantation* **1997**, *64*, 1650–1657. [CrossRef] [PubMed]

44. Belmar, N.A.; Lombardo, J.R.; Chao, D.T.; Li, O.; Ma, X.; Pong-Afar, M.; Law, D.A.; Starling, G.C. Dissociation of the efficacy and cytokine release mediated by an Fc-modified anti-CD3 mAb in a chronic experimental autoimmune encephalomyelitis model. *J. Neuroimmunol.* **2009**, *212*, 65–73. [CrossRef] [PubMed]
45. Clair, E.W.; Wagner, C.L.; Fasanmade, A.A.; Wang, B.; Schaible, T.; Kavanaugh, A.; Keystone, E.C. The relationship of serum infliximab concentrations to clinical improvement in rheumatoid arthritis: Results from ATTRACT, a multicenter, randomized, double-blind, placebo-controlled trial. *Arthritis Rheum.* **2002**, *46*, 1451–1459. [CrossRef] [PubMed]

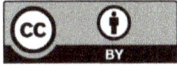

International Journal of
Molecular Sciences

MDPI

Review

Immunopathogenic Mechanisms and Novel Immune-Modulated Therapies in Rheumatoid Arthritis

Shyi-Jou Chen [1,2,3,4], Gu-Jiun Lin [5], Jing-Wun Chen [6], Kai-Chen Wang [7,8], Chiung-Hsi Tien [1,4], Chih-Fen Hu [1,4], Chia-Ning Chang [1,3], Wan-Fu Hsu [1,3], Hueng-Chuen Fan [1,9] and Huey-Kang Sytwu [2,4,6,10,*]

1   Department of Pediatrics, Tri-Service General Hospital, National Defense Medical Center, No. 325, Section 2, Chenggong Rd., Neihu District, Taipei City 114, Taiwan; pedneuchen@hotmail.com (S.-J.C.); tien.amoebia@msa.hinet.net (C.-H.T.); caperhu@gmail.com (C.-F.H.); Lizy0529@hotmail.com (C.-N.C.); kisetsu1110@gmail.com (W.-F.H.); fanhuengchuen@yahoo.com.tw (H.-C.F.)
2   Department of Microbiology and Immunology, National Defense Medical Center, No. 161, Section 6, MinChuan East Road, Neihu, Taipei City 114, Taiwan
3   Department of Pediatrics, Penghu Branch of Tri-Service General Hospital, National Defense Medical Center, No. 90, Qianliao, Magong City, Penghu County 880, Taiwan
4   Graduate Institute of Medical Sciences, National Defense Medical Center, No. 161, Section 6, MinChuan East Road, Neihu, Taipei City 114, Taiwan
5   Department of Biology and Anatomy, National Defense Medical Center, No. 161, Section 6, MinChuan East Road, Neihu, Taipei City 114, Taiwan; lingujiun@mail.ndmctsgh.edu.tw
6   Graduate Institute of Life Sciences, National Defense Medical Center, No. 161, Section 6, MinChuan East Road, Neihu, Taipei City 114, Taiwan; jiwechbmo@gmail.com
7   School of Medicine, National Yang-Ming University, No. 155, Section 2, Linong Street, Taipei City 112, Taiwan; kcwangtpe@gmail.com
8   Department of Neurology, Cheng Hsin General Hospital, No. 45, Cheng Hsin St., Pai-Tou, Taipei City 112, Taiwan
9   Department of Pediatrics, Tungs' Taichung MetroHarborHospital, No. 699, Section 8, Taiwan Blvd., Taichung City 435, Taiwan
10 National Institute of Infectious Diseases and Vaccinology, National Health Research Institutes, No. 35, Keyan Road, Zhunan, Miaoli County 350, Taiwan
*   Correspondence: sytwu@ndmctsgh.edu.tw; Tel.: +886-2-8792-3100 (ext. 18540); Fax: +886-2-8792-1774

Received: 5 January 2019; Accepted: 12 March 2019; Published: 16 March 2019

check for updates

Abstract: Rheumatoid arthritis (RA) is a chronic, inflammatory autoimmune disease of unknown etiology. It is characterized by the presence of rheumatoid factor and anticitrullinated peptide antibodies. The orchestra of the inflammatory process among various immune cells, cytokines, chemokines, proteases, matrix metalloproteinases (MMPs), and reactive oxidative stress play critical immunopathologic roles in the inflammatory cascade of the joint environment, leading to clinical impairment and RA. With the growing understanding of the immunopathogenic mechanisms, increasingly novel marked and potential biologic agents have merged for the treatment of RA in recent years. In this review, we focus on the current understanding of pathogenic mechanisms, highlight novel biologic disease-modifying antirheumatic drugs (DMRADs), targeted synthetic DMRADs, and immune-modulating agents, and identify the applicable immune-mediated therapeutic strategies of the near future. In conclusion, new therapeutic approaches are emerging through a better understanding of the immunopathophysiology of RA, which is improving disease outcomes better than ever.

Keywords: anticitrullinated peptide antibodies; antirheumatic drug; autoimmune; disease-modifying; immunology; pathology; rheumatoid factor

1. Introduction

Rheumatoid arthritis (RA) is one of the most widespread chronic immune-mediated inflammatory diseases, with a prevalence of 5–10 cases per 1000 people. It causes joint destruction, pain, and disability [1,2].

1.1. Characteristics

The initial symptoms of RA are swelling and pain in the joints of the hands and feet, especially in the metacarpophalangeal, metatarsophalangeal, and proximal interphalangeal joints. Large joints including the elbow, shoulder, ankle, and knee can also be involved [2]. Without adequate treatment, RA progresses to symmetric polyarthritis and destroys the diarthrodial joints of the hands and knees, leading to disability, inability, and mortality.

1.2. Current Therapeutics

Patients with RA should receive treatment with disease-modifying antirheumatic drugs (DMARDs). The definition of a DMARD is a medicine that interferes with signs and symptoms of RA, improves physical function, and inhibits the progression of joint damage [3]. Conventional synthetic DMARDs (csDMARDs) have been approved by licensing authorities via empiric clinical observation and have been used for more than 50 years. Methotrexate has been applied for treatment of RA for over 50 years, and even now, methotrexate is the most important of the csDMARDs. If intolerance, contraindications, adverse effects, or inadequate response occur in patients with RA treated with csDMARDs such as methotrexate, then a biologic DMARD and a targeted synthetic DMARD (tsDMARD) have superior efficacy when combined with methotrexate or another csDMARDs, compared with individual use [2]. Currently, IL-6R antibodies and JAK inhibitors are the most efficacious of the biologic DMARDs [4].

1.3. Limitations and Unmet Medical Needs

There are still unmet needs in RA treatment; full or stringent remission is not typical, nor is remission usually sustained without continuing treatment, which should now be the priority of research efforts [5]. Another concern is that biologic DMARDs and tsDMARDs are costly.

In this review, we focus on the current understanding of the immunopathogenic mechanisms that cause dysregulation of the inflammatory process leading to structural damage of bone and cartilage in patients with RA. Accordingly, understanding the immune-pathogenic mechanism is pivotal to the development of novel immune-mediated therapies.

2. Part I: Immunopathogenic Mechanisms in RA

In the inflammatory process of RA, the cascade responses of innate and adaptive immunity are the essential immune-pathogenic mechanisms [6]. This development is driven by a plethora of inflammatory cytokines and autoantibodies and is sustained by epigenetic changes in fibroblast-like synoviocytes, supporting further inflammation [7,8]. In the intermediate course, large numbers of different immune cells, including neutrophils, granulocytes, macrophages, B-cells, and T-cells invade the synovial membrane and fluid. This invasion results in tremendous releases of cytokines, chemokines, autoantibodies, and reactive oxidative stress (ROS) in the synovial membrane and space, leading to joint destruction. The serological hallmark of the disease is the presence of a high-titer of rheumatoid factor and anticitrullinated peptide antigen and antibodies (ACPAs) [9,10]. Additionally, Vande Walle et al. confirmed that the pathology of RA is strongly related to increased Nlrp3 inflammasome activation in vivo [11]. We discuss this complex mechanism further.

2.1. Role of Innate and Adaptive Immune Cells

Primary Immune Cells: Macrophages, Neutrophils, and Dendritic Cells in RA

Synovial membrane inflammation reflects consequent immune activation and is characterized by leukocyte invasion by innate immune cells such as monocytes, macrophages, dendritic cells, neutrophils, and adaptive immune cells including Th1, Th2, and Th17 cells, B-cells, and plasma cell lineages [5,12,13].

Both macrophages and neutrophils belong to the subset of phagocytes, which play the first defensive role against pathogens [12,14]. Macrophages contribute to the modulation of the immune response, which initiates immune-mediated inflammation leading to autoimmune disorders [15]. According to their microenvironment, macrophages can be divided into two distinct subsets with different physiological functions, one is proinflammatory subtype (M1), and the other is anti-inflammatory subtype (M2) [16,17].

Several proinflammatory cytokines such as IL-6, TNF-α, and IFN-γ are regulated at the transcriptional level and secreted through the endoplasmic reticulum/Golgi pathway. Interestingly, other proinflammatory cytokines including IL-1β and IL-18, are formed as cytosolic precursors, and their secretion is controlled by inflammatory caspases (caspase-1, -4, and -5) in humans [18]. These caspases are activated within cytosolic multimolecular complexes named inflammasomesin the milieu of the macrophage [19]. These intracellular inflammasomes that induce inflammatory responses in macrophages are activated by different types of ligands, leading tothe induction of inflammatory responses. The hallmark of inflammatory responses is the activation of inflammasomes—multiprotein oligomers containing intracellular pattern recognition receptors and inflammatory effectors—such as caspase recruitment domain (ASC) and pro-caspase-1and subsequently IL-1β andIL-18 is secreted from active macrophagein caspase-1-dependent manner [20].

And inflammasomes are classifiedinto three types: (1) 'canonical inflammsomes', such as nucleotide-bindingoligomerization domain (NOD)-like receptors (NLRs); (2) absentin melanoma 2 (AIM2) inflammasomes; (3): 'non-canonicalinflammasomes', such as caspase-4, -5, and -11 [21]. Remarkably, the nucleotide-binding oligomerization domain (NOD)-like receptor family pyrin domaincontaining 3 (NLRP3) inflammasone is emerging as an important factor in the inflammatory process of RA [19].

NLRP3 inflammasomes are highly activated in the infiltration of monocytes and macrophages in synovia but not in fibroblast-like synoviocytes from either RA patients or mice with collagen-induced arthritis (CIA). This activation pattern suggests a pathogenic role for NLRP3 inflammasomes in RA. The activation of NLRP3 inflammasomes was correlated with disease activity and IL-17A concentration in RA sera. Knockdown of NLRP3 suppressed Th17 differentiation MCC950, a selective NLRP3 inhibitor, had proven therapeutic effects in CIA in a murine RA model. MCC950-treated mice with CIA revealed significantly less severe joint inflammation and bone destruction. NLRP3 inflammasome activation in the synovia was significantly inhibited by MCC950, with reduced production of interleukin (IL)-1β [22]. Accordingly, the NLRP3 inflammasome could be a potential therapeutic target for the treatment of RA.

It is notable that the regulatory potential of caspase-11 in inflammatory responses during RA pathogenesis has been focused recently [20]. SinceLacey et al. disclosed the role of caspase-11 and its downstream effectors on inflammatory responses and infectious condition in the model of bacteria—induced inflammatory arthritis via caspase-11 knockout mice and proved that caspase-11 and caspase-1 induced proinflammatory cytokine production and joint inflammation in bacteria-infected arthritis mice, and delayed joint inflammation was observed in caspase-11 knockout mice alternatively. In addition, these results suggest that caspase-11 inflammasome in an IL-18-dependent manner induces the inflammatory responses and pathogenesisof joint inflammation in inflammatory arthritis [23].

Similar with canonical inflammasomes, non-canonical inflammasomesstimulate caspase-1 activation and GSDMD cleavage through the formation of cell membrane pores and caspase-1-mediated maturation and secretion of IL-1β and IL-18, suggesting that targeting of the non-canonical inflammasomes and their downstream effectors, such as caspase-11, caspase-1, GSDMD, and proinflammatory cytokines, could be considered as potential targets to suppress inflammatory responses, thus treat inflammatory diseases [20].

Given the existing evidence on the regulatory roles of either canonical or non-canonical inflammasomes during inflammatory responses, selective targeting of these inflammasomes by novel pharmacological approaches may potentially be applied clinically to prevent and treat various human inflammatory diseases including RA [20,24].

2.2. Dendritic Cells in RA

Dendritic cells in their role as antigen-presenting cells (APCs) are essential in inducing immunity and in mediating immune tolerance. Dendritic cells are now known to influence many different classes of lymphocytes (T, B, and NK cells) and many types of T-cell responses (Th1/Th2/Th17, regulatory T-cells, peripheral T-cell deletion) [25,26]. Dendritic cells have been investigated extensively in RA pathogenesis and have been implicated in RA [25]. The role of dendritic cells has been studied broadly in the pathogenesis of RA [27]. However, it remains unclear whether dendritic cells initiate autoimmunity in this disease [28].

Fully mature dendritic cells express high levels of MHC class II, costimulatory markers (CD86), proinflammatory cytokines (IL-12p70, IL-23, and tumor necrosis factor-α (TNF-α)), all of which are required for the efficient induction of T effector cell responses. Furthermore, the expression of chemokine receptors is controlled during the process of dendritic cell maturation, which enables dendritic cell migration toward lymphoid tissues to present antigen to naïve T-cells. For example, CCR5 is expressed on immature dendritic cells, which is down-regulated during cell maturation; alternatively, CCR7 is overexpressed in maturing dendritic cells [29]. On the other hand, specific repressive molecular patterns with immune suppressive compounds reveal a part of the maturation of dendritic cells with tolerogenic properties. These tolerogenic dendritic cells are considered "semi-mature." They may be phenotypically mature and exhibit high levels of MHC class II and costimulatory molecules but may express co-inhibitory molecules such as programmed death-ligands 1 and, 2, and immunoglobulin-like transcript 3; they may also characteristically produce immunosuppressive molecules including IL-10, TGF-β, and indoleamine 2,3-dioxygenase. Hence, they have plasticity regarding the functional maturation of dendritic cells, and environmental cues are essential for dendritic cells in the maturation process to determine whether they become immunogenic or tolerogenic [30–32]. Currently, tolerogenic dendritic cells are under investigation in clinical trials and could be applied clinically for RA treatment in the future [28,33].

2.2.1. T-Cells, B-Cells, and Cytokine Milieu in RA

T-cells also play a critical role in immune-mediated inflammation of RA. As the disease progresses, activated T-cells aggregate in inflamed joints in experimental CIA models of RA [34,35]. Naïve CD4 T helper (Th) cells can differentiate into distinct lineages (Th1, Th2, and Th17) that are characterized by lineage-specific expression of transcription factors and proinflammatory cytokines upon antigenic stimulation [36,37].

Before the era of proven Th17 cells, the imbalance of Th1 and Th2 was considered the central regulatory mechanism of adaptive immunity in autoimmune diseases including RA. Several studies have revealed that Th1 cells are found predominantly in RA joints [38]; alternatively, down-regulation of the Th1 response in experimental arthritis increased the Th2 response [39].

Since the discovery of Th17 cells more than one decade ago, their significance in RA has gradually emerged [40]. Human Th17 cell development is regulated by a transcription factor and RAR-related orphan receptor C. These cells express IL-17A, IL-17F, IL-21, IL-22, IL-26, TNF-α, GM-CSF, andCCL20 [41,42], which play specific roles in the immune response and exhibit synergetic effects [13,40]. The increased amounts of Th1, Th2, and Th17 cells are demonstrated [13,43], while that of regulatory T-cells (Tregs) suppresses disease severity in CIA [44]. In addition, Tregs are reduced in the blood of RA patients [45]. The dysregulation of CD4+ and CD8+ T-cells influences the autoimmune progression, depending on the presence of autoreactive Th1 and Th17 CD4+ T-cells, leading to RA immunopathology and disease development [45].

2.2.2. B-Cells in RA

Citrullinated antigen-directed B-cells of patients with RA and reacted with citrullinated antigens have a substantial in vitro effect [46]. This citrullinated antigen-directed B-cell response contributes to the initiation and persistence of the inflammatory process. Therefore, anticitrullinated protein antibody (ACPA) response is the primary humoral immune response associated with RA [10,47]. Accordingly, the biologic DMRADs for targeting B-cells was developed as the initial priority that is reviewed in this article.

Abnormal kinetics among immune cells results in an aberrant orchestra of activated T-cells, B-cells, mast cells, neutrophils, macrophages, and access APCs (i.e., dendritic cells), all of which contribute to the cellular immune responses of the RA disease process [48].

2.2.3. Immune-Mediated Inflammatory Milieu in RA

The initial effector cells of RA are neutrophils that release high levels of oxidants and cytotoxic products, such as ROS, and inflammatory agents including TNF-α, proteases, phospholipases, defensins, and myeloperoxidase at the site of acute RA in the affected joint. In chronic inflammation of RA, Th17 cells are involved in the induction of tissue inflammation by stimulation from recruited neutrophils. Reciprocally, these activated Th17 cells generate neutrophil chemoattractants such as IL-8 and TNF-α in the joint [49–52]. Neutrophils in the joint then facilitate the activation of Th17 cells through the secretion of Th17-maintaining chemokines CCL20 and CCL2 [53]. Likewise, neutrophils play a role in the activation of NK cells. The depletion of neutrophils can impair maturation, function, and homeostasis of NK cells [54]. Macrophages, while activated, play another crucial role in the inflammatory course of RA, and these cells, which are highly plastic, can polarize into either the M1 or M2 phenotype; M1 cells secrete proinflammatory cytokines, whereas M2 cells secrete anti-inflammatory cytokines [55,56].

M1 macrophages produce proinflammatory cytokines such as TNFα, IL-1β, IL-6, IL-12, IL-23, and low levels of IL-10 and inflammatory enzymes in the process of promoting acute RA. M1 macrophages also release inflammatory chemokines including CXCL5, CXCL8, CXCL9, CXCL10, and CXCL13 to recruit further leukocytes to the inflammatory site, and these cells produce more IL-1β, TNF-α IL-6, MMP, chemokine receptors, ROS, and inducible nitric oxide synthase in the joint, leading to joint destruction [49,57]. An evolutionary ancient inflammatory proteincalled high mobility group box 1 (HMGB1) rapidly activates APCs and activates innate and adaptive immune responses. This protein has been studied in patients with neuromyelitis optica and multiple sclerosis [58]. The risk factors associated with HMGB1 single nucleotide polymorphisms have been demonstrated in the development of RA disease among the Chinese Han population [59]. Thus, HMGB1 may be an emerging target for RA therapy.

The dominant function of M2 macrophages is anti-inflammation. Thus, M2 macrophages remodel and repair tissue by the production of IL-10, IL-12, and expression of CD163, and CD206, as well as releasing growth factors such as TGF-β and vascular endothelial growth factor (VEGF) during chronic inflammation [60,61]. Calreticulin (CRT), an endoplasmic reticulum residential glycoprotein, plays a crucial role in maintaining intracellular Ca^{2+} homeostasis. Soluble CRT accumulates in the blood of RA patients [62]. In addition, soluble oligomerized CRT could have a pathogenic function in autoimmune diseases through the induction of proinflammatory cytokines (e.g., TNF-α and IL-6) by macrophages via the MAPK-NF-κB signaling pathway [63]. This phenomenon implies soluble CRT has pathologic capability in RA, which could provide a strategy for a new therapeutic approach to RA.

The importance of the crosstalk between T-cells and monocytes in promoting inflammation is growing [64]. Remarkably, in RA, the receptors for IL-17 (IL-17RA and IL-17RC) are found in the synovium and are expressed on CD14+monocytes and macrophages, whereas synoviocytes bind with IL-17 to induce stimulation of further inflammation and production of IL-6 and MMPs in the synovium [61,65]. In addition, monocytes and macrophages from the synovial fluid of the inflamed arthritic joint can promote IL-17 production in CD4+ T-cells [66], suggesting that subsequently recruited CD4+T-cells in the rheumatoid joint can develop into a Th17 lineage in association with residential monocytes and macrophages. Consequently, a reciprocal synchronous loop between Th17 cells and monocytes and macrophages enables inflammation [13,67]. Regulatory T-cells (Tregs) are key participants in the regulation of various immune responses. Tregs have the potential to direct macrophages to develop into the M2 phenotype, with the functional and phenotypic characteristics of immune modulators [68]. Tregs express novel surface receptors Tregs such as neuropilin-1, CD83, and G protein-coupled receptor 83, which have advanced our understanding of Treg modulating mechanisms [69]. Thus, to target T-cell-macrophage interactions may have therapeutic potential in RA.

IL-6 and IL6R contribute to IL-6 blockade therapy currently on RA [70,71]. IL-6 is produced by a variety of cells such as endothelial cells, fibroblasts, keratinocytes, chondrocytes, some tumor cells, and immune cells including monocytes, macrophages, T-cells, and B-cells. IL-6 receptor is assembled from two subunits. One is IL-6-specific receptor (IL-6R), and the other is a signal transducer (gp130). Both the subunits exist in membrane-bound and soluble forms, named mIL-6R, sIL-6R, mgp130, and s130, respectively. However, mIL-6R is expressed only on some leukocytes while gp130 is found on many cells in body. IL-6 binds to mIL-6R, and the complex subsequently associates with signal transducing molecule gp130, which induces the activation of downstream signaling events in target cells via Janus kinase. This association leads to classic proinflammatory signaling. Alternatively, sIL-6R, without transmembrane and cytoplasmic regions converts to the anti-inflammatory pathway [8,72]. High levels of IL-6 have been detected in the blood and synovial fluid of most patients with RA. IL-6 facilities neutrophils to secrete ROS and proteolytic enzymes, which augment inflammation and eventually damage joints [73]. IL-6 causes inflammation and joint destruction by acting on neutrophils that secrete reactive oxygen intermediates and proteolytic enzymes. In addition, IL-6 stimulates osteoclast differentiation by activation of either RANKL-dependent or RANKL-independent mechanisms [74].

IL-6 enhances production of chemokines such as monocyte chemotactic protein-1 and IL-8 from endothelial cells, mononuclear cells, and fibroblast-like synoviocytes; it also induces adhesion molecules such as ICAM-1 in endothelial cells and induces increased adhesion of monocytes to endothelial cells in RA [75,76]. The synergistic effect of IL-6 with IL-1β and TNF-α stimulate the production of VEGF, which is an essential cytokine in the organization and maintenance of pannus [77].

Thus, knowledge and understanding of new and updated immunopathologic mechanisms could elicit the design and discovery of novel therapeutic and immune-modulatory agents to improve the life quality and disease control in RA.

3. Part II: Current Immune Target Therapy and on-Going Immune-Modulated Therapy in RA

By definition, DMARDs target inflammatory processes and lessen subsequent damage in diseasessuch asRA [5]. Monoclonal antibodies have been used extensively over the past two decades in clinical trials of RA treatments. TNFα–blocking monoclonal antibodies have been clinically proven and applied in patients with RA. However, the response period is limited [78]. Subsequently, many biologic and immune targeting agents have emerged with therapeutic effects in patients with RA. Furthermore, DMARDs cocktails mixed with several monoclonal antibodies or immune-modulated agents have been pre-clinically or clinically tested for inducing disease remission and maintenance [79].

Inspiringly, several biologic agents targeting cytokines and cytokine networks have achieved significant successes in RA treatment. Rituximab, a monoclonal antibody against the CD20 expressed on the surface of B-cells for depletion of B-cell, has been used in RA for more than one decade. Five TNF-α targeting biologic drugs are approved for treatment of RA, including etanercept, infliximab, adalimumab, certolizumab, pegol, and golimumab. Nonetheless, a substantial minority of patients with RA do not respond to these medications, which has necessitated the development of other biologic agents. Currently, tocilizumab, an anti-IL6R mAb; abatacept, a soluble fusion protein that consists of the extracellular domain of cytotoxic T-lymphocyte–associated antigen 4 linked to the modified Fc portion of IgG1, which interferes with T-cell activation; and tofacitinib, a Janus kinase class inhibitor that inhibits intracellular signaling are in clinical use [71].

We review the success of these therapeutic agents and potential strategies for RA treatment.

3.1. B-Cell Targeting Therapy

The first randomized, double-blind placebo-controlled trial of rituximab was completed in 2004 for patients with long-standing active RA, despite methotrexate treatment, or in combination with either cyclophosphamide or continued methotrexate, with significant improvement [80]. In addition, the efficacy and safety of different rituximab doses plus methotrexate, with or without glucocorticoids, in patients with active RA who did not respond to conventional DMARDs were tried in one clinical study. Either low or high dosages of rituximab were effective and well tolerated [81,82]. One concern is that serum sickness may occur following a first rituximab infusion without recurrence after the second infusion [83].

In patients with RA with an insufficient response to anti-TNF-α therapy, a single course of rituximab with methotrexate provided a significant improvement in disease activity and clinical progression of radiological damage [84]. An open-label prospective study further confirmed that rituximab is a treatment option for patients who do not respond to a single dose of TNF-α inhibitor, particularly for seropositive patients(patients with positive anti-CCP or RF) [85].

3.2. Anti-TNF-α Therapy

The strategy for blocking TNF-α was introduced to clinical practice at the end of the last century and revolutionized the treatment of RA as well as many other inflammatory conditions. Steeland et al. recently conducted an impressive review of successful anti-RA therapeutics with TNF-inhibitors (TNFi), including etanercept, infliximab, adalimumab, certolizumab, pegol, and golimumab [86]. Infliximab, adalimumab, and golimumab are full-length monoclonal antibodies, and thus, apart from their general TNF-blockage properties, they have Fc-effector activity as well. They can induce antibody-dependent cellular cytotoxicity (ADCC) and trigger the complement pathway leading to cell-dependent cytotoxicity (CDC) and apoptosis of target immune cells. Etanercept, a soluble TNF receptor, contains a truncated Fc-domain without the CH1 domain of IgG1; therefore, the potency of etanercept to induce ADCC and CDC is less than that of monoclonal antibodiessuch asinfliximab [87]. Certolizumab pegol, is a Fab' fragment, and its structure is incapable of inducing ADCC and CDC; therefore, its functioning mechanism is not dependent on the complement pathway [86,88].

Notably, Nguyen et al. demonstrated that adalimumab, but not etanercept, paradoxically promoted the interaction between monocytes and Tregs isolated from patients with RA. Adalimumab bound to monocyte membrane TNF and surprisingly enhanced its expression and its binding to TNF-RII expressed on Tregs. Consequently, adalimumab expanded functional Foxp3(+) T reg cells capable of suppressing Th17 cells through an IL-2/STAT5-dependent mechanism [89].

Total B-cell numbers are reduced in the blood of patients with RA vs. healthy controls but are significantly higher (normal levels) in patients undergoing anti–TNFα therapy. Cardiovascular disease, including heart failure and infections, represent the leading causes of disability and mortality in patients with RA [90]. Patients treated with anti–TNFα antibody alone or with methotrexate seem to be at further risk of severe infection such as tuberculosis [91,92]. As a result, the anti-TNFα treatment is contraindicated in all patients with heart failure and a substantial portion of patients with RA and impaired heart function who do not benefit from the treatment [93].

Nonetheless, anti–TNFα therapies are widely and successfully used despite the risk of serious adverse events. Presently, anti-TNF therapies are initiated as the standard-of-care in RA patients when methotrexate treatment fails to provide relief. TNF-inhibitors combined with methotrexate are used in the treatment of 70–80% of RA cases [86,94].

3.3. Anti-IL-12/IL-23 Therapy

TGF-β, IL-23, and proinflammatory cytokines function to drive and modulate human Th17 responses in RA [95,96]. Moreover, increased Th17 cell numbers and poor clinical outcomes in RA patients are associated with a genetic variant in the *IL4R* gene [97]. Accordingly, IL-12 and IL-23 are implicated in the pathogenesis of RA and may be considered candidate molecules for immune targeting in RA. Ustekinumab is a human monoclonal antibody targeting the IL-12/23 p40 subunit, which, in clinical trials, has inhibited both IL-12 and IL-23 activity and is effective in relieving moderate-to-severe psoriasis and active psoriatic arthritis [98,99].

Guselkumab is a new monoclonal antibody targeting IL-23 and is effective for psoriasis relief in a clinical trial [100]. The safety and efficacy of ustekinumab and guselkumab were studied in adults with active RA regardless of methotrexate therapy. However, targeting of IL-12/IL-23 p40 (ustekinumab) and IL-23 alone (guselkumab) were not proved yet in RA treatments [101].

3.4. Anti-IL6 Signaling Therapy

IL-6 is a kind of cytokine with multi-biological functions that include regulation of immune reaction, inflammation, and hematopoietic effects. IL-6 possesses quite a lot of proinflammatory characters, such as stimulating the production of chemokines and adhesion molecules in lymphocytes [4], and increasing neutrophil numbers in the blood [6].

Tocilizumab, humanized anti-IL-6 receptor (IL-6R) monoclonal antibody, is highly efficacious for the treatment of intractable autoimmune inflammatory diseases, including RA and juvenile idiopathic arthritis (JIA) in clinical trials [70].

Tofacitinib is a novel, oral Janus kinase (JAK) inhibitor-mediated by JAK1 and JAK3 to regulate STAT1 and STAT3 through the IL-6/gp130/STAT3 signaling pathway. Tofacitinib has been shown to amelirate arthritis symptoms effectively in patients with RA, and oral tofacitinib is Food and Drug Administration (FDA) approved for the treatment of RAand approved by the EMA [74,102]. Moreover, tofacitinib down-regulates the production of proinflammatory cytokines IL-17 and IFN-γ and the proliferation of CD4+ T-cells in patients with RA [103,104].

Global data has shown that patients with RA and inadequate response or intolerance to anti-TNFα therapy can often be effectively managed by switching to a drug with a novel mechanism of action, such as an IL-6R inhibitor [105]. Blockade of IL-6 signaling (via a monoclonal antibody to the IL-6 receptor, tocilizumab) reportedly boosts Tregs and inhibit monocyte IL-6 mRNA expression, inducing monocyte apoptosis [106–109]. Sarilumab, a fully human monoclonal antibody against IL-6R, has shown efficacy and safety in patients with active RA with an inadequate response to methotrexate in a randomized clinical trial [110,111]. Furthermore, in a phase III clinical trial, sarilumab has shown effectiveness in RA patients with an inadequate response to tumor necrosis factor inhibitor (TNFi). Sarilumab plus csDMARDs significantly decreased circulating biomarkers and synovial inflammation and bone resorption, including C1M, C3M, CXCL13, MMP-3 tRANKL levels, and sICAM-1 [112].

Baricitinib is a novel oral, once-daily targeted synthetic DMARD (tsDMARD) that inhibits JAK1 and JAK2. JAK1 and JAK2 are involved in the immunopathogenesis of RA by increasing the turnover of active, phosphorylated STAT1 and STAT3, and preventing chemotaxis toward IL-8. Baricitinib is approved in the FDA, EU and Japan for the treatment of patients with moderate or severe active RA who did not respond well or were intolerant of csDMARD(s) [48,113,114].

3.5. Anti-Cytotoxic T-Lymphocyte–Associated Antigen 4 Therapy

CTLA4-immunoglobulin (Ig) (abatacept) is a fusion protein containing components of IgG and cytotoxic T-lymphocyte–associated antigen 4 that inhibit costimulatory signals from APCs distinctively impairing T-cell costimulatory signals by binding to CD80 and CD86 receptors on APCs to target the interaction between monocytes and T-cells and prevent T-cell activation [115]. Abatacept significantly reduced disease severity and enhanced physical function in RA patients who experienced inadequate responses to methotrexate and TNFi [61,116]. Nonetheless, some patients did not respond to abatacept. They had an increased proportion of CD28-cells among CD4+ cells suggesting that CD4+ CD28+ Tfh-like cells could be targets of abatacept. Therefore, the presence of CD4+ CD28−cells may be a potential predictor of abatacept resistance [117].

3.6. Tolerogenic Dendritic Cells in RA

Tregs play an essential role in maintaining immune tolerance. Restoration of Treg function is a promising target for clinical intervention in autoimmune diseases. One treatment method is reloading the Treg pool in autoimmune patients with functional Tregs, either by treating the patients with drugs that selectively expand the Treg population in vivo or by generating new Tregs ex vivo before infusing them into the patient [118]. The challenge of Treg therapy is how to achieve the expansion of antigen-specific Tregs and how to determine the appropriate antigen(s) to activate the Tregs. One remarkable strategy that is developing is using tolerogenic dendritic cells to induce Tregs that are active against heat-shock proteins (HSPs) ubiquitously expressed in inflamed target tissues [119].

Interestingly, HSP 60 is expressed in the synovial membranes of patients with RA, and monoclonal antibodies that recognize mammalian HSP 60 were detected in patients with chronic arthritis. Similar results were noted for the HSP family members HSP 40 and HSP 70 in synovial fluid and on circulating T-cells of patients. The strategy is to pulse tolerogenic dendritic cells with targeted HSP peptides to generate HSP-specific T-cells from dendritic cells with stable tolerogenic function and to induce a regulatory effect on the specific antigen. Thus, such a combination therapy of tolerogenic dendritic cells and HSP peptide therapy could be the optimal solution for autoantigen(s) in autoimmune diseases such as RA [120,121].

Disease-specific ACPAs were found in a large population of RA patients and were strongly associated with HLA-DRB1 risk alleles [5]. Inspiringly, intradermal rheumavax, which is the first tolerogenic dendritic cell therapy in a clinical trial for the treatment of patients with RA with HLA risk genotype-positive and citrullinated peptide-specific autoimmunity, was usually well tolerated and considered safe [122].

Lack of vitamin D, especially vitamin D3, is regarded as a critical factor in autoimmune rheumatic disease, including initial disease development, and it is associated with poorer clinical outcomes [123,124]. The second trial of tolerogenic dendritic cells in RA was of dexamethasone and vitamin D3 for tolerogenic dendritic cell generation [125]. The generation of these cells with both dexamethasone and vitamin D3 had a synergistic effect on increasing IL-10 levels [126,127].

4. Clinical Trials and the Spotlight for RA in the Future

4.1. MicroRNA

MicroRNAs (miRNAs) are small non-coding RNAs that regulate gene expression by modulating the cell transcriptome directly [128,129]. miR-155 is a multifunctional miRNA with high production in immune cells and is essential for the immune response. Conversely, deregulation of miR-155 contributes to the progression of chronic inflammation in RA, and thus, miR-155 has potential as a therapeutic target for the treatment of RA [130]. Visfatin is a newly discovered adipocyte enzyme [131] that promotes the production of IL-6 and TNF-α via the inhibition of miR-199a-5p expression through the ERK, p38, and JNK pathways and is also a potential target for disease biomarker and drug development in inflammatory arthritis [132].

4.2. PI3Kγ Inhibitors

PI3Kγ mediates the modulation of chemokine-induced migration and enrollment of neutrophils, monocytes, and macrophages in patients with RA [133]. PI3Kγ is considered a potential target in the treatment of RA, though no drug has been developed yet to date [134]. In addition, pathogenic autoantibodies contribute significantly to antibody-initiated inflammation in RA progression. Targeting

IgG by glyco-engineering bacterial enzymes to specifically cleave IgG and alter N-linked Fc-glycans or blocking the downstream effector pathways offers a novel opportunity to develop therapeutics for RA treatment in the future [135]. Novel drugs targeting IL-12/IL-23 axis have been proven effective in the treatment of severe psoriasis and psoriatic arthritis (i.e., ustekinumab targeting the IL-12/23 p40 subunit that inhibits IL-12 and IL-23 activity and guselkumab targeting IL-23) [136]. The randomized phase II studies of ustekinumab and guselkumab in RA have shown convincing results, but infection is a primary concern [101].

The therapeutic design of TGFβ-transduced mesenchymal stem cells (MSCs) with enhanced immunomodulatory activity in experimental autoimmune arthritis reduces disease severity and modulates T-cell-mediated immune response. Thus, the use of gene-modified MSCs may be an avenue for new therapeutic development for RA treatment [137]. Several types of stem cells, such as hematopoietic stem cells, MSCs, and Tregs, are currently in clinical trials [138].

Attractively, novel anti-RA therapeutics had been developed currently such as antagonizing targets to histamine H4, histone deacetylase, LHRH (luteinizing hormone-releasing hormone), cadherin, MMP-9, CX3C ligand 1, and TLR4.

4.3. Histamine H4

Histamine H4 receptor (H4R) preserves immune-modulatory and chemotaxic potentials in various immune cells, andclozapine—a HR4 antagonist could protect mice from arthritis [139]. In addition, Yamaura et al. demonstrated that tJNJ77777120 (JNJ)—histamine4receptor (H4R) H4R antagonist exhibits significant anti-inflammatory and anti-arthritic activities in a mouse model of collagen antibody-induced arthritis (CAIA). Suggesting the apparent involvement of H4R antagonism in the pathogenesis and progression of RA and implying that H4R in synovial tissue play a role in cartilage and bone destruction by influencing the secretion of MMP-3 in RA patients [140].

4.4. Histone Deacetylase (HDAC)

Since histone deacetylase (HDAC) inhibitors repress the production of IL-6 in RA-FLS and macrophages by promoting mRNA decay [141]. Thus, the therapeutic potential of HDAC inhibitors had been investigated in RA and many HDAC inhibitors have been developed, e.g., the pan HDAC inhibitors, such as ITF 2357 and SAHA, inhibit all HDACs, and the selective HDAC inhibitors, such as Tubastatin A and Tubacin, inhibit HDAC6 specifically [142].

WhileHDAC3 powerfully regulates STAT1 activity in RA-FLS, indicating HDAC3 as a potential therapeutic target in the treatment of RA and type I IFN-driven autoimmune diseases [143].

Moreover, the therapeutic effect of a novel specific HDAC6 inhibitor, CKD-L, compared to the pan HDAC inhibitors, ITF 2357 or Tubastatin A on CIA and Treg cells isolated from RA patients. In the CIA model, CKD-L and Tubastatin A significantly ameliorated the arthritis severity. CKD-L increasedCTLA-4 expression in Foxp3+ T-cells and inhibited the T-cells proliferation in the suppression assay. InRA PBMC, CKD-L significantly increased IL-10, and inhibited TNF-α and IL-1β. These results suggest that CKD-L—a novel HDAC6 inhibitor may have a therapeutic effect of RA in the future [143].

4.5. Cadherins

Cadherin-11 expressed mainly in the synovial lining and FLS adhered to cadherin-11-Fc are first proved, supporting an important role for cadherin-11 in the specific adhesion of FLS and in synovial tissue organization and behavior in health and RA [144]. Furthermore, Lee et al. demonstrate cadherin-11-deficient mice with a hypoplastic synovial lining that display a disorganized synovial reaction to inflammation and resistant to inflammatory arthritis. Accordingly, synovial cadherin-11 determines the manner of synovial cells in their proinflammatory and destructive tissue effects in inflammatory arthritis [145].

In the joint, cadherin-11 is critical for synovial development. In synovial fibroblasts, cell surface cadherin-11 engagement with a recombinant soluble form of the cadherin-11 extracellular binding domain linked to immunoglobulin Fc tail induced MAPK and NF-κB activation, leading to significant IL-6, chemokines, and MMP expression [146]. Currently, a monoclonal antibody againstcadherin-11 is in early phases of clinical trials in patients with RA [147], and the result is expectable.

4.6. LHRH (Luteinizing Hormone-Releasing Hormone)

RA symptoms may develop or burst during stimulation of the hypothalamic-pituitary-gonadal axis, such as during the menopausal transition, postpartum, anti-estrogen treatment, or polycystic ovarian syndrome while GnRH and gonadotropin secretion increases [148].

GnRH-antagonism—cetrorelix produced rapid anti-inflammatory effects in terms of decreased TNF-α, IL-1β, IL-10, and CRP compared with placebo in RA patients with high gonadotropin levels [149]. Therefore, current developed GnRH-antagonism—cetrorelix has the positive effects in RA that addresses the potential therapeutic candidate in RA patients with high level GnRH.

4.7. MMP-9

High expression of transcription factor SOX5 was detected in RA-FLS and MMP-9 expression was inhibited from the knockdown model of SOX5 in CIA mice, suggesting thatSOX5 at least a part plays a pivotal role in mediating migration and invasion of FLS by regulating MMP-9 expression in RA that was confirmed inhibited in the joint tissue and reduced pannus migration and invasion into the cartilage [150].

Exposure of monocytes/macrophages to tocilizumab, etanercept or abatacept is resulted in a significant decrease of the PMA-induced superoxide anion production. The expression of PPARγ was significantly increased only by tocilizumab, while etanercept was the only one able to significantly reduce MMP-9 gene expression and inhibit the LPS-induced MMP-9 activity in monocytes. An uneven production of proinflammatory cytokines and MMP-9 in diseased articular joint tissues probably is affected by IL-17 through interacting with the macrophages in the rheumatoid synovium [151]. Thus, to block MMP-9 may be a potential strategy for developing novel therapeutics in RA.

4.8. CX3C Ligand 1

CX3CL1 is the member of t CX3C chemokines also named Fractalkine. CX3CL1 plays a role in monocyte chemotaxis and angiogenesis in the rheumatoid synoviumin RA. Increased MMP-2 production is detected from synovial fibroblasts upon CX3CL1 stimulation in vitro, suggesting a proinflammatory role of this Th1-type chemokine in RA [152]. Synergistic up-regulation of CX3CL1 protein also was observed after treatment with IL-1β and IFN-γ. The production of lung fibroblast-derived CX3CL1 were obviously reduced by specific inhibitors of the STAT-1 transcription factor, supporting the hypothesis that lung fibroblasts are an important cellular source of CX3CL1 and may contribute to causing pulmonary inflammation and fibrosis [153]. Recently, a clinical trial of an anti-CX3CL1 monoclonal antibody for the treatment of RA had been inaugurated in Japan. The multiple roles of CX3CL1 are in the pathogenesis of RA, to block CXCL1 may have a potential as a therapeutic target for this disease [154].

4.9. Toll-Like Receptors (TLRs)-TLR4

ACPA precede the onset of clinical and subclinical RA., ACPA fine profiling has the potential to identify RA patients with a predominantly TLR4-driven pathotype. Thus, TLR4 ligands may drive pathogenic processes of ACPA based on their target specificity in RA and thus address the potential therapeutic benefit when neutralizing TLR4 in the disease of RA [155]. Neutralization of TLR4 signaling was designed by using NI-0101, which is a TLR4 antagonism in terms of therapeutic and specific antibody to target TLR4. NI-0101-aTLR4 inhibition in an ex vivo model of RA pathogenesis can significantly amend cytokines release including IL1, IL-6, IL-8 and TNF-α.

Pharmacological inhibition of TLR4 and NF-κB activation blocked the HMGB1-dependent up-regulation of HIF-1α mRNA expression and its activity and HMGB1 stimulated expression of EGF, and inhibition of HIF-1α attenuated HMGB1-induced VEGF [156].

DFMG attenuates the activation of macrophages induced by co-culture with LPC-injured HUVE-12 cells via the TLR4/MyD88/NF-κB signaling pathway [157]. Predictably, the therapeutic design of TLR4 inhibition may be assumed as a therapeutic candidate for development in the treatment of RA soon or later.

4.10. Inflammasomes

Both hydroxychloroquine and VX740 are the potential candidates for the treatment of RA in the near future through modulation of inflammasomes [158]. Hydroxychloroquine (complex formationof the inflammasome) represses overexpression of TLR leading to inhibit the secretion of TNF-α. VX740—the inhibitor of caspase-1 inhibits CARD overexpression in RA and Decrease NLRP-3 and downstream proinflammatorycytokines. These novel approaches light on another therapeutic strategy in RA.

5. Conclusions

5.1. Challenge: Lessons from Targeted Interventions

Serious opportunistic infections rarely occur in long-term rituximab therapy. Nonetheless, patients and physicians must be aware that such opportunistic infections can occur. One example is the reactivation of the John Cunningham virus leading to progressive multifocal leukoencephalopathy, which has been reported in patients with autoimmune diseases. Patients must be informed of the risk of such adverse events with rituximab therapy [159,160]. Additionally, long-term rituximab therapy is related to hypogammaglobulinemia. Thus, basal immunoglobulin levels should be determined and carefully monitored to judge how rituximab therapy should be managed in light of IgG levels [161]. Additionally, late-onset neutropenia is a potential rituximab-related adverse event; thus, neutrophil levels should be carefully monitored [81,162].

A few biologic drugs such as TNF-α, IL6R, and CD20 inhibitors, can cause complications of neutropenia. Combination therapy of abatacept and G-CSF reduced such neutropenia [163].

The safety profile of oral tofacitinib seems acceptable, although some severe adverse effects have been observed, including serious and opportunistic infections (including tuberculosis and herpes zoster), malignancies, and cardiovascular events, which require strict monitoring irrespective of the duration of tofacitinib administration. As an oral drug, tofacitinib offers an alternative to subcutaneous or intravenous administration and should be recognized as a more convenient way of drug administration [163].

In RA, current immune-modulated therapies fail to maintain long-term physiological regulation in drug-free remission. Nonetheless, autologous conditioned tolerogenic dendritic cells with HSP-derived peptide antigen(s) could be used to restore immune tolerance. These treatments could either promote tolerance in pathologic T-cells or stimulate disease-suppressing Tregs in a dissimilarmanner [120].

5.2. Potential Targets for RA in the Future

Since a better understanding of the pathophysiology of RA, new therapeutic approaches are emerging (Table 1). Many novel approaches appear to have good therapeutic potential in the challenges of developing new treatments for RA [104]. We have summarized these potential targets in Table 2 including targets of microRNA (miR-155 and Visfatin) [164], PI3Kγ for chemokine-induced migration, histamine 4 receptor (H4R) through blocking H4R in synovial tissue to prevent the destruction cartilage and bone, histone deacetylase (HDAC), cadherin-11, LHRH (luteinizing hormone-releasing hormone), CX3CL1, TLR4, and activation of inflammasomes. (summarized in Table 2)

Table 1. Summary of novel treatment for RA.

Drug/Delivery	Target	Mechanism	Immune-Modulation
Target CD80/CD86 receptor on T cells			
Abatacept (Orencia®) /Intravenous delivery	Fc-fusion protein of the extracellular domain of human CTLA-4	block the binding reaction between CD80/CD86 and CD28, a costimulatory signal required for complete activation of T cells and inhibition of TNFα, and IFNγ production by activated T cells.	TNFα inducing the expression of innate cytokines IL-1β, IL-6 and IL-8, resulting in the rapid recruitment of neutrophils upon exposure to infection is blocked by and inhibition of TNFα, and IFNγ production by preveting T cells activation
Antagonist of IL-1			
Anakinra (Kineret®) / Subcutaneous injection	Block the reaction of IL-1 binding to IL-1RI	Block the reaction of IL-1 binding to IL-1RI resulting in intracellular signal transduction	Lessen the IL-1 effect on increasing the synovial fibroblast cytokine, chemokine, iNOS, PGs and MMPs release.
IL-6 receptor monoclonal antibody			
Sarilumab (Kevzara®)/Subcutaneous injection	a human IgG1 antibody, specifically binds to soluble and membrane-bound IL-6R (sIL-6Ra and mIL-6Ra)	Inhibit IL-6-mediated signalling involving ubiquitous signal transducing gp130 and STAT3	Interference the activator RANKL dependent or RANKL independent mechanismand also block the synergismwith IL-1β and TNF-α in producing VEGF
IL-12/IL-23 antibodies			
Ustekinumab (STELARA®)/ Subcutaneous injection	targeting the IL-12/23 p40 subunit, inhibiting both IL-12 and IL-23 activities	Bind to the IL-12 and IL-23, cytokines and down modulate lymphocyte function, including Th 1 and Th17 cell subsets	Inhibit IL-12-mediated signaling to reduce intracellular phosphorylation of STAT4 and STAT6 proteins, and impair the responses including cell surface molecule expression, NK cell activities and cytokine production, i.e., IFNγ
Guselkumab (Tremfya®)/ Subcutaneous injection	Specific targeting IL-23	Bind to IL-23 and repress induction of Th17 cell subsets IL-23, mainly produced by dendritic cells, macrophages	Block IL-23 target cells via either an IL-17-dependent or an IL-17-independent mechanism and decrease IL-23 secretion and inpair activation of producing Th17 cells via IL-23R and reduce cytokine such as IL-17 or IL-22
JAK inhibitor			
Tofacitinib (Xeljanz®)/ ORAL	the first-in-class JAK inhibitor, block JAK1 and JAK3 factor.	Interference the binding of IL-6 to the IL-6Rα/gp130 complex, STAT proteins	Tofacitinib block the pathway of JAK/STAT activation; due to JAK/STAT activation by IL-7 *versus* IL-6 or GM-CSF and the recruited to the cytokine/receptor complex
Baricitinib (Olumiant®) Decernotinib ORAL	Selective JAK1 and JAK2 inhibitor	Block with intracellular signal transduction , facilate the turnover of active, phosphorylated STAT1 and STAT3	inhibition of cytokine (IL-6) or thrombopoietin and reduce the expression of pathogenic Th1 and Th17 and prevent chemotaxis towards IL-8
Filgotinib/ORAL	selective JAK1 inhibitor	Block with intracellular signal transduction , facilate the turnover of active, phosphorylated STAT1	decrease IL-1β, IL-6, TNFα and MMP1 and MMP3, inhibit immune cell trafficking (CXCL10, ICAM-1 and VCAM-1) and VEGF. Also significantly decrease Th1 and Th17 cell subset differentiation and activity
Rheumavax®/ Intradermal injection	first-in-human trial for the treatment of RA generated tDC by NF-κB inhibition	InhibitNF-κB and prevent DC maturation to reduce the expression of CD40 and HLA-DR (a class II MHC molecule)	confers tolerogenic properties to DC including induction of T-cell anergy elevation of B220+ CD11c− B cells with a subpopulation of B-regulatory cells (Bregs)
Pulsing tlDCs with HSP peptides /Intravenous delivery with with HSP loaded tDCs	HSP 40 (dnaJB1): dnaJP1 HSP 60 (HspD1): DiaPep277 HSP 70 (HspA9): mB29a	Induce disease-suppressive regulatory T cells	induce IL-10 production and TGF-β

Table 2. Summary of potential targets for RA.

Drug or Compound	Target	Potential Mechanism	Immune-Modulation
Developing inhibitor of miR-155	miR-155	regulatory functions on the expression of genes by modulating the cell transcriptome directly	Inhibit TLR/cytokine receptor pathways and suppress the production of TNF, IL-1β, IL-6, and chemokines CCR7
Developing inhibitor of visfatin	Visfatin	Upregulation of miR-199a-5p expression through modulation of the ERK, p38, and JNK pathways	Decrease the production of IL-6 and TNF-α
Developing inhibitor of PI3Kγ	PI3Kγ	modulation of chemokine-induced migration	Control enrollment of inflammatory cells (i.e., neutrophils, monocytes, and macrophages)
andclozapine tJNJ77777120 (JNJ)	Histamine 4 receptor (H4R)	Block H4R in synovial tissue to prevent the destruction cartilage and bone	Immune-modulatory effect and repression of chemotaxic potentials by influencing the secretion of MMP-3
the pan HDAC inhibitors: ITF 2357 and SAHA HDAC6 inhibitors: Tubastatin A, Tubacin, and CKD-L	histone deacetylase (HDAC)	repress the production of IL-6 in RA FLS and macrophages by promoting mRNA decay	CKD-L increased CTLA-4 expression in Foxp3+ T cells and inhibited the T cells proliferation in the suppression assay. CKD-L significantly increased IL-10, and inhibited TNF-α and IL-1β
a monoclonal antibody against cadherin-11	cadherin-11	Block the reaction of engagement with a recombinant soluble form of the cadherin-11 extracellular binding domain linked to immunoglobulin Fc tail induced MAPK and NF-κB activation in SFL	Suppression the production of IL-6, chemokines, and MMP expression in SFL
GnRH-antagonism— cetrorelix	LHRH (luteinizing hormone-releasing hormone)	rapid anti-inflammatory effects	decreased TNF-α, IL-1β, IL-10, and CRP
knock-down model of SOX5	Block the MMP-9	Inhibit high expression of transcription factor SOX5 in RA-FLS	repressed IL-17 through interacting with the macrophages
anti-CX3CL1 monoclonal antibody	CX3CL1	Block monocyte chemotaxis and angiogenesis	Decreased MMP-2
NI-0101, a TLR4 antagonism	TLR4	block the HMGB1-dependent upregulation of HIF-1α mRNA expression	amend cytokines release including IL1, IL-6, IL-8 and TNF-α.
Hydroxychloroquine (complex formation of the inflammasome)	TLR overexpression	Inflammasome priming mechanism	Potential decreased TNF-α
VX 740	Caspace-1	Inhibit CARD8 overexpression	Decrease NLRP-3 and dwonstream cytokines

There is worth in studyingthe mechanisms of pathogenesis of RA and understanding causes of therapeutic failure in RA—for example, IL-1, IL-12, IL-17, IL-20, IL-21, IL-23, anti-CD4, anti-BAFF, and inhibitors of p38-MAPK and SYK [5]. The ultimate goal is todevelop cause-oriented, curative therapies; however, this willnot be easily achievable without better understanding of theexact cause(s) of RA.Nevertheless, through the development of early and precious diagnostic approaches and novel therapeuticsthat will provide more précised and efficient treatment of RA in the near future.

Funding: This work was supported by the Ministry of Science and Technology, Taiwan (MOST102-2314-B-016 -019 -MY3 and MOST106-2314-B-016 -041 -MY3 to S.-J. Chen) and by a research grant from Tri-Service GeneralHospital, Taiwan(TSGH-C101-009-S03 and TSGH-C107-008-S03 to S.-J. Chen), as well as, by the Penghu Branch of Tri-Service GeneralHospital, Taiwan, (TSGH-C104-PH-1 and TSGH-PH-105-1 to S.-J. Chen, TSGH-PH-106-1 to J.-N. Chang and TSGH-PH-107-7 to Wan-Fu Hsu). In addition, a part of research grants from Cheng Hsin General Hospital, Taiwan (CH-NDMC-107-05 to S.-J. Chen) and partly funded byNational Institute of Infectious Diseases and Vaccinology, National Health Research Institutes, Taiwan.

Conflicts of Interest: The authors declare no conflict of interest.

Abbreviations

ACPA	anticitrullinated protein antibody
TNFi	tumor necrosis factor inhibitor
APC	antigen-presenting cell
CRT	calreticulin
CIA	collagen-induced arthritis
DMARDs	disease-modifying antirheumatic drugs
csDMARD	conventional synthetic DMARD
tsDMARD	targeted synthetic DMARD
JAK	Janus kinase
MMP	matrix metalloproteinase
M1	type 1 macrophage
M2	type 2 macrophage
miRNA	microRNA
MSC	mesenchymal stem cell
NLRP3	nucleotide-binding oligomerization domain (NOD)-like receptor family pyrin domain containing 3
RA	rheumatoid arthritis
RANKL	receptor activator of NF-kappa B ligand;
ROS	reactive oxygen species
TNF-α	tumor necrosis factor-α
Th	T helper
TGF-β	tumor growth factor-β
Treg	regulatory T-cell
VEGF	vascular endothelial growth factor

References

1. Silman, A.J.; Pearson, J.E. Epidemiology andgenetics of rheumatoid arthritis. *Arthritis Res.* **2002**, *4*, S265–S272. [CrossRef]
2. Aletaha, D.; Smolen, J.S. Diagnosis and Management of Rheumatoid Arthritis: A Review. *JAMA* **2018**, *320*, 1360–1372. [CrossRef] [PubMed]
3. Smolen, J.S.; van der Heijde, D.; Machold, K.P.; Aletaha, D.; Landewe, R. Proposal fora new nomenclature of disease-modifying antirheumatic drugs. *Ann. Rheum. Dis.* **2014**, *73*, 3–5. [CrossRef] [PubMed]
4. Smolen, J.S.; Landewe, R.; Bijlsma, J.; Burmester, G.; Chatzidionysiou, K.; Dougados, M.; Nam, J.; Ramiro, S.; Voshaar, M.; van Vollenhoven, R.; et al. EULAR recommendations for the management of rheumatoid arthritis with synthetic and biological disease-modifying antirheumatic drugs: 2016 update. *Ann. Rheum. Dis.* **2017**, *76*, 960–977. [CrossRef]
5. Smolen, J.S.; Aletaha, D.; McInnes, I.B. Rheumatoid arthritis. *Lancet* **2016**, *388*, 2023–2038. [CrossRef]
6. Holmdahl, R.; Malmstrom, V.; Burkhardt, H. Autoimmune priming, tissue attack and chronic inflammation—The three stages of rheumatoid arthritis. *Eur. J. Immunol.* **2014**, *44*, 1593–1599. [CrossRef] [PubMed]
7. Harre, U.; Schett, G. Cellular and molecular pathways of structural damage in rheumatoid arthritis. *Semin. Immunopathol.* **2017**, *39*, 355–363. [CrossRef] [PubMed]
8. Mateen, S.; Zafar, A.; Moin, S.; Khan, A.Q.; Zubair, S. Understanding the role of cytokines in the pathogenesis of rheumatoid arthritis. *Clin. Chim. Acta* **2016**, *455*, 161–171. [CrossRef]
9. Cohen, E.; Nisonoff, A.; Hermes, P.; Norcross, B.M.; Lockie, L.M. Agglutination of sensitized alligator erythrocytes by rheumatoid factor(s). *Nature* **1961**, *190*, 552–553. [CrossRef]
10. Scherer, H.U.; Huizinga, T.W.J.; Kronke, G.; Schett, G.; Toes, R.E.M. The B cell response to citrullinated antigens in the development of rheumatoid arthritis. *Nat. Rev. Rheumatol.* **2018**, *14*, 157–169. [CrossRef]
11. Vande Walle, L.; Van Opdenbosch, N.; Jacques, P.; Fossoul, A.; Verheugen, E.; Vogel, P.; Beyaert, R.; Elewaut, D.; Kanneganti, T.D.; van Loo, G.; et al. Negative regulation of the NLRP3 inflammasome by A20 protects against arthritis. *Nature* **2014**, *512*, 69–73. [CrossRef]

12. Cuda, C.M.; Pope, R.M.; Perlman, H. The inflammatory role of phagocyte apoptotic pathways in rheumatic diseases. *Nat. Rev. Rheumatol.* **2016**, *12*, 543–558. [CrossRef]

13. Wang, S.P.; Lehman, C.W.; Lien, C.Z.; Lin, C.C.; Bazzazi, H.; Aghaei, M.; Memarian, A.; Asgarian-Omran, H.; Behnampour, N.; Yazdani, Y. Th1-Th17 Ratio as a New Insight in Rheumatoid Arthritis Disease. *Int. J. Mol. Sci.* **2018**, *17*, 68–77.

14. Kessenbrock, K.; Krumbholz, M.; Schonermarck, U.; Back, W.; Gross, W.L.; Werb, Z.; Grone, H.J.; Brinkmann, V.; Jenne, D.E. Netting neutrophils in autoimmune small-vessel vasculitis. *Nat. Med.* **2009**, *15*, 623–625. [CrossRef]

15. Orkin, S.H.; Zon, L.I. Hematopoiesis: An evolving paradigm for stem cell biology. *Cell* **2008**, *132*, 631–644. [CrossRef]

16. Wang, Y.; Han, C.C.; Cui, D.; Li, Y.; Ma, Y.; Wei, W. Is macrophage polarization important in rheumatoid arthritis? *Int. Immunopharmacol.* **2017**, *50*, 345–352. [CrossRef]

17. Jaguin, M.; Houlbert, N.; Fardel, O.; Lecureur, V. Polarization profiles of human M-CSF-generated macrophages and comparison of M1-markers in classically activated macrophages from GM-CSF and M-CSF origin. *Cell. Immunol.* **2013**, *281*, 51–61. [CrossRef]

18. Sidiropoulos, P.I.; Goulielmos, G.; Voloudakis, G.K.; Petraki, E.; Boumpas, D.T. Inflammasomes and rheumatic diseases: Evolving concepts. *Ann. Rheum. Dis.* **2008**, *67*, 1382–1389. [CrossRef]

19. Groslambert, M.; Py, B.F. Spotlight on the NLRP3 inflammasome pathway. *J. Inflamm. Res.* **2018**, *11*, 359–374. [CrossRef]

20. Yi, Y.S. Regulatory Roles of the Caspase-11 Non-Canonical Inflammasome in Inflammatory Diseases. *Immune Netw.* **2018**, *18*, e41. [CrossRef]

21. Yi, Y.S. Role of inflammasomes in inflammatory autoimmune rheumatic diseases. *Korean J. Physiol. Pharmacol.* **2018**, *22*, 1–15. [CrossRef]

22. Guo, C.; Fu, R.; Wang, S.; Huang, Y.; Li, X.; Zhou, M.; Zhao, J.; Yang, N. NLRP3 inflammasome activation contributes to the pathogenesis of rheumatoid arthritis. *Clin. Exp. Immunol.* **2018**, *194*, 231–243. [CrossRef]

23. Lacey, C.A.; Mitchell, W.J.; Dadelahi, A.S.; Skyberg, J.A. Caspases-1 and caspase-11 mediate pyroptosis, inflammation, and control of Brucella joint infection. *Infect. Immun.* **2018**, *86*, e00361-18. [CrossRef]

24. Shen, H.H.; Yang, Y.X.; Meng, X.; Luo, X.Y.; Li, X.M.; Shuai, Z.W.; Ye, D.Q.; Pan, H.F. NLRP3: A promising therapeutic target for autoimmune diseases. *Autoimmun. Rev.* **2018**, *17*, 694–702. [CrossRef]

25. Lebre, M.C.; Tak, P.P. Dendritic cell subsets: Their roles in rheumatoid arthritis. *Acta Reumatol. Port.* **2008**, *33*, 35–45.

26. Zhao, Y.; Zhang, A.; Du, H.; Guo, S.; Ning, B.; Yang, S. Tolerogenic dendritic cells and rheumatoid arthritis: Current status and perspectives. *Rheumatol. Int.* **2012**, *32*, 837–844. [CrossRef]

27. Schinnerling, K.; Soto, L.; Garcia-Gonzalez, P.; Catalan, D.; Aguillon, J.C. Skewing dendritic cell differentiation towards a tolerogenic state for recovery of tolerance in rheumatoid arthritis. *Autoimmun. Rev.* **2015**, *14*, 517–527. [CrossRef]

28. Khan, S.; Greenberg, J.D.; Bhardwaj, N. Dendritic cells as targets for therapy in rheumatoid arthritis. *Nat. Rev. Rheumatol.* **2009**, *5*, 566–571. [CrossRef]

29. Sallusto, F.; Schaerli, P.; Loetscher, P.; Schaniel, C.; Lenig, D.; Mackay, C.R.; Qin, S.; Lanzavecchia, A. Rapid and coordinated switch in chemokine receptor expression during dendritic cell maturation. *Eur. J. Immunol.* **1998**, *28*, 2760–2769. [CrossRef]

30. Van der Kleij, D.; Latz, E.; Brouwers, J.F.; Kruize, Y.C.; Schmitz, M.; Kurt-Jones, E.A.; Espevik, T.; de Jong, E.C.; Kapsenberg, M.L.; Golenbock, D.T.; et al. A novel host-parasite lipid cross-talk. Schistosomal lyso-phosphatidylserine activates toll-like receptor 2 and affects immune polarization. *J. Biol. Chem.* **2002**, *277*, 48122–48129. [CrossRef]

31. Steinbrink, K.; Jonuleit, H.; Muller, G.; Schuler, G.; Knop, J.; Enk, A.H. Interleukin-10-treated human dendritic cells induce a melanoma-antigen-specific anergy in CD8(+) T cells resulting in a failure to lyse tumor cells. *Blood* **1999**, *93*, 1634–1642.

32. Lan, Y.Y.; Wang, Z.; Raimondi, G.; Wu, W.; Colvin, B.L.; de Creus, A.; Thomson, A.W. "Alternatively activated" dendritic cells preferentially secrete IL-10, expand Foxp3+CD4+ T cells, and induce long-term organ allograft survival in combination with CTLA4-Ig. *J. Immunol.* **2006**, *177*, 5868–5877. [CrossRef]

33. Obregon, C.; Kumar, R.; Pascual, M.A.; Vassalli, G.; Golshayan, D. Update on Dendritic Cell-Induced Immunological and Clinical Tolerance. *Front. Immunol.* **2017**, *8*, 1514. [CrossRef]

34. Jung, S.M.; Lee, J.; Baek, S.Y.; Lee, J.; Jang, S.G.; Hong, S.M.; Park, J.S.; Cho, M.L.; Park, S.H.; Kwok, S.K. Fraxinellone Attenuates Rheumatoid Inflammation in Mice. *Int. J. Mol. Sci.* **2018**, *19*, 829. [CrossRef]

35. Myers, L.K.; Stuart, J.M.; Kang, A.H. A CD4 cell is capable of transferring suppression of collagen-induced arthritis. *J. Immunol.* **1989**, *143*, 3976–3980.

36. Chiocchia, G.; Boissier, M.C.; Ronziere, M.C.; Herbage, D.; Fournier, C. T cell regulation of collagen-induced arthritis in mice. I. Isolation of Type II collagen-reactive T cell hybridomas with specific cytotoxic function. *J. Immunol.* **1990**, *145*, 519–525.

37. Sakaguchi, S.; Benham, H.; Cope, A.P.; Thomas, R. T-cell receptor signaling and the pathogenesis of autoimmune arthritis: Insights from mouse and man. *Immunol. Cell Biol.* **2012**, *90*, 277–287. [CrossRef]

38. Miossec, P.; van den Berg, W. Th1/Th2 cytokine balance in arthritis. *Arthritis Rheum.* **1997**, *40*, 2105–2115. [CrossRef]

39. Mauri, C.; Feldmann, M.; Williams, R.O. Down-regulation of Th1-mediated pathology in experimental arthritis by stimulation of the Th2 arm of the immune response. *Arthritis Rheum.* **2003**, *48*, 839–845. [CrossRef]

40. Van Hamburg, J.P.; Tas, S.W. Molecular mechanisms underpinning T helper 17 cell heterogeneity and functions in rheumatoid arthritis. *J. Autoimmun.* **2018**, *87*, 69–81. [CrossRef]

41. Volin, M.V.; Shahrara, S. Role of TH-17 cells in rheumatic and other autoimmune diseases. *Rheumatology* **2011**, *1*. [CrossRef]

42. Ivanov, I.I.; McKenzie, B.S.; Zhou, L.; Tadokoro, C.E.; Lepelley, A.; Lafaille, J.J.; Cua, D.J.; Littman, D.R. The orphan nuclear receptor RORgammat directs the differentiation program of proinflammatory IL-17+ T helper cells. *Cell* **2006**, *126*, 1121–1133. [CrossRef]

43. Pollinger, B. IL-17 producing T cells in mouse models of multiple sclerosis and rheumatoid arthritis. *J. Mol. Med.* **2012**, *90*, 613–624. [CrossRef] [PubMed]

44. Kelchtermans, H.; Geboes, L.; Mitera, T.; Huskens, D.; Leclercq, G.; Matthys, P. Activated CD4+CD25+ regulatory T cells inhibit osteoclastogenesis and collagen-induced arthritis. *Ann. Rheum. Dis.* **2009**, *68*, 744–750. [CrossRef]

45. Dulic, S.; Vasarhelyi, Z.; Sava, F.; Berta, L.; Szalay, B.; Toldi, G.; Kovacs, L.; Balog, A. T-Cell Subsets in Rheumatoid Arthritis Patients on Long-Term Anti-TNF or IL-6 Receptor Blocker Therapy. *Mediat. Inflamm.* **2017**, *2017*, 6894374. [CrossRef] [PubMed]

46. Kerkman, P.F.; Rombouts, Y.; van der Voort, E.I.; Trouw, L.A.; Huizinga, T.W.; Toes, R.E.; Scherer, H.U. Circulating plasmablasts/plasmacells as a source of anticitrullinated protein antibodies in patients with rheumatoid arthritis. *Ann. Rheum. Dis.* **2013**, *72*, 1259–1263. [CrossRef]

47. Pelzek, A.J.; Gronwall, C.; Rosenthal, P.; Greenberg, J.D.; McGeachy, M.; Moreland, L.; Rigby, W.F.C.; Silverman, G.J. Persistence of Disease-Associated Anti-Citrullinated Protein Antibody-Expressing Memory B Cells in Rheumatoid Arthritis in Clinical Remission. *Arthritis Rheumatol.* **2017**, *69*, 1176–1186. [CrossRef]

48. Malemud, C.J. The role of the JAK/STAT signal pathway in rheumatoid arthritis. *Ther. Adv. Musculoskelet. Dis.* **2018**, *10*, 117–127. [CrossRef]

49. Navegantes, K.C.; de Souza Gomes, R.; Pereira, P.A.T.; Czaikoski, P.G.; Azevedo, C.H.M.; Monteiro, M.C. Immune modulation of some autoimmune diseases: The critical role of macrophages and neutrophils in the innate and adaptive immunity. *J. Transl. Med.* **2017**, *15*, 36. [CrossRef]

50. Milanova, V.; Ivanovska, N.; Dimitrova, P. TLR2 elicits IL-17-mediated RANKL expression, IL-17, and OPG production in neutrophils from arthritic mice. *Mediat. Inflamm.* **2014**, *2014*, 643406. [CrossRef]

51. Wright, H.L.; Chikura, B.; Bucknall, R.C.; Moots, R.J.; Edwards, S.W. Changes in expression of membrane TNF, NF-{kappa}B activation and neutrophil apoptosis during active and resolved inflammation. *Ann. Rheum. Dis.* **2011**, *70*, 537–543. [CrossRef]

52. Pelletier, M.; Maggi, L.; Micheletti, A.; Lazzeri, E.; Tamassia, N.; Costantini, C.; Cosmi, L.; Lunardi, C.; Annunziato, F.; Romagnani, S.; et al. Evidence for a cross-talk between human neutrophils and Th17 cells. *Blood* **2010**, *115*, 335–343. [CrossRef]

53. Cua, D.J.; Tato, C.M. Innate IL-17-producing cells: The sentinels of the immune system. *Nat. Rev. Immunol.* **2010**, *10*, 479–489. [CrossRef]

54. Jaeger, B.N.; Donadieu, J.; Cognet, C.; Bernat, C.; Ordonez-Rueda, D.; Barlogis, V.; Mahlaoui, N.; Fenis, A.; Narni-Mancinelli, E.; Beaupain, B.; et al. Neutrophil depletion impairs natural killer cell maturation, function, and homeostasis. *J. Exp. Med.* **2012**, *209*, 565–580. [CrossRef]

55. Mantovani, A.; Sozzani, S.; Locati, M.; Allavena, P.; Sica, A. Macrophage polarization: Tumor-associated macrophages as a paradigm for polarized M2 mononuclear phagocytes. *Trends Immunol.* **2002**, *23*, 549–555. [CrossRef]

56. Kennedy, A.; Fearon, U.; Veale, D.J.; Godson, C. Macrophages in synovial inflammation. *Front. Immunol.* **2011**, *2*, 52. [CrossRef]

57. Morand, E.F.; Leech, M. Macrophage migration inhibitory factor in rheumatoid arthritis. *Front. Biosci. A J. Virtual Libr.* **2005**, *10*, 12–22. [CrossRef]

58. Wang, K.C.; Tsai, C.P.; Lee, C.L.; Chen, S.Y.; Chin, L.T.; Chen, S.J. Elevated plasma high-mobility group box 1 protein is a potential marker for neuromyelitis optica. *Neuroscience* **2012**, *226*, 510–516. [CrossRef]

59. Wang, L.H.; Wu, M.H.; Chen, P.C.; Su, C.M.; Xu, G.; Huang, C.C.; Tsai, C.H.; Huang, Y.L.; Tang, C.H. Prognostic significance of high-mobility group box protein 1 genetic polymorphisms in rheumatoid arthritis disease outcome. *Int. J. Med Sci.* **2017**, *14*, 1382–1388. [CrossRef]

60. Wang, N.; Liang, H.; Zen, K. Molecular mechanisms that influence the macrophage m1-m2 polarization balance. *Front. Immunol.* **2014**, *5*, 614. [CrossRef]

61. Roberts, C.A.; Dickinson, A.K.; Taams, L.S. The Interplay Between Monocytes/Macrophages and CD4(+) T Cell Subsets in Rheumatoid Arthritis. *Front. Immunol.* **2015**, *6*, 571. [CrossRef]

62. Michalak, M.; Corbett, E.F.; Mesaeli, N.; Nakamura, K.; Opas, M. Calreticulin: One protein, one gene, many functions. *Biochem. J.* **1999**, *344*, 281–292. [CrossRef]

63. Duo, C.C.; Gong, F.Y.; He, X.Y.; Li, Y.M.; Wang, J.; Zhang, J.P.; Gao, X.M. Soluble calreticulin induces tumor necrosis factor-alpha (TNF-alpha) and interleukin (IL)-6 production by macrophages through mitogen-activated protein kinase (MAPK) and NFkappaB signaling pathways. *Int. J. Mol. Sci.* **2014**, *15*, 2916–2928. [CrossRef]

64. Burger, D.; Dayer, J.M. The role of human T-lymphocyte-monocyte contact in inflammation and tissue destruction. *Arthritis Res.* **2002**, *4*, S169–S176. [CrossRef]

65. Zrioual, S.; Toh, M.L.; Tournadre, A.; Zhou, Y.; Cazalis, M.A.; Pachot, A.; Miossec, V.; Miossec, P. IL-17RA and IL-17RC receptors are essential for IL-17A-induced ELR+ CXC chemokine expression in synoviocytes and are overexpressed in rheumatoid blood. *J. Immunol.* **2008**, *180*, 655–663. [CrossRef] [PubMed]

66. Evans, H.G.; Gullick, N.J.; Kelly, S.; Pitzalis, C.; Lord, G.M.; Kirkham, B.W.; Taams, L.S. In vivo activated monocytes from the site of inflammation in humans specifically promote Th17 responses. *Proc. Natl. Acad. Sci. USA* **2009**, *106*, 6232–6237. [CrossRef]

67. Alonso, M.N.; Wong, M.T.; Zhang, A.L.; Winer, D.; Suhoski, M.M.; Tolentino, L.L.; Gaitan, J.; Davidson, M.G.; Kung, T.H.; Galel, D.M.; et al. T(H)1, T(H)2, and T(H)17 cells instruct monocytes to differentiate into specialized dendritic cell subsets. *Blood* **2011**, *118*, 3311–3320. [CrossRef]

68. Brennan, F.M.; Foey, A.D.; Feldmann, M. The importance of T cell interactions with macrophages in rheumatoid cytokine production. *Curr. Top. Microbiol. Immunol.* **2006**, *305*, 177–194. [PubMed]

69. Hansen, W.; Westendorf, A.M.; Buer, J. Regulatory T cells as targets for immunotherapy of autoimmunity and inflammation. *Inflamm. Allergy Drug Targets* **2008**, *7*, 217–223. [CrossRef]

70. Kishimoto, T.; Kang, S.; Tanaka, T. IL-6: A New Era for the Treatment of Autoimmune Inflammatory Diseases. *Rheumatol. Int.* **2015**, 131–147.

71. Venuturupalli, S. Immune Mechanisms and Novel Targets in Rheumatoid Arthritis. *Immunol. Allergy Clin. North Am.* **2017**, *37*, 301–313. [CrossRef]

72. Rose-John, S. IL-6 trans-signaling via the soluble IL-6 receptor: Importance for the pro-inflammatory activities of IL-6. *Int. J. Biol. Sci.* **2012**, *8*, 1237–1247. [CrossRef]

73. Dayer, J.M.; Choy, E. Therapeutic targets in rheumatoid arthritis: The interleukin-6 receptor. *Rheumatology* **2010**, *49*, 15–24. [CrossRef]

74. Yoshida, Y.; Tanaka, T. Interleukin 6 and rheumatoid arthritis. *Biomed Res. Int.* **2014**, *2014*, 698313. [CrossRef]

75. Romano, M.; Sironi, M.; Toniatti, C.; Polentarutti, N.; Fruscella, P.; Ghezzi, P.; Faggioni, R.; Luini, W.; van Hinsbergh, V.; Sozzani, S.; et al. Role of IL-6 and its soluble receptor in induction of chemokines and leukocyte recruitment. *Immunity* **1997**, *6*, 315–325. [CrossRef]

76. Suzuki, M.; Hashizume, M.; Yoshida, H.; Mihara, M. Anti-inflammatory mechanism of tocilizumab, a humanized anti-IL-6R antibody: Effect on the expression of chemokine and adhesion molecule. *Rheumatol. Int.* **2010**, *30*, 309–315. [CrossRef]

77. Hashizume, M.; Mihara, M. The roles of interleukin-6 in the pathogenesis of rheumatoid arthritis. *Arthritis* **2011**, *2011*, 765624. [CrossRef]

78. Choy, E.H.; Panayi, G.S.; Kingsley, G.H. Therapeutic monoclonal antibodies. *Br. J. Rheumatol.* **1995**, *34*, 707–715. [CrossRef]

79. Serio, I.; Tovoli, F. Rheumatoid arthritis: New monoclonal antibodies. *Drugs Today* **2018**, *54*, 219–230. [CrossRef]

80. Edwards, J.C.; Szczepanski, L.; Szechinski, J.; Filipowicz-Sosnowska, A.; Emery, P.; Close, D.R.; Stevens, R.M.; Shaw, T. Efficacy of B-cell-targeted therapy with rituximab in patients with rheumatoid arthritis. *New Engl. J. Med.* **2004**, *350*, 2572–2581. [CrossRef]

81. Schioppo, T.; Ingegnoli, F. Current perspective on rituximab in rheumatic diseases. *Drug Des. Dev. Ther.* **2017**, *11*, 2891–2904. [CrossRef]

82. Emery, P.; Fleischmann, R.; Filipowicz-Sosnowska, A.; Schechtman, J.; Szczepanski, L.; Kavanaugh, A.; Racewicz, A.J.; van Vollenhoven, R.F.; Li, N.F.; Agarwal, S.; et al. The efficacy and safety of rituximab in patients with active rheumatoid arthritis despite methotrexate treatment: Results of a phase IIB randomized, double-blind, placebo-controlled, dose-ranging trial. *Arthritis Rheum.* **2006**, *54*, 1390–1400. [CrossRef] [PubMed]

83. Mehsen, N.; Yvon, C.M.; Richez, C.; Schaeverbeke, T. Serum sickness following a first rituximab infusion with no recurrence after the second one. *Clin. Exp. Rheumatol.* **2008**, *26*, 967. [PubMed]

84. Mease, P.J.; Cohen, S.; Gaylis, N.B.; Chubick, A.; Kaell, A.T.; Greenwald, M.; Agarwal, S.; Yin, M.; Kelman, A. Efficacy and safety of retreatment in patients with rheumatoid arthritis with previous inadequate response to tumor necrosis factor inhibitors: Results from the SUNRISE trial. *J. Rheumatol.* **2010**, *37*, 917–927. [CrossRef]

85. Emery, P.; Gottenberg, J.E.; Rubbert-Roth, A.; Sarzi-Puttini, P.; Choquette, D.; Taboada, V.M.; Barile-Fabris, L.; Moots, R.J.; Ostor, A.; Andrianakos, A.; et al. Rituximab versus an alternative TNF inhibitor in patients with rheumatoid arthritis who failed to respond to a single previous TNF inhibitor: SWITCH-RA, a global, observational, comparative effectiveness study. *Ann. Rheum. Dis.* **2015**, *74*, 979–984. [CrossRef]

86. Steeland, S.; Libert, C.; Vandenbroucke, R.E. A New Venue of TNF Targeting. *Int. J. Mol. Sci.* **2018**, *19*, 1442. [CrossRef] [PubMed]

87. Billmeier, U.; Dieterich, W.; Neurath, M.F.; Atreya, R. Molecular mechanism of action of anti-tumor necrosis factor antibodies in inflammatory bowel diseases. *World J. Gastroenterol.* **2016**, *22*, 9300–9313. [CrossRef]

88. Nesbitt, A.; Fossati, G.; Bergin, M.; Stephens, P.; Stephens, S.; Foulkes, R.; Brown, D.; Robinson, M.; Bourne, T. Mechanism of action of certolizumab pegol (CDP870): In vitro comparison with other anti-tumor necrosis factor alpha agents. *Inflamm. Bowel Dis.* **2007**, *13*, 1323–1332. [CrossRef]

89. Nguyen, D.X.; Ehrenstein, M.R. Anti-TNF drives regulatory T cell expansion by paradoxically promoting membrane TNF-TNF-RII binding in rheumatoid arthritis. *J. Exp. Med.* **2016**, *213*, 1241–1253. [CrossRef]

90. Levy, L.; Fautrel, B.; Barnetche, T.; Schaeverbeke, T. Incidence and risk of fatal myocardial infarction and stroke events in rheumatoid arthritis patients. A systematic review of the literature. *Clin. Exp. Rheumatol.* **2008**, *26*, 673–679.

91. Pala, O.; Diaz, A.; Blomberg, B.B.; Frasca, D. B Lymphocytes in Rheumatoid Arthritis and the Effects of Anti-TNF-alpha Agents on B Lymphocytes: A Review of the Literature. *Clin. Ther.* **2018**, *40*, 1034–1045. [CrossRef] [PubMed]

92. Kroesen, S.; Widmer, A.F.; Tyndall, A.; Hasler, P. Serious bacterial infections in patients with rheumatoid arthritis under anti-TNF-alpha therapy. *Rheumatology* **2003**, *42*, 617–621. [CrossRef]

93. Kotyla, P.J. Bimodal Function of Anti-TNF Treatment: Shall We Be Concerned about Anti-TNF Treatment in Patients with Rheumatoid Arthritis and Heart Failure? *Int. J. Mol. Sci.* **2018**, *19*, 1739. [CrossRef] [PubMed]

94. Monaco, C.; Nanchahal, J.; Taylor, P.; Feldmann, M. Anti-TNF therapy: Past, present and future. *Int. Immunol.* **2015**, *27*, 55–62. [CrossRef]

95. Volpe, E.; Servant, N.; Zollinger, R.; Bogiatzi, S.I.; Hupe, P.; Barillot, E.; Soumelis, V. A critical function for transforming growth factor-beta, interleukin 23 and proinflammatory cytokines in driving and modulating human T(H)-17 responses. *Nat. Immunol.* **2008**, *9*, 650–657. [CrossRef]

96. Kirkham, B.W.; Kavanaugh, A.; Reich, K. Interleukin-17A: A unique pathway in immune-mediated diseases: Psoriasis, psoriatic arthritis and rheumatoid arthritis. *Immunology* **2014**, *141*, 133–142. [CrossRef] [PubMed]

97. Leipe, J.; Schramm, M.A.; Prots, I.; Schulze-Koops, H.; Skapenko, A. Increased Th17 cell frequency and poor clinical outcome in rheumatoid arthritis are associated with a genetic variant in the IL4R gene, rs1805010. *Arthritis Rheumatol.* **2014**, *66*, 1165–1175. [CrossRef]

98. Leonardi, C.L.; Kimball, A.B.; Papp, K.A.; Yeilding, N.; Guzzo, C.; Wang, Y.; Li, S.; Dooley, L.T.; Gordon, K.B. PHOENIX 1 Study Investigators. Efficacy and safety of ustekinumab, a human interleukin-12/23 monoclonal antibody, in patients with psoriasis: 76-week results from a randomised, double-blind, placebo-controlled trial (PHOENIX 1). *Lancet* **2008**, *371*, 1665–1674. [CrossRef]

99. Papp, K.A.; Langley, R.G.; Lebwohl, M.; Krueger, G.G.; Szapary, P.; Yeilding, N.; Guzzo, C.; Hsu, M.C.; Wang, Y.; Li, S.; et al. Efficacy and safety of ustekinumab, a human interleukin-12/23 monoclonal antibody, in patients with psoriasis: 52-week results from a randomised, double-blind, placebo-controlled trial (PHOENIX 2). *Lancet* **2008**, *371*, 1675–1684. [CrossRef]

100. Gordon, K.B.; Duffin, K.C.; Bissonnette, R.; Prinz, J.C.; Wasfi, Y.; Li, S.; Shen, Y.K.; Szapary, P.; Randazzo, B.; Reich, K. A Phase 2 Trial of Guselkumab versus Adalimumab for Plaque Psoriasis. *N. Engl. J. Med.* **2015**, *373*, 136–144. [CrossRef]

101. Smolen, J.S.; Agarwal, S.K.; Ilivanova, E.; Xu, X.L.; Miao, Y.; Zhuang, Y.; Nnane, I.; Radziszewski, W.; Greenspan, A.; Beutler, A.; et al. A randomised phase II study evaluating the efficacy and safety of subcutaneously administered ustekinumab and guselkumab in patients with active rheumatoid arthritis despite treatment with methotrexate. *Ann. Rheum. Dis.* **2017**, *76*, 831–839. [CrossRef]

102. Traynor, K. FDA approves tofacitinib for rheumatoid arthritis. *Am. J. Health-Syst. Pharm.* **2012**, *69*, 2120. [CrossRef]

103. Gertel, S.; Mahagna, H.; Karmon, G.; Watad, A.; Amital, H. Tofacitinib attenuates arthritis manifestations and reduces the pathogenic CD4 T cells in adjuvant arthritis rats. *Clin. Immunol.* **2017**, *184*, 77–81. [CrossRef]

104. Cheung, T.T.; McInnes, I.B. Future therapeutic targets in rheumatoid arthritis? *Semin. Immunopathol.* **2017**, *39*, 487–500. [CrossRef]

105. Chastek, B.; Becker, L.K.; Chen, C.I.; Mahajan, P.; Curtis, J.R. Outcomes of tumor necrosis factor inhibitor cycling versus switching to a disease-modifying anti-rheumatic drug with a new mechanism of action among patients with rheumatoid arthritis. *J. Med Econ.* **2017**, *20*, 464–473. [CrossRef]

106. Samson, M.; Audia, S.; Janikashvili, N.; Ciudad, M.; Trad, M.; Fraszczak, J.; Ornetti, P.; Maillefert, J.F.; Miossec, P.; Bonnotte, B. Brief report: Inhibition of interleukin-6 function corrects Th17/Treg cell imbalance in patients with rheumatoid arthritis. *Arthritis Rheum.* **2012**, *64*, 2499–2503. [CrossRef]

107. Pesce, B.; Soto, L.; Sabugo, F.; Wurmann, P.; Cuchacovich, M.; Lopez, M.N.; Sotelo, P.H.; Molina, M.C.; Aguillon, J.C.; Catalan, D. Effect of interleukin-6 receptor blockade on the balance between regulatory T cells and T helper type 17 cells in rheumatoid arthritis patients. *Clin. Exp. Immunol.* **2013**, *171*, 237–242. [CrossRef]

108. Sarantopoulos, A.; Tselios, K.; Gkougkourelas, I.; Pantoura, M.; Georgiadou, A.M.; Boura, P. Tocilizumab treatment leads to a rapid and sustained increase in Treg cell levels in rheumatoid arthritis patients: Comment on the article by Thiolat et al. *Arthritis Rheumatol.* **2014**, *66*, 2638. [CrossRef]

109. Tono, T.; Aihara, S.; Hoshiyama, T.; Arinuma, Y.; Nagai, T.; Hirohata, S. Effects of anti-IL-6 receptor antibody on human monocytes. *Mod. Rheumatol.* **2015**, *25*, 79–84. [CrossRef]

110. Huizinga, T.W.; Fleischmann, R.M.; Jasson, M.; Radin, A.R.; van Adelsberg, J.; Fiore, S.; Huang, X.; Yancopoulos, G.D.; Stahl, N.; Genovese, M.C. Sarilumab, a fully human monoclonal antibody against IL-6Ralpha in patients with rheumatoid arthritis and an inadequate response to methotrexate: Efficacy and safety results from the randomised SARIL-RA-MOBILITY Part A trial. *Ann. Rheum. Dis.* **2014**, *73*, 1626–1634. [CrossRef]

111. Genovese, M.C.; Fleischmann, R.; Kivitz, A.J.; Rell-Bakalarska, M.; Martincova, R.; Fiore, S.; Rohane, P.; van Hoogstraten, H.; Garg, A.; Fan, C.; et al. Sarilumab Plus Methotrexate in Patients with Active Rheumatoid Arthritis and Inadequate Response to Methotrexate: Results of a Phase III Study. *Arthritis Rheumatol.* **2015**, *67*, 1424–1437. [CrossRef]

112. Gabay, C.; Msihid, J.; Zilberstein, M.; Paccard, C.; Lin, Y.; Graham, N.M.H.; Boyapati, A. Identification of sarilumab pharmacodynamic and predictive markers in patients with inadequate response to TNF inhibition: A biomarker substudy of the phase 3 TARGET study. *RMD Open* **2018**, *4*, e000607. [CrossRef]

113. Kubo, S.; Nakayamada, S.; Sakata, K.; Kitanaga, Y.; Ma, X.; Lee, S.; Ishii, A.; Yamagata, K.; Nakano, K.; Tanaka, Y. Janus Kinase Inhibitor Baricitinib Modulates Human Innate and Adaptive Immune System. *Front. Immunol.* **2018**, *9*, 1510. [CrossRef]

114. Al-Salama, Z.T.; Scott, L.J. Baricitinib: A Review in Rheumatoid Arthritis. *Drugs* **2018**, *78*, 761–772. [CrossRef]

115. Kaine, J.L. Abatacept for the treatment of rheumatoid arthritis: A review, Current therapeutic research. *Clin. Exp.* **2007**, *68*, 379–399.

116. Langdon, K.; Haleagrahara, N. Regulatory T-cell dynamics with abatacept treatment in rheumatoid arthritis. *Int. Rev. Immunol.* **2018**, *37*, 206–214. [CrossRef]

117. De Matteis, R.; Larghi, P.; Paroni, M.; Murgo, A.; De Lucia, O.; Pagani, M.; Pierannunzii, L.; Truzzi, M.; Ioan-Facsinay, A.; Abrignani, S.; et al. Abatacept therapy reduces CD28+CXCR5+ follicular helper-like T cells in patients with rheumatoid arthritis. *Arthritis Res. Ther.* **2017**, *35*, 562–570.

118. Trzonkowski, P.; Bacchetta, R.; Battaglia, M.; Berglund, D.; Bohnenkamp, H.R.; ten Brinke, A.; Bushell, A.; Cools, N.; Geissler, E.K.; Gregori, S.; et al. Hurdles in therapy with regulatory T cells. *Sci. Transl. Med.* **2015**, *7*, 304ps18. [CrossRef]

119. Jansen, M.A.A.; Spiering, R.; Broere, F.; van Laar, J.M.; Isaacs, J.D.; van Eden, W.; Hilkens, C.M.U. Targeting of tolerogenic dendritic cells towards heat-shock proteins: A novel therapeutic strategy for autoimmune diseases? *Immunology* **2018**, *153*, 51–59. [CrossRef]

120. Boog, C.J.; de Graeff-Meeder, E.R.; Lucassen, M.A.; van der Zee, R.; Voorhorst-Ogink, M.M.; van Kooten, P.J.; Geuze, H.J.; van Eden, W. Two monoclonal antibodies generated against human hsp60 show reactivity with synovial membranes of patients with juvenile chronic arthritis. *J. Exp. Med.* **1992**, *175*, 1805–1810. [CrossRef]

121. Schett, G.; Redlich, K.; Xu, Q.; Bizan, P.; Groger, M.; Tohidast-Akrad, M.; Kiener, H.; Smolen, J.; Steiner, G. Enhanced expression of heat shock protein 70 (hsp70) and heat shock factor 1 (HSF1) activation in rheumatoid arthritis synovial tissue. Differential regulation of hsp70 expression and hsf1 activation in synovial fibroblasts by proinflammatory cytokines, shear stress, and antiinflammatory drugs. *J. Clin. Investig.* **1998**, *102*, 302–311.

122. Benham, H.; Nel, H.J.; Law, S.C.; Mehdi, A.M.; Street, S.; Ramnoruth, N.; Pahau, H.; Lee, B.T.; Ng, J.; Brunck, M.E.; et al. Citrullinated peptide dendritic cell immunotherapy in HLA risk genotype-positive rheumatoid arthritis patients. *Sci. Transl. Med.* **2015**, *7*, 290ra87. [CrossRef]

123. Gatenby, P.; Lucas, R.; Swaminathan, A. Vitamin D deficiency and risk for rheumatic diseases: An update. *Curr. Opin. Rheumatol.* **2013**, *25*, 184–191. [CrossRef]

124. Ishikawa, L.L.W.; Colavite, P.M.; Fraga-Silva, T.F.C.; Mimura, L.A.N.; Franca, T.G.D.; Zorzella-Pezavento, S.F.G.; Chiuso-Minicucci, F.; Marcolino, L.D.; Penitenti, M.; Ikoma, M.R.V.; et al. Vitamin D Deficiency and Rheumatoid Arthritis. *Clin. Rev. Allergy Immunol.* **2017**, *52*, 373–388. [CrossRef]

125. Coutinho, A.E.; Chapman, K.E. The anti-inflammatory and immunosuppressive effects of glucocorticoids, recent developments and mechanistic insights. *Mol. Cell. Endocrinol.* **2011**, *335*, 2–13. [CrossRef]

126. Naranjo-Gomez, M.; Raich-Regue, D.; Onate, C.; Grau-Lopez, L.; Ramo-Tello, C.; Pujol-Borrell, R.; Martinez-Caceres, E.; Borras, F.E. Comparative study of clinical grade human tolerogenic dendritic cells. *J. Transl. Med.* **2011**, *9*, 89. [CrossRef]

127. Phillips, B.E.; Garciafigueroa, Y.; Trucco, M.; Giannoukakis, N. Clinical Tolerogenic Dendritic Cells: Exploring Therapeutic Impact on Human Autoimmune Disease. *Front. Immunol.* **2017**, *8*, 1279. [CrossRef]

128. Soltanzadeh-Yamchi, M.; Shahbazi, M.; Aslani, S.; Mohammadnia-Afrouzi, M. MicroRNA signature of regulatory T cells in health and autoimmunity. *Int. J. Mol. Sci.* **2018**, *100*, 316–323. [CrossRef]

129. Furer, V.; Greenberg, J.D.; Attur, M.; Abramson, S.B.; Pillinger, M.H. The role of microRNA in rheumatoid arthritis and other autoimmune diseases. *Clin. Immunol.* **2010**, *136*, 1–15. [CrossRef]

130. Alivernini, S.; Gremese, E.; McSharry, C.; Tolusso, B.; Ferraccioli, G.; McInnes, I.B.; Kurowska-Stolarska, M. MicroRNA-155-at the Critical Interface of Innate and Adaptive Immunity in Arthritis. *Front. Immunol.* **2017**, *8*, 1932. [CrossRef]

131. Fukuhara, A.; Matsuda, M.; Nishizawa, M.; Segawa, K.; Tanaka, M.; Kishimoto, K.; Matsuki, Y.; Murakami, M.; Ichisaka, T.; Murakami, H.; et al. Visfatin: A protein secreted by visceral fat that mimics the effects of insulin. *Science* **2005**, *307*, 426–430. [CrossRef]

132. Wu, M.H.; Tsai, C.H.; Huang, Y.L.; Fong, Y.C.; Tang, C.H. Visfatin Promotes IL-6 and TNF-α Production in Human Synovial Fibroblasts by Repressing miR-199a-5p through ERK, p38 and JNK Signaling Pathways. *Int. J. Mol. Sci.* **2018**, *19*, 190. [CrossRef]

133. Hayer, S.; Pundt, N.; Peters, M.A.; Wunrau, C.; Kuhnel, I.; Neugebauer, K.; Strietholt, S.; Zwerina, J.; Korb, A.; Penninger, J.; et al. PI3Kgamma regulates cartilage damage in chronic inflammatory arthritis. *FASEB J.* **2009**, *23*, 4288–4298. [CrossRef]

134. Rommel, C.; Camps, M.; Ji, H. PI3K delta and PI3K gamma: Partners in crime in inflammation in rheumatoid arthritis and beyond? *Nat. Rev. Immunol.* **2007**, *7*, 191–201. [CrossRef]
135. Nandakumar, K.S. Targeting IgG in Arthritis: Disease Pathways and Therapeutic Avenues. *Int. J. Mol. Sci.* **2018**, *19*, 677. [CrossRef]
136. Boutet, M.A.; Nerviani, A.; Gallo Afflitto, G.; Pitzalis, C. Role of the IL-23/IL-17 Axis in Psoriasis and Psoriatic Arthritis: The Clinical Importance of Its Divergence in Skin and Joints. *Int. J. Mol. Sci.* **2018**, *19*, 530. [CrossRef]
137. Park, M.J.; Park, H.S.; Cho, M.L.; Oh, H.J.; Cho, Y.G.; Min, S.Y.; Chung, B.H.; Lee, J.W.; Kim, H.Y.; Cho, S.G. Transforming growth factor beta-transduced mesenchymal stem cells ameliorate experimental autoimmune arthritis through reciprocal regulation of Treg/Th17 cells and osteoclastogenesis. *Arthritis Rheum.* **2011**, *63*, 1668–1680. [CrossRef]
138. Liu, R.; Zhao, P.; Tan, W.; Zhang, M. Cell therapies for refractory rheumatoid arthritis. *Clin. Exp. Rheumatol.* **2018**, *36*, 911–919.
139. Nent, E.; Frommholz, D.; Gajda, M.; Brauer, R.; Illges, H. Histamine 4 receptor plays an important role in auto-antibody-induced arthritis. *Int. Immunol.* **2013**, *25*, 437–443. [CrossRef]
140. Yamaura, K.; Oda, M.; Suzuki, M.; Ueno, K. Lower expression of histamine H(4) receptor in synovial tissues from patients with rheumatoid arthritis compared to those with osteoarthritis. *Rheumatol. Int.* **2012**, *32*, 3309–3313. [CrossRef]
141. Grabiec, A.M.; Korchynskyi, O.; Tak, P.P.; Reedquist, K.A. Histone deacetylase inhibitors suppress rheumatoid arthritis fibroblast-like synoviocyte and macrophage IL-6 production by accelerating mRNA decay. *Ann. Rheum. Dis.* **2012**, *71*, 424–431. [CrossRef] [PubMed]
142. Delcuve, G.P.; Khan, D.H.; Davie, J.R. Roles of histone deacetylases in epigenetic regulation: Emerging paradigms from studies with inhibitors. *Clin. Epigenetics* **2012**, *4*, 5. [CrossRef] [PubMed]
143. Angiolilli, C.; Kabala, P.A.; Grabiec, A.M.; Van Baarsen, I.M.; Ferguson, B.S.; Garcia, S.; Malvar Fernandez, B.; McKinsey, T.A.; Tak, P.P.; Fossati, G.; et al. Histone deacetylase 3 regulates the inflammatory gene expression programme of rheumatoid arthritis fibroblast-like synoviocytes. *Ann. Rheum. Dis.* **2017**, *76*, 277–285. [CrossRef] [PubMed]
144. Valencia, X.; Higgins, J.M.; Kiener, H.P.; Lee, D.M.; Podrebarac, T.A.; Dascher, C.C.; Watts, G.F.; Mizoguchi, E.; Simmons, B.; Patel, D.D.; et al. Cadherin-11 provides specific cellular adhesion between fibroblast-like synoviocytes. *J. Exp. Med.* **2004**, *200*, 1673–1679. [CrossRef] [PubMed]
145. Lee, D.M.; Kiener, H.P.; Agarwal, S.K.; Noss, E.H.; Watts, G.F.; Chisaka, O.; Takeichi, M.; Brenner, M.B. Cadherin-11 in synovial lining formation and pathology in arthritis. *Science* **2007**, *315*, 1006–1010. [CrossRef] [PubMed]
146. Noss, E.H.; Watts, G.F.; Zocco, D.; Keller, T.L.; Whitman, M.; Blobel, C.P.; Lee, D.M.; Brenner, M.B. Evidence for cadherin-11 cleavage in the synovium and partial characterization of its mechanism. *Arthritis Res. Ther.* **2015**, *17*, 126. [CrossRef]
147. Sfikakis, P.P.; Vlachogiannis, N.I.; Christopoulos, P.F. Cadherin-11 as a therapeutic target in chronic, inflammatory rheumatic diseases. *Clin. Immunol.* **2017**, *176*, 107–113. [CrossRef]
148. Tan, A.L.; Emery, P. Role of oestrogen in the development of joint symptoms? *Lancet Oncol.* **2008**, *9*, 817–818. [CrossRef]
149. Kass, A.; Hollan, I.; Fagerland, M.W.; Gulseth, H.C.; Torjesen, P.A.; Forre, O.T. Rapid Anti-Inflammatory Effects of Gonadotropin-Releasing Hormone Antagonism in Rheumatoid Arthritis Patients with High Gonadotropin Levels in the AGRA Trial. *PLoS ONE* **2015**, *10*, e0139439. [CrossRef]
150. Shi, Y.; Wu, Q.; Xuan, W.; Feng, X.; Wang, F.; Tsao, B.P.; Zhang, M.; Tan, W. Transcription Factor SOX5 Promotes the Migration and Invasion of Fibroblast-Like Synoviocytes in Part by Regulating MMP-9 Expression in Collagen-Induced Arthritis. *Front. Immunol.* **2018**, *9*, 749. [CrossRef]
151. Jovanovic, D.V.; Martel-Pelletier, J.; Di Battista, J.A.; Mineau, F.; Jolicoeur, F.C.; Benderdour, M.; Pelletier, J.P. Stimulation of 92-kd gelatinase (matrix metalloproteinase 9) production by interleukin-17 in human monocyte/macrophages: A possible role in rheumatoid arthritis. *Arthritis Rheum.* **2000**, *43*, 1134–1144. [CrossRef]
152. Blaschke, S.; Koziolek, M.; Schwarz, A.; Benohr, P.; Middel, P.; Schwarz, G.; Hummel, K.M.; Muller, G.A. Proinflammatory role of fractalkine (CX3CL1) in rheumatoid arthritis. *J. Rheumatol.* **2003**, *30*, 1918–1927.

153. Isozaki, T.; Otsuka, K.; Sato, M.; Takahashi, R.; Wakabayashi, K.; Yajima, N.; Miwa, Y.; Kasama, T. Synergistic induction of CX3CL1 by interleukin-1beta and interferon-gamma in human lung fibroblasts: Involvement of signal transducer and activator of transcription 1 signaling pathways. *Transl. Res. J. Lab. Clin. Med.* **2011**, *157*, 64–70. [CrossRef] [PubMed]

154. Nanki, T.; Imai, T.; Kawai, S. Fractalkine/CX3CL1 in rheumatoid arthritis. *Mod. Rheumatol.* **2017**, *27*, 392–397. [CrossRef]

155. Hatterer, E.; Shang, L.; Simonet, P.; Herren, S.; Daubeuf, B.; Teixeira, S.; Reilly, J.; Elson, G.; Nelson, R.; Gabay, C.; et al. A specific anti-citrullinated protein antibody profile identifies a group of rheumatoid arthritis patients with a toll-like receptor 4-mediated disease. *Arthritis Res. Ther.* **2016**, *18*, 224. [CrossRef]

156. Park, S.Y.; Lee, S.W.; Kim, H.Y.; Lee, W.S.; Hong, K.W.; Kim, C.D. HMGB1 induces angiogenesis in rheumatoid arthritis via HIF-1alpha activation. *Eur. J. Immunol.* **2015**, *45*, 1216–1227. [CrossRef] [PubMed]

157. Cong, L.; Yang, S.; Zhang, Y.; Cao, J.; Fu, X. DFMG attenuates the activation of macrophages induced by coculture with LPCinjured HUVE12 cells via the TLR4/MyD88/NFkappaB signaling pathway. *Int. J. Mol. Med.* **2018**, *41*, 2619–2628. [PubMed]

158. Deuteraiou, K.; Kitas, G.; Garyfallos, A.; Dimitroulas, T. Novel insights into the role of inflammasomes in autoimmune and metabolic rheumatic diseases. *Rheumatol. Int.* **2018**, *38*, 1345–1354. [CrossRef] [PubMed]

159. Borie, D.; Kremer, J.M. Considerations on the appropriateness of the John Cunningham virus antibody assay use in patients with rheumatoid arthritis. *Semin. Arthritis Rheum.* **2015**, *45*, 163–166. [CrossRef] [PubMed]

160. Ishikawa, Y.; Kasuya, T.; Ishikawa, J.; Fujiwara, M.; Kita, Y. A case of developing progressive multifocal leukoencephalopathy while using rituximab and mycophenolate mofetil in refractory systemic lupus erythematosus. *Ther. Clin. Risk Manag.* **2018**, *14*, 1149–1153. [CrossRef]

161. Casulo, C.; Maragulia, J.; Zelenetz, A.D. Incidence of hypogammaglobulinemia in patients receiving rituximab and the use of intravenous immunoglobulin for recurrent infections. *Clin. Lymphoma Myeloma Leuk.* **2013**, *13*, 106–111. [CrossRef] [PubMed]

162. Breuer, G.S.; Ehrenfeld, M.; Rosner, I.; Balbir-Gurman, A.; Zisman, D.; Oren, S.; Paran, D. Late-onset neutropenia following rituximab treatment for rheumatologic conditions. *Clin. Rheumatol.* **2014**, *33*, 1337–1340. [CrossRef]

163. Priora, M.; Parisi, S.; Scarati, M.; Borrelli, R.; Peroni, C.L.; Fusaro, E. Abatacept and granulocyte-colony stimulating factor in a patient with rheumatoid arthritis and neutropenia. *Immunotherapy* **2017**, *9*, 1055–1059. [CrossRef] [PubMed]

164. Li, X.; Tian, F.; Wang, F. Rheumatoid arthritis-associated microRNA-155 targets SOCS1 and upregulates TNF-alpha and IL-1beta in PBMCs. *Int. J. Mol. Sci.* **2013**, *14*, 23910–23921. [CrossRef] [PubMed]

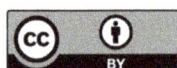

International Journal of
Molecular Sciences

MDPI

Review

Structural Biology of the TNFα Antagonists Used in the Treatment of Rheumatoid Arthritis

Heejin Lim, Sang Hyung Lee, Hyun Tae Lee, Jee Un Lee, Ji Young Son, Woori Shin and Yong-Seok Heo *

Department of Chemistry, Konkuk University, 120 Neungdong-ro, Gwangjin-gu, Seoul 05029, Korea; gmlwls454@naver.com (H.L.); dltkdgud92@naver.com (S.H.L.); hst2649@naver.com (H.T.L.); jaspersky@naver.com (J.U.L.); jieyson@hanmail.net (J.Y.S.); woolishin@nate.com (W.S.)
* Correspondence: ysheo@konkuk.ac.kr; Tel.: +82-2-450-3408; Fax: +82-2-3436-5382

Received: 8 February 2018; Accepted: 6 March 2018; Published: 7 March 2018

Abstract: The binding of the tumor necrosis factor α (TNFα) to its cognate receptor initiates many immune and inflammatory processes. The drugs, etanercept (Enbrel®), infliximab (Remicade®), adalimumab (Humira®), certolizumab-pegol (Cimzia®), and golimumab (Simponi®), are anti-TNFα agents. These drugs block TNFα from interacting with its receptors and have enabled the development of breakthrough therapies for the treatment of several autoimmune inflammatory diseases, including rheumatoid arthritis, Crohn's disease, and psoriatic arthritis. In this review, we describe the latest works on the structural characterization of TNFα–TNFα antagonist interactions related to their therapeutic efficacy at the atomic level. A comprehensive comparison of the interactions of the TNFα blockers would provide a better understanding of the molecular mechanisms by which they neutralize TNFα. In addition, an enhanced understanding of the higher order complex structures and quinary structures of the TNFα antagonists can support the development of better biologics with the improved pharmacokinetic properties. Accumulation of these structural studies can provide a basis for the improvement of therapeutic agents against TNFα for the treatment of rheumatoid arthritis and other autoimmune inflammatory diseases in which TNFα plays an important role in pathogenesis.

Keywords: TNFα; etanercept; infliximab; adalimumab; certolizumab pegol; golimumab; rheumatoid arthritis; therapeutic antibody; structure

1. Introduction

Tumor necrosis factor superfamily (TNFSF) proteins and their receptors (TNFRSF) play critical roles in mammalian biology, including cell growth, survival, and apoptosis, immune responses, and organogenesis of the immune, ectodermal, and nervous systems [1]. It has been known that there are more than 35 specific ligand-receptor pairs between TNFSF and TNFRSF [2]. Among them, TNFα is a major inflammatory cytokine that exerts pleiotropic effects on various cell types by activating intracellular signaling through interactions with its cognate receptors. Therefore, TNFα plays a crucial role in the pathogenesis of inflammatory autoimmune diseases [3]. TNFα is mainly expressed in activated macrophages and natural killer cells as a 26 kDa transmembrane precursor, which is cleaved by a metalloproteinase, TNFα-converting enzyme (TACE), into a soluble form of 157 amino acid residues. Both soluble and transmembrane TNFα exist as homotrimers and bind to type 1 and 2 TNF receptors (TNFR1 and TNFR2) in order to mediate the signaling processes of apoptosis, cell proliferation, and cytokine production [4–10].

TNFα antagonists have been developed for the treatment of rheumatoid arthritis (RA), psoriatic arthritis, juvenile idiopathic arthritis, ankylosing spondylitis, Crohn's disease, and ulcerative colitis [11–14]. It is well known that the elevated concentration of TNFα at the site of inflammation is driving pathology of these inflammatory autoimmune diseases. Therefore, the removal or neutralization of excess TNFα from sites of inflammation was expected to be promising to achieve a therapeutic goal. Among the five FDA-approved TNFα antagonists, infliximab, adalimumab, certolizumab-pegol, and golimumab are antibody-based drugs, and etanercept is an Fc-fusion protein of TNFR2 [15–19]. The crucial mechanism of action of these TNFα antagonists is their neutralizing activities against soluble TNFα are [19–21]. Rrecent studies have shown that these biologics also act on transmembrane TNFα and Fcγ receptors (FcγR) [22–33]. Unfortunately, blocking TNFα-mediated signaling often causes side effects including bacterial or viral infection and the development of lymphoma [34–36]. Therefore, a more thorough investigation of the interactions between TNFα and its receptor or antagonists is essential for the rational design of improved anti-TNFα therapeutics in future.

The crystal structures of lymphotoxin α (LTα)-TNFR1 and TNFα–TNFR2 complexes have established the foundations of our understanding of the cytokine-receptor interactions. These structures have provided invaluable information for understanding the molecular mechanisms of TNF signaling [37,38]. Additionally, the crystal structures of TNFα in complex with anti-TNFα antibodies have aided the elucidation of the precise epitopes that were involved and the structural basis of TNFα neutralization by these antibodies [39–41]. Here, we focus on the structural features of the interactions of the FDA-approved TNFα antagonists related to their clinical efficacies. We also describe the unique quinary structure of infliximab and the recent electron microscopy (EM) study of the higher order complex structures of TNFα with therapeutic antibodies [42–44].

2. TNFα Antagonists for the Treatment of Inflammatory Autoimmune Diseases

Human TNFα is generated as a precursor protein called transmembrane TNFα consisting of 233 amino acid residues, which is expressed on the cell surface of macrophages and lymphocytes as well as other cell types [45–51]. After being cleaved by TACE between residues Ala76 and Val77, soluble TNFα is released and binds to TNFR1 or TNFR2, thereby mediating inflammatory signaling (Figure 1). Transmembrane TNFα also binds to both TNFR1 and TNFR2, but TNFR2 is thought to be the major receptor for mediating the biological activities of transmembrane TNFα [52]. TNFR1 is expressed on almost all the nucleated cells, whereas TNFR2 is mainly expressed on endothelial cells and hematopoietic cells [53,54]. Both receptors are preassembled as homotrimers and are capable of binding to intracellular adaptor proteins to activate the pleiotropic effects of TNFα [55,56].

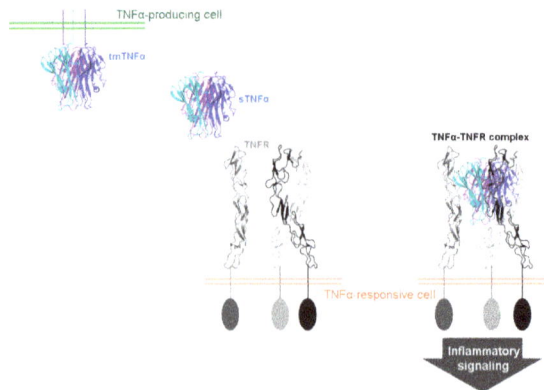

Figure 1. Biology of tumor necrosis factor α (TNFα). A soluble TNFα (sTNFα) trimer is released from its transmembrane form (tmTNFα) and binds to a preassembled trimer of TNF receptor (TNFR), thereby mediating inflammatory signaling. Each protomer of TNFα homotrimer is colored blue, cyan, and purple. The green and pale red bars indicate membranes of a TNFα-producing and TNFα-responsive cells, respectively.

Receptor-mediated effects of TNFα can lead alternatively to activation of nuclear factor kappa-B or to apoptosis, depending on the metabolic state of the cell. Transmembrane TNFα acts as a ligand and as a receptor. Transmembrane TNFα-expressing cells transduce intracellular signaling via direct interaction with TNFR-bearing cells, in which it is referred to as "outside-to-inside signal" or "reverse signal" [21]. This transmembrane TNFα-mediated reverse signal is also thought to contribute to the pleiotropic effects of TNFα [57]. The biology of TNFα gains complexity from the different signaling pathways mediated by TNFR1, TNFR2, soluble TNFα, and transmembrane TNFα.

The FDA has approved five TNFα blockers, including etanercept, infliximab, adalimumab, certolizumab-pegol, and golimumab, for the treatment of inflammatory diseases, including RA, juvenile idiopathic arthritis, psoriatic arthritis, psoriasis, Crohn's disease (CD), ulcerative colitis (UC), ankylosing spondylitis, and Behçet's disease (Table 1). Each of these drugs have shown excellent efficacy, with similar rates of response, although the similarity is somewhat controversial owing to the lack of a head-to-head comparative studies [20]. As the patents of etanercept, infliximab, and adalimumab expired, there are several biosimilar (also known as follow-on biologic or subsequent entry biologic) drugs that are available, which are almost identical to the original product of these TNFα antagonists.

Table 1. FDA-approved TNFα antagonists.

TNFα Antagonist	Original Product	Biosimilar Product	Type
Etanercept	Enbrel® (1998)	Erelzi® (2016)	TNFR2 ectodomain fused to IgG1 Fc
Infliximab	Remicade® (1998)	Inflectra® (2016), Ixifi® (2017)	Chimeric murine/human IgG1
Adalimumab	Humira® (2002)	Amjevita® (2016), Cyltezo® (2017)	Fully Human IgG1
Certolizumab-pegol	Cimzia® (2008)		Humanized, PEGylated Fab′
Golimumab	Simponi® (2009)		Fully Human IgG1

Values in parentheses indicate the dates of FDA approval.

Etanercept is a genetically engineered fusion protein that is composed of two identical TNFR2 extracellular region linked to the Fc fragment of human IgG1. Infliximab is a chimeric monoclonal antibody (mAb) consisting of a murine variable region and a human IgG1 constant region. Adalimumab and golimumab are fully human IgG1 isotype anti-TNFα antibodies. Certolizumab-pegol is a monovalent Fab fragment of a humanized anti-TNFα antibody and lacks the Fc region [58]. The hinge region of certolizumab is attached to two cross-linked chains of a 20 kDa polyethylene glycol (PEG) and named the certolizumab-pegol [59]. Despite the lack of the Fc region, PEGylation increases the plasma half-life and solubility and reduces the immunogenicity and protease sensitivity [60]. Although the main mechanism of action of these TNFα antagonists is through the neutralization of soluble TNFα, they also bind to transmembrane TNFα homotrimers, providing additional mechanisms. Additionally, with the exception of the Fc region-lacking certolizumab-pegol, these drugs show potent activities of complement-dependent cytotoxicity (CDC) and antibody-dependent cell-mediated cytotoxicity (ADCC) toward transmembrane TNFα-bearing cells [26,32]. The full-length IgG1 antibodies, including infliximab, adalimumab, and golimumab, can induce apoptosis and cell cycle G0/G1 arrest by forming a 1:2 complex between IgG and the transmembrane TNFα trimer, thereby inhibiting TNFα-producing cells and leading to an anti-inflammatory response [27,61].

3. Interactions between TNFα and FDA-Approved TNFα Antagonists

Recent structural studies have revealed the interactions between TNFα and its antagonists (Table 2). The interactions between TNFα and etanercept can be deduced from the crystal structure of TNFα in complex with the extracellular domain TNFR2. This is possible because etanercept is an Fc-fusion protein of the extracellular domain of TNFR2, implying the pharmacological efficacy of etanercept results from completely occupying the TNFα receptor binding site [38]. The extracellular portion of TNFR2 is composed of cysteine-rich domains (CRDs) with three internal disulfide bonds. In the complex structure of TNFα–TNFR2, one TNFR2 molecule interacts with the two neighboring

TNFα protomers in the homotrimer, and the CRD2 and CRD3 domains of TNFR2 mediated major interactions with TNFα (Figure 2A). The crystal structures of TNFα in complex with the Fab fragments of the therapeutic antibodies, including infliximab, adalimumab, and certolizumab, have also been determined [39–41]. All of the structures contain a 3:3 complex between TNFα and the Fab fragments with a three-fold symmetry (Figure 2). When viewed along the three-fold axis, the trimeric complexes have a shape that resembles a three-bladed propeller, with each protomer representing one blade. The pseudo two-fold axes of the bound Fab fragments relating the heavy and light chains intersected the three-fold axis of the TNFα homotrimer with an approximate angle of 30°–50° downward from a plane perpendicular to the 3-fold axis. When we consider a cell with a transmembrane TNFα precursor attached, this plane represents the cell membrane (Figure 2). In this binding orientation, the antibody drugs can bind both soluble and transmembrane TNFα. This structural feature is consistent with the characteristics of the antibody drugs, which target both soluble TNFα and transmembrane TNFα [62].

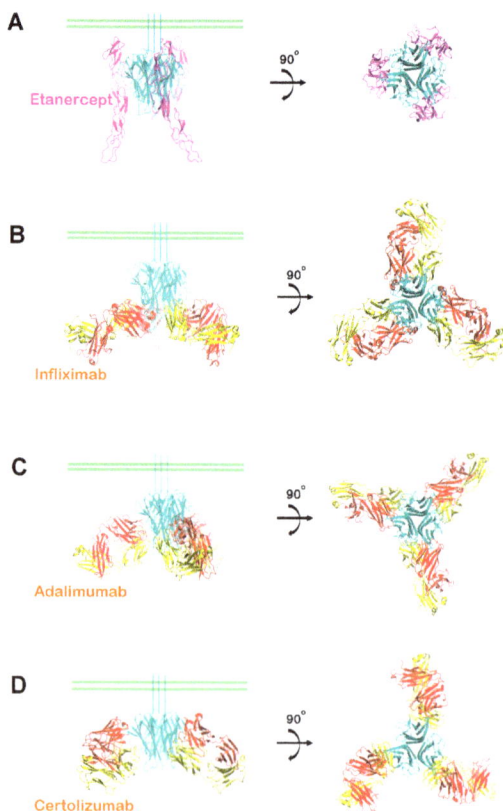

Figure 2. Overall structures of TNFα in complex with antagonists. (**A**) Ribbon representation of TNFα (cyan) in complex with the extracellular domain of TNFR2 (purple) in two orientations; (**B**) The structure of the TNFα trimer (cyan) in complex with the infliximab Fab fragment (heavy chain: red; light chain: yellow); (**C**) The structure of the TNFα trimer (cyan) in complex with the adalimumab Fab fragment (heavy chain: red; light chain: yellow); and, (**D**) The structure of the TNFα trimer (cyan) in complex with the certolizumab Fab fragment (heavy chain: red; light chain: yellow). The green bars indicate a putative membrane of a TNFα-producing cell if the TNFα trimer is a precursor form of transmembrane TNFα.

Table 2. List of the TNFα antagonists related structures.

TNFα Antagonist	Protein/Complex	Method	PDB ID	References
Etanercept	TNFR2 ectodomain in complex with TNFα	X-ray	3ALQ	[38]
Infliximab	Fab fragment in complex with TNFα	X-ray	4G3Y	[39]
	Fab fragment	X-ray	5VH3	[42]
	Fab fragment	X-ray	5VH4	[42]
	Fc fragment	X-ray	5VH5	[42]
	1:1, 1:2, 2:2, 3:2 complex	Cryo-EM		[44]
Adalimumab	Fab fragment in complex with TNFα	X-ray	3WD5	[40]
	Fab fragment	X-ray	4NYL	to be published
	1:1, 1:2, 2:2, 3:2 complex	Cryo-EM		[44]
Certolizumab-pegol	Fab fragment in complex with TNFα	X-ray	5WUX	[41]
	Fab fragment	X-ray	5WUV	[41]

The epitopes revealed from analysis of the complex structures imply that TNFα neutralization by these antagonists occurs through outcompeting TNFRs for binding to TNFα, through partially or completely occupying the receptor binding site of TNFα due to higher affinity or avidity (Figure 3). However, a comprehensive comparison of the interactions of each TNFα antagonist with TNFα can provide a better understanding of their mechanisms of action. In the complex structure with adalimumab, one Fab fragment of adalimumab interacts with two neighboring protomers of the TNFα homotrimer, like the TNFα–TNFR2 complex [40]. In contrast, the Fab fragments of infliximab and certolizumab interact with only one protomer of the TNFα homotrimer [39]. The E-F loop of TNFα plays a crucial role in the interaction with the adalimumab and infliximab Fab fragments [39,40]. On the other hand, this region is completely unobservable in the complex structures of TNFα with TNFR2 or certolizumab, indicating that the E-F loop is flexible and is not involved in these interactions [38,41]. Interestingly, the interaction of certolizumab induced a conformational change of the D-E loop of TNFα [41]. In the structure of TNFα in complex with TNFR2, the residues of the D-E loop were optimally accommodated into a pocket on the surface of TNFR2, and thereby contributing to the binding energy of the TNFα–TNFR2 interaction [38]. However, the structural change induced by certolizumab binding was incompatible with TNFR2 binding, as this conformational alteration of the D-E loop would cause steric collision with TNFR2. Thus, the conformational change of the D-E loop also appears to contribute to the neutralizing effect of certolizumab.

At physiological concentrations, the TNFα homotrimer slowly dissociates into monomers and trimerizes reversibly [63–65]. It has been reported that etanercept, adalimumab, and infliximab abrogated this monomer exchange reaction of the TNFα homotrimer, while certolizumab and golimumab were unable to prevent it [66]. As adalimumab and etanercept simultaneously interact with two adjacent TNFα protomers, they could stabilize the interactions between the protomers in the TNFα homotrimer [38,40]. Although the interactions that are mediated by the infliximab Fab fragments involved only one protomer of the TNFα homotrimer, the E-F loop provided key interactions through taking on a unique conformation. This may contribute to the stabilization of TNFα homotrimer via the productive communication between the E-F loops of the TNFα homotrimer in the unique conformation [39]. The lack of trimer stabilization by certolizumab can be explained by the structural features of the TNFα-certolizumab interaction, which only involves a single protomer without influencing the conformation of the E-F loop in the TNFα homotrimer [41]. The monomer exchange behavior of golimumab is like that of certolizumab, so golimumab is expected to bind to an epitope composed of only a single protomer without interacting with the E-F loop of TNFα.

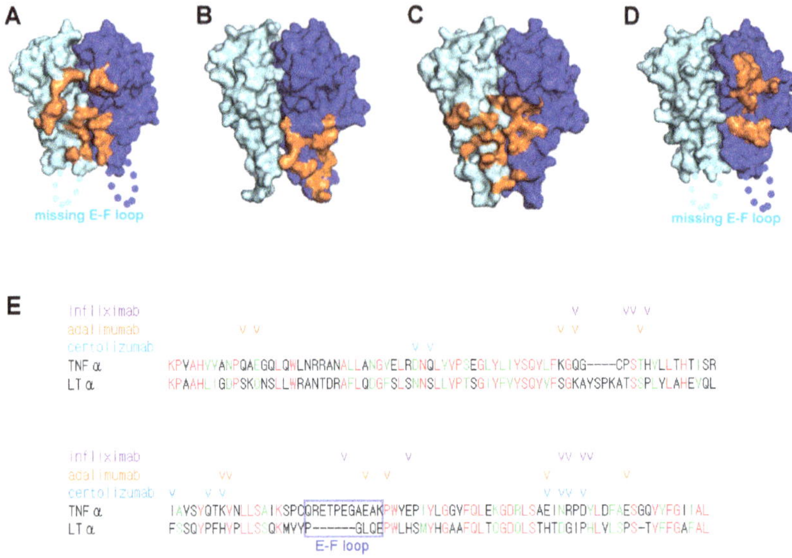

Figure 3. The binding interfaces between TNFα and its antagonists. (**A**) The TNFR2 binding site on the surface of the TNFα trimer (cyan and blue for each protomer) is colored orange; (**B**) The infliximab epitope on the surface of the TNFα trimer (cyan and blue for each protomer) is colored orange; (**C**) The adalimumab epitope on the surface of the TNFα trimer (cyan and blue for each protomer) is colored orange; (**D**) The certolizumab epitope on the surface of the TNFα trimer (cyan and blue for each protomer) is colored orange. The E-F loop, which is missing in the structures of TNFα–TNFR2 and the TNFα-certolizumab complex owing to a lack of interactions, is labeled; (**E**) Structure-based sequence alignment of TNFα and LTα (lymphotoxin α). The identical and homologous residues are colored red and green, respectively. The E-F loop region is indicated with a blue box and labeled. The TNFα residues involved in the interaction with anti-TNFα antibodies are indicated with check marks colored purple, orange, and cyan for infliximab, adalimumab, and certolizumab, respectively.

4. Selectivity of TNFα Antagonists against Lymphotoxin α

Lymphotoxin α (LTα, formerly called TNFβ) and LTβ are two related TNF superfamilies produced by activated cells of the innate and adaptive immune response [67]. The homotrimer of LTα (LTα3) and heterotrimer of two LTα and one LTβ (LTα2β1) bind both TNFR1 and TNFR2, probably due to the high similarities of amino acid sequences between LTα and TNFα. Of the FDA-approved TNFα antagonists, only etanercept can neutralize LTα3 and LTα2β1 [22,28,53]. LTα3 activates the inflammatory environment and mediates cytokine secretion in RA patients [68]. Although the blocking of LTα alone is not effective against RA, the neutralization of both TNFα and LTα by etanercept is clinically beneficial in RA patients [69]. The epitopes of the anti-TNFα antibodies revealed by structural studies explain their lack of binding to LTα (Figure 3). When comparing the amino acid sequences of TNFα and LTα, many residues of TNFα involved in anti-TNFα antibody interactions are not conserved in LTα (Figure 3E). In addition, the short E-F loop within LTα might contribute to the selective binding to TNFα but not to LTα, especially in infliximab and adalimumab, due to the involvement of the E-F loop in their binding to TNFα.

5. Structural Rigidity of the CDR Loops within Anti-TNFα Antibodies

The crystal structures of the uncomplexed Fab fragments of anti-TNFα antibodies were also determined (Table 2) [41,42]. They presented a canonical immunoglobulin fold and four intramolecular disulfide bonds in the structures, as expected. The electron densities of the structures of the uncomplexed Fab fragments were clear throughout the entire structure, including the complementarity-determining regions (CDRs). These results imply that the CDR loops are structurally rigid despite the absence of the binding partner (TNFα). Structural comparison of the CDR loops of the anti-TNFα antibodies before and after binding to TNFα showed little conformational deviation and minor adjustments in the side chains that are involved in the interaction with TNFα. This implies that these antibodies maintain the CDR loops in productive conformations prior to binding to TNFα, ultimately contributing to the high-affinity binding to TNFα (Figure 4). According to a Kabat sequence database search, the CDR loops of the anti-TNFα antibodies have an ordinary length without unusual residues [70]. All six CDR loops of adalimumab and infliximab were involved in the interaction with TNFα, whereas certolizumab utilized all the three heavy chain CDRs and only CDR2 of the light chain [39–41]. The interaction of the light chain of certolizumab mediated only by the LCDR2 loop represents a novel and unique finding as the LCDR2 region of antibodies is generally not involved in antigen binding [71].

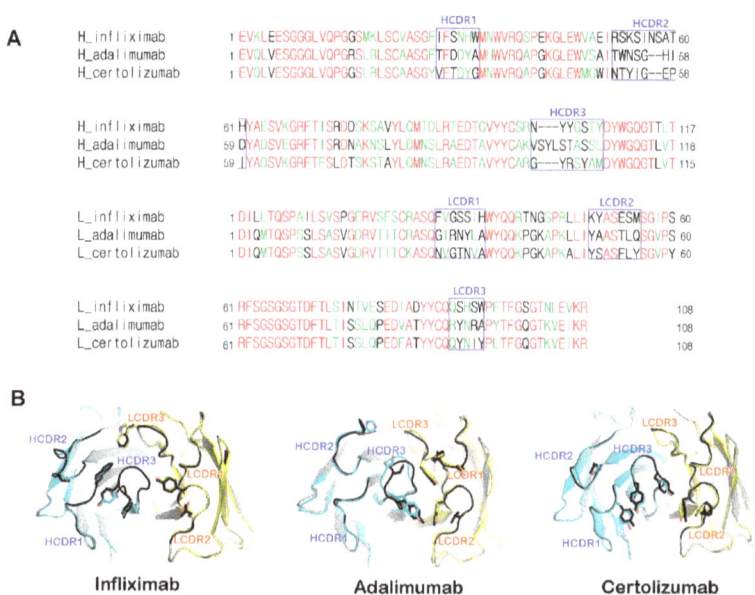

Figure 4. Complementarity-determining regions (CDR) loops within anti-TNFα antibodies. (**A**) Sequence comparison of the anti-TNFα antibodies. CDRs are indicated with boxes and labeled. Identical and homologous residues are colored red and green, respectively; (**B**) Superposition of the free Fab fragments of anti-TNFα antibodies (gray; CDR regions: black) onto the Fab fragment extracted from the complexes with TNFα (heavy chain: cyan; light chain: yellow).

6. Higher Order Structures of Antibody-TNFα Complexes

Given that the anti-TNFα antibodies of the IgG form are bivalent and that TNFα also provides three epitopes for therapeutic antibodies, they may form higher order complex structures. It has been reported that a stable complex of adalimumab and TNFα with a molecular weight of about 598 kDa was formed after overnight incubation at 37 °C [72,73]. In contrast, etanercept forms only 1:1 complex with TNFα trimer through a bidentate interaction of the two TNFR2 domains with a single TNFα trimer [22]. Although the crystal structures elucidated the detailed interactions between TNFα and the Fab fragments of the therapeutic antibodies, the higher order complex structures that were formed by full-length anti-TNFα IgG form antibodies were not clear. In addition to X-ray crystallography, EM techniques have been successfully used to determine antigen-antibody complex structures. Very recently, the structures of TNFα in complex with the full-length infliximab and adalimumab were described using a cryo-EM technique (Table 2) [44]. Adalimumab-TNFα and infliximab-TNFα formed a variety of higher order structures consisting of 1:1, 1:2, 2:2, and 3:2 complexes between IgG and TNFα trimer molecule (Figure 5). In 1:1 and 1:2 complexes, one or both Fab arms of IgG were bound to one or two TNFα trimers. The 2:2 complexes had a diamond shaped structure through the interactions of the four Fab arms of two IgGs with two TNFα trimers. In 3:2 complexes, the residual one face of 3:2 complex was occupied by a third IgG molecule, retaining the structural features recognized in the 2:2 complexes. Additional analytical ultracentrifugation and size exclusion chromatography showed that the stable complex of about 598 kDa corresponds to the 3:2 complex, suggesting that this 3:2 complex is the major form present upon extended incubation.

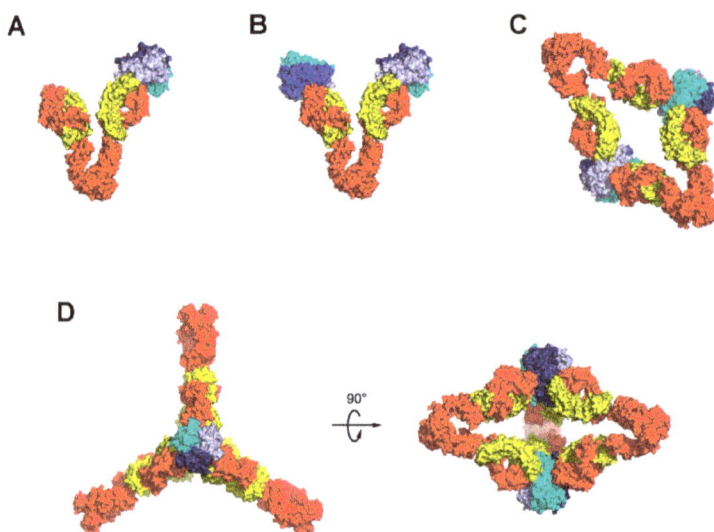

Figure 5. Models of the complexes of full-length adalimumab and TNFα trimers. The models are derived by fitting a TNFα trimer (blue, pale blue, and cyan) and bound Fab fragments (heavy chain: red, light chain: yellow) of PDB ID 3WD5 to the cryo EM electron density. (**A**) 1:1 complex; (**B**) 1:2 complex; (**C**) 2:2 complex; (**D**) 3:3 complex.

7. The Quinary Structure of Infliximab

Oligomerization and aggregation of therapeutic proteins can lead to inactivity or undesired risk for an immunogenetic response by generating anti-drug antibodies. Although many researchers try to predict and prevent aggregation of biotherapeutics through rational design and diverse formulation, the aggregation mechanisms of many therapeutic proteins remain poorly understood. The corresponding physiochemical properties of a given protein originate from its quinary structure. The quinary structure is defined as the association of quaternary structures, an example of which is the oligomerization of the hemoglobin structure causing sickle cell anemia. Many studies have revealed diverse aggregation mechanisms of monoclonal antibodies [74]. For instance, acid-induced aggregation of nivolumab, an anti-PD1 antibody, is dependent on the Fc fragment of the monoclonal antibody [75]. Several analytical methods, including gel filtration chromatography, multi-angle light scattering, circular dichroism, and NMR, revealed that infliximab was in monomer-oligomer equilibrium and its self-association was dependent on the Fab fragment [42,43]. A recent X-ray crystallographic study revealed the Fab fragment of infliximab and provided a potential self-association mechanism that is mediated by the infliximab Fab fragment (Table 2) [42]. Crystals of the infliximab Fab fragment belong to two distinct space groups, $I2_12_12_1$ and $C222_1$ (Figure 6). Both crystal forms contain two copies of the Fab fragment in the asymmetric unit. Although details of the packing interactions in the asymmetric unit are distinct between the two crystal forms due to an elbow rotation of ~40°, the interactions are mediated exclusively via the light chains in a head-to-tail orientation in both crystal structures with contact areas of 1083 Å^2 and 1066 Å^2 in the $I2_12_12_1$ and $C222_1$ forms, respectively. When considering the interfaces of heavy chains in the Fc fragment of IgG are ~1000 Å^2, the interactions by the light chains of infliximab in both crystal forms may mediate putative interfaces of infliximab self-association in solution.

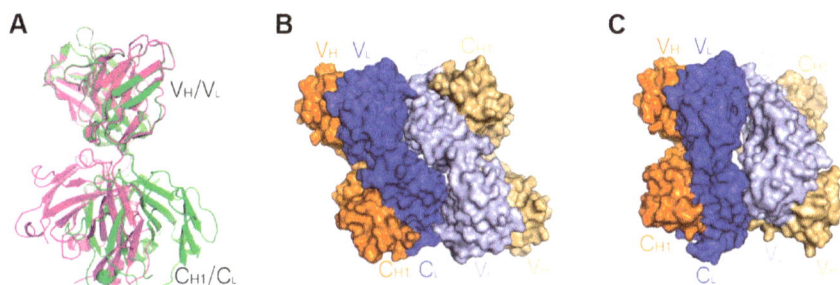

Figure 6. Self-association of infliximab mediated by the light chains. (**A**) An elbow rotation of Fab structures of ~40° in the $I2_12_12_1$ (green) and $C222_1$ (purple) forms indicates the flexibility between the variable (V_H/V_L) and constant (C_{H1}/C_L) regions of the infliximab Fab.; (**B**) Head-to tail interaction mediated by the light chains of two Fab fragments in the $I2_12_12_1$ form; (**C**) Head-to tail interaction mediated by the light chains of two Fab fragments in the $C222_1$ form. In (**B,C**), the heavy chains are colored orange and pale orange, and the light chains are colored blue and pale blue.

The monomer-dimer dissociation constant of infliximab self-association (21 μM) was determined by a sedimentation equilibrium analytical ultracentrifugation experiment [42]. In addition, self-association of infliximab is not observed in the TNFα-infliximab complex because the strong interaction between TNFα and infliximab precludes the head-to-tail orientation observed in the structures of the infliximab Fab fragment. There has been no known immunogenicity issue associated with infliximab self-association, probably due to the low affinity of the self-association, which does not affect the TNFα interaction. However, enhanced understanding of the quinary structures of therapeutic antibodies can support the development of better biologics with the improved pharmacokinetic properties.

8. Conclusions

The structures of TNFα in complex with its antagonists allow for us to elucidate the molecular mechanisms underlying the therapeutic activities of these biologics. The structure of TNFα–TNFR2 complex revealed the molecular basis of the cytokine-receptor recognition and provides a better understanding of the mechanism of signal initiation by TNFα. The epitopes and binding modes of the FDA-approved anti-TNFα antibodies can be references for the development of other antibodies in future. Given that the binding affinity of therapeutic antibodies is one of the most important determinants for their development, these structures can aid in improving the surface complementarity of the interface between antibodies and target molecules, and thereby enhancing the binding affinity through altering the paratopes of the antibodies. Moreover, a comprehensive analysis of the complex structures could provide useful information with which to improve the current TNFα-targeting biological agents for the treatment of inflammatory autoimmune diseases. Different mechanisms of action can lead to different therapeutic results. Therefore, elucidation of the mechanisms of action therapeutic antibodies through structural studies can provide logic for a design of combination therapy to achieve clinical synergy. Once a new antibody is characterized as being promising in an early stage of development, a structural study to investigate its precise epitope and mechanism of action may be helpful in making decisions before proceeding with costly clinical trials. Structural studies on the interactions between TNFα and its antagonists can provide insight into the design of small molecules targeting TNFα, as their potency can be enhanced by mimicking the diverse interactions of these antagonists. We also believe that the investigation of the higher order complex structures and quinary structures of therapeutic antibodies might be helpful for fine-tuning of their physicochemical properties for maximal therapeutic efficacy. Accumulation of such structural studies will provide invaluable information for developing next-generation therapeutic antibodies, such as antibody drug conjugates (ADCs) and bi-specific antibodies, and for coping with any possible antigen mutational escape of TNFα in future.

Acknowledgments: This paper was supported by Konkuk University in 2014.

Author Contributions: Heejin Lim, Sang Hyung Lee, Hyun Tae Lee, Jee Un Lee, Woori Shin, Ji Young Son, and Yong-Seok Heo collected information and Yong-Seok Heo wrote the manuscript.

Conflicts of Interest: The authors declare no conflict of interest.

References

1. Locksley, R.M.; Killeen, N.; Lenardo, M.J. The TNF and TNF receptor superfamilies: Integrating mammalian biology. *Cell* **2001**, *104*, 487–501. [CrossRef]
2. Wiens, G.D.; Glenney, G.W. Origin and evolution of TNF and TNF receptor superfamilies. *Dev. Comp. Immunol.* **2011**, *35*, 1324–1335. [CrossRef] [PubMed]
3. Chen, G.; Goeddel, D.V. TNF-R1 signaling: A beautiful pathway. *Science* **2002**, *296*, 1634–1635. [CrossRef] [PubMed]
4. Pennica, D.; Nedwin, G.E.; Hayflick, J.S.; Seeburg, P.H.; Derynck, R.; Palladino, M.A.; Kohr, W.J.; Aggarwal, B.B.; Goeddel, D.V. Human tumor necrosis factor: Precursor structure, cDNA cloning, expression, and homology to lymphotoxin. *Nature* **1984**, *312*, 724–729. [CrossRef] [PubMed]
5. Luettiq, B.; Decker, T.; Lohmann-Matthes, M.L. Evidence for the existence of two forms of membrane tumor necrosis factor: An integral protein and a molecule attached to its receptor. *J. Immunol.* **1989**, *143*, 4034–4038.
6. Kriegler, M.; Perez, C.; DeFay, K.; Albert, I.; Lu, S.D. A novel form of TNF/cachectin is a cell surface cytotoxic transmembrane protein: Ramifications for the complex physiology of TNF. *Cell* **1988**, *53*, 45–53. [CrossRef]
7. Vandenabeele, P.; Declercq, W.; Beyaert, R.; Fiers, W. Two tumour necrosis factor receptors: Structure and function. *Trends Cell Biol.* **1995**, *5*, 392–399. [CrossRef]
8. Bazzoni, F.; Beutler, B. The tumor necrosis factor ligand and receptor families. *N. Engl. J. Med.* **1996**, *334*, 1717–1725. [CrossRef] [PubMed]
9. Black, R.A.; Rauch, C.T.; Kozlosky, C.J.; Peschon, J.J.; Slack, J.L.; Wolfson, M.F.; Castner, B.J.; Stocking, K.L.; Reddy, P.; Srinivasan, S.; et al. A metalloproteinase disintegrin that releases tumour-necrosis factor-alpha from cells. *Nature* **1997**, *385*, 729–733. [CrossRef] [PubMed]
10. Moss, M.L.; Jin, S.-L.C.; Milla, M.E.; Burkhart, W.; Carter, H.L.; Chen, W.-J.; Clay, W.C.; Didsbury, J.R.; Hassler, D.; Hoffman, C.R.; et al. Cloning of a disintegrin metalloproteinase that processes precursor tumour-necrosis factor-alpha. *Nature* **1997**, *385*, 733–736. [CrossRef] [PubMed]
11. Elliott, M.J.; Maini, R.N.; Feldmann, M.; Kalden, J.R.; Antoni, C.; Smolen, J.S.; Leeb, B.; Breedveld, F.C.; Macfarlane, J.D.; Bijl, J.A.; et al. Randomised double-blind comparison of chimeric monoclonal antibody to tumour necrosis factor alpha (cA2) versus placebo in rheumatoid arthritis. *Lancet* **1994**, *344*, 1105–1110. [CrossRef]
12. Weinblatt, M.E.; Keystone, E.C.; Furst, D.E.; Moreland, L.W.; Weisman, M.H.; Birbara, C.A.; Teoh, L.A.; Fischkoff, S.A.; Chartash, E.K. Adalimumab, a fully human anti-tumor necrosis factor alpha monoclonal antibody, for the treatment of rheumatoid arthritis in patients taking concomitant methotrexate: The ARMADA trial. *Arthritis Rheum.* **2003**, *48*, 35–45. [CrossRef] [PubMed]

13. Hanauer, S.B.; Sandborn, W.J.; Rutgeerts, P.; Fedorak, R.N.; Lukas, M.; MacIntosh, D.; Panaccione, R.; Wolf, D.; Pollack, P. Human anti-tumor necrosis factor monoclonal antibody (adalimumab) in Crohn's disease: The CLASSIC-I trial. *Gastroenterology* **2006**, *130*, 323–333. [CrossRef] [PubMed]

14. Murdaca, G.; Colombo, B.M.; Cagnati, P.; Gulli, R.; Spanò, F.; Puppo, F. Update upon efficacy and safety of TNF-alpha inhibitors. *Expert Opin. Drug Saf.* **2012**, *11*, 1–5. [CrossRef] [PubMed]

15. Ducharme, E.; Weinberg, J.M. Etanercept. *Expert Opin. Biol. Ther.* **2008**, *8*, 491–502. [CrossRef] [PubMed]

16. Taylor, P.C. Pharmacology of TNF blockade in rheumatoid arthritis and other chronic inflammatory diseases. *Curr. Opin. Pharmacol.* **2010**, *10*, 308–315. [CrossRef] [PubMed]

17. De Simone, C.; Amerio, P.; Amoruso, G.; Bardazzi, F.; Campanati, A.; Conti, A.; Gisondi, P.; Gualdi, G.; Guarneri, C.; Leoni, L.; et al. Immunogenicity of anti-TNFα therapy in psoriasis: A clinical issue? *Expert Opin. Biol. Ther.* **2013**, *13*, 1673–1682. [CrossRef] [PubMed]

18. Cohen, M.D.; Keystone, E.C. Intravenous golimumab in rheumatoid arthritis. *Expert Rev. Clin. Immunol.* **2014**, *10*, 823–830. [CrossRef] [PubMed]

19. Deeks, E.D. Certolizumab Pegol: A Review in Inflammatory Autoimmune Diseases. *BioDrugs* **2016**, *30*, 607–617. [CrossRef] [PubMed]

20. Mitoma, H.; Horiuchi, T.; Tsukamoto, H.; Ueda, N. Molecular mechanisms of action of anti-TNF-α agents—Comparison among therapeutic TNF-α antagonists. *Cytokine* **2018**, *101*, 56–63. [CrossRef] [PubMed]

21. Horiuchi, T.; Mitoma, H.; Harashima, S.; Tsukamoto, H.; Shimoda, T. Transmembrane TNF-alpha: Structure, function and interaction with anti-TNF agents. *Rheumatology (Oxford)* **2010**, *49*, 1215–1228. [CrossRef] [PubMed]

22. Scallon, B.; Cai, A.; Solowski, N.; Rosenberg, A.; Song, X.Y.; Shealy, D.; Wagner, C. Binding and functional comparisons of two types of tumor necrosis factor antagonists. *J. Pharmacol. Exp. Ther.* **2002**, *301*, 418–426. [CrossRef] [PubMed]

23. Ringheanu, M.; Daum, F.; Markowitz, J.; Levine, J.; Katz, S.; Lin, X.; Silver, J. Effects of infliximab on apoptosis and reverse signaling of monocytes from healthy individuals and patients with Crohn's disease. *Inflamm. Bowel Dis.* **2004**, *10*, 801–810. [CrossRef] [PubMed]

24. Mitoma, H.; Horiuchi, T.; Tsukamoto, H.; Tamimoto, Y.; Kimoto, Y.; Uchino, A.; To, K.; Harashima, S.; Hatta, N.; Harada, M. Mechanisms for cytotoxic effects of anti-tumor necrosis factor agents on transmembrane tumor necrosis factor alpha-expressing cells: Comparison among infliximab, etanercept, and adalimumab. *Arthritis Rheum.* **2008**, *58*, 1248–1257. [CrossRef] [PubMed]

25. Van den Brande, J.M.; Braat, H.; van den Brink, G.R.; Versteeg, H.H.; Bauer, C.A.; Hoedemaeker, I.; van Montfrans, C.; Hommes, D.W.; Peppelenbosch, M.P.; van Deventer, S.J. Infliximab but not etanercept induces apoptosis in lamina propria T-lymphocytes from patients with Crohn's disease. *Gastroenterology* **2003**, *124*, 1774–1785. [CrossRef]

26. Nesbitt, A.; Fossati, G.; Bergin, M.; Stephens, P.; Stephens, S.; Foulkes, R.; Brown, D.; Robinson, M.; Bourne, T. Mechanism of action of certolizumab pegol (CDP870): In vitro comparison with other anti-tumor necrosis factor alpha agents. *Inflamm. Bowel Dis.* **2007**, *13*, 1323–1332. [CrossRef] [PubMed]

27. Mitoma, H.; Horiuchi, T.; Hatta, N.; Tsukamoto, H.; Harashima, S.-I.; Kikuchi, Y.; Otsuka, J.; Okamura, S.; Fujita, S.; Harada, M. Infliximab induces potent anti-inflammatory responses by outside-to-inside signals through transmembrane TNF-alpha. *Gastroenterology* **2005**, *128*, 376–392. [CrossRef] [PubMed]

28. Kaymakcalan, Z.; Sakorafas, P.; Bose, S.; Scesney, S.; Xiong, L.; Hanzatian, D.K.; Salfeld, J.; Sasso, E.H. Comparisons of affinities, avidities, and complement activation of adalimumab, infliximab, and etanercept in binding to soluble and membrane tumor necrosis factor. *Clin. Immunol.* **2009**, *131*, 308–316. [CrossRef] [PubMed]

29. Shealy, D.J.; Cai, A.; Staquet, K.; Baker, A.; Lacy, E.R.; Johns, L.; Vafa, O.; Gunn, G.; Tam, S.; Sague, S.; et al. Characterization of golimumab, a human monoclonal antibody specific for human tumor necrosis factor α. *MAbs* **2010**, *2*, 428–439. [CrossRef] [PubMed]

30. Vos, A.C.; Wildenberg, M.E.; Duijvestein, M.; Verhaar, A.P.; van den Brink, G.R.; Hommes, D.W. Anti-tumor necrosis factor-α antibodies induce regulatory macrophages in an Fc region-dependent manner. *Gastroenterology* **2011**, *140*, 221–230. [CrossRef] [PubMed]

31. Wojtal, K.A.; Rogler, G.; Scharl, M.; Biedermann, L.; Frei, P.; Fried, M.; Weber, A.; Eloranta, J.J.; Kullak-Ublick, G.A.; Vavricka, S.R. Fc gamma receptor CD64 modulates the inhibitory activity of infliximab. *PLoS ONE* **2012**, *7*, e43361. [CrossRef] [PubMed]

32. Ueda, N.; Tsukamoto, H.; Mitoma, H.; Ayano, M.; Tanaka, A.; Ohta, S.; Inoue, Y.; Arinobu, Y.; Niiro, H.; Akashi, K.; et al. The cytotoxic effects of certolizumab pegol and golimumab mediated by transmembrane tumor necrosis factor α. *Inflamm. Bowel Dis.* **2013**, *19*, 1224–1231. [CrossRef] [PubMed]

33. Derer, S.; Till, A.; Haesler, R.; Sina, C.; Grabe, N.; Jung, S.; Nikolaus, S.; Kuehbacher, T.; Groetzinger, J.; Rose-John, S.; et al. mTNF reverse signalling induced by TNFα antagonists involves a GDF-1 dependent pathway: Implications for Crohn's disease. *Gut* **2013**, *62*, 376–386. [CrossRef] [PubMed]

34. Lubel, J.S.; Testro, A.G.; Angus, P.W. Hepatitis B virus reactivation following immunosuppressive therapy: Guidelines for prevention and management. *Intern. Med. J.* **2007**, *37*, 705–712. [CrossRef] [PubMed]

35. Gómez-Reino, J.J.; Carmona, L.; Valverde, V.R.; Mola, E.M.; Montero, M.D.; BIOBADASER Group. Treatment of rheumatoid arthritis with tumor necrosis factor inhibitors may predispose to significant increase in tuberculosis risk: A multicenter active-surveillance report. *Arthritis Rheum.* **2003**, *48*, 2122–2127.

36. Brown, S.L.; Greene, M.H.; Gershon, S.K.; Edwards, E.T.; Braun, M.M. Tumor necrosis factor antagonist therapy and lymphoma development: Twenty-six cases reported to the Food and Drug Administration. *Arthritis Rheum.* **2002**, *46*, 3151–3158. [CrossRef] [PubMed]

37. Banner, D.W.; D'Arcy, A.; Janes, W.; Gentz, R.; Schoenfeld, H.J.; Broger, C.; Loetscher, H.; Lesslauer, W. Crystal structure of the soluble human 55 kd TNF receptor-human TNF beta complex: Implications for TNF receptor activation. *Cell* **1993**, *73*, 431–445. [CrossRef]

38. Mukai, Y.; Nakamura, T.; Yoshikawa, M.; Yoshioka, Y.; Tsunoda, S.; Nakagawa, S.; Yamagata, Y.; Tsutsumi, Y. Solution of the structure of the TNF-TNFR2 complex. *Sci. Signal.* **2010**, *3*, ra83. [CrossRef] [PubMed]

39. Liang, S.; Dai, J.; Hou, S.; Su, L.; Zhang, D.; Guo, H.; Hu, S.; Wang, H.; Rao, Z.; Guo, Y.; et al. Structural basis for treating tumor necrosis factor α (TNFα)-associated diseases with the therapeutic antibody infliximab. *J. Biol. Chem.* **2013**, *288*, 13799–13807. [CrossRef] [PubMed]

40. Hu, S.; Liang, S.; Guo, H.; Zhang, D.; Li, H.; Wang, X.; Yang, W.; Qian, W.; Hou, S.; Wang, H.; et al. Comparison of the inhibition mechanisms of adalimumab and infliximab in treating tumor necrosis factor α-associated diseases from a molecular view. *J. Biol. Chem.* **2013**, *288*, 27059–27067. [CrossRef] [PubMed]

41. Lee, J.U.; Shin, W.; Son, J.Y.; Yoo, K.Y.; Heo, Y.S. Molecular Basis for the Neutralization of Tumor Necrosis Factor α by Certolizumab Pegol in the Treatment of Inflammatory Autoimmune Diseases. *Int. J. Mol. Sci.* **2017**, *18*, 228. [CrossRef] [PubMed]

42. Lerch, T.F.; Sharpe, P.; Mayclin, S.J.; Edwards, T.E.; Lee, E.; Conlon, H.D.; Polleck, S.; Rouse, J.C.; Luo, Y.; Zou, Q. Infliximab crystal structures reveal insights into self-association. *MAbs* **2017**, *9*, 874–883. [CrossRef] [PubMed]

43. Chen, K.; Long, D.S.; Lute, S.C.; Levy, M.J.; Brorson, K.A.; Keire, D.A. Simple NMR methods for evaluating higher order structures of monoclonal antibody therapeutics with quinary structure. *J. Pharm. Biomed. Anal.* **2016**, *128*, 398–407. [CrossRef] [PubMed]

44. Tran, B.N.; Chan, S.L.; Ng, C.; Shi, J.; Correia, I.; Radziejewski, C.; Matsudaira, P. Higher order structures of Adalimumab, Infliximab and their complexes with TNFα revealed by electron microscopy. *Protein Sci.* **2017**, *26*, 2392–2398. [CrossRef] [PubMed]

45. Agostini, C.; Sancetta, R.; Cerutti, A.; Semenzato, G. Alveolar macrophages as a cell source of cytokine hyperproduction in HIV-related interstitial lung disease. *J. Leukoc. Biol.* **1995**, *58*, 495–500. [CrossRef] [PubMed]

46. Caron, G.; Delneste, Y.; Aubry, J.P.; Magistrelli, G.; Herbault, N.; Blaecke, A.; Meager, A.; Bonnefoy, J.Y.; Jeannin, P. Human NK cells constitutively express membrane TNF-alpha (mTNFalpha) and present mTNFalpha-dependent cytotoxic activity. *Eur. J. Immunol.* **1999**, *29*, 3588–3595. [CrossRef]

47. Fishman, M. Cytolytic activities of activated macrophages versus paraformaldehyde-fixed macrophages; soluble versus membrane-associated TNF. *Cell Immunol.* **1991**, *137*, 164–174. [CrossRef]

48. Armstrong, L.; Thickett, D.R.; Christie, S.J.; Kendall, H.; Millar, A.B. Increased expression of functionally active membrane-associated tumor necrosis factor in acute respiratory distress syndrome. *Am. J. Respir. Cell Mol. Biol.* **2000**, *22*, 68–74. [CrossRef] [PubMed]

49. Kresse, M.; Latta, M.; Künstle, G.; Riehle, H.M.; van Rooijen, N.; Hentze, H.; Tiegs, G.; Biburger, M.; Lucas, R.; Wendel, A. Kupffer cell-expressed membrane-bound TNF mediates melphalan hepatotoxicity via activation of both TNF receptors. *J. Immunol.* **2005**, *175*, 4076–4083. [CrossRef] [PubMed]

50. Peck, R.; Brockhaus, M.; Frey, J.R. Cell surface tumor necrosis factor (TNF) accounts for monocyte- and lymphocyte-mediated killing of TNF-resistant target cells. *Cell Immunol.* **1989**, *122*, 1–10. [CrossRef]

51. Horiuchi, T.; Morita, C.; Tsukamoto, H.; Mitoma, H.; Sawabe, T.; Harashima, S.; Kashiwagi, Y.; Okamura, S. Increased expression of membrane TNF-alpha on activated peripheral CD8+ T cells in systemic lupus erythematosus. *Int. J. Mol. Med.* **2006**, *17*, 875–879. [PubMed]

52. Grell, M.; Douni, E.; Wajant, H.; Löhden, M.; Clauss, M.; Maxeiner, B.; Georgopoulos, S.; Lesslauer, W.; Kollias, G.; Pfizenmaier, K.; et al. The transmembrane form of tumor necrosis factor is the prime activating ligand of the 80 kDa tumor necrosis factor receptor. *Cell* **1995**, *83*, 793–802. [CrossRef]

53. Tracey, D.; Klareskog, L.; Sasso, E.H.; Salfeld, J.G.; Tak, P.P. Tumor necrosis factor antagonist mechanisms of action: A comprehensive review. *Pharmacol. Ther.* **2008**, *117*, 244–279. [CrossRef] [PubMed]

54. Kaufman, D.R.; Choi, Y. Signaling by tumor necrosis factor receptors: pathways, paradigms and targets for therapeutic modulation. *Int. Rev. Immunol.* **1999**, *18*, 405–427. [CrossRef] [PubMed]

55. Chan, F.K.; Chun, H.J.; Zheng, L.; Siegel, R.M.; Bui, K.L.; Lenardo, M.J. A domain in TNF receptors that mediates ligand-independent receptor assembly and signaling. *Science* **2000**, *288*, 2351–2354. [CrossRef] [PubMed]

56. MacEwan, D.J. TNF ligands and receptors-a matter of life and death. *Br. J. Pharmacol.* **2002**, *135*, 855–875. [CrossRef] [PubMed]

57. Eissner, G.; Kolch, W.; Scheurich, P. Ligands working as receptors: Reverse signaling by members of the TNF superfamily enhance the plasticity of the immune system. *Cytokine Growth Factor Rev.* **2004**, *15*, 353–366. [CrossRef] [PubMed]

58. Rivkin, A. Certolizumab pegol for the management of Crohn's disease in adults. *Clin. Ther.* **2009**, *31*, 1158–1176. [CrossRef] [PubMed]

59. Bourne, T.; Fossati, G.; Nesbitt, A. A PEGylated Fab' fragment against tumor necrosis factor for the treatment of Crohn disease: Exploring a new mechanism of action. *BioDrugs* **2008**, *22*, 331–337. [CrossRef] [PubMed]

60. Pasut, G. Pegylation of biological molecules and potential benefits: Pharmacological properties of certolizumab pegol. *BioDrugs* **2014**, *28* (Suppl. 1), S15–S23. [CrossRef] [PubMed]

61. Arora, T.; Padaki, R.; Liu, L.; Hamburger, A.E.; Ellison, A.R.; Stevens, S.R.; Louie, J.S.; Kohno, T. Differences in binding and effector functions between classes of TNF antagonists. *Cytokine* **2009**, *45*, 124–131. [CrossRef] [PubMed]

62. Lis, K.; Kuzawińska, O.; Bałkowiec-Iskra, E. Tumor necrosis factor inhibitors—State of knowledge. *Arch. Med. Sci.* **2014**, *10*, 1175–1185. [CrossRef] [PubMed]

63. Narhi, L.O.; Arakawa, T. Dissociation of recombinant tumor necrosis factor-α studied by gel permeation chromatography. *Biochem. Biophys. Res. Commun.* **1987**, *147*, 740–746. [CrossRef]

64. Corti, A.; Fassina, G.; Marcucci, F.; Barbanti, E.; Cassani, G. Oligomeric tumour necrosis factor α slowly converts into inactive forms at bioactive levels. *Biochem. J.* **1992**, *284*, 905–910. [CrossRef] [PubMed]

65. Hlodan, R.; Pain, R.H. The folding and assembly pathway of tumour necrosis factor TNFα, a globular trimeric protein. *Eur. J. Biochem.* **1995**, *231*, 381–387. [CrossRef] [PubMed]

66. Van Schie, K.A.; Ooijevaar-de Heer, P.; Dijk, L.; Kruithof, S.; Wolbink, G.; Rispens, T. Therapeutic TNF inhibitors can differentially stabilize trimeric TNF by inhibiting monomer exchange. *Sci. Rep.* **2016**, *6*, 32747. [CrossRef] [PubMed]

67. Browning, J.L.; Miatkowski, K.; Griffiths, D.A.; Bourdon, P.R.; Hession, C.; Ambrose, C.M.; Meier, W. Preparation and characterization of soluble recombinant heterotrimeric complexes of human lymphotoxins alpha and beta. *J. Biol. Chem.* **1996**, *271*, 8618–8626. [CrossRef] [PubMed]

68. Calmon-Hamaty, F.; Combe, B.; Hahne, M.; Morel, J. Lymphotoxin α stimulates proliferation and pro-inflammatory cytokine secretion of rheumatoid arthritis synovial fibroblasts. *Cytokine* **2011**, *53*, 207–214. [CrossRef] [PubMed]

69. Buhrmann, C.; Shayan, P.; Aggarwal, B.B.; Shakibaei, M. Evidence that TNF-β (lymphotoxin α) can activate the inflammatory environment in human chondrocytes. *Arthritis Res. Ther.* **2013**, *15*, R202. [CrossRef] [PubMed]

70. Martin, A.C. Accessing the Kabat antibody sequence database by computer. *Proteins* **1996**, *25*, 130–133. [CrossRef]

71. Wilson, I.A.; Stanfield, R.L. Antibody-antigen interactions: New structures and new conformational changes. *Curr. Opin. Struct. Biol.* **1994**, *4*, 857–867. [CrossRef]

72. Kohno, T.; Tam, L.T.; Stevens, S.R.; Louie, J.S. Binding characteristics of tumor necrosis factor receptor-Fc fusion proteins vs anti-tumor necrosis factor mAbs. *J. Investig. Dermatol. Symp. Proc.* **2007**, *12*, 5–8. [CrossRef] [PubMed]

73. Santora, L.C.; Kaymakcalan, Z.; Sakorafas, P.; Krull, I.S.; Grant, K. Characterization of noncovalent complexes of recombinant human monoclonal antibody and antigen using cation exchange, size exclusion chromatography, and BIAcore. *Anal. Biochem.* **2001**, *299*, 119–129. [CrossRef] [PubMed]

74. Kalonia, C.; Toprani, V.; Toth, R.; Wahome, N.; Gabel, I.; Middaugh, C.R.; Volkin, D.B. Effects of Protein Conformation, Apparent Solubility, and Protein-Protein Interactions on the Rates and Mechanisms of Aggregation for an IgG1Monoclonal Antibody. *J. Phys. Chem. B* **2016**, *120*, 7062–7075. [CrossRef] [PubMed]

75. Liu, B.; Guo, H.; Xu, J.; Qin, T.; Xu, L.; Zhang, J.; Guo, Q.; Zhang, D.; Qian, W.; Li, B.; et al. Acid-induced aggregation propensity of nivolumab is dependent on the Fc. *MAbs* **2016**, *8*, 1107–1117. [CrossRef] [PubMed]

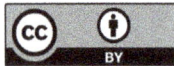

International Journal of
Molecular Sciences

MDPI

Review

Targeting IgG in Arthritis: Disease Pathways and Therapeutic Avenues

Kutty Selva Nandakumar [1,2]

[1] School of Pharmaceutical Sciences, Southern Medical University, Guangzhou 510000, China;
nandakumar@smu.edu.cn
[2] Department of Medical Biochemistry and Biophysics, Karolinska Institute, 17177 Stockholm, Sweden

Received: 31 December 2017; Accepted: 22 February 2018; Published: 28 February 2018

Abstract: Rheumatoid arthritis (RA) is a polygenic and multifactorial syndrome. Many complex immunological and genetic interactions are involved in the final outcome of the clinical disease. Autoantibodies (rheumatoid factors, anti-citrullinated peptide/protein antibodies) are present in RA patients' sera for a long time before the onset of clinical disease. Prior to arthritis onset, in the autoantibody response, epitope spreading, avidity maturation, and changes towards a pro-inflammatory Fc glycosylation phenotype occurs. Genetic association of epitope specific autoantibody responses and the induction of inflammation dependent and independent changes in the cartilage by pathogenic autoantibodies emphasize the crucial contribution of antibody-initiated inflammation in RA development. Targeting IgG by glyco-engineering, bacterial enzymes to specifically cleave IgG/alter N-linked Fc-glycans at Asn 297 or blocking the downstream effector pathways offers new avenues to develop novel therapeutics for arthritis treatment.

Keywords: rheumatoid arthritis; antibodies; collagen; glycosylation; disease pathways; therapy; experimental arthritis

---

1. Introduction

Rheumatoid arthritis (RA) in the articular joints involves a multicellular inflammatory process; infiltration of lymphocytes and granulocytes into the articular cartilage, proliferation of synovial cells, leukocyte extravasation, and, neo-vascularization of the synovial lining surrounding the joints [1]. This proliferative process not only induces swelling, erythema, and pain of multiple joints, but also progresses to the destruction and loss of cartilage and bone architecture. Many cellular components (macrophages, dendritic cells, synovial cells, mast cells, neutrophils, T cells, and B cells), cell surface molecules (co-receptors, adhesion molecules, and integrins), signaling components (ZAP70, PTPN22, JAK, MAPK and Stat1), metabolic components, and humoral mediators (antibodies, cytokines, chemokines, metalloproteinases, serine proteases, and aggrecanases) interact and aid in the disease progression, leading to the digestion of extracellular matrix and the destruction of articular structures [2].

Several theories on the pathogenesis of RA have been put forward that are based on autoantibodies and immune complexes, T cell mediated antigen specific immune responses, cytokine deregulations, and aggressive tumor-like behavior of the rheumatoid synovia. Improved understanding of the cellular and molecular events occurring in the rheumatoid joints during the pathogenesis of the disease is particularly important to find new or better combination of therapeutics for RA [3].

The major genetic factor that is consistently associated with RA is human leukocyte antigens (*HLA*), located on chromosome 6 in the major histocompatibility complex (*MHC*) class II region, which participate in the antigen presentation. *DR* genes, including *DR4* and *DR1* are associated with RA. The susceptibility epitope is glutamine-leucine-arginine-alanine-alanine (QKRAA) or glutamine-arginine-arginine-alanine-alanine (QRRAA), the so-called shared epitope identified in amino acids 70 through 74 in the third hypervariable region of the DRβ chain [2]. In addition, Raychaudhuri et al. have identified the amino acids (leucine or valine variants at amino acid position 11) that are located in the base of the antigen binding groove as further possible explanation for antigen selection [4]. The predominance of *HLA* and prominent infiltration of T cells to the rheumatoid synovia have suggested a key role for T cells in RA. Specific peptides that bind to these DR proteins in RA patients may promote arthritis, however, so far no such dominant peptides have been identified. It is possible that the susceptibility epitope is closely linked to other genes in the MHC region, and, T cells might drive the inflammation by their cellular interactions and cytokine production [5].

On the other hand, B cells contribute to the disease pathogenesis as antigen presenting cells, through co-stimulatory functions by supporting neo-lymphogenesis as well through the secretion of antibodies [6]. In RA, autoantibodies (rheumatoid factors (RFs), anti-citrullinated protein/peptide antibodies (ACPAs)) provide diagnostic and prognostic criteria, and serve as surrogate markers for disease activity), and may play a requisite role in the disease pathogenesis (anti-CII and anti-GPI antibodies) as well. RFs have been consistently associated with RA (60–80% sero-positivity), but it has also been reported to be present in normal individuals as well as under other chronic inflammatory conditions [7]. The contributions of antibodies to the disease are not solely dependent upon their direct binding to their respective antigens, but also through indirect mechanisms, including immune complex formation, deposition, and activation of complement components and FcγRs. Modulation of circulating ICs and pathogenic antibodies by removal using therapeutic plasmapheresis [8] or depleting B cells with the antibody rituximab proved to be beneficial for RA patients [9].

Most likely candidate autoantigens in RA are the joint derived macromolecules. Arthritis can be induced in animals by immunization with different components of cartilage; collagen type II (CII), collagen type IX (CIX), and collagen type XI (CXI), proteoglycan (PG), cartilage link protein (CLP), and chitinase 3-like protein 2 (CHI3L2/YKL-39). CII, a homo-trimer composed of α1(II) chains, is the most abundant fibrillar protein that is found in the articular cartilage and constitutes 80–85% of the total collagen. Autoimmunity to CII occurs in RA, target of inflammatory attack and CII has been proposed to be the driving force in arthritis [10].

Immunization of susceptible rodents with CII emulsified in adjuvant induced polyarthritis (so called, collagen induced arthritis, CIA), which resembles RA in several aspects. It has been well documented that both T and B cells are important in the disease pathogenesis, as demonstrated by the resistance of mice for arthritis induction that are deficient in these cell populations [11,12]. Similar to RA, susceptibility to CIA in rodents is closely associated with the expression of specific class II molecules of the *MHC* that are involved in the specific recognition of T cell receptor (TCR) and in binding and presenting antigenic peptides to it. Mice having H2^q and H2^r haplotypes are the most susceptible to arthritis [13]. Various humanized *HLA* transgenic mice having *HLA-DQ8* [14], *DR1* [15], or *DR4* and *CD4* [16] developed severe arthritis after CII immunization. In the H-2^q context, the dominant heterologous T cell epitope resides in the amino acids position 260–270 [17,18]. Substitution of amino acids at positions 260-264 and 266 appeared to be critical for T cell recognition [19,20]. Interestingly, epitope glycosylation is important for T cell recognition of CII in CIA [21,22].

On the other hand, major B cell epitopes well defined so far (C1, J1, U1, D3, F4, and E8) are spread over the entire triple helical CII molecule. CII reactive B cells were shown to be neither negatively selected, somatically mutated, nor tolerized [23,24]. Native but not the denatured CII induces arthritis suggests the requirement of triple helical confirmation of CII for disease induction [25,26]. In CIA, antibodies play a major role in the immuno-pathology of autoimmune arthritis, and IgG and C3 depositions were detected in the inflamed joints [27,28]. Antibodies against C1, J1, and U1 epitopes were detected in CII immunized chronic arthritis mice [29], and these CII epitopes are conserved across the species [30]. However, DBA/1 mice deficient in the *RAG1* gene still developed some synovial hyperplasia, pannus, and erosions of cartilage and bone [31], demonstrating that arthritis development is still possible even in the absence of mature T and B lymphocytes.

2. CII-Specific Antibodies

Germ line encoded antibodies are important in the pathogenesis of antibody mediated autoimmune diseases [32]. Genetic control of autoantibody responses [33,34] and the association of epitope-specific antibody response with specific *VH* alleles were identified earlier [35]. Antibodies either directly or as constituents of immune complexes, play a central role in triggering inflammation in a number of autoimmune diseases [6,36]. In experimental arthritis, disease can be passively induced in naive mice using serum from arthritic mice [27,37], RA patients [38,39], with a combination of CII specific mAbs [40–44] or single mAb [45]. Arthritis produced by passive transfer of CII mAb, so called collagen antibody induced arthritis (CAIA), resembles actively induced CIA, with a much more rapid onset (24–48 h), but in acute form (Figure 1). LPS (ligand for toll-like receptors, TLR4/TLR2) [41,46] or lipomannan (ligand for TLR2) [47] enhances the incidence and severity of the antibody initiated disease by decreasing the threshold for arthritis induction. Disease susceptibility is independent of MHC alleles [27,42] and severe combined immunodeficient (SCID) mice developed arthritis [48], as well as T or B cell deficient mice [49], but the T and B cell double deficient mice had less severe arthritis [49], suggesting a regulatory role for these cells at the effector level [50–52]. CAIA is an acute arthritis that is triggered by antibody binding and neutrophils/macrophages, but bypassing the adaptive immune responses.

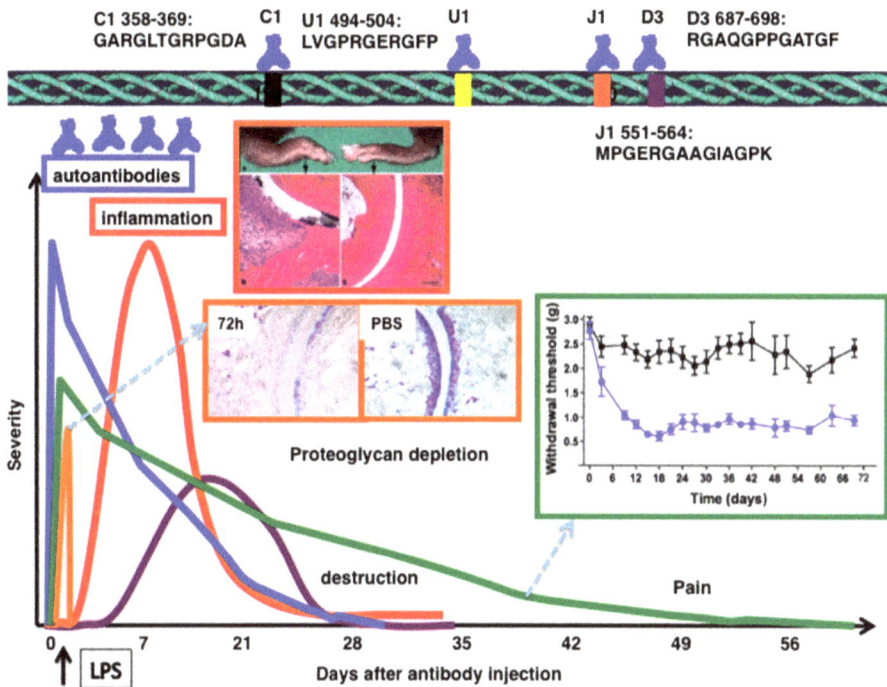

Figure 1. Schematic diagram of acute form of collagen antibody induced arthritis. Autoantibodies binding to well defined epitopes are transferred at day 0, followed by injection of lipopolysaccharide from *E. coli* 05:B55 as the secondary stimulus at day 3. Significant level of proteoglycan depletion was observed 72 h after antibody injection. Inflammation (red and swollenness) and, cartilage and bone erosions between arthritis and control mouse are shown. HE stained joint morphology of arthritis and control mice. Magnification, 10×. Pain (withdrawal threshold levels) started even before inflammation began and prolonged even after resolution of inflammation. Dotted arrows indicate the inserted figures.

For CAIA induction, IL-1β, TNF-α and MIP-1α are required, but not IL-6 [48]. IL-4 [53,54] and IL-10 [55] promoted the disease. Several complement components and their receptors [28,56–61] are involved. The complement factor 5 (C5) break down product, C5a is the most potent anaphylatoxin and a powerful chemo-attractant for neutrophils and monocytes, with the ability to promote margination, extravasation, and activation of these cells [62]. C5a levels are markedly elevated in the synovial fluids of patients with RA [63], and a selective C5a receptor antagonist is inhibitory to immune complex–induced inflammation [64]. Hence, C5a plays a crucial role in antibody mediated arthritis [65] and a recombinant vaccine, which induced C5a-specific neutralizing antibodies attenuated CAIA development [66]. Similarly, a fusion protein containing synovial-homing peptide and anti-C5 neutralizing antibody, which specifically targeted inflamed joints attenuated antibody initiated arthritis [67]. Presumably, inflammatory cell recruitment to the joint by C5a or by other complement-induced chemotactic factors are required for the disease initiation.

Interestingly, C5a binding to C5aR induces the expression of activating FcγRIII, while down modulating inhibitory FcγRII on macrophages, which demonstrates how these two key components of acute inflammation can interact with each other in vivo [68]. Mice lacking the common γ-chain of FcRs are highly resistant [45,69] to CAIA, but are only partially resistant in FcγRIII deficient mice [69]. The absence of FcγRII in DBA/1 mice exacerbates the disease [45], but not so in the BALB/c background [69]. More rapid and severe arthritis was observed with an injection of single anti-CII antibody in FcγIIa transgenic mice [70]. Recent observations also highlight the difference in effector functions of IgG Fc engaged to the complement components and FcγRs [71]. There are several factors that could influence the relative contributions of complement versus FcR dependent inflammatory pathways to the immune complex-triggered inflammatory responses. These include antibody isotype, titer as well as the site of immune complex deposition. With respect to Ig isotype, FcR mechanisms could predominate with immune complexes comprised of non-complement-fixing antibodies or after deposition in sites with abundant resident FcR-bearing inflammatory cells. Conversely, complement-driven inflammation may dominate when immune complexes containing Ig-constant regions poorly bound by FcR or when leukocytes must be attracted to an inflammatory site. In addition, antibody titer may influence the humoral pathways of inflammation [72] and subsequent antibody synthesis by feedback regulation [73]. It has also been shown that C5a can down modulate TLR4 induced immune responses [74], indicating the complexity of interactions occurring during antibody initiated inflammation. In essence, IgG mediated inflammation is mainly dependent on age, sex, FcγRs, complement factors, cytokines (IL-1β, IL-4, IL-10, TNF-α, IFN-β and -γ), chemokines, neutrophils, macrophages, different types of proteases, and other inflammatory mediators, like prostaglandins, leukotrienes, etc. [75–77] (Figure 2).

Interestingly, apart from the above described inflammatory phase, antibodies could be pathogenic to the cartilage independent of inflammatory cells and factors [78]. Anti-CII antibodies could be pathogenic to chondrocytes, even in the absence of inflammatory mediators, like involvement in impaired cartilage formation [79], strong inhibition of collagen fibrillogenesis [80], and disorganization of CII fibrils in the extracellular matrix (ECM) with or without increased matrix synthesis [81]. In addition, these pathogenic monoclonal antibodies (mAbs) also induce deleterious effects on cartilage [82–84] and inhibit CII self-assembly, which suggests that pathogenic antibodies could possibly interfere with the crucial epitopes at sites essential for the stabilization of the polymeric CII fibrils, leading to disturbances in the integrity of the cartilage matrix. Hence, it is plausible that autoantibodies after binding to the cartilage could initiate unwinding of the triple helical structure of CII, which in turn could lead to proteoglycan depletion [85], allowing more enzymes, inflammatory cells to penetrate into the cartilage architecture to induce further damage. But, direct evidence for these suggested initial pathological events is still not available. Surprisingly, instead of LPS or lipomannan, when mannan from *Saccharomyces cerevisiae* was used as the secondary stimulus after anti-CII antibodies transfer, chronic arthritis phenotype developed in mice having low levels of reactive oxygen species [86] suggesting that under certain in vivo conditions, antibodies could also contribute to chronic disease manifestations and disease relapses in RA.

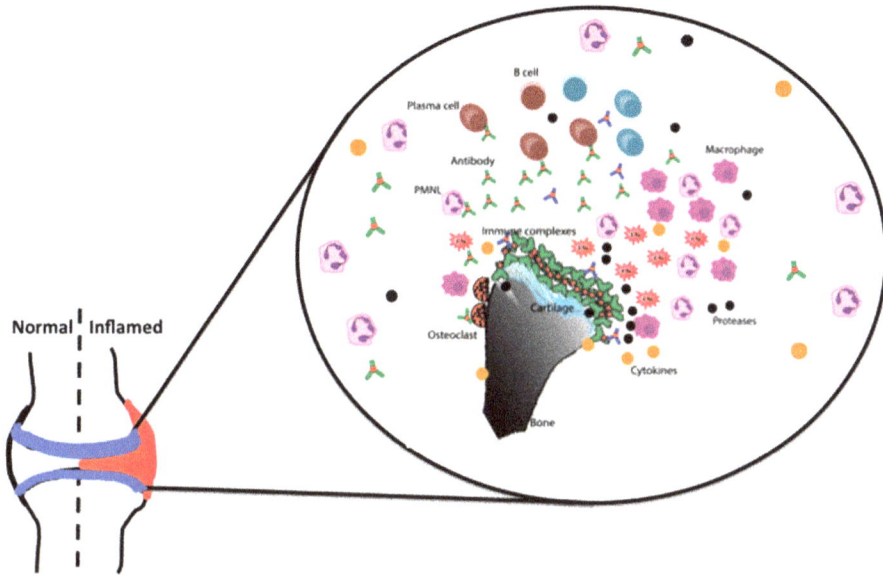

Figure 2. IgG dependent effector phase of arthritis. Binding of antibodies to epitopes present on the cartilage surface forms immune complexes leading to the activation of complement cascades and formation of anaphylatoxin, C5a, which attracts immune cells to the inflammatory foci. Antibodies also interact with FcγR bearing granulocytes, which secrete pro-inflammatory cytokines and proteases damaging cartilage and bone.

3. COMP-Specific Antibodies

Cartilage oligomeric matrix protein (COMP) is a structural cartilage protein synthesized by chondrocytes and composed of 5 identical subunits, with disulfide bonds near the N-terminal, and with a globular domain at the C-terminal end [87,88]. Immunization with COMP leads to induction of arthritis in rats [89] and mice [90]. Polyclonal antibodies binding to COMP upon passive transfer induced arthritis, albeit at a lower level of severity [90] as compared to CAIA. Subsequently, mAbs to COMP were generated and shown to induce arthritis in mice [91]. In addition, anti-COMP mAbs enhanced arthritis when co-administered with a sub-arthritogenic dose of CII-specific mAb [91].

4. Anti-GPI Antibodies

The F1 progeny (KBN) of the KRN TCR (recognizing bovine RNase presented by A^k) transgenic mice and the non-obese diabetic (NOD) mice carrying MHC class II allele $A\beta^{g7}$ spontaneously developed severe peripheral arthritis beginning at about three weeks of age [92]. T and B cell autoimmunity to the ubiquitous glycolytic enzyme glucose-6-phosphate isomerase (GPI) is the deriving force in this disease model [93]. The KRN TCR recognizes a peptide derived from GPI (residues 282–294), in the context of $A\beta^{g7}$ [94]. After the initiation, the disease proceeds due to the presence of high levels of anti-GPI antibodies that are present in the KBN serum. Injection of recombinant hGPI [95] or hG6PI (325–339) peptide [96] induced arthritis in mice.

Naïve mice injected with KBN serum [97], affinity-purified anti-GPI antibodies [93], or a combination of two or more anti-GPI mAbs [98] induced arthritis. Purified anti-GPI antibodies transferred into the mice localized specifically to distal joints in the front and rear limbs within minutes of injection, saturated within 20 min and remained localized for at least 24 h [99], and the accumulation of immune complexes seems to be possible due to a lack of decay-accelerating factor (DAF) in this tissue [100] and caused macromolecular vasopermeability localized to joints, thus augmenting its severity [101]. The predominant isotype of the antibodies that are present in the KBN serum is γ1 and severe arthritis is maintained if repeated injections of serum are given [97]. Degranulation of mast cells was apparent within an hour [102] and an influx of neutrophils was prominent within 1–2 days [103]; synovial hyperplasia and mononuclear cell infiltration, with pannus formation and erosions of bone and cartilage, began within a week [97,103].

Similar to CAIA, arthritis caused by KBN serum transfer is *MHC* independent. Also, T and B cells are not required since arthritis developed in recombination activating gene 1 (*RAG1*) deficient mice [97] but IL-17-producing T cells can augment this autoantibody-induced arthritis [104]. A single injection of anti-GPI antibody caused prolonged and more severe arthritis in B cell-deficient KBN mice [97]. Mice depleted of neutrophils using anti-Gr-1 antibodies are resistant [103] and neutrophil FcγR, C5aR, and CD11a/LFA-1 are critical components [105]. Interestingly, CpG-oligodeoxynucleotides induced cross talk between $CD8\alpha^+$ dendritic cells and NK cells, which resulted in the suppression of neutrophil recruitment to the joint [106]; mice lacking macrophage-like synoviocytes (op/op) are not susceptible [107]. Similarly, mice that were depleted of macrophages by clodronate liposomes were completely resistant. Reconstituting these mice with macrophages from naive animals reversed this resistance [108]. Intravenous immunoglobulins (IVIG) induced expression of FcγRIIB in macrophages but not in neutrophils protected the mice from the disease [107]. Mice having mutations in the stem cell factor (SCF) receptor, c-kit (*W/Wv*) or its ligand, SCF (*Sl/Sld*), leading to mast cells deficiency, are resistant, and susceptibility can be restored by reconstitution with mast cell precursors [102,109]. Subsequently, it was shown that mast cells contribute to the antibody initiated arthritis via IL-1 [110]. TNF-α and IL-1R, but not IL-6 deficient mice were resistant to disease induction [111,112], but TNFR1 and TNFR2 deficient mice were susceptible [113]. IL-4 is dispensable [114] and a genetic polymorphism in IL-1β gene was shown to be of importance [115]. Gene-disrupted or congenic mice were used to delineate the roles of complement components: factor B, C3, C5 and C5aR are essential, but not C1q, C4, MBL-1, C6, CR1, 2, and 3 [113]. Thus, it has been concluded that activation through the alternative pathway leading to the generation of C5a is important in the serum transfer arthritis. Mice lacking the common γ-chain of FcRs are more resistant than those lacking only FcγRIII [113]. But, different results were obtained with FcγRII deficient mice, either they had no effect [113], or they had an earlier onset and greater severity of disease [109]. The neonatal MHC-like FcR (FcRn), associated with the half-life of transferred antibodies, is required [116]. NKT cells promoted this antibody-mediated inflammation [117]. Interestingly, IVIG treatment or ant-murine albumin antibodies protected mice against KBN serum induced arthritis [118], suggesting the importance of antibody-FcR interactions in arthritis pathogenesis.

5. Immune-Complex Mediated Arthritis

Immune-complex arthritis (ICA) was elicited in naive mice using a non-self-antigen [119]. Mice injected intravenously with heat-inactivated polyclonal rabbit anti-lysozyme serum, followed by an injection with poly-L-lysine-coupled lysozyme in the joint developed arthritis. Disease featuring a massive influx of neutrophils is evident within a day and wanes over the course of a week. Antigen is deposited on the articular surface, presumably in complex with specific antibody [119]. Local depletion of macrophage-like synoviocytes prevents disease [120]. IL-1 is required for inflammation and cartilage destruction, but TNF-α may be dispensable. In this model, FcγRIII is required for inflammation and cartilage breakdown, but FcγRI seems to be only important in cartilage loss [121], whereas IFN-γ bypasses the dependence on FcγRIII [122]. FcγRII plays a suppressive role, since inflammation and cartilage breakdown are enhanced in FcγRII deficient mice [121]. Chondrocyte death in $FcγRI^{-/-}$ mice was completely abrogated, whereas matrix metalloproteinases (MMPs) mediated cartilage destruction was significantly diminished [121]. Local adenoviral overexpression of IFN-γ in the knee joint prior to the onset of IC-mediated arthritis aggravated severe cartilage destruction. IFN-γ stimulated ICA showed pronounced chondrocyte death that was also completely mediated by FcγRI [123]. Thus, during ICA, synovial macrophages seem to be the dominant factor in the induction of severe cartilage destruction [124].

6. Anti-Citrullinated Peptide/Protein Antibodies

Several citrullinated autoantigens (α-enolase, fibrinogen, filaggrin, vimentin, and CII) are used as targets of ACPAs in the diagnostic assays [125]. Around 70% of RA patients sera contain antibodies binding to cyclic citrullinated peptides (CCP2), and these ACPAs are reported to be associated with more severe arthritis [126]. ACPAs are included as one of the classification criteria for RA by American College of Rheumatology/European League Against Rheumatism (ACR/EULAR) consortium [127]. ACPAs are present in the RA sera decades before the onset of clinical disease [128], possibly suggesting that the triggering for autoimmunity may occur at other locations in the body than the joints [129]. Prior to arthritis onset, epitope spreading [130], avidity maturation [131], and changes towards a pro-inflammatory Fc glycosylation phenotype [132] occurs in the ACPA response.

ACPAs activate osteoclasts [133], leading to bone loss even before the onset of clinical disease [134] and the glycosylation status of IgG determines osteoclast differentiation and bone loss [135]. Thus, autoantibodies could have direct influence on osteoclastogenesis by binding to certain activating FcγRs present on immature osteoclasts leading to enhanced osteoclast generation and bone destruction [136]. Binding of ACPAs to osteoclasts releases IL-8, leading to bone erosion [137] and pain [138], which in turn, could lead to pro-inflammatory processes [139]. Furthermore, ACPAs induce macrophages to secrete TNF-α, mediate activation of complement cascades [140], and FcγRIIa-dependent activation of platelets [141]. ACPAs are also shown to be pathogenic in experimental arthritis [142,143]. Hence, it is plausible that ACPAs may play a crucial part in RA pathogenesis [144].

7. Antibody Induced Pain

Autoantibodies binding to target tissues can induce pain through Fc, Fab-dependent mechanisms [145] possibly via inflammatory mediators like high mobility group box-1 protein (HMGB1) [146] or chemokines released from osteoclasts [138]. Arthralgia in RA patients' may precede joint inflammation, may not correlate with the degree of inflammation, and may persist even after successful treatment of inflammation. In this context, KBN serum transfer induced persistent pain and TNF-α/prostaglandin inhibitors attenuated the allodynia induced during inflammation [147]. Experiments with CII-specific pathogenic IgG antibodies demonstrated time-dependent prostaglandin and spinal glial contribution to antibody-induced pain [148]. Spinal HMGB1 also contributes to nociceptive signal transmission via the activation of TLR4 in antibody induced inflammation [146].

8. Protective Autoantibodies

Interestingly, not all the antibodies are pathogenic in nature. Some of them could be protective, which suggests the possible regulation at the effector level of arthritis. One of the anti-CII antibodies, named CIIF4 binding to the CII epitope, F4 (ERGLKGHRGFT, amino acids Gly926-Phe936) has a protective role against arthritis, when given in combination with arthritogenic antibodies [85,149]. Cartilage explant studies showed that CIIF4 penetrated the extracellular matrix during culture, remained bound to the tissue [82], induced negligible loss of proteoglycan, minimal chemical changes in the composition of the matrix [85], and allowed matrix regeneration, which required viable chondrocytes [150]. Similarly, one of the ACPA mAbs binding to citrullinated fibrinogen [132,151] was found to be protective [152]. However, the mechanisms (for example, steric hindrance for pathogenic antibody binding to the cartilage, blocking of MMP cleavage sites and/or having protective IgG N-glycome profile) of antibody protection are still not clear.

9. Targeting IgG to Treat Antibody Dependent Pathologies

At the effector level of arthritis, apart from targeting effector molecules, like C5 [67,153] and its break down product C5a [65,154,155], receptors (FcRs [156], TLRs [157]), transcription factors [158,159]), and cytokines, using different strategies and drugs [160–162], methods for direct targeting of pathogenic IgG antibodies could be attractive and optimal for therapeutic applications.

IgG molecules at Asn-297 of the CH2 domain of IgG Fc part are glycosylated with variable galactosylation and limited sialylation [163]. Changes in N-glycome alter Fc conformation with direct effects on IgG effector functions [164,165] and have important immunoregulatory functions [166]. For example, increasing afucosylated glycoforms by glyco-engineering have significantly increased the cell mediated cytotoxicity of the target bound anti-CD20 antibody [167]. It is clear that sialylation of the of the Fc fragment confers anti-inflammatory properties [168,169]. Anti-inflammatory property of intravenous IgGs (IVIGs) is mainly attributed to sialylated glycans present in the Fc part of IgG [169,170]. Abrogation of the arthritis activity of KBN sera was observed when sialic acids attached to the penultimate galactose of IgG Fc by α2,6 linkages were cleaved using sialidase or after administration of sialic acid enriched Fc fragments [171]. Sialylated Fcs bind to a specific C-type lectin receptors, SIGN-R1 expressed on macrophages [172], leading to the up-regulation of the inhibitory FcγRIIb on inflammatory cells and inhibition of autoantibody initiated inflammation [173,174] via production of IL-33 and, IL-4 [175] acting on IL-4α [176]. Interestingly, sialylation of anti-CII antibodies and ACPAs attenuates arthritogenic activity and leads to suppression of CIA [177]. Recently, several methods have been developed to modulate the glycan pattern of an antibody for therapeutic benefits (for recent review, see [178]).

Bacterial enzymes to specifically cleave IgG at the hinge region or remove specific carbohydrate moieties linked to the N-glycans of the Fc core polysaccharides could also be used for inhibition of antibody induced inflammation (Figure 3). Endo-β-*N*-acetylglucosaminidase (EndoS) is a member of the GlcNAc polymer hydrolyzing glycosyl hydrolases of family 18-glycosyl hydrolase secreted by group A β-hemolytic *Streptococcus pyogenes*. It exclusively hydrolyses the β-1,4-di-*N*-acetylchitobiose core of the N-linked complex type glycan on Asn-297 of the γ-chains of IgG [179]. EndoS treatment of antibodies did not affect binding of IgG to CII and complement activation, but reduced binding to FcγRs and formation of stable immune complexes [180]. EndoS treatment of KBN serum decreased inflammation induced by anti-GPI antibodies [181]. Similarly, pathogenic potential of IgG molecules were attenuated in other inflammatory conditions as well [182]. EndoS is extremely potent in disrupting larger immune complex lattice formation on the cartilage surface possibly through the destabilization of Fc-Fc interactions [183]. Treatment of mice with EndoS has suppressed many antibody mediated experimental autoimmune diseases (thrombocytopenic purpura [184], arthritis [181], glomerulonephritis [185,186], encephalomyelitis [187], hemolytic anemia [188], and epidermolysis bullosa acquisita [189]). Recent studies also showed that treatment with EndoS reduced Fc/FcγR interactions through Fc deglycosylation, which led to reduction in immune complex-mediated neutrophil activation [190].

Another enzyme secreted by *S. pyogenes* is the IgG-degrading enzyme (IdeS), a cysteine endopeptidase, which cleaves the heavy chains of IgG with a unique specificity [191]. By removing the Fc part from the antigen recognizing Fab, immune responses such as complement activation and Fc dependent effector mechanisms are eliminated. IdeS completely blocked antibody-induced arthritis, reduced CIA disease severity, and inhibited antibody initiated arthritis relapses [192]. Similarly, IdeS is effective in ameliorating other IgG dependent pathologies [182]. Recently, IdeS was shown to reduce/eliminate donor specific antibodies and permitted *HLA*-incompatible transplantation in patients [193]. Interestingly, IdeS can also cleave IgG type B cell receptors, leading to abolished receptor mediated signal transduction and memory B cell activation, temporarily [194].

A **216**   IdeS   **250**
EPKSCDKTHT CPPCPAPELL GGP SV FLFPPKPKDT

B
NeuAc α2—6 Gal β1—4 GlcNAc β1—2 Man α1

Fucose1

GlcNAc β1—4 Man β1—4 GlcNAc β1—4 GlcNAc—Asn-297

NeuAc α2—6 Gal β1—4 GlcNAc β1—2 Man α1

EndoS

C

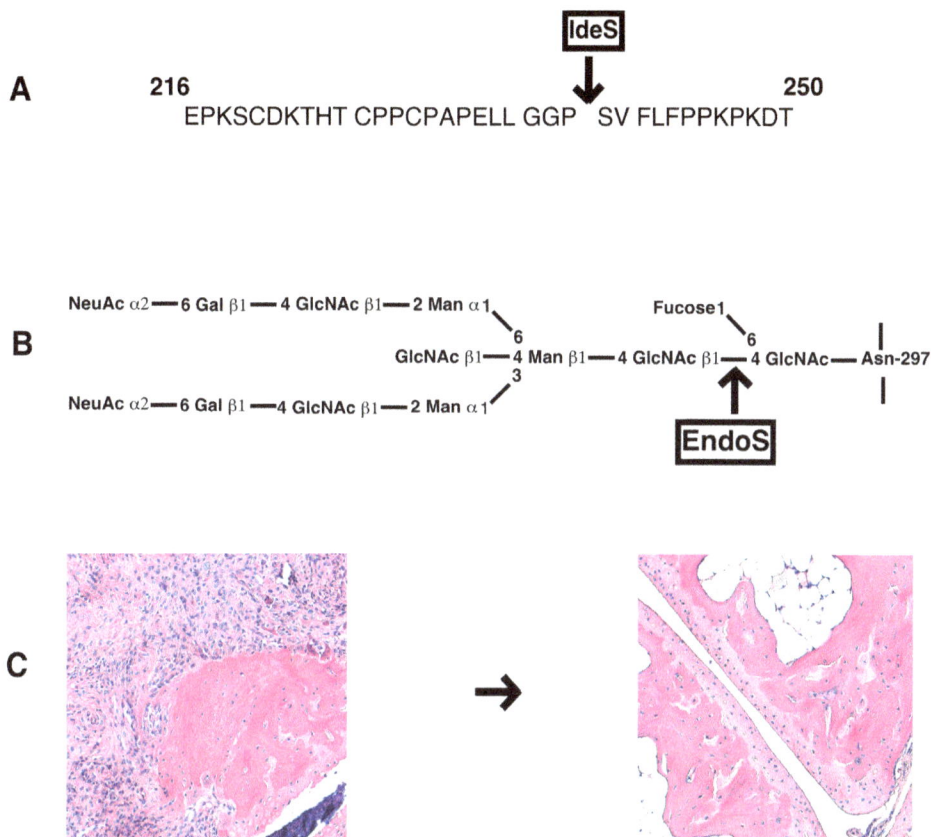

Figure 3. Bacterial enzymes as therapeutics for IgG dependent diseases. *Streptococcus pyogenes* secreted IdeS (**A**) cleaves IgG molecules at the hinge region and EndoS (**B**) cleaves N-linked carbohydrates specifically present on Fc region. Arthritis is ameliorated either after IgG-degrading enzyme (IdeS) or Endo-β-*N*-acetylglucosaminidase (EndoS) cleavage of pathogenic IgG (**C**). HE stained joint morphology of mouse with and without arthritis after treatment. Magnification, 10×.

Thus, glyco-engineering of IgG molecules [195], use of bacterial enzymes to specifically cleave IgG or remove certain carbohydrate moieties [78,182], or blocking the downstream effector pathways [65] to ameliorate IgG dependent pathologies offer new avenues for novel drug development. It is of interest to note that several modifications have been reported that could modulate the therapeutic capability of IgG antibodies [196] and designing of antibodies for improving their therapeutic potency has been reviewed recently [197].

10. Conclusions

At the IgG mediated effector level of arthritis, different pathways of complement activation, FcγR engagement, activation of residential, and infiltrated immune cells in the synovia, various cytokine and chemokine secretion are essential for the development of clinical disease. Requirement for the APC derived cytokines, TNF-α and IL-1β for arthritis induction and perpetuation is obvious. Whereas, T cell secreted cytokines could be detrimental or protective to the joints, depending on the phase of the clinical disease and in situ conditions. Effector cells of the innate immune system (neutrophils, macrophages, and mast cells) drawn to the inflammatory foci by different chemokines and chemo-attractants are actively engaged to induce inflammation, inflict damage to the cartilage, and perpetuate the ongoing immune responses by secreting cytokines and proteases. Once the stimuli (pathogenic IgG molecules) are eliminated, the inflammation subsides. However, if epitope spreading and release of unexposed antigens or antigenic modifications in the presence of strong immune stimuli (for example, mannan) are continuing within the joint, it could drive the acute disease into chronic inflammation under certain conditions with a complete disruption of joint architecture. Hence, it would be valuable to dissect the fine specificity of the molecules taking part in the pathogenesis, as well as understanding both the upstream and downstream molecular events that are involved in the antibody mediated disease process for effective development of therapeutic strategies. With the recent advances in our knowledge and techniques in various scientific disciplines, the possibility of developing such novel therapies for RA is all the more promising.

Acknowledgments: The author acknowledges the project grant from Southern Medical University, Guangzhou, China (No. C1034211).

Conflicts of Interest: The author declares no conflict of interest.

References

1. Orr, C.; Vieira-Sousa, E.; Boyle, D.L.; Buch, M.H.; Buckley, C.D.; Cañete, J.D.; Catrina, A.I.; Choy, E.H.S.; Emery, P.; Fearon, U.; et al. Synovial tissue research: A state-of-the-art review. *Nat. Rev. Rheumatol.* **2017**, *13*, 463–475. [CrossRef] [PubMed]
2. Firestein, G.S.; McInnes, I.B. Immunopathogenesis of Rheumatoid Arthritis. *Immunity* **2017**, *46*, 183–196. [CrossRef] [PubMed]
3. McInnes, I.B.; Schett, G. Pathogenetic insights from the treatment of rheumatoid arthritis. *Lancet* **2017**, *389*, 2328–2337. [CrossRef]
4. Raychaudhuri, S.; Sandor, C.; Stahl, E.A.; Freudenberg, J.; Lee, H.-S.; Jia, X.; Alfredsson, L.; Padyukov, L.; Klareskog, L.; Worthington, J.; et al. Five amino acids in three HLA proteins explain most of the association between MHC and seropositive rheumatoid arthritis. *Nat. Genet.* **2012**, *44*, 291–296. [CrossRef] [PubMed]
5. McInnes, I.B.; Buckley, C.D.; Isaacs, J.D. Cytokines in rheumatoid arthritis—Shaping the immunological landscape. *Nat. Rev. Rheumatol.* **2016**, *12*, 63–68. [CrossRef] [PubMed]
6. Martin, F.; Chan, A.C. B cell immunobiology in disease: Evolving concepts from the clinic. *Annu. Rev. Immunol.* **2006**, *24*, 467–496. [CrossRef] [PubMed]
7. Steiner, G.; Smolen, J. Autoantibodies in rheumatoid arthritis and their clinical significance. *Arthritis Res.* **2002**, *4* (Suppl. 2), S1–S5. [CrossRef] [PubMed]
8. Cheng, Y.; Yang, F.; Huang, C.; Huang, J.; Wang, Q.; Chen, Y.; Du, Y.; Zhao, L.; Gao, M.; Wang, F. Plasmapheresis therapy in combination with TNF-α inhibitor and DMARDs: A multitarget method for the treatment of rheumatoid arthritis. *Mod. Rheumatol.* **2017**, *27*, 576–581. [CrossRef] [PubMed]
9. Nam, J.L.; Takase-Minegishi, K.; Ramiro, S.; Chatzidionysiou, K.; Smolen, J.S.; van der Heijde, D.; Bijlsma, J.W.; Burmester, G.R.; Dougados, M.; Scholte-Voshaar, M.; et al. Efficacy of biological disease-modifying antirheumatic drugs: A systematic literature review informing the 2016 update of the EULAR recommendations for the management of rheumatoid arthritis. *Ann. Rheum. Dis.* **2017**, *76*, 1113–1136. [CrossRef] [PubMed]
10. Holmdahl, R.; Andersson, M.; Goldschmidt, T.J.; Gustafsson, K.; Jansson, L.; Mo, J.A. Type II collagen autoimmunity in animals and provocations leading to arthritis. *Immunol. Rev.* **1990**, *118*, 193–232. [CrossRef] [PubMed]
11. Svensson, L.; Jirholt, J.; Holmdahl, R.; Jansson, L. B cell-deficient mice do not develop type II collagen-induced arthritis (CIA). *Clin. Exp. Immunol.* **1998**, *111*, 521–526. [CrossRef] [PubMed]
12. Corthay, A.; Johansson, A.; Vestberg, M.; Holmdahl, R. Collagen-induced arthritis development requires alpha beta T cells but not gamma delta T cells: Studies with T cell-deficient (TCR mutant) mice. *Int. Immunol.* **1999**, *11*, 1065–1073. [CrossRef] [PubMed]
13. Wooley, P.H.; Luthra, H.S.; Griffiths, M.M.; Stuart, J.M.; Huse, A.; David, C.S. Type II collagen-induced arthritis in mice. IV. Variations in immunogenetic regulation provide evidence for multiple arthritogenic epitopes on the collagen molecule. *J. Immunol.* **1985**, *135*, 2443–2451. [PubMed]

14. Nabozny, G.H.; Baisch, J.M.; Cheng, S.; Cosgrove, D.; Griffiths, M.M.; Luthra, H.S.; David, C.S. HLA-DQ8 transgenic mice are highly susceptible to collagen-induced arthritis: A novel model for human polyarthritis. *J. Exp. Med.* **1996**, *183*, 27–37. [CrossRef] [PubMed]

15. Rosloniec, E.F.; Brand, D.D.; Myers, L.K.; Whittington, K.B.; Gumanovskaya, M.; Zaller, D.M.; Woods, A.; Altmann, D.M.; Stuart, J.M.; Kang, A.H. An HLA-DR1 transgene confers susceptibility to collagen-induced arthritis elicited with human type II collagen. *J. Exp. Med.* **1997**, *185*, 1113–1122. [CrossRef] [PubMed]

16. Andersson, E.C.; Hansen, B.E.; Jacobsen, H.; Madsen, L.S.; Andersen, C.B.; Engberg, J.; Rothbard, J.B.; McDevitt, G.S.; Malmström, V.; Holmdahl, R.; et al. Definition of MHC and T cell receptor contacts in the HLA-DR4restricted immunodominant epitope in type II collagen and characterization of collagen-induced arthritis in HLA-DR4 and human CD4 transgenic mice. *Proc. Natl. Acad. Sci. USA* **1998**, *95*, 7574–7579. [CrossRef] [PubMed]

17. Michaëlsson, E.; Andersson, M.; Engström, A.; Holmdahl, R. Identification of an immunodominant type-II collagen peptide recognized by T cells in H-2q mice: Self tolerance at the level of determinant selection. *Eur. J. Immunol.* **1992**, *22*, 1819–1825. [CrossRef] [PubMed]

18. Rosloniec, E.F.; Whittington, K.B.; Brand, D.D.; Myers, L.K.; Stuart, J.M. Identification of MHC class II and TCR binding residues in the type II collagen immunodominant determinant mediating collagen-induced arthritis. *Cell. Immunol.* **1996**, *172*, 21–28. [CrossRef] [PubMed]

19. Lambert, L.E.; Berling, J.S. Structural requirements for recognition of a type II collagen peptide by murine T cell hybridomas. *Cell. Immunol.* **1994**, *153*, 171–183. [CrossRef] [PubMed]

20. Michaëlsson, E.; Broddefalk, J.; Engström, A.; Kihlberg, J.; Holmdahl, R. Antigen processing and presentation of a naturally glycosylated protein elicits major histocompatibility complex class II-restricted, carbohydrate-specific T cells. *Eur. J. Immunol.* **1996**, *26*, 1906–1910. [CrossRef] [PubMed]

21. Michaëlsson, E.; Malmström, V.; Reis, S.; Engström, A.; Burkhardt, H.; Holmdahl, R. T cell recognition of carbohydrates on type II collagen. *J. Exp. Med.* **1994**, *180*, 745–749. [CrossRef] [PubMed]

22. Corthay, A.; Bäcklund, J.; Broddefalk, J.; Michaëlsson, E.; Goldschmidt, T.J.; Kihlberg, J.; Holmdahl, R. Epitope glycosylation plays a critical role for T cell recognition of type II collagen in collagen-induced arthritis. *Eur. J. Immunol.* **1998**, *28*, 2580–2590. [CrossRef]

23. Mo, J.A.; Bona, C.A.; Holmdahl, R. Variable region gene selection of immunoglobulin G-expressing B cells with specificity for a defined epitope on type II collagen. *Eur. J. Immunol.* **1993**, *23*, 2503–2510. [CrossRef] [PubMed]

24. Cao, D.; Khmaladze, I.; Jia, H.; Bajtner, E.; Nandakumar, K.S.; Blom, T.; Mo, J.A.; Holmdahl, R. Pathogenic autoreactive B cells are not negatively selected toward matrix protein collagen II. *J. Immunol.* **2011**, *187*, 4451–4458. [CrossRef] [PubMed]

25. Trentham, D.E.; Townes, A.S.; Kang, A.H. Autoimmunity to type II collagen an experimental model of arthritis. *J. Exp. Med.* **1977**, *146*, 857–868. [CrossRef] [PubMed]

26. Terato, K.; Hasty, K.A.; Cremer, M.A.; Stuart, J.M.; Townes, A.S.; Kang, A.H. Collagen-induced arthritis in mice. Localization of an arthritogenic determinant to a fragment of the type II collagen molecule. *J. Exp. Med.* **1985**, *162*, 637–646. [CrossRef] [PubMed]

27. Stuart, J.M.; Dixon, F.J. Serum transfer of collagen-induced arthritis in mice. *J. Exp. Med.* **1983**, *158*, 378–392. [CrossRef] [PubMed]

28. Wang, Y.; Kristan, J.; Hao, L.; Lenkoski, C.S.; Shen, Y.; Matis, L.A. A role for complement in antibody-mediated inflammation: C5-deficient DBA/1 mice are resistant to collagen-induced arthritis. *J. Immunol.* **2000**, *164*, 4340–4347. [CrossRef] [PubMed]

29. Bajtner, E.; Nandakumar, K.S.; Engström, A.; Holmdahl, R. Chronic development of collagen-induced arthritis is associated with arthritogenic antibodies against specific epitopes on type II collagen. *Arthritis Res. Ther.* **2005**, *7*, R1148–R1157. [CrossRef] [PubMed]

30. Lindh, I.; Snir, O.; Lönnblom, E.; Uysal, H.; Andersson, I.; Nandakumar, K.S.; Vierboom, M.; 't Hart, B.; Malmström, V.; Holmdahl, R. Type II collagen antibody response is enriched in the synovial fluid of rheumatoid joints and directed to the same major epitopes as in collagen induced arthritis in primates and mice. *Arthritis Res. Ther.* **2014**, *16*, R143. [CrossRef] [PubMed]

31. Plows, D.; Kontogeorgos, G.; Kollias, G. Mice lacking mature T and B lymphocytes develop arthritic lesions after immunization with type II collagen. *J. Immunol.* **1999**, *162*, 1018–1023. [PubMed]

32. Mo, J.A.; Holmdahl, R. The B cell response to autologous type II collagen: Biased V gene repertoire with V gene sharing and epitope shift. *J. Immunol.* **1996**, *157*, 2440–2448. [PubMed]

33. Nandakumar, K.S.; Lindqvist, A.-K.B.; Holmdahl, R. A dominant suppressive MHC class II haplotype interacting with autosomal genes controls autoantibody production and chronicity of arthritis. *Ann. Rheum. Dis.* **2011**, *70*, 1664–1670. [CrossRef] [PubMed]

34. Förster, M.; Raposo, B.; Ekman, D.; Klaczkowska, D.; Popovic, M.; Nandakumar, K.S.; Lindvall, T.; Hultqvist, M.; Teneva, I.; Johannesson, M.; et al. Genetic control of antibody production during collagen-induced arthritis development in heterogeneous stock mice. *Arthritis Rheum.* **2012**, *64*, 3594–3603. [CrossRef] [PubMed]

35. Raposo, B.; Dobritzsch, D.; Ge, C.; Ekman, D.; Xu, B.; Lindh, I.; Förster, M.; Uysal, H.; Nandakumar, K.S.; Schneider, G.; et al. Epitope-specific antibody response is controlled by immunoglobulin V(H) polymorphisms. *J. Exp. Med.* **2014**, *211*, 405–411. [CrossRef] [PubMed]

36. Ludwig, R.J.; Vanhoorelbeke, K.; Leypoldt, F.; Kaya, Z.; Bieber, K.; McLachlan, S.M.; Komorowski, L.; Luo, J.; Cabral-Marques, O.; Hammers, C.M.; et al. Mechanisms of Autoantibody-Induced Pathology. *Front. Immunol.* **2017**, *8*, 603. [CrossRef] [PubMed]

37. Holmdahl, R.; Jansson, L.; Larsson, A.; Jonsson, R. Arthritis in DBA/1 mice induced with passively transferred type II collagen immune serum. Immunohistopathology and serum levels of anti-type II collagen auto-antibodies. *Scand. J. Immunol.* **1990**, *31*, 147–157. [CrossRef] [PubMed]

38. Wooley, P.H.; Luthra, H.S.; Singh, S.K.; Huse, A.R.; Stuart, J.M.; David, C.S. Passive transfer of arthritis to mice by injection of human anti-type II collagen antibody. *Mayo Clin. Proc.* **1984**, *59*, 737–743. [CrossRef]

39. Petkova, S.B.; Konstantinov, K.N.; Sproule, T.J.; Lyons, B.L.; Awwami, M.A.; Roopenian, D.C. Human antibodies induce arthritis in mice deficient in the low-affinity inhibitory IgG receptor Fc gamma RIIB. *J. Exp. Med.* **2006**, *203*, 275–280. [CrossRef] [PubMed]

40. Terato, K.; Hasty, K.A.; Reife, R.A.; Cremer, M.A.; Kang, A.H.; Stuart, J.M. Induction of arthritis with monoclonal antibodies to collagen. *J. Immunol.* **1992**, *148*, 2103–2108. [PubMed]

41. Terato, K.; Harper, D.S.; Griffiths, M.M.; Hasty, D.L.; Ye, X.J.; Cremer, M.A.; Seyer, J.M. Collagen-induced arthritis in mice: Synergistic effect of E. coli lipopolysaccharide bypasses epitope specificity in the induction of arthritis with monoclonal antibodies to type II collagen. *Autoimmunity* **1995**, *22*, 137–147. [CrossRef] [PubMed]

42. Nandakumar, K.S.; Svensson, L.; Holmdahl, R. Collagen type II-specific monoclonal antibody-induced arthritis in mice: Description of the disease and the influence of age, sex, and genes. *Am. J. Pathol.* **2003**, *163*, 1827–1837. [CrossRef]

43. Nandakumar, K.S.; Holmdahl, R. Efficient promotion of collagen antibody induced arthritis (CAIA) using four monoclonal antibodies specific for the major epitopes recognized in both collagen induced arthritis and rheumatoid arthritis. *J. Immunol. Methods* **2005**, *304*, 126–136. [CrossRef] [PubMed]

44. Hutamekalin, P.; Saito, T.; Yamaki, K.; Mizutani, N.; Brand, D.D.; Waritani, T.; Terato, K.; Yoshino, S. Collagen antibody-induced arthritis in mice: Development of a new arthritogenic 5-clone cocktail of monoclonal anti-type II collagen antibodies. *J. Immunol. Methods* **2009**, *343*, 49–55. [CrossRef] [PubMed]

45. Nandakumar, K.S.; Andrén, M.; Martinsson, P.; Bajtner, E.; Hellström, S.; Holmdahl, R.; Kleinau, S. Induction of arthritis by single monoclonal IgG anti-collagen type II antibodies and enhancement of arthritis in mice lacking inhibitory Fcgamma RIIB. *Eur. J. Immunol.* **2003**, *33*, 2269–2277. [CrossRef] [PubMed]

46. Lee, E.-K.; Kang, S.-M.; Paik, D.-J.; Kim, J.M.; Youn, J. Essential roles of Toll-like receptor-4 signaling in arthritis induced by type II collagen antibody and LPS. *Int. Immunol.* **2005**, *17*, 325–333. [CrossRef] [PubMed]

47. Kelkka, T.; Hultqvist, M.; Nandakumar, K.S.; Holmdahl, R. Enhancement of antibody-induced arthritis via Toll-like receptor 2 stimulation is regulated by granulocyte reactive oxygen species. *Am. J. Pathol.* **2012**, *181*, 141–150. [CrossRef] [PubMed]

48. Kagari, T.; Doi, H.; Shimozato, T. The importance of IL-1 beta and TNF-alpha, and the noninvolvement of IL-6, in the development of monoclonal antibody-induced arthritis. *J. Immunol.* **2002**, *169*, 1459–1466. [CrossRef] [PubMed]

49. Nandakumar, K.S.; Bäcklund, J.; Vestberg, M.; Holmdahl, R. Collagen type II (CII)-specific antibodies induce arthritis in the absence of T or B cells but the arthritis progression is enhanced by CII-reactive T cells. *Arthritis Res. Ther.* **2004**, *6*, R544–R550. [CrossRef] [PubMed]

50. Wang, J.; Fathman, J.W.; Lugo-Villarino, G.; Scimone, L.; von Andrian, U.; Dorfman, D.M.; Glimcher, L.H. Transcription factor T-bet regulates inflammatory arthritis through its function in dendritic cells. *J. Clin. Investig.* **2006**, *116*, 414–421. [CrossRef] [PubMed]

51. Mitamura, M.; Nakano, N.; Yonekawa, T.; Shan, L.; Kaise, T.; Kobayashi, T.; Yamashita, K.; Kikkawa, H.; Kinoshita, M. T cells are involved in the development of arthritis induced by anti-type II collagen antibody. *Int. Immunopharmacol.* **2007**, *7*, 1360–1368. [CrossRef] [PubMed]

52. Park, J.-S.; Oh, Y.; Park, O.; Foss, C.A.; Lim, S.M.; Jo, D.-G.; Na, D.H.; Pomper, M.G.; Lee, K.C.; Lee, S. PEGylated TRAIL ameliorates experimental inflammatory arthritis by regulation of Th17 cells and regulatory T cells. *J. Control. Release* **2017**, *267*, 163–171. [CrossRef] [PubMed]

53. Svensson, L.; Nandakumar, K.S.; Johansson, A.; Jansson, L.; Holmdahl, R. IL-4-deficient mice develop less acute but more chronic relapsing collagen-induced arthritis. *Eur. J. Immunol.* **2002**, *32*, 2944–2953. [CrossRef]

54. Nandakumar, K.S.; Holmdahl, R. Arthritis induced with cartilage-specific antibodiesis IL-4-dependent. *Eur. J. Immunol.* **2006**, *36*, 1608–1618. [CrossRef] [PubMed]

55. Johansson, A.C.; Hansson, A.S.; Nandakumar, K.S.; Bäcklund, J.; Holmdahl, R. IL-10-deficient B10.Q mice develop more severe collagen-induced arthritis, but are protected from arthritis induced with anti-type II collagen antibodies. *J. Immunol.* **2001**, *167*, 3505–3512. [CrossRef] [PubMed]

56. Hietala, M.A.; Nandakumar, K.S.; Person, L.; Fahlen, S.; Holmdahl, R.; Pekna, M. Complement activation by both classical and alternative pathways is critical for the effector phase of arthritis. *Mol. Immunol.* **2003**, *40*, 190. [CrossRef] [PubMed]

57. Banda, N.K.; Thurman, J.M.; Kraus, D.; Wood, A.; Carroll, M.C.; Arend, W.P.; Holers, V.M. Alternative complement pathway activation is essential for inflammation and joint destruction in the passive transfer model of collagen-induced arthritis. *J. Immunol.* **2006**, *177*, 1904–1912. [CrossRef] [PubMed]

58. Banda, N.K.; Levitt, B.; Glogowska, M.J.; Thurman, J.M.; Takahashi, K.; Stahl, G.L.; Tomlinson, S.; Arend, W.P.; Holers, V.M. Targeted inhibition of the complement alternative pathway with complement receptor 2 and factor H attenuates collagen antibody-induced arthritis in mice. *J. Immunol.* **2009**, *183*, 5928–5937. [CrossRef] [PubMed]

59. Banda, N.K.; Hyatt, S.; Antonioli, A.H.; White, J.T.; Glogowska, M.; Takahashi, K.; Merkel, T.J.; Stahl, G.L.; Mueller-Ortiz, S.; Wetsel, R.; et al. Role of C3a receptors, C5a receptors, and complement protein C6 deficiency in collagen antibody-induced arthritis in mice. *J. Immunol.* **2012**, *188*, 1469–1478. [CrossRef] [PubMed]

60. Banda, N.K.; Mehta, G.; Ferreira, V.P.; Cortes, C.; Pickering, M.C.; Pangburn, M.K.; Arend, W.P.; Holers, V.M. Essential role of surface-bound complement factor H in controlling immune complex-induced arthritis. *J. Immunol.* **2013**, *190*, 3560–3569. [CrossRef] [PubMed]

61. Banda, N.K.; Acharya, S.; Scheinman, R.I.; Mehta, G.; Takahashi, M.; Endo, Y.; Zhou, W.; Farrar, C.A.; Sacks, S.H.; Fujita, T.; et al. Deconstructing the Lectin Pathway in the Pathogenesis of Experimental Inflammatory Arthritis: Essential Role of the Lectin Ficolin B and Mannose-Binding Protein-Associated Serine Protease 2. *J. Immunol.* **2017**, *199*, 1835–1845. [CrossRef] [PubMed]

62. Gerard, C.; Gerard, N.P. C5A anaphylatoxin and its seven transmembrane-segment receptor. *Annu. Rev. Immunol.* **1994**, *12*, 775–808. [CrossRef] [PubMed]

63. Jose, P.J.; Moss, I.K.; Maini, R.N.; Williams, T.J. Measurement of the chemotactic complement fragment C5a in rheumatoid synovial fluids by radioimmunoassay: Role of C5a in the acute inflammatory phase. *Ann. Rheum. Dis.* **1990**, *49*, 747–752. [CrossRef] [PubMed]

64. Heller, T.; Hennecke, M.; Baumann, U.; Gessner, J.E.; zu Vilsendorf, A.M.; Baensch, M.; Boulay, F.; Kola, A.; Klos, A.; Bautsch, W.; et al. Selection of a C5a receptor antagonist from phage libraries attenuating the inflammatory response in immune complex disease and ischemia/reperfusion injury. *J. Immunol.* **1999**, *163*, 985–994. [PubMed]

65. Woodruff, T.M.; Nandakumar, K.S.; Tedesco, F. Inhibiting the C5-C5a receptor axis. *Mol. Immunol.* **2011**, *48*, 1631–1642. [CrossRef] [PubMed]

66. Nandakumar, K.S.; Jansson, Å.; Xu, B.; Rydell, N.; Blom, A.M. A Recombinant Vaccine Effectively Induces C5a-Specific Neutralizing Antibodies and Prevents Arthritis. *PLoS ONE* **2010**, *6*. [CrossRef] [PubMed]

67. Macor, P.; Durigutto, P.; De Maso, L.; Garrovo, C.; Biffi, S.; Cortini, A.; Fischetti, F.; Sblattero, D.; Pitzalis, C.; Marzari, R.; et al. Treatment of experimental arthritis by targeting synovial endothelium with a neutralizing recombinant antibody to C5. *Arthritis Rheum.* **2012**, *64*, 2559–2567. [CrossRef] [PubMed]

68. Shushakova, N.; Skokowa, J.; Schulman, J.; Baumann, U.; Zwirner, J.; Schmidt, R.E.; Gessner, J.E. C5a anaphylatoxin is a major regulator of activating versus inhibitory FcgammaRs in immune complex-induced lung disease. *J. Clin. Investig.* **2002**, *110*, 1823–1830. [CrossRef] [PubMed]

69. Kagari, T.; Tanaka, D.; Doi, H.; Shimozato, T. Essential role of Fc gamma receptors in anti-type II collagen antibody-induced arthritis. *J. Immunol.* **2003**, *170*, 4318–4324. [CrossRef] [PubMed]

70. Tan Sardjono, C.; Mottram, P.L.; van de Velde, N.C.; Powell, M.S.; Power, D.; Slocombe, R.F.; Wicks, I.P.; Campbell, I.K.; McKenzie, S.E.; Brooks, M.; et al. Development of spontaneous multisystem autoimmune disease and hypersensitivity to antibody-induced inflammation in Fcgamma receptor IIa-transgenic mice. *Arthritis Rheum.* **2005**, *52*, 3220–3229. [CrossRef] [PubMed]

71. Lee, C.-H.; Romain, G.; Yan, W.; Watanabe, M.; Charab, W.; Todorova, B.; Lee, J.; Triplett, K.; Donkor, M.; Lungu, O.I.; et al. IgG Fc domains that bind C1q but not effector Fcγ receptors delineate the importance of complement-mediated effector functions. *Nat. Immunol.* **2017**, *18*, 889–898. [CrossRef] [PubMed]

72. Quigg, R.J.; Lim, A.; Haas, M.; Alexander, J.J.; He, C.; Carroll, M.C. Immune complex glomerulonephritis in C4- and C3-deficient mice. *Kidney Int.* **1998**, *53*, 320–330. [CrossRef] [PubMed]

73. Hjelm, F.; Carlsson, F.; Getahun, A.; Heyman, B. Antibody-mediated regulation of the immune response. *Scand. J. Immunol.* **2006**, *64*, 177–184. [CrossRef] [PubMed]

74. Hawlisch, H.; Belkaid, Y.; Baelder, R.; Hildeman, D.; Gerard, C.; Köhl, J. C5a negatively regulates toll-like receptor 4-induced immune responses. *Immunity* **2005**, *22*, 415–426. [CrossRef] [PubMed]

75. Nandakumar, K.S.; Holmdahl, R. Antibody-induced arthritis: Disease mechanisms and genes involved at the effector phase of arthritis. *Arthritis Res. Ther.* **2006**, *8*, 223. [CrossRef] [PubMed]

76. Rowley, M.J.; Nandakumar, K.S.; Holmdahl, R. The role of collagen antibodies in mediating arthritis. *Mod. Rheumatol.* **2008**, *18*, 429–441. [CrossRef] [PubMed]

77. Nandakumar, K.S. Pathogenic antibody recognition of cartilage. *Cell Tissue Res.* **2010**, *339*, 213–220. [CrossRef] [PubMed]

78. Nandakumar, K.S.; Holmdahl, R. Therapeutic cleavage of IgG: New avenues for treating inflammation. *Trends Immunol.* **2008**, *29*, 173–178. [CrossRef] [PubMed]

79. Amirahmadi, S.F.; Pho, M.H.; Gray, R.E.; Crombie, D.E.; Whittingham, S.F.; Zuasti, B.B.; van Damme, M.-P.; Rowley, M.J. An arthritogenic monoclonal antibody to type II collagen, CII-C1, impairs cartilage formation by cultured chondrocytes. *Immunol. Cell Biol.* **2004**, *82*, 427–434. [CrossRef] [PubMed]

80. Gray, R.E.; Seng, N.; Mackay, I.R.; Rowley, M.J. Measurement of antibodies to collagen II by inhibition of collagen fibril formation in vitro. *J. Immunol. Methods* **2004**, *285*, 55–61. [CrossRef] [PubMed]

81. Amirahmadi, S.F.; Whittingham, S.; Crombie, D.E.; Nandakumar, K.S.; Holmdahl, R.; Mackay, I.R.; van Damme, M.-P.; Rowley, M.J. Arthritogenic anti-type II collagen antibodies are pathogenic for cartilage-derived chondrocytes independent of inflammatory cells. *Arthritis Rheum.* **2005**, *52*, 1897–1906. [CrossRef] [PubMed]

82. Crombie, D.E.; Turer, M.; Zuasti, B.B.; Wood, B.; McNaughton, D.; Nandakumar, K.S.; Holmdahl, R.; van Damme, M.-P.; Rowley, M.J. Destructive effects of murine arthritogenic antibodies to type II collagen on cartilage explants in vitro. *Arthritis Res. Ther.* **2005**, *7*, R927–R937. [CrossRef] [PubMed]

83. Croxford, A.M.; Nandakumar, K.S.; Holmdahl, R.; Tobin, M.J.; McNaughton, D.; Rowley, M.J. Chemical changes demonstrated in cartilage by synchrotron infrared microspectroscopy in an antibody-induced murine model of rheumatoid arthritis. *J. Biomed. Opt.* **2011**, *16*, 066004. [CrossRef] [PubMed]

84. Croxford, A.M.; Whittingham, S.; McNaughton, D.; Nandakumar, K.S.; Holmdahl, R.; Rowley, M.J. Type II collagen–specific antibodies induce cartilage damage in mice independent of inflammation. *Arthritis Rheum.* **2013**, *65*, 650–659. [CrossRef] [PubMed]

85. Nandakumar, K.S.; Bajtner, E.; Hill, L.; Böhm, B.; Rowley, M.J.; Burkhardt, H.; Holmdahl, R. Arthritogenic antibodies specific for a major type II collagen triple-helical epitope bind and destabilize cartilage independent of inflammation. *Arthritis Rheum.* **2008**, *58*, 184–196. [CrossRef] [PubMed]

86. Hagert, C.; Sareila, O.; Kelkka, T.; Nandakumar, K.S.; Collin, M.; Xu, B.; Guerard, S.; Bäcklund, J.; Jalkanen, S.; Holmdahl, R. Chronic active arthritis driven by macrophages without involvement of T cells. *Arthritis Rheum.* **2002**, *4* (Suppl. 3), S197–S211.

87. Mörgelin, M.; Heinegård, D.; Engel, J.; Paulsson, M. Electron microscopy of native cartilage oligomeric matrix protein purified from the Swarm rat chondrosarcoma reveals a five-armed structure. *J. Biol. Chem.* **1992**, *267*, 6137–6141. [PubMed]

88. Oldberg, A.; Antonsson, P.; Lindblom, K.; Heinegård, D. COMP (cartilage oligomeric matrix protein) is structurally related to the thrombospondins. *J. Biol. Chem.* **1992**, *267*, 22346–22350. [PubMed]

89. Carlsén, S.; Hansson, A.S.; Olsson, H.; Heinegård, D.; Holmdahl, R. Cartilage oligomeric matrix protein (COMP)-induced arthritis in rats. *Clin. Exp. Immunol.* **1998**, *114*, 477–484. [CrossRef] [PubMed]

90. Carlsen, S.; Nandakumar, K.S.; Bäcklund, J.; Holmberg, J.; Hultqvist, M.; Vestberg, M.; Holmdahl, R. Cartilage oligomeric matrix protein induction of chronic arthritis in mice. *Arthritis Rheum.* **2008**, *58*, 2000–2011. [CrossRef] [PubMed]

91. Geng, H.; Nandakumar, K.S.; Pramhed, A.; Aspberg, A.; Mattsson, R.; Holmdahl, R. Cartilage oligomeric matrix protein specific antibodies are pathogenic. *Arthritis Res. Ther.* **2012**, *14*, R191. [CrossRef] [PubMed]

92. Kouskoff, V.; Korganow, A.S.; Duchatelle, V.; Degott, C.; Benoist, C.; Mathis, D. Organ-specific disease provoked by systemic autoimmunity. *Cell* **1996**, *87*, 811–822. [CrossRef]

93. Matsumoto, I.; Staub, A.; Benoist, C.; Mathis, D. Arthritis provoked by linked T and B cell recognition of a glycolytic enzyme. *Science* **1999**, *286*, 1732–1735. [CrossRef] [PubMed]

94. Basu, D.; Horvath, S.; Matsumoto, I.; Fremont, D.H.; Allen, P.M. Molecular basis for recognition of an arthritic peptide and a foreign epitope on distinct MHC molecules by a single TCR. *J. Immunol.* **2000**, *164*, 5788–5796. [CrossRef] [PubMed]

95. Schubert, D.; Maier, B.; Morawietz, L.; Krenn, V.; Kamradt, T. Immunization with glucose-6-phosphate isomerase induces T cell-dependent peripheral polyarthritis in genetically unaltered mice. *J. Immunol.* **2004**, *172*, 4503–4509. [CrossRef] [PubMed]

96. Iwanami, K.; Matsumoto, I.; Tanaka, Y.; Inoue, A.; Goto, D.; Ito, S.; Tsutsumi, A.; Sumida, T. Arthritogenic T cell epitope in glucose-6-phosphate isomerase-induced arthritis. *Arthritis Res. Ther.* **2008**, *10*, R130. [CrossRef] [PubMed]

97. Korganow, A.S.; Ji, H.; Mangialaio, S.; Duchatelle, V.; Pelanda, R.; Martin, T.; Degott, C.; Kikutani, H.; Rajewsky, K.; Pasquali, J.L.; et al. From systemic T cell self-reactivity to organ-specific autoimmune disease via immunoglobulins. *Immunity* **1999**, *10*, 451–461. [CrossRef]

98. Maccioni, M.; Zeder-Lutz, G.; Huang, H.; Ebel, C.; Gerber, P.; Hergueux, J.; Marchal, P.; Duchatelle, V.; Degott, C.; van Regenmortel, M.; et al. Arthritogenic monoclonal antibodies from K/BxN mice. *J. Exp. Med.* **2002**, *195*, 1071–1077. [CrossRef] [PubMed]

99. Wipke, B.T.; Wang, Z.; Kim, J.; McCarthy, T.J.; Allen, P.M. Dynamic visualization of a joint-specific autoimmune response through positron emission tomography. *Nat. Immunol.* **2002**, *3*, 366–372. [CrossRef] [PubMed]

100. Wipke, B.T.; Wang, Z.; Nagengast, W.; Reichert, D.E.; Allen, P.M. Staging the initiation of autoantibody-induced arthritis: A critical role for immune complexes. *J. Immunol.* **2004**, *172*, 7694–7702. [CrossRef] [PubMed]

101. Binstadt, B.A.; Patel, P.R.; Alencar, H.; Nigrovic, P.A.; Lee, D.M.; Mahmood, U.; Weissleder, R.; Mathis, D.; Benoist, C. Particularities of the vasculature can promote the organ specificity of autoimmune attack. *Nat. Immunol.* **2006**, *7*, 284–292. [CrossRef] [PubMed]

102. Lee, D.M.; Friend, D.S.; Gurish, M.F.; Benoist, C.; Mathis, D.; Brenner, M.B. Mast cells: A cellular link between autoantibodies and inflammatory arthritis. *Science* **2002**, *297*, 1689–1692. [CrossRef] [PubMed]

103. Wipke, B.T.; Allen, P.M. Essential role of neutrophils in the initiation and progression of a murine model of rheumatoid arthritis. *J. Immunol.* **2001**, *167*, 1601–1608. [CrossRef] [PubMed]

104. Jacobs, J.P.; Wu, H.-J.; Benoist, C.; Mathis, D. IL-17-producing T cells can augment autoantibody-induced arthritis. *Proc. Natl. Acad. Sci. USA* **2009**, *106*, 21789–21794. [CrossRef] [PubMed]

105. Monach, P.A.; Nigrovic, P.A.; Chen, M.; Hock, H.; Lee, D.M.; Benoist, C.; Mathis, D. Neutrophils in a mouse model of autoantibody-mediated arthritis: Critical producers of Fc receptor gamma, the receptor for C5a, and lymphocyte function-associated antigen 1. *Arthritis Rheum.* **2010**, *62*, 753–764. [CrossRef] [PubMed]

106. Wu, H.-J.; Sawaya, H.; Binstadt, B.; Brickelmaier, M.; Blasius, A.; Gorelik, L.; Mahmood, U.; Weissleder, R.; Carulli, J.; Benoist, C.; et al. Inflammatory arthritis can be reined in by CpG-induced DC-NK cell cross talk. *J. Exp. Med.* **2007**, *204*, 1911–1922. [CrossRef] [PubMed]

107. Bruhns, P.; Samuelsson, A.; Pollard, J.W.; Ravetch, J.V. Colony-stimulating factor-1-dependent macrophages are responsible for IVIG protection in antibody-induced autoimmune disease. *Immunity* **2003**, *18*, 573–581. [CrossRef]

108. Solomon, S.; Rajasekaran, N.; Jeisy-Walder, E.; Snapper, S.B.; Illges, H. A crucial role for macrophages in the pathology of K/B x N serum-induced arthritis. *Eur. J. Immunol.* **2005**, *35*, 3064–3073. [CrossRef] [PubMed]

109. Corr, M.; Crain, B. The role of FcgammaR signaling in the K/B x N serum transfer model of arthritis. *J. Immunol.* **2002**, *169*, 6604–6609. [CrossRef] [PubMed]

110. Nigrovic, P.A.; Binstadt, B.A.; Monach, P.A.; Johnsen, A.; Gurish, M.; Iwakura, Y.; Benoist, C.; Mathis, D.; Lee, D.M. Mast cells contribute to initiation of autoantibody-mediated arthritis via IL-1. *Proc. Natl. Acad. Sci. USA* **2007**, *104*, 2325–2330. [CrossRef] [PubMed]

111. Ji, H.; Pettit, A.; Ohmura, K.; Ortiz-Lopez, A.; Duchatelle, V.; Degott, C.; Gravallese, E.; Mathis, D.; Benoist, C. Critical roles for interleukin 1 and tumor necrosis factor alpha in antibody-induced arthritis. *J. Exp. Med.* **2002**, *196*, 77–85. [CrossRef] [PubMed]

112. Choe, J.-Y.; Crain, B.; Wu, S.R.; Corr, M. Interleukin 1 receptor dependence of serum transferred arthritis can be circumvented by toll-like receptor 4 signaling. *J. Exp. Med.* **2003**, *197*, 537–542. [CrossRef] [PubMed]

113. Ji, H.; Ohmura, K.; Mahmood, U.; Lee, D.M.; Hofhuis, F.M.A.; Boackle, S.A.; Takahashi, K.; Holers, V.M.; Walport, M.; Gerard, C.; et al. Arthritis critically dependent on innate immune system players. *Immunity* **2002**, *16*, 157–168. [CrossRef]

114. Ohmura, K.; Nguyen, L.T.; Locksley, R.M.; Mathis, D.; Benoist, C. Interleukin-4 can be a key positive regulator of inflammatory arthritis. *Arthritis Rheum.* **2005**, *52*, 1866–1875. [CrossRef] [PubMed]

115. Ohmura, K.; Johnsen, A.; Ortiz-Lopez, A.; Desany, P.; Roy, M.; Besse, W.; Rogus, J.; Bogue, M.; Puech, A.; Lathrop, M.; et al. Variation in IL-1beta gene expression is a major determinant of genetic differences in arthritis aggressivity in mice. *Proc. Natl. Acad. Sci. USA* **2005**, *102*, 12489–12494. [CrossRef] [PubMed]

116. Akilesh, S.; Petkova, S.; Sproule, T.J.; Shaffer, D.J.; Christianson, G.J.; Roopenian, D. The MHC class I-like Fc receptor promotes humorally mediated autoimmune disease. *J. Clin. Investig.* **2004**, *113*, 1328–1333. [PubMed]

117. Kim, H.Y.; Kim, H.J.; Min, H.S.; Kim, S.; Park, W.S.; Park, S.H.; Chung, D.H. NKT cells promote antibody-induced joint inflammation by suppressing transforming growth factor beta1 production. *J. Exp. Med.* **2005**, *201*, 41–47. [CrossRef] [PubMed]

118. Siragam, V.; Brinc, D.; Crow, A.R.; Song, S.; Freedman, J.; Lazarus, A.H. Can antibodies with specificity for soluble antigens mimic the therapeutic effects of intravenous IgG in the treatment of autoimmune disease? *J. Clin. Investig.* **2005**, *115*, 155–160. [CrossRef] [PubMed]

119. Van Lent, P.L.; van den Bersselaar, L.A.; van den Hoek, A.E.; van de Loo, A.A.; van den Berg, W.B. Cationic immune complex arthritis in mice—A new model. Synergistic effect of complement and interleukin-1. *Am. J. Pathol.* **1992**, *140*, 1451–1461. [PubMed]

120. Van Lent, P.L.; van den Hoek, A.E.; van den Bersselaar, L.A.; Spanjaards, M.F.; Van Rooijen, N.; Dijkstra, C.D.; Van de Putte, L.B.; van den Berg, W.B. In vivo role of phagocytic synovial lining cells in onset of experimental arthritis. *Am. J. Pathol.* **1993**, *143*, 1226–1237. [PubMed]

121. Nabbe, K.C.A.M.; Blom, A.B.; Holthuysen, A.E.M.; Boross, P.; Roth, J.; Verbeek, S.; van Lent, P.L.E.M.; van den Berg, W.B. Coordinate expression of activating Fc gamma receptors I and III and inhibiting Fc gamma receptor type II in the determination of joint inflammation and cartilage destruction during immune complex-mediated arthritis. *Arthritis Rheum.* **2003**, *48*, 255–265. [CrossRef] [PubMed]

122. Nabbe, K.C.A.M.; Boross, P.; Holthuysen, A.E.M.; Sloëtjes, A.W.; Kolls, J.K.; Verbeek, S.; van Lent, P.L.E.M.; van den Berg, W.B. Joint inflammation and chondrocyte death become independent of Fcgamma receptor type III by local overexpression of interferon-gamma during immune complex-mediated arthritis. *Arthritis Rheum.* **2005**, *52*, 967–974. [CrossRef] [PubMed]

123. Nabbe, K.C.; van Lent, P.L.; Holthuysen, A.E.; Kolls, J.K.; Verbeek, S.; van den Berg, W.B. FcgammaRI up-regulation induced by local adenoviral-mediated interferon-gamma production aggravates chondrocyte death during immune complex-mediated arthritis. *Am. J. Pathol.* **2003**, *163*, 743–752. [CrossRef]

124. Van Lent, P.L.; Licht, R.; Dijkman, H.; Holthuysen, A.E.; Berden, J.H.; van den Berg, W.B. Uptake of apoptotic leukocytes by synovial lining macrophages inhibits immune complex-mediated arthritis. *J. Leukoc. Biol.* **2001**, *70*, 708–714. [PubMed]

125. Burska, A.N.; Hunt, L.; Boissinot, M.; Strollo, R.; Ryan, B.J.; Vital, E.; Nissim, A.; Winyard, P.G.; Emery, P.; Ponchel, F. Autoantibodies to posttranslational modifications in rheumatoid arthritis. *Mediat. Inflamm.* **2014**, *2014*, 492873. [CrossRef] [PubMed]

126. Van Gaalen, F.A.; Linn-Rasker, S.P.; van Venrooij, W.J.; de Jong, B.A.; Breedveld, F.C.; Verweij, C.L.; Toes, R.E.M.; Huizinga, T.W.J. Autoantibodies to cyclic citrullinated peptides predict progression to rheumatoid arthritis in patients with undifferentiated arthritis: A prospective cohort study. *Arthritis Rheum.* **2004**, *50*, 709–715. [CrossRef] [PubMed]

127. Aletaha, D.; Neogi, T.; Silman, A.J.; Funovits, J.; Felson, D.T.; Bingham, C.O.; Birnbaum, N.S.; Burmester, G.R.; Bykerk, V.P.; Cohen, M.D.; et al. 2010 Rheumatoid arthritis classification criteria: An American College of Rheumatology/European League Against Rheumatism collaborative initiative. *Arthritis Rheum.* **2010**, *62*, 2569–2581. [CrossRef] [PubMed]

128. McInnes, I.B.; Schett, G. The pathogenesis of rheumatoid arthritis. *N. Engl. J. Med.* **2011**, *365*, 2205–2219. [CrossRef] [PubMed]

129. Malmström, V.; Catrina, A.I.; Klareskog, L. The immunopathogenesis of seropositive rheumatoid arthritis: From triggering to targeting. *Nat. Rev. Immunol.* **2017**, *17*, 60–75. [CrossRef] [PubMed]

130. Van der Woude, D.; Rantapää-Dahlqvist, S.; Ioan-Facsinay, A.; Onnekink, C.; Schwarte, C.M.; Verpoort, K.N.; Drijfhout, J.W.; Huizinga, T.W.J.; Toes, R.E.M.; Pruijn, G.J.M. Epitope spreading of the anti-citrullinated protein antibody response occurs before disease onset and is associated with the disease course of early arthritis. *Ann. Rheum. Dis.* **2010**, *69*, 1554–1561. [CrossRef] [PubMed]

131. Suwannalai, P.; van de Stadt, L.A.; Radner, H.; Steiner, G.; El-Gabalawy, H.S.; Zijde, C.M.J.-V.D.; van Tol, M.J.; van Schaardenburg, D.; Huizinga, T.W.J.; Toes, R.E.M.; et al. Avidity maturation of anti-citrullinated protein antibodies in rheumatoid arthritis. *Arthritis Rheum.* **2012**, *64*, 1323–1328. [CrossRef] [PubMed]

132. Rombouts, Y.; Ewing, E.; van de Stadt, L.A.; Selman, M.H.J.; Trouw, L.A.; Deelder, A.M.; Huizinga, T.W.J.; Wuhrer, M.; van Schaardenburg, D.; Toes, R.E.M.; et al. Anti-citrullinated protein antibodies acquire a pro-inflammatory Fc glycosylation phenotype prior to the onset of rheumatoid arthritis. *Ann. Rheum. Dis.* **2015**, *74*, 234–241. [CrossRef] [PubMed]

133. Harre, U.; Georgess, D.; Bang, H.; Bozec, A.; Axmann, R.; Ossipova, E.; Jakobsson, P.-J.; Baum, W.; Nimmerjahn, F.; Szarka, E.; et al. Induction of osteoclastogenesis and bone loss by human autoantibodies against citrullinated vimentin. *J. Clin. Investig.* **2012**, *122*, 1791–1802. [CrossRef] [PubMed]

134. Kleyer, A.; Finzel, S.; Rech, J.; Manger, B.; Krieter, M.; Faustini, F.; Araujo, E.; Hueber, A.J.; Harre, U.; Engelke, K.; et al. Bone loss before the clinical onset of rheumatoid arthritis in subjects with anticitrullinated protein antibodies. *Ann. Rheum. Dis.* **2014**, *73*, 854–860. [CrossRef] [PubMed]

135. Harre, U.; Lang, S.C.; Pfeifle, R.; Rombouts, Y.; Frühbeißer, S.; Amara, K.; Bang, H.; Lux, A.; Koeleman, C.A.; Baum, W.; et al. Glycosylation of immunoglobulin G determines osteoclast differentiation and bone loss. *Nat. Commun.* **2015**, *6*, 6651. [CrossRef] [PubMed]

136. Seeling, M.; Hillenhoff, U.; David, J.P.; Schett, G.; Tuckermann, J.; Lux, A.; Nimmerjahn, F. Inflammatory monocytes and Fcγ receptor IV on osteoclasts are critical for bone destruction during inflammatory arthritis in mice. *Proc. Natl. Acad. Sci. USA* **2013**, *110*, 10729–10734. [CrossRef] [PubMed]

137. Krishnamurthy, A.; Joshua, V.; Haj Hensvold, A.; Jin, T.; Sun, M.; Vivar, N.; Ytterberg, A.J.; Engström, M.; Fernandes-Cerqueira, C.; Amara, K.; et al. Identification of a novel chemokine-dependent molecular mechanism underlying rheumatoid arthritis-associated autoantibody-mediated bone loss. *Ann. Rheum. Dis.* **2016**, *75*, 721–729. [CrossRef] [PubMed]

138. Wigerblad, G.; Bas, D.B.; Fernades-Cerqueira, C.; Krishnamurthy, A.; Nandakumar, K.S.; Rogoz, K.; Kato, J.; Sandor, K.; Su, J.; Jimenez-Andrade, J.M.; et al. Autoantibodies to citrullinated proteins induce joint pain independent of inflammation via a chemokine-dependent mechanism. *Ann. Rheum. Dis.* **2016**, *75*, 730–738. [CrossRef] [PubMed]

139. Catrina, A.I.; Svensson, C.I.; Malmström, V.; Schett, G.; Klareskog, L. Mechanisms leading from systemic autoimmunity to joint-specific disease in rheumatoid arthritis. *Nat. Rev. Rheumatol.* **2017**, *13*, 79–86. [CrossRef] [PubMed]

140. Trouw, L.A.; Haisma, E.M.; Levarht, E.W.N.; van der Woude, D.; Ioan-Facsinay, A.; Daha, M.R.; Huizinga, T.W.J.; Toes, R.E. Anti-cyclic citrullinated peptide antibodies from rheumatoid arthritis patients activate complement via both the classical and alternative pathways. *Arthritis Rheum.* **2009**, *60*, 1923–1931. [CrossRef] [PubMed]

141. Habets, K.L.L.; Trouw, L.A.; Levarht, E.W.N.; Korporaal, S.J.A.; Habets, P.A.M.; de Groot, P.; Huizinga, T.W.J.; Toes, R.E.M. Anti-citrullinated protein antibodies contribute to platelet activation in rheumatoid arthritis. *Arthritis Res. Ther.* **2015**, *17*, 209. [CrossRef] [PubMed]

142. Uysal, H.; Bockermann, R.; Nandakumar, K.S.; Sehnert, B.; Bajtner, E.; Engström, A.; Serre, G.; Burkhardt, H.; Thunnissen, M.M.G.M.; Holmdahl, R. Structure and pathogenicity of antibodies specific for citrullinated collagen type II in experimental arthritis. *J. Exp. Med.* **2009**, *206*, 449–462. [CrossRef] [PubMed]

143. Uysal, H.; Nandakumar, K.S.; Kessel, C.; Haag, S.; Carlsen, S.; Burkhardt, H.; Holmdahl, R. Antibodies to citrullinated proteins: Molecular interactions and arthritogenicity. *Immunol. Rev.* **2010**, *233*, 9–33. [CrossRef] [PubMed]

144. Klareskog, L.; Rönnelid, J.; Lundberg, K.; Padyukov, L.; Alfredsson, L. Immunity to citrullinated proteins in rheumatoid arthritis. *Annu. Rev. Immunol.* **2008**, *26*, 651–675. [CrossRef] [PubMed]

145. Goebel, A. Autoantibody pain. *Autoimmun. Rev.* **2016**, *15*, 552–557. [CrossRef] [PubMed]

146. Agalave, N.M.; Larsson, M.; Abdelmoaty, S.; Su, J.; Baharpoor, A.; Lundbäck, P.; Palmblad, K.; Andersson, U.; Harris, H.; Svensson, C.I. Spinal HMGB1 induces TLR4-mediated long-lasting hypersensitivity and glial activation and regulates pain-like behavior in experimental arthritis. *Pain* **2014**, *155*, 1802–1813. [CrossRef] [PubMed]

147. Christianson, C.A.; Corr, M.; Firestein, G.S.; Mobargha, A.; Yaksh, T.L.; Svensson, C.I. Characterization of the acute and persistent pain state present in K/BxN serum transfer arthritis. *Pain* **2010**, *151*, 394–403. [CrossRef] [PubMed]

148. Bas, D.B.; Su, J.; Sandor, K.; Agalave, N.M.; Lundberg, J.; Codeluppi, S.; Baharpoor, A.; Nandakumar, K.S.; Holmdahl, R.; Svensson, C.I. Collagen antibody-induced arthritis evokes persistent pain with spinal glial involvement and transient prostaglandin dependency. *Arthritis Rheum.* **2012**, *64*, 3886–3896. [CrossRef] [PubMed]

149. Burkhardt, H.; Koller, T.; Engström, A.; Nandakumar, K.S.; Turnay, J.; Kraetsch, H.G.; Kalden, J.R.; Holmdahl, R. Epitope-specific recognition of type II collagen by rheumatoid arthritis antibodies is shared with recognition by antibodies that are arthritogenic in collagen-induced arthritis in the mouse. *Arthritis Rheum.* **2002**, *46*, 2339–2348. [CrossRef] [PubMed]

150. Croxford, A.M.; Crombie, D.; McNaughton, D.; Holmdahl, R.; Nandakumar, K.S.; Rowley, M.J. Specific antibody protection of the extracellular cartilage matrix against collagen antibody-induced damage. *Arthritis Rheum.* **2010**, *62*, 3374–3384. [CrossRef] [PubMed]

151. Van de Stadt, L.A.; van Schouwenburg, P.A.; Bryde, S.; Kruithof, S.; van Schaardenburg, D.; Hamann, D.; Wolbink, G.; Rispens, T. Monoclonal anti-citrullinated protein antibodies selected on citrullinated fibrinogen have distinct targets with different cross-reactivity patterns. *Rheumatology* **2013**, *52*, 631–635. [CrossRef] [PubMed]

152. Ge, C.; Xu, B.; liang, B.; Nandakumar, K.S.; Tong, D.; Lundqvist, C.; Urbonaviciute, V.; Lönnblom, E.; Ayoglu, B.; Nilsson, P.; et al. Autoantibodies specific for a citrulline side chain protect against arthritis. *Ann. Rheum. Dis.* **2018**. in review.

153. Durigutto, P.; Macor, P.; Ziller, F.; De Maso, L.; Fischetti, F.; Marzari, R.; Sblattero, D.; Tedesco, F. Prevention of arthritis by locally synthesized recombinant antibody neutralizing complement component C5. *PLoS ONE* **2013**, *8*, e58696. [CrossRef] [PubMed]

154. Nandakumar, K.S.; Jansson, A.; Xu, B.; Rydell, N.; Ahooghalandari, P.; Hellman, L.; Blom, A.M.; Holmdahl, R. A recombinant vaccine effectively induces c5a-specific neutralizing antibodies and prevents arthritis. *PLoS ONE* **2010**, *5*, e13511. [CrossRef] [PubMed]

155. Mehta, G.; Scheinman, R.I.; Holers, V.M.; Banda, N.K. A New Approach for the Treatment of Arthritis in Mice with a Novel Conjugate of an Anti-C5aR1 Antibody and C5 Small Interfering RNA. *J. Immunol.* **2015**, *194*, 5446–5454. [CrossRef] [PubMed]

156. Nimmerjahn, F.; Ravetch, J.V. Fcgamma receptors as regulators of immune responses. *Nat. Rev. Immunol.* **2008**, *8*, 34–47. [CrossRef] [PubMed]

157. Zhu, G.; Xu, Y.; Cen, X.; Nandakumar, K.S.; Liu, S.; Cheng, K. Targeting pattern-recognition receptors to discover new small molecule immune modulators. *Eur. J. Med. Chem.* **2018**, *144*, 82–92. [CrossRef] [PubMed]

158. Son, D.J.; Kim, D.H.; Nah, S.-S.; Park, M.H.; Lee, H.P.; Han, S.B.; Venkatareddy, U.; Gann, B.; Rodriguez, K.; Burt, S.R.; et al. Novel synthetic (E)-2-methoxy-4-(3-(4-methoxyphenyl) prop-1-en-1-yl) phenol inhibits arthritis by targeting signal transducer and activator of transcription 3. *Sci. Rep.* **2016**, *6*, 36852. [CrossRef] [PubMed]

159. Ahmad, S.F.; Ansari, M.A.; Nadeem, A.; Zoheir, K.M.A.; Bakheet, S.A.; Alsaad, A.M.S.; Al-Shabanah, O.A.; Attia, S.M. STA-21, a STAT-3 inhibitor, attenuates the development and progression of inflammation in collagen antibody-induced arthritis. *Immunobiology* **2017**, *222*, 206–217. [CrossRef] [PubMed]

160. Hultqvist, M.; Nandakumar, K.S.; Björklund, U.; Holmdahl, R. The novel small molecule drug Rabeximod is effective in reducing disease severity of mouse models of autoimmune disorders. *Ann. Rheum. Dis.* **2009**, *68*, 130–135. [CrossRef] [PubMed]

161. Hultqvist, M.; Nandakumar, K.S.; Björklund, U.; Holmdahl, R. Rabeximod reduces arthritis severity in mice by decreasing activation of inflammatory cells. *Ann. Rheum. Dis.* **2010**, *69*, 1527–1532. [CrossRef] [PubMed]

162. Sim, J.H.; Lee, W.K.; Lee, Y.S.; Kang, J.S. Assessment of collagen antibody-induced arthritis in BALB/c mice using bioimaging analysis and histopathological examination. *Lab. Anim. Res.* **2016**, *32*, 135–143. [CrossRef] [PubMed]

163. Arnold, J.N.; Wormald, M.R.; Sim, R.B.; Rudd, P.M.; Dwek, R.A. The impact of glycosylation on the biological function and structure of human immunoglobulins. *Annu. Rev. Immunol.* **2007**, *25*, 21–50. [CrossRef] [PubMed]

164. Jefferis, R.; Lund, J.; Pound, J.D. IgG-Fc-mediated effector functions: Molecular definition of interaction sites for effector ligands and the role of glycosylation. *Immunol. Rev.* **1998**, *163*, 59–76. [CrossRef] [PubMed]

165. Ferrara, C.; Grau, S.; Jäger, C.; Sondermann, P.; Brünker, P.; Waldhauer, I.; Hennig, M.; Ruf, A.; Rufer, A.C.; Stihle, M.; et al. Unique carbohydrate-carbohydrate interactions are required for high affinity binding between FcgammaRIII and antibodies lacking core fucose. *Proc. Natl. Acad. Sci. USA* **2011**, *108*, 12669–12674. [CrossRef] [PubMed]

166. Jennewein, M.F.; Alter, G. The Immunoregulatory Roles of Antibody Glycosylation. *Trends Immunol.* **2017**, *38*, 358–372. [CrossRef] [PubMed]

167. Mössner, E.; Brünker, P.; Moser, S.; Püntener, U.; Schmidt, C.; Herter, S.; Grau, R.; Gerdes, C.; Nopora, A.; van Puijenbroek, E.; et al. Increasing the efficacy of CD20 antibody therapy through the engineering of a new type II anti-CD20 antibody with enhanced direct and immune effector cell-mediated B-cell cytotoxicity. *Blood* **2010**, *115*, 4393–4402. [CrossRef] [PubMed]

168. Kaneko, Y.; Nimmerjahn, F.; Ravetch, J.V. Anti-inflammatory activity of immunoglobulin G resulting from Fc sialylation. *Science* **2006**, *313*, 670–673. [CrossRef] [PubMed]

169. Nimmerjahn, F.; Ravetch, J.V. The antiinflammatory activity of IgG: The intravenous IgG paradox. *J. Exp. Med.* **2007**, *204*, 11–15. [CrossRef] [PubMed]

170. Schwab, I.; Nimmerjahn, F. Intravenous immunoglobulin therapy: How does IgG modulate the immune system? *Nat. Rev. Immunol.* **2013**, *13*, 176–189. [CrossRef] [PubMed]

171. Anthony, R.M.; Nimmerjahn, F.; Ashline, D.J.; Reinhold, V.N.; Paulson, J.C.; Ravetch, J.V. Recapitulation of IVIG anti-inflammatory activity with a recombinant IgG Fc. *Science* **2008**, *320*, 373–376. [CrossRef] [PubMed]

172. Anthony, R.M.; Wermeling, F.; Karlsson, M.C.I.; Ravetch, J.V. Identification of a receptor required for the anti-inflammatory activity of IVIG. *Proc. Natl. Acad. Sci. USA* **2008**, *105*, 19571–19578. [CrossRef] [PubMed]

173. Nimmerjahn, F.; Ravetch, J.V. Anti-inflammatory actions of intravenous immunoglobulin. *Annu. Rev. Immunol.* **2008**, *26*, 513–533. [CrossRef] [PubMed]

174. Anthony, R.M.; Ravetch, J.V. A novel role for the IgG Fc glycan: The anti-inflammatory activity of sialylated IgG Fcs. *J. Clin. Immunol.* **2010**, *30* (Suppl. 1), S9–S14. [CrossRef] [PubMed]

175. Anthony, R.M.; Kobayashi, T.; Wermeling, F.; Ravetch, J.V. Intravenous gammaglobulin suppresses inflammation through a novel T(H)2 pathway. *Nature* **2011**, *475*, 110–113. [CrossRef] [PubMed]

176. Wermeling, F.; Anthony, R.M.; Brombacher, F.; Ravetch, J.V. Acute inflammation primes myeloid effector cells for anti-inflammatory STAT6 signaling. *Proc. Natl. Acad. Sci. USA* **2013**, *110*, 13487–13491. [CrossRef] [PubMed]

177. Ohmi, Y.; Ise, W.; Harazono, A.; Takakura, D.; Fukuyama, H.; Baba, Y.; Narazaki, M.; Shoda, H.; Takahashi, N.; Ohkawa, Y.; et al. Sialylation converts arthritogenic IgG into inhibitors of collagen-induced arthritis. *Nat. Commun.* **2016**, *7*, 11205. [CrossRef] [PubMed]

178. Cymer, F.; Beck, H.; Rohde, A.; Reusch, D. Therapeutic monoclonal antibody *N*-glycosylation—Structure, function and therapeutic potential. *Biologicals* **2017**, in press. [CrossRef] [PubMed]

179. Collin, M.; Olsén, A. EndoS, a novel secreted protein from Streptococcus pyogenes with endoglycosidase activity on human IgG. *EMBO J.* **2001**, *20*, 3046–3055. [CrossRef] [PubMed]

180. Nandakumar, K.S.; Collin, M.; Olsén, A.; Nimmerjahn, F.; Blom, A.M.; Ravetch, J.V.; Holmdahl, R. Endoglycosidase treatment abrogates IgG arthritogenicity: Importance of IgG glycosylation in arthritis. *Eur. J. Immunol.* **2007**, *37*, 2973–2982. [CrossRef] [PubMed]

181. Albert, H.; Collin, M.; Dudziak, D.; Ravetch, J.V.; Nimmerjahn, F. In vivo enzymatic modulation of IgG glycosylation inhibits autoimmune disease in an IgG subclass-dependent manner. *Proc. Natl. Acad. Sci. USA* **2008**, *105*, 15005–15009. [CrossRef] [PubMed]

182. Collin, M.; Björck, L. Toward Clinical use of the IgG Specific Enzymes IdeS and EndoS against Antibody-Mediated Diseases. *Methods Mol. Biol.* **2017**, *1535*, 339–351. [PubMed]

183. Nandakumar, K.S.; Collin, M.; Happonen, K.E.; Lundstrom, S.L.; Croxford, A.M.; Xu, B.; Zubarev, R.A.; Rowley, M.J.; Blom, A.M.; Kjellman, C.; et al. Streptococcal endo-β-N-acetylglucosaminidase within IgG immune complexes potently suppress inflammation in vivo. *Front. Immunol.* In review.

184. Collin, M.; Shannon, O.; Björck, L. IgG glycan hydrolysis by a bacterial enzyme as a therapy against autoimmune conditions. *Proc. Natl. Acad. Sci. USA* **2008**, *105*, 4265–4270. [CrossRef] [PubMed]

185. Van Timmeren, M.M.; van der Veen, B.S.; Stegeman, C.A.; Petersen, A.H.; Hellmark, T.; Collin, M.; Heeringa, P. IgG glycan hydrolysis attenuates ANCA-mediated glomerulonephritis. *J. Am. Soc. Nephrol.* **2010**, *21*, 1103–1114. [CrossRef] [PubMed]

186. Yang, R.; Otten, M.A.; Hellmark, T.; Collin, M.; Björck, L.; Zhao, M.-H.; Daha, M.R.; Segelmark, M. Successful treatment of experimental glomerulonephritis with IdeS and EndoS, IgG-degrading streptococcal enzymes. *Nephrol. Dial. Transplant.* **2010**, *25*, 2479–2486. [CrossRef] [PubMed]

187. Benkhoucha, M.; Molnarfi, N.; Santiago-Raber, M.-L.; Weber, M.S.; Merkler, D.; Collin, M.; Lalive, P.H. IgG glycan hydrolysis by EndoS inhibits experimental autoimmune encephalomyelitis. *J. Neuroinflamm.* **2012**, *9*, 209. [CrossRef] [PubMed]

188. Allhorn, M.; Briceño, J.G.; Baudino, L.; Lood, C.; Olsson, M.L.; Izui, S.; Collin, M. The IgG-specific endoglycosidase EndoS inhibits both cellular and complement-mediated autoimmune hemolysis. *Blood* **2010**, *115*, 5080–5088. [CrossRef] [PubMed]

189. Hirose, M.; Vafia, K.; Kalies, K.; Groth, S.; Westermann, J.; Zillikens, D.; Ludwig, R.J.; Collin, M.; Schmidt, E. Enzymatic autoantibody glycan hydrolysis alleviates autoimmunity against type VII collagen. *J. Autoimmun.* **2012**, *39*, 304–314. [CrossRef] [PubMed]

190. Yu, X.; Zheng, J.; Collin, M.; Schmidt, E.; Zillikens, D.; Petersen, F. EndoS reduces the pathogenicity of anti-mCOL7 IgG through reduced binding of immune complexes to neutrophils. *PLoS ONE* **2014**, *9*, e85317. [CrossRef] [PubMed]

191. von Pawel-Rammingen, U.; Johansson, B.P.; Björck, L. IdeS, a novel streptococcal cysteine proteinase with unique specificity for immunoglobulin G. *EMBO J.* **2002**, *21*, 1607–1615. [CrossRef] [PubMed]

192. Nandakumar, K.S.; Johansson, B.P.; Björck, L.; Holmdahl, R. Blocking of experimental arthritis by cleavage of IgG antibodies in vivo. *Arthritis Rheum.* **2007**, *56*, 3253–3260. [CrossRef] [PubMed]

193. Jordan, S.C.; Lorant, T.; Choi, J.; Kjellman, C.; Winstedt, L.; Bengtsson, M.; Zhang, X.; Eich, T.; Toyoda, M.; Eriksson, B.-M.; et al. IgG Endopeptidase in Highly Sensitized Patients Undergoing Transplantation. *N. Engl. J. Med.* **2017**, *377*, 442–453. [CrossRef] [PubMed]

194. Järnum, S.; Bockermann, R.; Runström, A.; Winstedt, L.; Kjellman, C. The Bacterial Enzyme IdeS Cleaves the IgG-Type of B Cell Receptor (BCR), Abolishes BCR-Mediated Cell Signaling, and Inhibits Memory B Cell Activation. *J. Immunol.* **2015**, *195*, 5592–5601. [CrossRef] [PubMed]

195. Pagan, J.D.; Kitaoka, M.; Anthony, R.M. Engineered Sialylation of Pathogenic Antibodies In Vivo Attenuates Autoimmune Disease. *Cell* **2018**, *172*, 564–577. [CrossRef] [PubMed]

196. Liu, H.; Ponniah, G.; Zhang, H.-M.; Nowak, C.; Neill, A.; Gonzalez-Lopez, N.; Patel, R.; Cheng, G.; Kita, A.Z.; Andrien, B. In vitro and in vivo modifications of recombinant and human IgG antibodies. *MAbs* **2014**, *6*, 1145–1154. [CrossRef] [PubMed]

197. Tiller, K.E.; Tessier, P.M. Advances in Antibody Design. *Annu. Rev. Biomed. Eng.* **2015**, *17*, 191–216. [CrossRef] [PubMed]

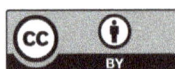

International Journal of
Molecular Sciences

MDPI

Review

The Effect of Triptolide in Rheumatoid Arthritis: From Basic Research towards Clinical Translation

Danping Fan [1], Qingqing Guo [1,2], Jiawen Shen [1,3], Kang Zheng [1,2], Cheng Lu [1], Ge Zhang [2], Aiping Lu [2,4] and Xiaojuan He [1,2,*]

[1]   Institute of Basic Research in Clinical Medicine, China Academy of Chinese Medical Sciences, Beijing 100700, China; fdp0406@gmail.com (D.F.); qingqingguo@hkbu.edu.hk (Q.G.); shenjiawen23@gmail.com (J.S.); zhengkang@hkbu.edu.hk (K.Z.); lcheng0816@gmail.com (C.L.)
[2]   Law Sau Fai Institute for Advancing Translational Medicine in Bone and Joint Diseases, School of Chinese Medicine, Hong Kong Baptist University, Kowloon Tong, Hong Kong; zhangge@hkbu.edu.hk (G.Z.); aipinglu@hkbu.edu.hk (A.L.)
[3]   School of Life Sciences and Engineering, Southwest Jiaotong University, Chengdu 610031, China
[4]   School of Basic Medical Sciences, Shanghai University of Traditional Chinese Medicine, Shanghai 201203, China
*   Correspondence: hxjuan19@gmail.com; Tel.: +86-10-6409-3073

Received: 27 December 2017; Accepted: 23 January 2018; Published: 26 January 2018

Abstract: Triptolide (TP), a major extract of the herb *Tripterygium wilfordii* Hook F (TWHF), has been shown to exert potent pharmacological effects, especially an immunosuppressive effect in the treatment of rheumatoid arthritis (RA). However, its multiorgan toxicity prevents it from being widely used in clinical practice. Recently, several attempts are being performed to reduce TP toxicity. In this review, recent progress in the use of TP for RA, including its pharmacological effects and toxicity, is summarized. Meanwhile, strategies relying on chemical structural modifications, innovative delivery systems, and drug combinations to alleviate the disadvantages of TP are also reviewed. Furthermore, we also discuss the challenges and perspectives in their clinical translation.

Keywords: triptolide; rheumatoid arthritis; basic research; clinical translation

---

1. Introduction

Rheumatoid arthritis (RA) is an immune-related disease that generally gives rise to continuous joint destruction, decreased expectancy of life and work ability, considerable disability, and even raised mortality [1]. Disease-modifying anti-rheumatic drugs (DMARDs), such as conventional synthetic DMARDs (csDMARDs) and biological DMARDs (bDMARDs), are currently the most commonly used drugs for treating RA. However, these drugs can not cure RA completely and often bring about severe side effects, such as infection and malignancies. Moreover, bDMARDs have low cost-effectiveness and bring a huge financial burden to the patients. Thus, it is still an imperative mission for researchers to find safer and more cost-effective medications.

Traditional Chinese medicine (TCM), as an important kind of complementary and alternative medicine, is a precious resource for finding cost-efficient drugs, such as artemisinin. As for RA, there are many Chinese herbs with excellent immunosuppressive and anti-inflammatory functions [2]. *Tripterygium wilfordii* Hook F (TWHF) is a case in point. Tripterygium glycosides, extracted from TWHF, have been widely used to treat RA in China [3]. As the main active ingredient in Tripterygium glycosides, Triptolide (TP, a dierpene triepoxide in chemical structure, see Figure 1) has been considered as a promising anti-RA drug [4]. Increasing experimental evidence has verified its anti-RA effect. TP can significantly alleviate the severity of collagen-induced arthritis (CIA) in rats, with not only a potent anti-inflammatory effect but also the ability to prevent bone destruction [5,6]. Because of its outstanding anti-RA effect, TP has a great application potential in the clinic. Nonetheless, TP also exerts extreme toxicity and has poor water solubility, which impede its clinical application. Fortunately, many promising attempts for its clinical translation have been performed by researchers.

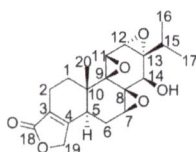

Figure 1. Chemical structure of (Triptolide)TP.

Thus, on the one hand, in order to gain a comprehensive and deep understanding of TP's pharmacodynamic effect and toxicity in RA, related studies were summarized and reviewed in this paper; on the other hand, we also focused on the clinical translation researches of TP in RA hoping to get a better grasp of the progress in this area and provide proper directions and suggestions for its further study.

2. Effect and Mechanisms of Triptolide (TP) in Rheumatoid Arthritis (RA)

As a chronic immune-mediated inflammatory disease, immune regulatory factors play vital roles in the pathogenesis of RA. Until now, the anti-RA properties of TP in this condition have been attributed to its immunosupressive and antiproliferative effect (Figure 2).

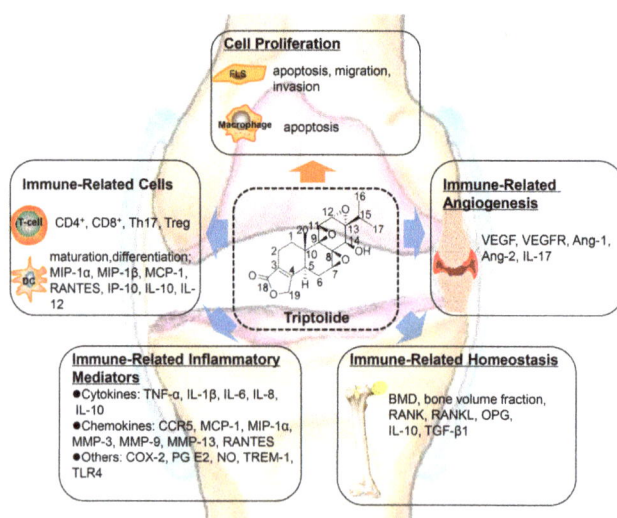

Figure 2. Schematic illustration of TP properties in the treatment of rheumatoid arthritis (RA). The anti-RA properties of TP have been attributed to its immunosupressive and antiproliferative effect. MIP: macrophage inflammatory protein; MCP: monocyte chemoattractant protein; RANTES: regulated upon activation normal T cell expressed and secreted; IP: interferon-induced protein; IL: interleukin; VEGF: vascular endothelial growth factor; VEGFR: vascular endothelial growth factor receptor; Ang: angiopoietin; TNF: tumor necrosis factor; CCR: C-C chemokine receptor; MMP: matrix metalloproteinase; COX: cyclooxygenase; PG: prostaglandin; NO: nitric oxide; TREM: triggering receptors expressed on myeloid cells-1; TLR: toll-like receptor; BMD: bone mineral density; RANK: receptor activator of nuclear factor-κB; RNAKL: receptor activator of nuclear factor-κB ligand; OPG: osteoprotegerin; TGF: transforming growth factor.

2.1. Regulation of Immunological Functions

2.1.1. Regulation of Immune-Related Cells

T cells are among the key regulators of synovial inflammation in the development of RA, having both stimulatory and inhibitory roles [7] and playing a destructive or a protective role in bone metabolism in a context- and subtype-dependent manner [8]. TP was effective in preventing T cells proliferation [9]. CD4[+] T cells play an important role in the induction and development of CIA, and CD8[+] T cells might have a suppressive role in the etiology of CIA [10]. Previous studies showed that TP could increase CD8[+] cells, while it decreased CD4[+] cells in the Peyer's patch. Therefore, the effect of TP on Peyer's patch immune cells might partially explain some of the immunosuppressive activities of TP [11,12]. In addition, the overexpression of T cell receptor (TCR) variable gene (V gene) fragments can cause the activation and infiltration of autoreactive T cells. Nevertheless, TP was found to decrease the expression levels of TCR BV15 and TCR BV19. These changes might help explain the effectiveness of TP in the treatment of RA [13].

Th17 cells, a more recently characterized subset of CD4[+] T cells, were shown to be more osteoclastogenic [8] and play an important role in the pathogenesis of RA through the production of Th17 signature cytokines [14]. Interleukin (IL)-6 and transforming growth factor (TGF)-β in mice or TGF-β and inflammatory cytokines in human are recognized as crucial factors necessary for the differentiation of naïve T cells into Th17 cells [14,15]. In vivo, TP significantly suppressed the production of Th17 cells from murine splenocytes and purified CD4[+] T cells. Importantly, TP could inhibit the transcription of IL-17 mRNA and IL-6-induced phosphorylation of signal transducers and activators of transcription (STAT)3, which is a key signaling molecule involved in the development of Th17 cells. In vitro, TP reduced the production of collagen type II (CII)-specific IL-17 and the percentages of CII-specific IL-17[+] CD4[+] T cells in draining lymph nodes and spleens in CIA mice [16].

The dendritic cell (DC) is the most potent professional antigen-presenting cell (APC). Immature DCs (iDCs) have the ability to capture and process antigens in inflammatory tissues and undergo phenotypic and functional maturation implying the production of cytokines and chemokines in inflammatory microenvironments. Mature DCs produce multiple chemokines which act as chemoattractants for T cells, B cells, natural killer (NK) cells, and even neutrophils [17–19]. Therefore, DC is also regarded as an important target of immunosuppressants. Recently, research indicated that TP treatment inhibited lipopolysaccharide (LPS)-induced phenotypic changes and maturation of DCs [20,21]. TP also prevented the differentiation of immature human monocytes (MoDC) by inhibiting CD1a, CD40, CD80, and CD86 expression and upregulating CD14 expression [22]. In addition, the ability of DCs to stimulate allogeneic T cell responses was also impaired by TP. Furthermore, the production of IL-10 and IL-12 by DCs was modulated after TP treatment [20]. Yan et al. study indicated that TP might induce splenic DCs to CD11c[low] differentiation, followed by shifting of Th1 to Th2 in vitro [23]. Cao et al. [24] conducted a study to investigate whether TP can inhibit DC-mediated chemoattraction of immune cells, because DC and chemokines are all important mediators in linking innate immunity and adaptive immunity. They found that TP impaired DC-mediated chemoattraction of neutrophils and T cells. Additionally, TP inhibited LPS-induced DC production of chemokines such as macrophage inflammatory protein (MIP)-1α, MIP-1β, monocyte chemoattractant protein (MCP)-1, regulated upon activation normal T cell expressed and secreted (RANTES), and interferon-induced protein 10 (IP-10) via suppression of nuclear factor kappa-light-chain-enhancer of activated B cells (NF-κB) activation and STAT3 phosphorylation. These data provided new insights into TP immunopharmacology.

2.1.2. Regulation of Immune-Related Inflammatory Mediators

As RA is a complicated disease caused by a variety of factors, the inflammatory response has been considered as the main protracted cause of RA. The process of inflammation is usually tightly regulated by both mediators that initiate and maintain inflammation and mediators that shut the process down [25]. In states of chronic inflammation, an imbalance between the two types of mediators leaves inflammation unchecked, which leads to cellular damage. Previous studies have demonstrated that proinflammatory cytokines and chemokines produced by infiltrating immune cells and synoviocytes are implicated in the pathogenesis of RA. Meanwhile, plenty of cytokines and chemokines are also found in the synovial fluid of RA patients [26]. These cytokines and chemokines play an essential role in synovitis, pannus formation, and joint destruction caused by RA [27–30]. Previous studies showed that TP could lower the level of tumour necrosis factor (TNF)-α, IL-1β, IL-6, nuclear factor (NF)-κB, and cyclooxygenase (COX)-2 in ankle joints and serum in CIA rats [5,31]. Meanwhile, in LPS-induced mouse macrophages, TP could induce the reduction of toll-like receptor 4 (TLR4) proteins and of TIR-domain-containing adapter-inducing interferon-β (TRIF) adapter proteins in the MyD88-independent pathway of TLR4, confirming that both MyD88- and TRIF-mediated NF-κB activation might be suppressed by TP [32]. Moreover, TP decreased C-C chemokine receptor type 5 (CCR5) protein and mRNA levels in synovial tissue of adjuvant-induced arthritis (AIA) rats [33]. Except for CCR5, the overexpression of MCP-1, MIP-1α, and RANTES were also downregulated in TP-treated AIA rats [34]. Additionally, TP could inhibit prostaglandin (PG) E [2] production via a selective suppression of the production and gene expression of COX-2 in CIA rats [35]. Simultaneously, Wang et al. reported that TP could inhibit the production of nitric oxide (NO) by decreasing inducible NO synthase gene transcription [36]. Triggering receptor expressed on myeloid cells (TREM)-1 is a member of the Ig superfamily, and its activation can result in an inflammatory reaction [37,38]. We learned that the expression of TREM-1 could be activated by TLR through LPS, which could further lead to the production of proinflammatory cytokines via the NF-κB pathway [39,40]. Our study indicated that TP could significantly inhibit TREM-1 expressions in CIA rats, as well as decrease the production of TREM-1 in LPS-stimulated U937 cells, which demonstrated that TP could modulate the TREM-1 signaling pathway to inhibit the inflammatory response in RA [5]. TP suppressed TNF-α-induced expression of the IL-1β, IL-6, and IL-8 in fibroblast-like synoviocytes (FLSs) [41]. Treatment with TP also decreased the activation of matrix metalloproteinase (MMP)-3, MMP-9, MMP-13, and the cytoskeleton rearrangement of RA FLSs [42,43]. Moreover, TP not only decreased the IL-1α-induced production of proMMP-1 and 3, but also suppressed their messenger RNA (mRNA) levels in human RA FLSs. Conversely, the expression of tissue inhibitors of metalloproteinases (TIMPs) 1 and 2 induced by IL-1α was augmented by TP in the synovial cells [44]. In phorbol 12-myristate 13-acetate (PMA)-stimulated RA, the expression of IL-18 and IL-18 receptor (IL-18R) at protein and gene levels FLSs were also reduced by TP [45].

While some cytokines initiate and maintain the inflammatory process, others dampen it. The two best studied anti-inflammatory cytokines are IL-10 and IL-4. These cytokines cooperate to inhibit the production of inflammatory cytokines in vitro [46,47]. Xu et al. reported that TP could enhance the expression of IL-10 in regulatory T cells (Tregs) and further suppress osteoclast formation and bone resorption [6], and in vivo data revealed that the level of IL-10 was increased in the TP treatment group compared with the CIA group [13].

2.1.3. Regulation of Immune-Related Angiogenesis

In the development of RA, blood vessel proliferation is common because of the influence of angiogenesis factors and angiogenic activators, like vascular endothelial growth factor (VEGF), fibroblast growth factor (FGF)-2, and hepatocyte growth factor in the inflamed and hypoxic environment. Angiogenesis is indispensable in perpetuating immune and inflammatory responses and can foster the infiltration of inflammatory cells into the joints, resulting in synovial hyperplasia and progressive bone destruction [48–51]. Previous studies suggested that TP could markedly reduce the capillary and the small, medium, and large vessel density in synovial membrane tissues of inflamed joints, and inhibit the expression of VEGF in the sera of CIA rats. The levels of VEGF, vascular endothelial growth factor receptor (VEGFR), Angiopoietin (Ang)-1, Ang-2, and IL-17 in the supernatants of human RA FLSs and human umbilical vein endothelial cells (HUVEC) were also decreased after TP treatment. These results implied that TP might possess an anti-angiogenic effect in RA both in vivo and in in vitro assay systems [52,53].

2.1.4. Regulation of Immune-Related Bone Homeostasis

As an autoimmune disease characterized by inflammation and bone loss, bone homeostasis, which involves bone formation mediated by osteoblasts and bone resorption regulated by osteoclasts, is disrupted in the pathological condition of RA. The bone loss and joint destruction are mediated by immunological insults by various immune cells and inflammatory cytokines. The bone destruction that occurs in RA is also regulated by the receptor activator of nuclear factor-κB (RANK) and its ligand (RANKL), simultaneously [8]. Liu et al. found that TP could upregulate the bone mineral density (BMD), bone volume fraction, and trabecular thickness of inflamed joints and downregulate the trabecular separation, which suggests a protective role of TP on the volume and quality of the preserved trabecular bone despite joint inflammation [54]. Meanwhile, TP could significantly reduce the expression of RANKL and RANK, enhance the level of osteoprotegerin (OPG) in joints and sera of CIA rats, as well as decrease RANKL and RANK level and increase OPG production in the coculture system of human FLSs and peripheral blood mononuclear cells (PBMCs), which further revealed that TP might attenuate RA in part by preventing bone destruction, and inhibit osteoclast formation by regulating the RANKL–RANK–OPG signaling pathway [54]. Another study showed that the protective effects of TP on the joint destruction seen in RA might be associated with its inhibitory effect on the aggression of RA FLSs by blocking c-Jun N-terminal kinase (JNK) activation [42]. Furthermore, Tregs secrete cytokines like IL-10 and TGF-β1 that appear to play a key role in suppressing the differentiation of osteoclasts and the resorption of bone [55]. Research by Xu et al. indicated that TP could enhance the expression of IL-10 and TGF-β1 secreted by Tregs in vitro, which further inhibit osteoclast formation and bone resorption [6]. In another study, TP was found be able to reverse TNF-α-associated suppression of osteoblast differentiation, suggesting that TP might have a positive effect on bone remodeling [56].

2.2. Regulation of Cell Proliferation

Accumulating research suggests that FLSs contribute to synovial inflammation and joint destruction [57–59]. They play a crucial part in the initial stages of synovitis through the local production of proinflammatory cytokines and small-molecule mediators of inflammation [7,59]. TP could inhibit the proliferation of FLSs, arrest the cycle of FLSs, and induce apoptosis of FLSs [41,60]. In addition, the migration of FLSs to the cartilage and bone is regarded as a critical process in cartilage destruction in RA [59]. Yang et al. demonstrated that TP could suppress the migration and invasion of RA FLSs by partially blocking the phosphorylation of the JNK pathway [42].

Macrophages are found in the synovial membrane and are central effectors of synovitis. Macrophages act through the release of cytokines such as TNF-α and IL-1 [7]. TP treatment could result in macrophage apoptosis, while no obvious necrosis occurred [61]. The level of TNF-α in LPS-induced macrophages could be decreased by TP [62].

3. Mechanisms of TP Toxicity

Despite TP remarkable effect on RA, an increasing number of studies demonstrated that TP could induce toxicity, including hepatotoxicity, nephrotoxicity, reproductive toxicity, and so on.

3.1. Hepatotoxicity

To evaluate the liver injury effect of TP, the serum activities of alanine transaminase (ALT), aspartate transaminase (AST), and lactic dehydrogenase (LDH) were used as biochemical markers. One study on C57BL/6 mice reported the time-dependent hepatotoxicity of TP, accompanied by an increasing trend of AST and ALT in the serum at 6 and 12 h, a peak at 24 h after TP (600 mg/kg) administration, and a decrease after 24 h [63]. Another study showed that ALT, AST, and LDH activities in serum were multiplied by 9.1, 9.8, and 3.0, respectively, which occurred in BALB/C mice treated only with TP (1.0 mg/kg) but not in control groups [64]. Additionally, the livers of TP-treated (0.5 mg/kg) mice showed hyperemic, mottled, fragile, and fuzzy structures, hepatocytes' nuclei displayed pyknosis and ruptures, and cytoplasmic staining was uneven with slight cell damage [65]. In contrast, after giving TP (0.1, 0.3 mg/kg) through intravenous administration once daily for 14 days, AST activity in the serum of Wistar rats significantly decreased as the TP dose increased, but there was no significant change in ALT [66]. Moreover, TP (200–400 μg/kg, 28 days) induced mitochondrial membrane depolarization in female Sprague Dawley (SD) rats, resulting in liver damage with microvesicular steatosis and hyperlactacidaemia, and was accompanied by an augmentation in reactive oxygen species (ROS) [67]. In addition, an abnormal immune response can induce organ or tissue damage influenced by CD4$^+$ T cells such as Th17 and Tregs. Recently, Wang et al. reported that TP (500 μg/kg for 24 h) elevated the Th17/Treg ratio, which was positively correlated with ALT and AST in the serum, as well as acute liver injury of female C57BL/6 mice [63]. Recently, Yang and her colleagues found that the intragastric administration of TP (400 μg/kg body weight, 28 days) increased serum total bile acid and ALP levels and suppressed hepatic gluconeogenesis in Wistar rats, indicating that TP induced hepatotoxicity, and this hepatotoxicity was related to the sirtuin (Sirt1)/farnesoid X receptor (FXR) signaling pathway [68]. Simultaneously, Lu et al. suggested that TP could cause hepatotoxicity by reducing substrate affinity, activity, and expression of the CYP450 isoforms 3A, 2C9, 2C19, and 2E1 [69].

3.2. Nephrotoxicity

To estimate the nephrotoxicity of TP, blood urea nitrogen (BUN) and creatinine (Cr), which are important biochemical parameters in the serum, were used. Yang et al. reported that TP could cause a significant reduction of renal function characterized by a remarkable upregulation of Cr and BUN concentrations. Research about the relationship between TP-induced nephrotoxicity and oxidative stress indicated that TP caused serious oxidative stress after a single dose of 1 mg/kg in male SD rats, decreased the activities of renal superoxide dismutase (SOD) and glutathione (GSH), increased the level of malondialdehyde (MDA) and BUN, and caused structural damage [70]. In the meantime, TP induced severe damage in the renal structure, characterized by tubular epithelial cell detachment, necrosis, and tubular obstruction [71]. Furthermore, renal glomeruli were hyperemic, swelling, scattered, and necrotic after TP treatment [65].

3.3. Reproductive Toxicity

Except for hepatotoxicity and nephrotoxicity, toxicity for the reproductive system and an antifertility effect were also obvious. In female reproductive toxicity studies, TP caused prolonged estrous cycles and reduced the relative weights of the ovary and uterus [72]. In male reproductive toxicity studies, after treating with TP, the testis and epididymis weights were severely decreased. The cauda epididymis sperm content and motility even decreased to zero [73]. Studies have demonstrated that TP toxicity to the reproduction system emerged mainly through a disruption of the normal androgen and estrogen signaling [74]. Estrogen synthesis enzymes, aromatase and steroidogenic regulatory protein, play important roles in estradiol synthesis and estrogen signaling. TP could disrupt the expression of these three key proteins leading to estradiol synthesis reduction and reproductive dysfunction [75]. Intracellular ROS, glutathione peroxidase (GPx), and SOD are very important for testosterone generation. Studies found that TP had an influence on ROS, GPx, and SOD resulting in testosterone reduction. It was also found that TP could induce direct cytotoxicity in Leydig cells [76].

3.4. Further Toxicity

It is widely known that TP could cause reproductive toxicity, liver damage, and renal injury. However, TP could also lead to damage in other organs. TP acute poisoning could cause acute myocardial damage, such as myocardium swelling, denaturation, cytolysis, and contraction band necrosis. This toxicological effect of TP might be closely related to mitochondria and cell membrane functions [77]. Furthermore, there was also injury to the spleen after long-term TP administration. As an inflammation inhibitor, a long-time usage of TP could cause immunotoxicity in the spleen. Increased spleen index, spleen volume, and spleen weight could be seen in impaired spleens [66]. Gastrointestinal tract symptoms, such as nausea, anorexia, vomiting, diarrhea, gastrointestinal ulcers, and bleeding, were also a result of adverse reactions to TP [78]. In the meantime, TP could induce hematologic toxicity. In hepatic P450-deficient mice, the total number of platelets (PLT) and the number of white blood cells were reduced after TP treatment (0.5, 1.0 mg/kg). TP also decreased the absolute number and percent of lymphocytes, while it increased the absolute number and percent of neutrophils to a concentration of 1.0 mg/kg. There was no difference in the levels of red blood cells (RBC) or hemoglobin (Hb) after TP treatment [79]. Scientists confirmed that P450s was responsible for the metabolism of TP in the liver. P450s deficiency might cause an increase in the bioavailability and toxicity of TP [79]. In the study of Liu et al., TP (200 and 400 mg/kg/day for 28 days) showed a reduced toxicity and a higher metabolic rate in male SD rats linked to CYP3A2 which was the main metabolic isozyme in male rats, revealing the importance of CYP3A2 on the sex-based differences in TP toxicity [80]. Although there was no clear explanation of the effects of TP toxicity on RA, this research provided novel directions for further studies on TP toxicity.

4. Translational Research of TP

As mentioned above, the potent immunosuppressive and antiproliferative effects make TP a promising drug for clinical RA therapy. At the same time, its high toxicity as well as its poor water solubility greatly hinder TP's clinical applications [73,81]. In order to improve the characteristics of TP, strategies relying on chemical structural modifications, innovative delivery systems, and drug combinations are increasingly employed by researchers [65,82,83].

4.1. Chemical Structural Modifications of TP

Many drugs like TP exert excellent therapeutic effects while simultaneously causing dramatic toxicity and displaying poor water solubility. Certain chemical properties of a compound can be changed by modifying its chemical structure. These modifications may be employed to increase water solubility or decrease the toxicity of a drug, thus making it available for clinical use. Over the past decades, several TP analogs (Table 1) have been developed and evaluated, mainly including (5R)-5-hydroxytriptolide (LLDT-8) [84], PG490-88 [85], LLDT-67 [86], LLDT-288 [87], and so on. Among these derivatives, LLDT-8 has comparable immunosuppressive and anti-inflammatory functions and a much lower toxicity compared to TP [88]. Its effects on RA have been proved by preclinical tests and Phase I clinical trials in RA patients [88,89]. With regard to its mechanism of action, LLDT-8 is thought to inhibit the activation of macrophages and regulate T cells proliferation and function [90,91].

Table 1. Main derivatives of TP.

No.	Compound Name	Chemical Structure	Modification Sites	Improved Characteristics Compared with TP	References
1	(5R)-5-hydroxytriptolide (LLDT-8)		C-5 site	much lower toxicity	[88]
2	LLDT-67		C-14 site	low toxicity	[86]
3	LLDT-288		C-14 site	low toxicity	[87]
4	PG490-88		C-14-hydroxyl site	Water soluble	[85]
5	Minnelide		C-14-hydroxyl site	Water soluble	[92]
6	MRx102	——	——	low toxicity	[93]

Note: "——"means that there are no corresponding chemical structure and modification site in the literature we cited.

4.2. Innovative Delivery System

Drugs with poor solubility in water have trouble dissolving in the gastrointestinal tract, engendering a low bioavailability. Some innovative delivery systems, like those obtained through nanotechnology and microemulsions, can be employed to enhance the delivery efficiency of medications [94,95]. Hence, studies of TP delivered by liposomes, nanoparticles, solid lipid nanoparticles, and microemulsions are summarized below and listed in Table 2.

Table 2. Innovative delivery system studies of TP.

Drug Carrier	In Vivo/In Vitro	Advantages	References
liposome hydrogel patch	CIA rats	improves bioavailability of TP; bypasses hepatic first-pass metabolism, and reduces the incidence or severity of gastrointestinal reactions	[96]
nanodrug carrier system (γ-PGA-L-PAE-TP (PPT))	normal C57/B6 mice/RAW264.7 cell lines	reduces free TP toxicity in vitro and in vivo	[97]
poly(D,L-lactic acid) (PLA) nanoparticles	AIA rats	improve bioavailability of TP	[98]
poly(D,L-lactic acid) (PLA) nanoparticles	normal SD rats	abate the renal toxicity caused by TP	[99]

Table 2. *Cont.*

Drug Carrier	In Vivo/In Vitro	Advantages	References
solid lipid nanoparticle hydrogel	carrageenan-induced rats	improves safety and minimizes the toxicity induced by TP	[100]
solid lipid nanoparticle/microemulsions	carrageenan-induced rats and AIA rats	increase therapeutic index	[101]
solid lipid nanoparticles	carrageenan-induced rats	enhance the anti-inflammatory activity of TP have a protective effect against TP-induced hepatotoxicity	[102]
solid lipid nanoparticles	normal SD rats	reduce gastric irritation	[78]
solid lipid nanoparticles	normal SD rats	enhance efficacy, decrease reproductive toxicity	[103]
nanostructured lipid carriers	normal SD rats	reduce subacute toxicity in male rats	[104]
hydrogel-thickened microemulsion	normal rabbits, mice, beagle dogs, guinea pigs	no obvious toxicities	[105]

Note: CIA: collagen-induced arthritis; AIA: adjuvant-induced arthritis; SD: Sprague Dawley; TP: triptolide.

4.2.1. Liposomes

Chen et al. [96] developed a TP-loaded liposome hydrogel patch (TP-LHP) which was proved to improve the bioavailability of TP because of its stable and long-term release. Similar to TP, TP-LHP showed significant efficacy in CIA rats. Moreover, TP was delivered transdermally in this study, which can avoid the first-pass effects on the liver and abate gastrointestinal toxicity.

4.2.2. Nanoparticles

Nanocarriers can reduce the side effects and increase the delivery efficiency of many drugs. Poly-γ-glutamic acid (γ-PGA) has been reported to be a promising drug carrier. Zhang and his colleagues created a nanodrug carrier system called γ-PGA-L-PAE-TP (PPT) by wrapping TP in a poly-γ-glutamicacid-grafted L-phenylalanine ethylester copolymer. PPT demonstrated controlled release behavior. This research indicated that PPT could alleviate free TP toxicity on murine macrophage RAW264.7 cells and normal C57/B6 mice. The nanodrug carrier system showed broad application prospects in RA treatment [97].

Poly(D,L-lacticacid) nanoparticles were used as TP carrier by Liu group. They fabricated TP-loaded poly(D,L-lacticacid) nanoparticles (TP-PLA-NPs) through the spontaneous emulsification solvent diffusion method with modifications. This delivery system caused TP to be burst-released initially and slow-released subsequently. In vivo tests demonstrated the significant inhibition effect of TP-PLA-NPs on AIA rats [98]. Furthermore, another study demonstrated that TP-PLA-NPs could effectively lower renal toxicity in rats [99].

4.2.3. Solid Lipid Nanoparticles

Solid lipid nanoparticles (SLNs) were introduced as an innovative drug delivery system at the beginning of the 1990s. This system has become a promising alternative to liposomes, polymeric nanoparticles, and so on because of its merits, like nontoxicity, excellent biocompatibility, as well as large-scale production possibilities [106]. The solid matrix of SLNs can protect the loaded drug from degrading in the gastrointestinal tract [78,107]. SLNs can be employed in both topical application and oral administration. Mei et al. [100–102] found that SLNs could efficiently promote TP penetration into the skin. Furthermore, they also confirmed the anti-inflammatory effect of SLNs on carrageenan-induced rats as well as AIA rats, with improved safety and minimized toxicity compared to TP. Another research group compared the toxicokinetics and tissue distribution of TP-SLN versus free TP in rats, and the results suggested that TP-SLN enhanced TP absorption, with a slow release which may contribute to boost TP efficacy. Tissue distribution results showed that TP-SLN was more distributed in the lung and spleen than in plasma, liver, kidney, and testes. This explained why TP-SLN could mitigate the genital toxicity of TP [103].

4.2.4. Microemulsions

Microemulsions are increasingly used for the transdermal delivery of drugs because of their several advantages, such as enhanced efficacy in transdermal applications over conventional formulations, elevated drug solubility, and ease of manufacturing [108]. A previous study prepared TP-loaded microemulsions and proved that they could penetrate in vitro through the mouse skin without obvious irritation to the skin [109]. Furthermore, Xu et al. [105] developed a kind of TP-loaded hydrogel-thickened microemulsion (TP-MTH) to treat RA through transdermal delivery. They testified its good effects without apparent local and systemic toxicities.

4.3. Drug Combinations

In the clinic, it has been found that drug combinations could be a good choice to solve drug toxicity. Drug combinations use several drugs that interact with multiple targets in the molecular networks of a disease and, in practice, may achieve better efficacy and lower toxicity than monotherapies. Thus, drug combinations can produce a synergistic effect without increased toxicity [110]. To solve TP toxicity, scientists have already found some drug, such as glycyrrhetinic acid and silymarin, which could produce a synergistic therapeutic effect, detoxication, or both.

4.3.1. Glycyrrhetinic Acid

During the process of RA treatment, Licorice (*Glycyrrhiza glabra* L.) was often used combined with TWHF or TWHF preparations to reduce the latter's adverse effects. Glycyrrhizin (GL) was considered a main active component of Licorice. Research showed that a combination of GL and TP could reduce the side effects of TP. The detoxifying effect of GL on TP was considered inseparable from GL's selective influence on cytochrome P4503A (CYP3A). CYP3A, a major Phase I xenobiotic metabolizing enzyme, is responsible for regulating the metabolism of TP in the liver, avoiding the accumulation of TP [111]. By activating CYP3A, GL could accelerate the metabolism of TP and reduce the body exposure to TP. This suggested a significant protective action against chronic liver injury in rats [82]. In addition, many studies have reported that both GL and TP have an anti-inflammatory effect [112,113]. Furthermore, GL combined with TP produced a synergistic anti-inflammatory effect [114].

GL dissolves in water and transforms into glycyrrhetinic acid (GA), which is an important active ingredient with pharmacological properties [115]. Pharmacokinetic studies found that an extensive accumulation of TP in the liver caused liver damage [116]. This kind of liver damage could be reduced by the combination of GA and TP. The possible mechanism is that GA could reduce TP accumulation by promoting TP hepatic metabolic clearance. Several studies proved that GA could promote TP hepatic metabolic clearance, and this action was closely related to P-glycoprotein (P-gp) [117–119].

4.3.2. Silymarin

The excessive release of inflammatory mediators could lead to immunological injury. TP combined with silymarin produced synergistic anti-inflammatory effects when treating inflammatory diseases like RA [35]. Silymarin is an active ingredient of *Silybum marianum* and it was reported to have various pharmacological functions. Silymarin was often used, alone or as a major component of various pharmaceutical preparations, as a hepatoprotective agent clinically. Additionally, silymarin has also exhibited protective effects against inflammation [120]. Short-term oral administration of silymarin exerted protective effects on TP-induced liver injury. The combination of silymarin and TP could produce a synergistic immunosuppressive effect by reducing the excessive expression of proinflammatory cytokines and inhibiting inflammatory signaling [121].

Int. J. Mol. Sci. **2018**, *19*, 376

5. Discussion and Further Perspectives

Here, in this review, we examined the research on the pharmacodynamic effects, toxicity, and clinical translation of TP in RA. An increasing number of preclinical studies have testified the immunosuppressant, anti-inflammatory, and antiproliferative effects of TP which scientifically explain its good clinical effect on RA. Additionally, TP toxicity in RA is also increasingly studied. By analyzing a series of reports, we speculated that the potential primary effect of TP in RA might be achieved via its immunosuppressive property. As RA is a systemic disease, the effective and toxic mechanisms of TP in RA still need deep investigation. Perhaps, bioinformatic methods rising recently can be exploited to explore TP pharmacodynamics and toxicological mechanisms from a more systematic point of view.

In terms of the clinical translation of TP, several problems should be raised here. Firstly, we found that several derivatives of TP were synthesized and proven to possess effects comparable to those of TP and are even currently able to enter clinical trials. However, most of the derivatives are studied for cancer with only one of them used to treat RA. Furthermore, only LLDT-8 is still awaiting the outcomes of the clinical tests, although it showed promising anti-RA effects in preclinical studies. In addition, with regard to innovative delivery systems, targeted drug deliveries are becoming more and more popular because of their specific targeting of certain organs or cells. Nevertheless, the current targeted delivery systems of TP are mostly renal-targeted and tumor-targeted. For example, 3,5-dipentadecyloxybenzamidine hydrochloride (TRX-20)-modified liposomes [122], PF-A299–585 [123], 2-Glucosamine [124], and lysozyme [125] were reported to specifically deliver TP to the kidney. Carbonic anhydrase IX (CA IX) [126], AS1411 [127], and nanoformulations coated with folate [128] were used to specifically deliver TP to lung cancer, pancreatic cancer, and hepatocellular carcinoma cells, respectively. Investigations using targeted delivery system for TP to treat RA are still scarce. Thus, more research is needed to advance the application of TP in RA.

Acknowledgments: This study was supported by the Hong Kong Baptist University Strategic Development Fund (SDF15-0324-P02(b)).

Author Contributions: Danping Fan wrote the manuscript; Qingqing Guo, Jiawen Shen, Kang Zheng, and Cheng Lu contributed to the literature research for the manuscript ; Ge Zhang and Aiping Lu revised the manuscript; Xiaojuan He revised and approved the manuscript.

Conflicts of Interest: The authors declare no conflict of interest.

References

1. Burmester, G.R.; Pope, J.E. Novel treatment strategies in rheumatoid arthritis. *Lancet* **2017**, *389*, 2338–2348. [CrossRef]
2. Lu, S.; Wang, Q.; Li, G.; Sun, S.; Guo, Y.; Kuang, H. The treatment of rheumatoid arthritis using Chinese medicinal plants: From pharmacology to potential molecular mechanisms. *J. Ethnopharmacol.* **2015**, *176*, 177–206. [CrossRef] [PubMed]
3. Wang, J.; Chu, Y.; Zhou, X. Inhibitory effect of Triperygium wilfordii polyglucoside on dipeptidyl peptidase I in vivo and in vitro. *Biomed. Pharmacother.* **2017**, *96*, 466–470. [CrossRef] [PubMed]
4. Han, R.; Rostami-Yazdi, M.; Gerdes, S.; Mrowietz, U. Triptolide in the treatment of psoriasis and other immune-mediated inflammatory diseases. *Br. J. Clin. Pharmacol.* **2012**, *74*, 424–436. [CrossRef] [PubMed]
5. Fan, D.; He, X.; Bian, Y.; Guo, Q.; Zheng, K.; Zhao, Y.; Lu, C.; Liu, B.; Xu, X.; Zhang, G. Triptolide Modulates TREM-1 Signal Pathway to Inhibit the Inflammatory Response in Rheumatoid Arthritis. *Int. J. Mol. Sci.* **2016**, *17*, 498. [CrossRef] [PubMed]
6. Xu, H.; Zhao, H.; Lu, C. Triptolide Inhibits Osteoclast Differentiation and Bone Resorption In Vitro via Enhancing the Production of IL-10 and TGF-β1 by Regulatory T Cells. *Mediat. Inflamm.* **2016**, *2016*, 8048170. [CrossRef] [PubMed]
7. McInnes, I.B.; Schett, G. The pathogenesis of rheumatoid arthritis. *N. Engl. J. Med.* **2011**, *365*, 2205–2219. [CrossRef] [PubMed]
8. Jung, S.M.; Kim, K.W.; Yang, C.W.; Park, S.H.; Ju, J.H. Cytokine-mediated bone destruction in rheumatoid arthritis. *J. Immunol. Res.* **2014**, *2014*, 263625. [CrossRef] [PubMed]

9.   Chan, M.A.; Kohlmeier, J.E.; Branden, M.; Jung, M.; Benedict, S.H. Triptolide is more effective in preventing T cell proliferation and interferon-gamma production than is FK506. *Phytother. Res.* **1999**, *13*, 464–467. [CrossRef]

10.   Mellado, M.; Martinez-Munoz, L.; Cascio, G.; Lucas, P.; Pablos, J.L.; Rodriguez-Frade, J.M. T Cell Migration in Rheumatoid Arthritis. *Front. Immunol.* **2015**, *6*, 384. [CrossRef] [PubMed]

11.   Xiao, C.; Zhao, L.; Liu, Z.; Lu, C.; Zhao, N.; Yang, D.; Chen, S.; Tang, J.C.; Chan, A.; Lu, A.P. The effect of triptolide on CD4+ and CD8+ cells in the Peyer's patch of DA rats with collagen induced arthritis. *Nat. Prod. Res.* **2009**, *23*, 1699–1706. [CrossRef] [PubMed]

12.   Zhou, J.; Xiao, C.; Zhao, L.; Jia, H.; Zhao, N.; Lu, C.; Yang, D.; Tang, J.C.; Chan, A.S.; Lu, A.P. The effect of triptolide on CD4+ and CD8+ cells in Peyer's patch of SD rats with collagen induced arthritis. *Int. Immunopharmacol.* **2006**, *6*, 198–203. [CrossRef] [PubMed]

13.   Wang, J.; Wang, A.; Zeng, H.; Liu, L.; Jiang, W.; Zhu, Y.; Xu, Y. Effect of triptolide on T-cell receptor beta variable gene mRNA expression in rats with collagen-induced arthritis. *Anal. Rec.* **2012**, *295*, 922–927. [CrossRef] [PubMed]

14.   Miossec, P.; Korn, T.; Kuchroo, V.K. Interleukin-17 and type 17 helper T cells. *N. Engl. J. Med.* **2009**, *361*, 888–898. [CrossRef] [PubMed]

15.   Volpe, E.; Servant, N.; Zollinger, R.; Bogiatzi, S.I.; Hupe, P.; Barillot, E.; Soumelis, V. A critical function for transforming growth factor-β, interleukin 23 and proinflammatory cytokines in driving and modulating human T(H)-17 responses. *Nat. Immunol.* **2008**, *9*, 650–657. [CrossRef] [PubMed]

16.   Wang, Y.; Jia, L.; Wu, C.Y. Triptolide inhibits the differentiation of Th17 cells and suppresses collagen-induced arthritis. *Scand. J. Immunol.* **2008**, *68*, 383–390. [CrossRef] [PubMed]

17.   Morelli, A.E.; Thomson, A.W. Dendritic cells: Regulators of alloimmunity and opportunities for tolerance induction. *Immunol. Rev.* **2003**, *196*, 125–146. [CrossRef] [PubMed]

18.   Banchereau, J.; Steinman, R.M. Dendritic cells and the control of immunity. *Nature* **1998**, *392*, 245–252. [CrossRef] [PubMed]

19.   Banchereau, J.; Briere, F.; Caux, C.; Davoust, J.; Lebecque, S.; Liu, Y.J.; Pulendran, B.; Palucka, K. Immunobiology of dendritic cells. *Annu. Rev. Immunol.* **2000**, *18*, 767–811. [CrossRef] [PubMed]

20.   Liu, Y.; Chen, Y.; Lamb, J.R.; Tam, P.K. Triptolide, a component of Chinese herbal medicine, modulates the functional phenotype of dendritic cells. *Transplantation* **2007**, *84*, 1517–1526. [CrossRef] [PubMed]

21.   Chen, X.; Murakami, T.; Oppenheim, J.J.; Howard, O.M. Triptolide, a constituent of immunosuppressive Chinese herbal medicine, is a potent suppressor of dendritic-cell maturation and trafficking. *Blood* **2005**, *106*, 2409–2416. [CrossRef] [PubMed]

22.   Zhu, K.J.; Shen, Q.Y.; Cheng, H.; Mao, X.H.; Lao, L.M.; Hao, G.L. Triptolide affects the differentiation, maturation and function of human dendritic cells. *Int. Immunopharmacol.* **2005**, *5*, 1415–1426. [CrossRef] [PubMed]

23.   Yan, Y.H.; Shang, P.Z.; Lu, Q.J.; Wu, X. Triptolide regulates T cell-mediated immunity via induction of CD11c(low) dendritic cell differentiation. *Food Chem. Toxicol.* **2012**, *50*, 2560–2564. [CrossRef] [PubMed]

24.   Liu, Q.; Chen, T.; Chen, G.; Li, N.; Wang, J.; Ma, P.; Cao, X. Immunosuppressant triptolide inhibits dendritic cell-mediated chemoattraction of neutrophils and T cells through inhibiting Stat3 phosphorylation and NF-κB activation. *Biochem. Biophys. Res. Commun.* **2006**, *345*, 1122–1130. [CrossRef] [PubMed]

25.   Choy, E.H.; Panayi, G.S. Cytokine pathways and joint inflammation in rheumatoid arthritis. *N. Engl. J. Med.* **2001**, *344*, 907–916. [CrossRef] [PubMed]

26.   Iwamoto, T.; Okamoto, H.; Toyama, Y.; Momohara, S. Molecular aspects of rheumatoid arthritis: Chemokines in the joints of patients. *FEBS J.* **2008**, *275*, 4448–4455. [CrossRef] [PubMed]

27.   Kim, W.U.; Kwok, S.K.; Hong, K.H.; Yoo, S.A.; Kong, J.S.; Choe, J.; Cho, C.S. Soluble Fas ligand inhibits angiogenesis in rheumatoid arthritis. *Arthritis Res. Ther.* **2007**, *9*, R42. [CrossRef] [PubMed]

28.   Harris, E.D., Jr. Rheumatoid arthritis. Pathophysiology and implications for therapy. *N. Engl. J. Med.* **1990**, *322*, 1277–1289. [PubMed]

29.   Sivalingam, S.P.; Thumboo, J.; Vasoo, S.; Thio, S.T.; Tse, C.; Fong, K.Y. In vivo pro- and anti-inflammatory cytokines in normal and patients with rheumatoid arthritis. *Ann. Acad. Med. Singap.* **2007**, *36*, 96–99. [PubMed]

30.   Koch, A.E. Angiogenesis as a target in rheumatoid arthritis. *Ann. Rheum. Dis.* **2003**, *62*, ii60–ii67. [CrossRef] [PubMed]

31. Xiao, C.; Zhou, J.; He, Y.; Jia, H.; Zhao, L.; Zhao, N.; Lu, A. Effects of triptolide from Radix *Tripterygium wilfordii* (Leigongteng) on cartilage cytokines and transcription factor NF-κB: A study on induced arthritis in rats. *Chin. Med.* **2009**, *4*, 13. [CrossRef] [PubMed]

32. Premkumar, V.; Dey, M.; Dorn, R.; Raskin, I. MyD88-dependent and independent pathways of Toll-Like Receptors are engaged in biological activity of Triptolide in ligand-stimulated macrophages. *BMC Chem. Biol.* **2010**, *10*, 3. [CrossRef] [PubMed]

33. Yifan, W.; Dengming, W.; Zheng, L.; Yanping, L.; Junkan, S. Triptolide inhibits CCR5 expressed in synovial tissue of rat adjuvant-induced arthritis. *Pharmacol. Rep.* **2007**, *59*, 795–799. [PubMed]

34. Wang, Y.; Wei, D.; Lai, Z.; Le, Y. Triptolide inhibits CC chemokines expressed in rat adjuvant-induced arthritis. *Int. Immunopharmacol.* **2006**, *6*, 1825–1832. [CrossRef] [PubMed]

35. Lin, N.; Liu, C.; Xiao, C.; Jia, H.; Imada, K.; Wu, H.; Ito, A. Triptolide, a diterpenoid triepoxide, suppresses inflammation and cartilage destruction in collagen-induced arthritis mice. *Biochem. Pharmacol.* **2007**, *73*, 136–146. [CrossRef] [PubMed]

36. Wang, B.; Ma, L.; Tao, X.; Lipsky, P.E. Triptolide, an active component of the Chinese herbal remedy Tripterygium wilfordii Hook F, inhibits production of nitric oxide by decreasing inducible nitric oxide synthase gene transcription. *Arthritis Rheum.* **2004**, *50*, 2995–3003. [CrossRef] [PubMed]

37. Bleharski, J.R.; Kiessler, V.; Buonsanti, C.; Sieling, P.A.; Stenger, S.; Colonna, M.; Modlin, R.L. A role for triggering receptor expressed on myeloid cells-1 in host defense during the early-induced and adaptive phases of the immune response. *J. Immunol.* **2003**, *170*, 3812–3818. [CrossRef] [PubMed]

38. Bouchon, A.; Dietrich, J.; Colonna, M. Cutting edge: Inflammatory responses can be triggered by TREM-1, a novel receptor expressed on neutrophils and monocytes. *J. Immunol.* **2000**, *164*, 4991–4995. [CrossRef] [PubMed]

39. Choi, S.T.; Kang, E.J.; Ha, Y.J.; Song, J.S. Levels of plasma-soluble triggering receptor expressed on myeloid cells-1 (sTREM-1) are correlated with disease activity in rheumatoid arthritis. *J. Rheumatol.* **2012**, *39*, 933–938. [CrossRef] [PubMed]

40. Fortin, C.F.; Lesur, O.; Fulop, T., Jr. Effects of TREM-1 activation in human neutrophils: Activation of signaling pathways, recruitment into lipid rafts and association with TLR4. *Int. Immunol.* **2007**, *19*, 41–50. [CrossRef] [PubMed]

41. Su, Z.; Sun, H.; Ao, M.; Zhao, C. Atomic Force Microscopy Study of the Anti-inflammatory Effects of Triptolide on Rheumatoid Arthritis Fibroblast-like Synoviocytes. *Microsc. Microanal.* **2017**, *23*, 1002–1012. [CrossRef] [PubMed]

42. Yang, Y.; Ye, Y.; Qiu, Q.; Xiao, Y.; Huang, M.; Shi, M.; Liang, L.; Yang, X.; Xu, H. Triptolide inhibits the migration and invasion of rheumatoid fibroblast-like synoviocytes by blocking the activation of the JNK MAPK pathway. *Int. Immunopharmacol.* **2016**, *41*, 8–16. [CrossRef] [PubMed]

43. Liacini, A.; Sylvester, J.; Zafarullah, M. Triptolide suppresses proinflammatory cytokine-induced matrix metalloproteinase and aggrecanase-1 gene expression in chondrocytes. *Biochem. Biophys. Res. Commun.* **2005**, *327*, 320–327. [CrossRef] [PubMed]

44. Lin, N.; Sato, T.; Ito, A. Triptolide, a novel diterpenoid triepoxide from Tripterygium wilfordii Hook. f., suppresses the production and gene expression of pro-matrix metalloproteinases 1 and 3 and augments those of tissue inhibitors of metalloproteinases 1 and 2 in human synovial fibroblasts. *Arthritis Rheum.* **2001**, *44*, 2193–2200. [PubMed]

45. Lu, Y.; Wang, W.J.; Leng, J.H.; Cheng, L.F.; Feng, L.; Yao, H.P. Inhibitory effect of triptolide on interleukin-18 and its receptor in rheumatoid arthritis synovial fibroblasts. *Inflamm. Res.* **2008**, *57*, 260–265. [CrossRef] [PubMed]

46. Van Roon, J.A.; van Roy, J.L.; Gmelig-Meyling, F.H.; Lafeber, F.P.; Bijlsma, J.W. Prevention and reversal of cartilage degradation in rheumatoid arthritis by interleukin-10 and interleukin-4. *Arthritis Rheum.* **1996**, *39*, 829–835. [CrossRef] [PubMed]

47. Sugiyama, E.; Kuroda, A.; Taki, H.; Ikemoto, M.; Hori, T.; Yamashita, N.; Maruyama, M.; Kobayashi, M. Interleukin 10 cooperates with interleukin 4 to suppress inflammatory cytokine production by freshly prepared adherent rheumatoid synovial cells. *J. Rheumatol.* **1995**, *22*, 2020–2026. [PubMed]

48. Szekanecz, Z.; Koch, A.E. Vascular involvement in rheumatic diseases: "vascular rheumatology". *Arthritis Res. Ther.* **2008**, *10*, 224. [CrossRef] [PubMed]

49. Lainer-Carr, D.; Brahn, E. Angiogenesis inhibition as a therapeutic approach for inflammatory synovitis. *Nat. Clin. Pract. Rheumatol.* **2007**, *3*, 434–442. [CrossRef] [PubMed]
50. Koch, A.E. Review: Angiogenesis: Implications for rheumatoid arthritis. *Arthritis Rheum.* **1998**, *41*, 951–962. [CrossRef]
51. Veale, D.J.; Fearon, U. Inhibition of angiogenic pathways in rheumatoid arthritis: Potential for therapeutic targeting. *Best Pract. Res. Clin. Rheumatol.* **2006**, *20*, 941–947. [CrossRef] [PubMed]
52. Kong, X.; Zhang, Y.; Liu, C.; Guo, W.; Li, X.; Su, X.; Wan, H.; Sun, Y.; Lin, N. Anti-angiogenic effect of triptolide in rheumatoid arthritis by targeting angiogenic cascade. *PLoS ONE* **2013**, *8*, e77513. [CrossRef] [PubMed]
53. He, M.F.; Huang, Y.H.; Wu, L.W.; Ge, W.; Shaw, P.C.; But, P.P. Triptolide functions as a potent angiogenesis inhibitor. *Int. J. Cancer* **2010**, *126*, 266–278. [CrossRef] [PubMed]
54. Liu, C.; Zhang, Y.; Kong, X.; Zhu, L.; Pang, J.; Xu, Y.; Chen, W.; Zhan, H.; Lu, A.; Lin, N. Triptolide Prevents Bone Destruction in the Collagen-Induced Arthritis Model of Rheumatoid Arthritis by Targeting RANKL/RANK/OPG Signal Pathway. *Evid. Based Complement. Altern. Med.* **2013**, *2013*, 626038. [CrossRef] [PubMed]
55. Luo, C.Y.; Wang, L.; Sun, C.; Li, D.J. Estrogen enhances the functions of CD4$^+$CD25$^+$Foxp3$^+$ regulatory T cells that suppress osteoclast differentiation and bone resorption in vitro. *Cell. Mol. Immunol.* **2011**, *8*, 50–58. [CrossRef] [PubMed]
56. Liu, S.P.; Wang, G.D.; Du, X.J.; Wan, G.; Wu, J.T.; Miao, L.B.; Liang, Q.D. Triptolide inhibits the function of TNF-α in osteoblast differentiation by inhibiting the NF-κB signaling pathway. *Exp. Ther. Med.* **2017**, *14*, 2235–2240. [CrossRef] [PubMed]
57. Cooles, F.A.; Isaacs, J.D. Pathophysiology of rheumatoid arthritis. *Curr. Opin. Rheumatol.* **2011**, *23*, 233–240. [CrossRef] [PubMed]
58. Noss, E.H.; Brenner, M.B. The role and therapeutic implications of fibroblast-like synoviocytes in inflammation and cartilage erosion in rheumatoid arthritis. *Immunol. Rev.* **2008**, *223*, 252–270. [CrossRef] [PubMed]
59. Bartok, B.; Firestein, G.S. Fibroblast-like synoviocytes: Key effector cells in rheumatoid arthritis. *Immunol. Rev.* **2010**, *233*, 233–255. [CrossRef] [PubMed]
60. Kusunoki, N.; Yamazaki, R.; Kitasato, H.; Beppu, M.; Aoki, H.; Kawai, S. Triptolide, an active compound identified in a traditional Chinese herb, induces apoptosis of rheumatoid synovial fibroblasts. *BMC Pharmacol.* **2004**, *4*, 2. [CrossRef] [PubMed]
61. Bao, X.; Cui, J.; Wu, Y.; Han, X.; Gao, C.; Hua, Z.; Shen, P. The roles of endogenous reactive oxygen species and nitric oxide in triptolide-induced apoptotic cell death in macrophages. *J. Mol. Med.* **2007**, *85*, 85–98. [CrossRef] [PubMed]
62. Yang, F.; Bai, X.J.; Hu, D.; Li, Z.F.; Liu, K.J. Effect of triptolide on secretion of inflammatory cellular factors TNF-α and IL-8 in peritoneal macrophages of mice activated by lipopolysaccharide. *World J. Emerg. Med.* **2010**, *1*, 70–74. [PubMed]
63. Wang, X.; Jiang, Z.; Cao, W.; Yuan, Z.; Sun, L.; Zhang, L. Th17/Treg imbalance in triptolide-induced liver injury. *Fitoterapia* **2014**, *93*, 245–251. [CrossRef] [PubMed]
64. Li, J.; Shen, F.; Guan, C.; Wang, W.; Sun, X.; Fu, X.; Huang, M.; Jin, J.; Huang, Z. Activation of Nrf2 protects against triptolide-induced hepatotoxicity. *PLoS ONE* **2014**, *9*, e100685. [CrossRef] [PubMed]
65. Lu, J.; Jiang, F.; Lu, A.; Zhang, G. Linkers Having a Crucial Role in Antibody-Drug Conjugates. *Int. J. Mol. Sci.* **2016**, *17*, 561. [CrossRef] [PubMed]
66. Xu, L.; Qiu, Y.; Xu, H.; Ao, W.; Lam, W.; Yang, X. Acute and subacute toxicity studies on triptolide and triptolide-loaded polymeric micelles following intravenous administration in rodents. *Food Chem. Toxicol.* **2013**, *57*, 371–379. [CrossRef] [PubMed]
67. Fu, Q.; Huang, X.; Shu, B.; Xue, M.; Zhang, P.; Wang, T.; Liu, L.; Jiang, Z.; Zhang, L. Inhibition of mitochondrial respiratory chain is involved in triptolide-induced liver injury. *Fitoterapia* **2011**, *82*, 1241–1248. [CrossRef] [PubMed]
68. Yang, J.; Sun, L.; Wang, L.; Hassan, H.M.; Wang, X.; Hylemon, P.B.; Wang, T.; Zhou, H.; Zhang, L.; Jiang, Z. Activation of Sirt1/FXR Signaling Pathway Attenuates Triptolide-Induced Hepatotoxicity in Rats. *Front. Pharmacol.* **2017**, *8*, 260. [CrossRef] [PubMed]

69. Lu, Y.; Xie, T.; Zhang, Y.; Zhou, F.; Ruan, J.; Zhu, W.; Zhu, H.; Feng, Z.; Zhou, X. Triptolide Induces hepatotoxicity via inhibition of CYP450s in Rat liver microsomes. *BMC Complement. Altern. Med.* **2017**, *17*, 15. [CrossRef] [PubMed]

70. Yang, F.; Ren, L.; Zhuo, L.; Ananda, S.; Liu, L. Involvement of oxidative stress in the mechanism of triptolide-induced acute nephrotoxicity in rats. *Exp. Toxicol. Pathol.* **2012**, *64*, 905–911. [CrossRef] [PubMed]

71. Yang, F.; Zhuo, L.; Ananda, S.; Sun, T.; Li, S.; Liu, L. Role of reactive oxygen species in triptolide-induced apoptosis of renal tubular cells and renal injury in rats. *J. Huazhong Univ. Sci. Technol.* **2011**, *31*, 335–341. [CrossRef] [PubMed]

72. Liu, J.; Jiang, Z.; Liu, L.; Zhang, Y.; Zhang, S.; Xiao, J.; Ma, M.; Zhang, L. Triptolide induces adverse effect on reproductive parameters of female Sprague-Dawley rats. *Drug Chem. Toxicol.* **2011**, *34*, 1–7. [CrossRef] [PubMed]

73. Ni, B.; Jiang, Z.; Huang, X.; Xu, F.; Zhang, R.; Zhang, Z.; Tian, Y.; Wang, T.; Zhu, T.; Liu, J.; et al. Male Reproductive Toxicity and Toxicokinetics of Triptolide in Rats. *Arzneimittelforschung* **2008**, *58*, 673–680. [CrossRef] [PubMed]

74. Zhang, J.; Liu, L.; Mu, X.; Jiang, Z.; Zhang, L. Effect of triptolide on estradiol release from cultured rat granulosa cells. *Endocr. J.* **2012**, *59*, 473–481. [CrossRef] [PubMed]

75. Zhang, J.; Jiang, Z.; Mu, X.; Wen, J.; Su, Y.; Zhang, L. Effect of triptolide on progesterone production from cultured rat granulosa cells. *Arzneimittelforschung* **2012**, *62*, 301–306. [CrossRef] [PubMed]

76. Guo, W.; Hu, S.; Elgehama, A.; Shao, F.; Ren, R.; Liu, W.; Zhang, W.; Wang, X.; Tan, R.; Xu, Q.; et al. Fumigaclavine C ameliorates dextran sulfate sodium-induced murine experimental colitis via NLRP3 inflammasome inhibition. *J. Pharmacol. Sci.* **2015**, *129*, 101–106. [CrossRef] [PubMed]

77. Wang, H.; Huang, G.Z.; Zheng, N.; Liu, L. Injury of myocadium of rats by acute triptolide poisoning. *ICI World J.* **2010**, *24*, 460–465.

78. Zhang, C.; Gu, C.; Peng, F.; Liu, W.; Wan, J.; Xu, H.; Lam, W.C.; Yang, X. Preparation and Optimization of Triptolide-Loaded Solid Lipid Nanoparticles for Oral Delivery with Reduced Gastric Irritation. *Molecules* **2013**, *18*, 13340–13356. [CrossRef] [PubMed]

79. Xue, X.; Gong, L.; Qi, X.; Wu, Y.; Xing, G.; Yao, J.; Luan, Y.; Xiao, Y.; Li, Y.; Wu, X.; et al. Knockout of hepatic P450 reductase aggravates triptolide-induced toxicity. *Toxicol. Lett.* **2011**, *205*, 47–54. [CrossRef] [PubMed]

80. Liu, L.; Jiang, Z.; Liu, J.; Huang, X.; Wang, T.; Liu, J.; Zhang, Y.; Zhou, Z.; Guo, J.; Yang, L.; et al. Sex differences in subacute toxicity and hepatic microsomal metabolism of triptolide in rats. *Toxicology* **2010**, *271*, 57–63. [CrossRef] [PubMed]

81. Liu, Q. Triptolide and its expanding multiple pharmacological functions. *Int. Immunopharmacol.* **2011**, *11*, 377–383. [CrossRef] [PubMed]

82. Tai, T.; Huang, X.; Su, Y.; Ji, J.; Su, Y.; Jiang, Z.; Zhang, L. Glycyrrhizin accelerates the metabolism of triptolide through induction of CYP3A in rats. *J. Ethnopharmacol.* **2014**, *152*, 358–363. [CrossRef] [PubMed]

83. Zhang, C.; Sun, P.P.; Guo, H.T.; Liu, Y.; Li, J.; He, X.J.; Lu, A.P. Corrigendum: Safety Profiles of Tripterygium wilfordii Hook F: A Systematic Review and Meta-Analysis. *Front. Pharmacol.* **2017**, *8*, 59. [CrossRef] [PubMed]

84. Wang, L.; Xu, Y.; Fu, L.; Li, Y.; Lou, L. (5R)-5-hydroxytriptolide (LLDT-8), a novel immunosuppressant in clinical trials, exhibits potent antitumor activity via transcription inhibition. *Cancer Lett.* **2012**, *324*, 75–82. [CrossRef] [PubMed]

85. Fidler, J.M.; Li, K.; Chung, C.; Wei, K.; Ross, J.A.; Gao, M.; Rosen, G.D. PG490-88, a derivative of triptolide, causes tumor regression and sensitizes tumors to chemotherapy. *Mol. Cancer Ther.* **2003**, *2*, 855–862. [PubMed]

86. Wu, D.D.; Huang, L.; Zhang, L.; Wu, L.-Y.; Li, Y.-C.; Feng, L. LLDT-67 attenuates MPTP-induced neurotoxicity in mice by up-regulating NGF expression. *Acta Pharmacol. Sin.* **2012**, *33*, 1187–1194. [CrossRef] [PubMed]

87. Xu, H.; Fan, X.; Zhang, G.; Liu, X.; Li, Z.; Li, Y.; Jiang, B. LLDT-288, a novel triptolide analogue exhibits potent antitumor activity in vitro and in vivo. *Biomed. Pharmacother.* **2017**, *93*, 1004–1009. [CrossRef] [PubMed]

88. Tang, W.; Zuo, J.P. Immunosuppressant discovery from Tripterygium wilfordii Hook f: The novel triptolide analog (5R)-5-hydroxytriptolide (LLDT-8). *Acta Pharmacol. Sin.* **2012**, *33*, 1112–1118. [CrossRef] [PubMed]

89. Zhou, R.; Tang, W.; Ren, Y.-X.; He, P.-L.; Zhang, F.; Shi, L.-P.; Fu, Y.-F.; Li, Y.-C.; Ono, S.; Fujiwara, H.; et al. (5R)-5-hydroxytriptolide attenuated collagen-induced arthritis in DBA/1 mice via suppressing interferon-γ production and its related signaling. *J. Pharmacol. Exp. Ther.* **2006**, *318*, 35–44. [CrossRef] [PubMed]

90. Zhou, R.; Tang, W.; He, P.-L.; Li, X.-Y.; Yang, Y.-F.; Li, Y.-C.; Geng, J.-G.; Zuo, J.-P. Inhibition of inducible nitric-oxide synthase expression by (5R)-5-hydroxytriptolide in interferon-γ- and bacterial lipopolysaccharide-stimulated macrophages. *J. Pharmacol. Exp. Ther.* **2006**, *316*, 121–128. [CrossRef] [PubMed]

91. Fu, Y.F.; Ni, J.; Zhong, X.-G.; Tang, W.; Zhou, R.; Zhou, Y.; Dong, J.-R.; He, P.-L.; Wan, H.; Li, Y.-C.; et al. (5R)-5-hydroxytriptolide (LLDT-8), a novel triptolide derivative, prevents experimental autoimmune encephalomyelitis via inhibiting T cell activation. *J. Neuroimmunol.* **2006**, *175*, 142–151. [CrossRef] [PubMed]

92. Banerjee, S.; Modi, S.; McGinn, O.; Zhao, X.; Dudeja, V.; Ramakrishnan, S.; Saluja, A.K. Impaired Synthesis of Stromal Components in Response to Minnelide Improves Vascular Function, Drug Delivery, and Survival in Pancreatic Cancer. *Clin. Cancer Res.* **2016**, *22*, 415–425. [CrossRef] [PubMed]

93. Carter, B.Z.; Shi, Y.; Fidler, J.M.; Chen, R.; Ling, X.; Plunkett, W.; Andreeff, M. MRx102, a triptolide derivative, has potent antileukemic activity in vitro and in a murine model of AML. *Leukemia* **2012**, *26*, 443–450. [CrossRef] [PubMed]

94. Lin, C.H.; Chen, C.H.; Lin, Z.C.; Fang, J.Y. Recent advances in oral delivery of drugs and bioactive natural products using solid lipid nanoparticles as the carriers. *J. Food Drug Anal.* **2017**, *25*, 219–234. [CrossRef] [PubMed]

95. Callender, S.P.; Mathews, J.A.; Kobernyk, K.; Wettig, S.D. Microemulsion utility in pharmaceuticals: Implications for multi-drug delivery. *Int. J. Pharm.* **2017**, *526*, 425–442. [CrossRef] [PubMed]

96. Chen, G.; Hao, B.; Ju, D.; Liu, M.; Zhao, H.; Du, Z.; Xia, J. Pharmacokinetic and pharmacodynamic study of triptolide-loaded liposome hydrogel patch under microneedles on rats with collagen-induced arthritis. *Acta Pharm. Sin. B* **2015**, *5*, 569–576. [CrossRef] [PubMed]

97. Zhang, L.; Wang, T.; Li, Q.; Huang, J.; Xu, H.; Li, J.; Wang, Y.; Liang, Q. Fabrication of novel vesicles of triptolide for antirheumatoid activity with reduced toxicity in vitro and in vivo. *Int. J. Nanomed.* **2016**, *11*, 2663–2673.

98. Liu, M.; Dong, J.; Yang, Y.; Yang, X.; Xu, H. Anti-inflammatory effects of triptolide loaded poly(D,L-lactic acid) nanoparticles on adjuvant-induced arthritis in rats. *J. Ethnopharmacol.* **2005**, *97*, 219–225. [CrossRef] [PubMed]

99. Liu, M.; Dong, J.; Yang, Y.; Yang, X.; Xu, H. Effect of poly(D,L-lactic acid) nanoparticles as triptolide carrier on abating rats renal toxicity by NMR-based metabolic analysis. *J. Nanosci. Nanotechnol.* **2008**, *8*, 3493–3499. [CrossRef] [PubMed]

100. Mei, Z.; Wu, Q.; Hu, S.; Li, X.; Yang, X. Triptolide loaded solid lipid nanoparticle hydrogel for topical application. *Drug Dev. Ind. Pharm.* **2005**, *31*, 161–168. [CrossRef] [PubMed]

101. Mei, Z.; Chen, H.; Weng, T.; Yang, Y.; Yang, X. Solid lipid nanoparticle and microemulsion for topical delivery of triptolide. *Eur. J. Pharm. Biopharm.* **2003**, *56*, 189–196. [CrossRef]

102. Mei, Z.; Li, X.; Wu, Q.; Hu, S.; Yang, X. The research on the anti-inflammatory activity and hepatotoxicity of triptolide-loaded solid lipid nanoparticle. *Pharmacol. Res.* **2005**, *51*, 345–351. [CrossRef] [PubMed]

103. Xue, M.; Zhao, Y.; Li, X.-J.; Jiang, Z.-Z.; Zhang, L.; Liu, S.-H.; Li, X.-M.; Zhang, L.-Y.; Yang, S.-Y. Comparison of toxicokinetic and tissue distribution of triptolide-loaded solid lipid nanoparticles vs free triptolide in rats. *Eur. J. Pharm. Sci.* **2012**, *47*, 713–717. [CrossRef] [PubMed]

104. Zhang, C.; Peng, F.; Liu, W.; Wan, J.; Wan, C.; Xu, H.; Lam, C.W.; Yang, X. Nanostructured lipid carriers as a novel oral delivery system for triptolide: Induced changes in pharmacokinetics profile associated with reduced toxicity in male rats. *Int. J. Nanomed.* **2014**, *9*, 1049–1063.

105. Xu, L.; Pan, J.; Chen, Q.; Yu, Q.; Chen, H.; Xu, H.; Qiu, Y.; Yang, X. In vivo evaluation of the safety of triptolide-loaded hydrogel-thickened microemulsion. *Food Chem. Toxicol.* **2008**, *46*, 3792–3799. [CrossRef] [PubMed]

106. Mehnert, W.; Mader, K. Solid lipid nanoparticles: Production, characterization and applications. *Adv. Drug Deliv. Rev.* **2001**, *47*, 165–196. [CrossRef]

107. zur Muhlen, A.; Schwarz, C.; Mehnert, W. Solid lipid nanoparticles (SLN) for controlled drug delivery—Drug release and release mechanism. *Eur. J. Pharm. Biopharm.* **1998**, *45*, 149–155. [CrossRef]

108. Kogan, A.; Garti, N. Microemulsions as transdermal drug delivery vehicles. *Adv. Colloid Interface Sci.* **2006**, *123–126*, 369–385. [CrossRef] [PubMed]

109. Chen, H.; Chang, X.; Weng, T.; Zhao, X.; Gao, Z.; Yang, Y.; Xu, H.; Yang, X. A study of microemulsion systems for transdermal delivery of triptolide. *J. Control Release* **2004**, *98*, 427–436. [CrossRef] [PubMed]

110. He, B.; Lu, C.; Zheng, G.; He, X.; Wang, M.; Chen, G.; Zhang, G.; Lu, A. Combination therapeutics in complex diseases. *J. Cell. Mol. Med.* **2016**, *20*, 2231–2240. [CrossRef] [PubMed]

111. Ye, X.; Li, W.; Yan, Y.; Mao, C.; Cai, R.; Xu, H.; Yang, X. Effects of cytochrome P4503A inducer dexamethasone on the metabolism and toxicity of triptolide in rat. *Toxicol. Lett.* **2010**, *192*, 212–220. [CrossRef] [PubMed]

112. Cao, L.; Ding, W.; Jia, R.; Du, J.; Wang, T.; Zhang, C.; Gu, Z.; Yin, G. Anti-inflammatory and hepatoprotective effects of glycyrrhetinic acid on CCl4-induced damage in precision-cut liver slices from Jian carp (Cyprinus carpio var. jian) through inhibition of the NF-κB pathway. *Fish Shellfish Immunol.* **2017**, *64*, 234–242. [CrossRef] [PubMed]

113. Qiu, D.; Kao, P.N. Immunosuppressive and anti-inflammatory mechanisms of triptolide, the principal active diterpenoid from the Chinese medicinal herb *Tripterygium wilfordii* Hook. f. *Drugs R D* **2003**, *4*, 1–18. [CrossRef] [PubMed]

114. Chen, B.J. Triptolide, a novel immunosuppressive and anti-inflammatory agent purified from a Chinese herb Tripterygium wilfordii Hook F. *Leuk. Lymphoma* **2001**, *42*, 253–265. [CrossRef] [PubMed]

115. Feng, X.; Ding, L.; Qiu, F. Potential drug interactions associated with glycyrrhizin and glycyrrhetinic acid. *Drug Metab. Rev.* **2015**, *47*, 229–238. [CrossRef] [PubMed]

116. Shao, F.; Wang, G.; Xie, H.; Zhu, X.; Sun, J.; A, J. Pharmacokinetic study of triptolide, a constituent of immunosuppressive chinese herb medicine, in rats. *Biol. Pharm. Bull.* **2007**, *30*, 702–707. [CrossRef] [PubMed]

117. Kong, L.-L.; zhuang, X.-M.; Yang, H.-Y.; Yuan, M.; Xu, L.; Li, H. Inhibition of P-glycoprotein Gene Expression and Function Enhances Triptolide-induced Hepatotoxicity in Mice. *Sci. Rep.* **2015**, *5*, 11747. [CrossRef] [PubMed]

118. Han, F.M.; Peng, Z.H.; Wang, J.J.; Chen, Y. In vivo effect of triptolide combined with glycyrrhetinic acid on rat cytochrome P450 enzymes. *Yao Xue Xue Bao* **2013**, *48*, 1136–1141. [PubMed]

119. Li, Z.; Yan, M.; Cao, L.; Fang, P.; Guo, Z.; Hou, Z.; Zhang, B. Glycyrrhetinic Acid Accelerates the Clearance of Triptolide through P-gp In Vitro. *Phytother. Res.* **2017**, *31*, 1090–1096. [CrossRef] [PubMed]

120. Arafa, H.M. Uroprotective effects of curcumin in cyclophosphamide-induced haemorrhagic cystitis paradigm. *Basic Clin. Pharmacol. Toxicol.* **2009**, *104*, 393–399. [CrossRef] [PubMed]

121. Wang, L.; Huang, Q.H.; Li, Y.X.; Huang, Y.F.; Xie, J.H.; Xu, L.Q.; Dou, Y.X.; Su, Z.R.; Zeng, H.F.; Chen, J.N. Protective effects of silymarin on triptolide-induced acute hepatotoxicity in rats. *Mol. Med. Rep.* **2018**, *17*, 789–800. [CrossRef] [PubMed]

122. Yuan, Z.X.; Jia, L.; Lim, L.Y.; Lin, J.C.; Shu, G.; Zhao, L.; Ye, G.; Liang, X.X.; Ji, H.; Fu, H.L. Renal-targeted delivery of triptolide by entrapment in pegylated TRX-20-modified liposomes. *Int. J. Nanomed.* **2017**, *12*, 5673–5686. [CrossRef] [PubMed]

123. Yuan, Z.X.; Wu, X.J.; Mo, J.; Wang, Y.L.; Xu, C.Q.; Lim, L.Y. Renal targeted delivery of triptolide by conjugation to the fragment peptide of human serum albumin. *Eur. J. Pharm. Biopharm.* **2015**, *94*, 363–371. [CrossRef] [PubMed]

124. Fu, Y.; Lin, Q.; Gong, T.; Sun, X.; Zhang, Z.R. Renal-targeting triptolide-glucosamine conjugate exhibits lower toxicity and superior efficacy in attenuation of ischemia/reperfusion renal injury in rats. *Acta Pharmacol. Sin.* **2016**, *37*, 1467–1480. [CrossRef] [PubMed]

125. Zhang, Z.; Zheng, Q.; Han, J.; Gao, G.; Liu, J.; Gong, T.; Gu, Z.; Huang, Y.; Sun, X.; He, Q. The targeting of 14-succinate triptolide-lysozyme conjugate to proximal renal tubular epithelial cells. *Biomaterials* **2009**, *30*, 1372–1381. [CrossRef] [PubMed]

126. Lin, C.; Wong, B.C.K.; Chen, H.; Bian, Z.; Zhang, G.; Zhang, X.; Kashif Riaz, M.; Tyagi, D.; Lin, G.; Zhang, Y.; et al. Pulmonary delivery of triptolide-loaded liposomes decorated with anti-carbonic anhydrase IX antibody for lung cancer therapy. *Sci. Rep.* **2017**, *7*, 1097. [CrossRef] [PubMed]

127. Wang, C.; Liu, B.; Xu, X.; Zhuang, B.; Li, H.; Yin, J.; Cong, M.; Xu, W.; Lu, A. Toward targeted therapy in chemotherapy-resistant pancreatic cancer with a smart triptolide nanomedicine. *Oncotarget* **2016**, *7*, 8360–8372. [CrossRef] [PubMed]

128. Ling, D.; Xia, H.; Park, W.; Hackett, M.J.; Song, C.; Na, K.; Hui, K.M.; Hyeon, T. pH-sensitive nanoformulated triptolide as a targeted therapeutic strategy for hepatocellular carcinoma. *ACS Nano* **2014**, *8*, 8027–8039. [CrossRef] [PubMed]

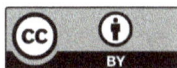

International Journal of
Molecular Sciences

MDPI

Review

The Biological Enhancement of Spinal Fusion for Spinal Degenerative Disease

Takahiro Makino, Hiroyuki Tsukazaki, Yuichiro Ukon, Daisuke Tateiwa, Hideki Yoshikawa and Takashi Kaito *

Department of Orthopedic Surgery, Osaka University Graduate School of Medicine, 2-2 Yamadaoka, Suita, Osaka 565-0871, Japan; t-makino@za2.so-net.ne.jp (T.M.); tsukazaki.hiroyuki@gmail.com (H.T.); gonza721ukon@yahoo.co.jp (Y.U.); tateiwa.daisuke1@gmail.com (D.T.); yhideki@ort.med.osaka-u.ac.jp (H.Y.)
* Correspondence: takashikaito@ort.med.osaka-u.ac.jp; Tel.: +81-6-6879-3552

Received: 7 June 2018; Accepted: 14 August 2018; Published: 17 August 2018

check for
updates

Abstract: In this era of aging societies, the number of elderly individuals who undergo spinal arthrodesis for various degenerative diseases is increasing. Poor bone quality and osteogenic ability in older patients, due to osteoporosis, often interfere with achieving bone fusion after spinal arthrodesis. Enhancement of bone fusion requires shifting bone homeostasis toward increased bone formation and reduced resorption. Several biological enhancement strategies of bone formation have been conducted in animal models of spinal arthrodesis and human clinical trials. Pharmacological agents for osteoporosis have also been shown to be effective in enhancing bone fusion. Cytokines, which activate bone formation, such as bone morphogenetic proteins, have already been clinically used to enhance bone fusion for spinal arthrodesis. Recently, stem cells have attracted considerable attention as a cell source of osteoblasts, promising effects in enhancing bone fusion. Drug delivery systems will also need to be further developed to assure the safe delivery of bone-enhancing agents to the site of spinal arthrodesis. Our aim in this review is to appraise the current state of knowledge and evidence regarding bone enhancement strategies for spinal fusion for degenerative spinal disorders, and to identify future directions for biological bone enhancement strategies, including pharmacological, cell and gene therapy approaches.

Keywords: spinal fusion; biological; osteoblast; osteoclast; bisphosphonate; parathyroid hormone; bone morphogenetic protein; receptor activator of nuclear factor κB; stem cell; drug delivery system

1. Introduction

Spinal arthrodesis is one of the most common surgical procedures used for the treatment of various spinal pathologies, such as spinal deformity, spondylolisthesis, foraminal stenosis, or disc disease. A nationwide epidemiological study in the United States reported a 2.4-fold increase in the number of spinal fusion surgeries performed between 1998 and 2008 [1]. Various techniques were reported for performing spinal arthrodesis, including different surgical approaches, graft materials used, and the instrumentation method. However, whichever spinal arthrodesis technique is performed, the fundamental aim is to achieve bony fusion at a mobile segment after the transplantation of autologous, allogeneic or artificial bone graft, and to induce bone modeling and remodeling. The insufficiency of bony fusion or pseudoarthrosis/non-union after spinal arthrodesis can cause a loss of correction and instrumentation failure or deterioration of patients' quality of life (QOL) [2–6]. Thus, early and successful bony fusion can provide better radiological and clinical outcomes.

In many countries, the segment of the general population over the age of 60 years have been continuously growing [7]. In these aging societies, the prevalence of degenerative spinal disorders is increasing, and the number of older patients who undergo spinal fusion surgeries is also increasing.

Deyo et al. [8] reported that the rates of lumbar fusion surgery among patients over the age of 60 years have increased by 230% between 1988 and 2001 in the United States. Rajaee et al. [1] also reported that the rate of spinal fusion surgery among patients over the age of 65 years has increased by 239.2% between 1998 and 2008 in the United States. In these older individuals, low bone quality or osteoporosis is a great concern for achieving bone fusion after spinal arthrodesis. Instrumentation failure and the low osteogenic quality of autologous bone grafts due to osteoporosis may prevent achieving bone fusion.

The process of bone fusion after spinal arthrodesis relies principally on bone remodeling, following adequate bone grafting at fusion sites to prove the scaffold. This process progresses through a complex bone metabolism and relies heavily on osteoblasts, osteoclasts, and osteocytes, with the balance of activity between these two cell types being auto-regulated by metabolic, endocrine, and mechanical signaling pathways, similar to the fracture healing process (Figure 1) [9–11]. Boden et al. [12] reported that the histological bone fusion process of posterolateral fusion in rabbits, stating that the membranous bone formation began primarily, and increased volume of woven bone and endochondral ossification were seen subsequently at the bone grafted site. As for vertebral interbody fusion, the local environment of intervertebral space is originally hypo-vascular and of a low nutrient condition. Furthermore, this unfavorable environment becomes exacerbated by degenerative changes. Therefore, the accomplishment of bone fusion at intervertebral space is more demanding biologically compared to posterolateral fusion.

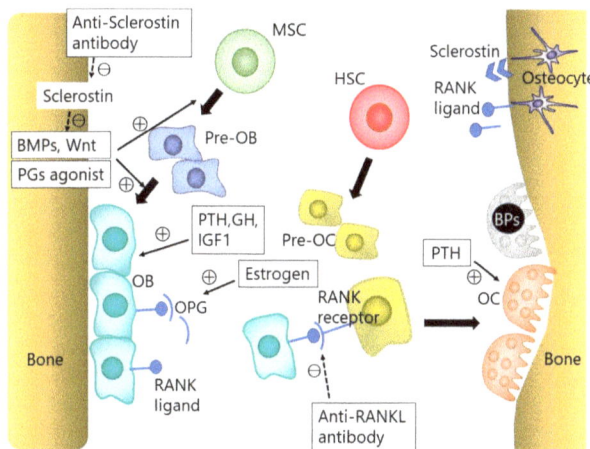

Figure 1. The osteoblast (OB) and osteoclast (OC) lineage cells. Bone homeostasis is maintained by the interaction between osteoblasts, osteoclasts, and osteocytes. Osteoblasts arise from mesenchymal stem cells (MSCs), and osteoclasts from hematopoietic stem cells (HSCs). Osteoblasts can also become osteocytes. Bone morphogenetic proteins (BMPs) and Wnt signaling play an important role in osteoblastogenesis. The receptor activator of nuclear factor κB ligand (RANKL)-RANK interaction is essential for osteoclast differentiation. The RANKL produced by osteoblasts and osteocytes binds to RANK on the osteoclast precursor cells, which triggers the differentiations into osteoclasts. Osteoblast lineage cells also express osteoprotegerin (OPG), which is a soluble decoy receptor of RANKL, blocking RANKL by binding to its cellular receptor RANK. This RANKL-RANK-OPG system plays an important role in bone homeostasis. BP indicates bisphosphonate; GH, growth hormone; IGF1, insulin-like growth factor 1; PG, prostaglandin; PTH, parathyroid hormone.

Osteoblasts are derived from undifferentiated mesenchymal cells. Runt-related transcription factor 2 (Runx2), also described as the core-binding factor subunit alpha-1 (Cbfa1), is necessary to differentiate osteoblasts from undifferentiated mesenchymal precursor cells [13]. Bone morphogenetic proteins (BMPs), Wnt, and the Notch signaling pathways all play important roles in the differentiation of osteoblasts, by regulating the transcription of Runx2 [14–16]. BMP signaling, particularly by BMP2 and BMP4, stimulates osteoblast differentiation and function by the activation of Runx2 via SMAD1/5/8. Wnt signaling also stimulates osteoblast differentiation by the activation of Runx2 through either β-catenin stabilization or protein kinase Cδ (PKCδ) (Figure 2). In contrast, Notch signaling inhibits the activity of Runx2 and osteoblast differentiation. Besides these local regulatory signal pathways, osteoblast lineage cell development is also regulated by systemic signals such as Leptin, the parathyroid hormone (PTH), growth hormone, or insulin-like growth factor 1, and sex hormones.

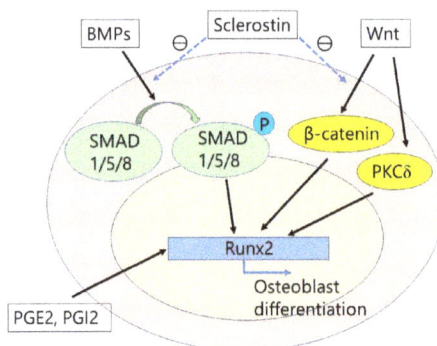

Figure 2. The integration of bone morphogenetic proteins (BMPs) and Wnt signaling. BMPs stimulate osteoblast differentiation by activation of Runx2 via SMAD proteins. Wnt signaling also stimulates osteoblast differentiation by activation of Runx2 through either β-catenin stabilization or protein kinase Cδ (PKCδ). Prostaglandins (PGs), particularly PGE2 and PGI2, also activates Runx2, which results in osteoblast differentiation. In contrast, sclerostin inhibits BMP signaling and Wnt/β-catenin signaling. Therefore, the anti-sclerostin antibody can stimulate osteoblast differentiation.

Osteoclasts are giant multinucleated cells which resorb the calcified matrix by secreting acids and collagenolytic enzymes. Osteoclasts are differentiated from hematopoietic cells. The bone marrow is considered to be the site of osteoclast generation, whereas the exact process of osteoclast generation in vivo is still unclear [17]. The receptor activator of nuclear factor κB ligand (RANKL)-RANK interaction is essential for osteoclast differentiation. The RANKL produced by osteoblasts and osteocytes binds to RANK on the osteoclast precursor cells, which triggers the differentiations into osteoclasts. Osteoblast lineage cells also express osteoprotegerin (OPG), which is a soluble decoy receptor of RANKL by blocking RANKL binding to its cellular receptor RANK [18]. Thus, the overexpression of OPG inhibits osteoclastogenesis by RANKL-RANK interaction. This RANKL-RANK-OPG system plays an important role in bone homeostasis through osteoclast regulation (Figure 1) [19].

Bone fusion after spinal arthrodesis can be achieved when the balance of bone homeostasis shifts into an increased bone formation and reduced resorption at the site of bone grafting, though many factors such as age, sex, the spinal fusion procedure, and pre-existing co-morbidities can affect the progress of bone fusion clinically. Therefore, promoting osteoblast activity and/or inhibiting osteoclast activity through the use of biological agents is a feasible approach for promoting successful fusion after spinal arthrodesis, particularly for osteoporotic patients, in addition to the development of biomaterials with high osteogenic properties and improvement in spinal operative and instrumentation techniques. This review is designed to appraise the current methods, and future directions, for the biological enhancement of spinal fusion for degenerative spinal disorders, including pharmacological, cell and gene therapy approaches (Table 1).

Table 1. The summary of approaches for biological enhancement of spinal fusion identified in this review.

	Mechanism of Action	Effect on Bone Metabolism	Clinical Trials for Human Spinal Fusion	Effect on Fusion in Animal Models	Effect on Fusion in Human
Bisphosphonates	Involved in osteoclasts and induction of apoptosis of osteoclasts	Inhibition of bone resorption	Yes	Yes	Controversial
Anti-RANKL monoclonal antibody	Prevention of the interaction between RANKL and RANK receptor on osteoclasts and osteoclast precursors by binding RANKL	Inhibition of bone resorption	No	N/A	N/A
PTH1-34	Stimulation of osteoblast differentiation by intermittent PTH (PTH1-34)	Activation of bone formation (intermittent PTH1-34) Activation of bone resorption (continuous PTH1-34)	Yes	Yes	Yes
BMPs	Activation of Runx2 expression and induction of osteoblast differentiation	Activation of bone formation	Yes	Yes	Yes
Anti-sclerostin antibody	Inhibition of sclerostin which interferes BMP and Wnt signaling	Activation of bone formation	No	N/A	N/A
Prostaglandins agonist	Activation of Runx2 expression	Activation of bone formation	No	Yes (combined use with BMP)	N/A
Stem cell	Induction of mesenchymal stem cells (bone marrow stem cells, adipose-derived stem cells, and bone marrow aspiration)	Supplementation of cell source for osteoblast	Yes	Yes	Yes
Gene therapy	Delivery of osteoinductive genes locally around the sites of fusion	Activation of bone formation	No	N/A	N/A

RANKL indicates Receptor activator of nuclear factor κB ligand; N/A, not available; PTH, parathyroid hormone; BMP, bone morphogenetic protein; Runx2, Runt-related transcription factor-2.

2. Bisphosphonates

2.1. Mechanism of Action

Bisphosphonates are pyrophosphate analogs that strongly bind to hydroxyapatite and have been shown to reduce the bone turnover rate, increase the bone mineral density (BMD), and prevent fragility fractures [20–22]. Bisphosphonates are classified into 2 groups, non-nitrogen-containing and nitrogen-containing, which work differently in bone metabolisms. Etidronate, clodronate, and tiludronate are non-nitrogen-containing bisphosphonates which inhibit adenosine triphosphate (ATP) in cellular metabolism and, therefore, lead to the apoptosis of osteoclasts (Figure 1) [23]. They not only decrease bone resorption but also calcification and, therefore, their long-term use is a potential risk for osteomalacia [24]. On the other hand, pamidronate, alendronate, risedronate, ibandronate, and zoledronate are nitrogen-containing bisphosphonates which have 1000 times more antiresorptive potencies than non-nitrogen-containing bisphosphonates [25]. Nitrogen-containing bisphosphonates block farnesyl pyrophosphate synthase, which is an enzyme of the mevalonate pathway that inhibits protein prenylation and results in the inhibition of the ruffled border formation [26,27]. It has been long discussed whether bisphosphonates help or harm the bone healing process [28], and the effect of bisphosphonates for spinal fusion has also been controversial.

2.2. Experimental Studies in Animal Models of Spinal Fusion

There have been many studies regarding the efficacy of bisphosphonate on spinal fusion in animal models. Several authors have reported on the negative effect of alendronate on the progression of spinal fusion [29,30]. Nakao et al. [31] subcutaneously administered alendronate to ovariectomized rats and showed that alendronate inhibited osteoclasts activity around the bone graft. On histology, the ingrowth of newly developed bone was also found to be greater in rats with alendronate than those without. Other studies have provided evidence of a positive effect of bisphosphonates for spinal arthrodesis. Yasen et al. [32] performed spinal fusion in ovariectomized rats and administered zoledronate at various concentrations after surgery. They found that zoledronate did not accelerate the spinal fusion at the clinical dose or lower, but did increase the fusion rate significantly at doses higher than the clinical dose.

2.3. Clinical Trials for Human Spinal Fusion

In a clinical trial of patients with osteoporosis, alendronate reportedly increased the fusion rate and decreased the risk of cage subsidence and postoperative vertebral compression fractures after spinal fusion surgery [33]. A recent study demonstrated the clinical usefulness of zoledronate, which has a 10-fold higher potency in preventing bone loss than alendronate in the ovariectomized rat model [34]. Furthermore, several authors have reported that zoledronate shortened the duration of time to fusion and improved the clinical and radiological outcomes [35,36]. Tu et al. [36] reported that solid fusion after spinal arthrodesis was achieved in 75% of patients who received an intravenous injection of zoledronate, compared to a rate of 56% in those who did not receive zoledronate. Therefore, these authors proposed that zoledronate could reduce the incidence of the subsequent vertebral compression fractures, pedicle screw loosening and cage subsidence at the 2-year follow up. While these studies demonstrate a positive effect of bisphosphonates, Buerba et al. [37] concluded that there were no statistically significant differences in the fusion rate and screw loosening between patients treated with bisphosphonates and those without after spinal arthrodesis in their review.

2.4. Side Effects

In 2003, a first case report was published describing bisphosphonate-related osteonecrosis of the jaw (BRONJ) [38]. The pathology of BRONJ is uncertain, but Santini et al. [39] found that bisphosphonates could lead to osteonecrosis through its effects on blood vessels in the bone by inhibiting the vascular endothelial growth factor. Rasmusson et al. [40] reviewed that exposed bone and subsequent bacterial contamination, typically after dental extraction, seem to trigger BRONJ. Atypical femoral fracture is another serious adverse effect of bisphosphonate, with the risk of atypical femoral fracture increasing as a function of the duration of with bisphosphonate therapy [41].

3. Anti-RANKL Monoclonal Antibody

3.1. Mechanism of Action

RANKL and its co-stimulatory signals, as well as macrophage colony-stimulating factor, can mediate osteoclastogenic signals. For example, osteopetrosis which is characterized by a high bone mass and a defect in bone-marrow formation can be induced by the congenital lack of osteoclasts [42]. Denosumab, a fully human monoclonal antibody to RANKL, interferes with the interaction between RANKL and RANK receptor on osteoclasts and osteoclast precursors by binding RANKL. Thus, denosumab reversibly inhibits osteoclast-mediated bone resorption (Figure 1) [43]. Denosumab has been recently used for the treatment of severe osteoporosis and its effect on the increase in BMD was reportedly larger than that of bisphosphonates [44,45]. Although bisphosphonates and denosumab are both classified as bone-modifying agents that particularly target osteoclast activity, some differences between these two agents. Kostenuik et al. [46] reported that denosumab significantly reduces cortical porosity compared to bisphosphonates. This difference in bone structure between bisphosphonates and denosumab is attributed to the fact that denosumab acts without binding to bone surfaces, unlike bisphosphonates which are absorbed into bone surfaces [47].

3.2. Side Effects

Significant and serious side effects of denosumab include hypocalcemia, osteonecrosis of the jaw and atypical femoral fracture, these side effects being similar to those of bisphosphonate [48–50]. Zhou et al. [51] reported that denosumab significantly reduced the risk for fractures except for vertebral fractures. In contrast, they also reported that denosumab could increase the risk of serious adverse events related to infection in postmenopausal women with osteoporosis compared to a placebo group; however, there was no significant difference with regard to safety between denosumab and bisphosphonates.

3.3. Experimental Studies in Animal Models of Spinal Fusion and Clinical Trials for Human Spinal Fusion

There has been no report on the use of denosumab in a clinical trial for enhancing bone fusion in spinal surgery. However, denosumab has the potential to enhance spinal fusion through its dual effect in inhibiting bone resorption and promoting bone formation. Further studies need to clarify whether denosumab could play a positive role in spinal fusion.

4. PTH

4.1. Mechanism of Action

PTH is an 84-amino acid polypeptide that is secreted by the parathyroid glands in response to a decrease in plasma calcium. The regulation of serum calcium is the major effect of PTH, which acts directly on osteoblasts, as well as indirectly increasing the differentiation and function of osteoclasts through its interaction with the RANKL of an osteoblast with the RANK receptor of an intermediate osteoclast cell. Finally, PTH enhances the release of calcium by bone resorption. Thus, PTH is involved in bone remodeling, which is an ongoing process where mature bone tissue is removed by osteoclasts (bone resorption) and new bone tissue is formed by osteoblasts (bone formation) (Figure 1). Teriparatide is a recombinant deoxyribonucleic acid form of PTH that has an identical sequence to the biologically active region on the skeleton (the first N-terminal 34 amino acids: rhPTH1-34).

It has been well known that the continuous infusion of PTH1-34 is associated with a catabolic effect, but that an intermittent administration promotes an anabolic effect on bone [52–54]. The mechanism underlying the anabolic and catabolic effect of PTH1-34 on bone metabolism is still unclear. However, we do know that the intermittent exposure to PTH1-34 induces expression of interleukin-11 which, in turn, suppresses Dickopf and, consequently, activates the Wnt signal pathway [16]. Therefore, the expression of bone-formation markers increases before that of bone-resorption markers with intermittent PTH1-34 administration [55,56]. Horwitz et al. [57] developed a seven-day continuous infusion model of PTH1-34 in healthy human adult volunteers and demonstrated that the continuous exposure to PTH1-34 in vivo activated bone resorption. On the other hand, numerous studies have reported on the possible benefit of an intermittent program of administration of PTH1-34. In an experimental animal model, Sato et al. [58] demonstrated, using cortical bone analyses after intermittent PTH1-34 administration in aged ovariectomized rats, that PTH1-34 stimulated the endosteal and periosteal bone formation, with a resulting increase in cortical thickness, a moment of inertia, strength, and stiffness of the femur. Jerome et al. [59] further demonstrated that intermittent PTH1-34 administration increased cancellous bone volume and improved trabecular architecture in ovariectomized cynomolgus monkeys.

Regarding the frequency of administration, the daily but not weekly administration of PTH1-34 caused cortical porosity and endosteal naïve bone formation in a rabbit model [60,61]. In a clinical study, the EUROFORS study, Graff et al. [62] demonstrated that a daily intermittent PTH1-34 administration increased most vertebral microstructural variables and BMD. Furthermore, several clinical studies showed that the treatment of osteoporosis with daily intermittent PTH1-34 administration decreased the risk of fractures and increased BMD [63,64]. As well, several recent reports have revealed an enhancement of bone healing via the anabolic effect of PTH1-34. In animal experimental models, the intermittent PTH1-34 treatment increased callus formation and accelerated bone healing, which resulted in an increase of the mechanical strength of healed bones [65,66]. Zhang et al. [67] demonstrated that weekly PTH1-34 injections promoted bone fracture healing to the same extent as daily injections in a rat model. Furthermore, Andreassen et al. [68] reported an increase in the guided bone regeneration of calvarial bone defects in a rat model with a daily intermittent PTH1-34 administration. A randomized double-blind placebo-controlled study reported the shortening of the time-to-healing of distal radial fractures, after closed reduction and immobilization, using a daily dose of PTH1-34 compared to a placebo group [69].

4.2. Experimental Studies in Animal Models of Spinal Fusion

Several reports have been published regarding the effect of intermittent PTH1-34 on spinal fusion in animal models. Abe et al. [70] reported an enhancement of graft bone healing by intermittent administration of PTH1-34 in a rat model of spinal arthrodesis with autograft. The intermittent administration of PTH1-34 was also reported to improve the fusion rate and decrease the time required for bone graft healing, in the same rat model, providing a structurally superior fusion mass [71]. O'Loughlin et al. [71] reported on the effect of a daily administration of PTH1-34 in a rabbit model of posterolateral spinal fusion with autograft and showed that intermittent PTH1-34 administration promoted a successful fusion using volumetric and histological analyses. Lehman et al. [72] also confirmed an increase in the rate of histological fusion of 86.7% with the intermittent PTH1-34 administration in a rabbit model of posterolateral spinal fusion model, compared to the control autograft only control group (50%). Moreover, there was a strong trend of the superior rate of radiological fusion (85.7%) with PTH1-34 compared to the calcitonin group (56.3%).

4.3. Combination Therapy of PTH1-34 and Anti-RANKL Monoclonal Antibody

The combination therapy of denosumab and PTH1-34 has been considered to be effective due to the potential effect of this combination in inhibiting bone resorption and promoting new bone formation, even in spinal arthrodesis. In an ovariectomized mouse model, a significant increase in BMD of the distal femur and femoral shaft was reported with the use of denosumab and PTH1-34 compared to the use of only denosumab [73]. Tsai et al. [74] evaluated the outcomes of a 2-year program of combined administration of denosumab and PTH1-34 in postmenopausal women with osteoporosis, showing that concomitant PTH1-34 and denosumab therapy increased BMD to a greater extent than either medication used individually. Kitaguchi et al. [75] demonstrated the positive effects of combination therapy of PTH1-34 and denosumab on bone defect regeneration in mice, with this combination accelerating the regeneration of cancellous bone in bone defects in the early phase of bone regeneration and increasing the cancellous bone mass more effectively than either agent individually used. Such a combination therapy could offer a positive impact on spinal arthrodesis, even in humans.

4.4. Clinical Trials for Human Spinal Fusion

Several clinical studies on the role of PTH1-34 for spinal fusion have been reported. In their prospective study, Ohtori et al. [76] reported a shorter average delay to fusion after lumbar posterolateral fusion in women with postmenopausal osteoporosis with PTH1-34 than with the use of bisphosphonates. In a further study on spinal fusion among postmenopausal women with osteoporosis, the same authors reported a significantly lower incidence rate of pedicle screw loosening in the subgroup treated with the daily administration of PTH1-34, compared to the risedronate or no medication groups [77]. In a retrospective case series analysis, the authors further confirmed that daily PTH1-34 administration for a period of >6 months was effective in promoting bone union after lumbar posterolateral fusion surgery and, therefore, decreasing the period of treatment [78]. Cho et al. [79] compared the effect of PTH1-34 and bisphosphonate administration on posterior lumbar interbody fusion in patients with osteoporosis through a prospective cohort study and concluded that there was no significant improvement in the overall fusion rate at 24 months after surgery and clinical outcome between the two groups, although the PTH1-34 group showed faster bony union than the bisphosphonate group. Ebata et al. [80] reported that bone fusion, evaluated on CT images, after posterior or transforaminal lumbar interbody fusion in patients with osteoporosis was significantly higher in patients using PTH1-34 than the no PTH1-34 group, both at 4 and 6 months postoperatively. Although the positive effect of PTH1-34 on bone fusion has been described in both animal models and clinical studies, the specific effect of PTH1-34 for bone fusion after spinal arthrodesis remains to be fully clarified.

5. BMP

5.1. Mechanism of Action

BMPs are a family of dimeric growth factors that belong to the transforming growth factor superfamily and are critical for skeletal development and bone formation. In 1965, Urist [81] was the first to report on the activity of BMPs as proteins present in the demineralized bone matrix that are capable of osteoinduction in ectopic sites in rats. However, it was not until the late 1980s that the first BMPs were characterized and cloned [82]. Since then, several BMP family members have been isolated, and to date, approximately 20 BMPs have been discovered. Of all, BMP2 and BMP7 significantly induce bone and cartilage formation. While BMP4, BMP5, BMP6, BMP8, BMP9, and BMP10 also contribute to bone formation, BMP3 and BMP13 are BMP inhibitors [83]. BMPs initiate their signaling transduction by binding to a heterodimeric complex of two transmembrane serine–threonine kinase receptors, BMP receptor type I (BMPRI) and type II (BMPR II). Activated receptors phosphorylate SMAD1, 5, and 8, which are specific for the BMP signaling pathway. Then heterodimeric complexes are formed by the phosphorylated SMADs with SMAD4 in the nucleus and regulate the transcription of target genes (Figures 1 and 2) [84].

5.2. Clinical Trials for Human Spinal Fusion

Iliac crest autologous bone grafting (ICBG) has been the "gold standard" choice for autologous grafts because of its structural lattice that facilitates cell migration, proliferation, and tissue regeneration, using growth factors and osteoprogenitor cells [85]. However, ICBG has several disadvantages, including postoperative donor site pain, extended operating time, high intra-operative blood loss, the risk of infection, and limited availability of graft, particularly in elderly individuals [86]. Thus, BMPs have been considered as a replacement for ICBG. Among the several recombinant forms of BMP, the US Food and Drug Administration (FDA) has sanctioned two recombinant human (rh)BMPs: rhBMP-2 and rhBMP-7 [also known as osteogenic protein-1]. rhBMP-2 has been approved for use in the single-level anterior lumbar interbody fusion. At present, rhBMP-2 is marketed as an absorbable collagen sponge (ACS) that functions as a carrier for the protein. In contrast, rhBMP-7 has been approved as an alternative to autografts in compromised patients through the Humanitarian Device Exemption process. Two clinical trials compared rhBMP-2/ACS treatment against the standard ICBG for anterior lumbar interbody fusion procedures, reporting higher fusion rates for the rhBMP-2/ACS group [87,88]. Recently, a meta-analysis, conducted by the Yale University Open Data Access project, reported that rhBMP-2 enhanced the fusion rates in spinal surgery, compared to ICBG; however, it also highlighted concerns associated with the safety of rhBMP-2 [89].

5.3. Side Effects

The efficacy of BMPs resulted in their frequent "off-label" use in spinal fusion procedures [90]. However, the rapid increase in their use led to the emergence of a series of reports regarding the possible side effects of BMPs, including inflammation, ectopic/heterotopic bone formation, dysphagia in cervical spinal fusions, and vertebral bone resorption (osteolysis) [91,92]. Eventually, the 2008 FDA Public Health Notification published an alert regarding safety concerns for BMPs, which led to a gradual decline in their use. Therefore, despite having excellent osteoinductive capabilities, a series of potential side effects have restricted the widespread use of BMPs. The side effects of BMPs' could be attributed to the administration of high-dose BMPs to induce sufficient fusion because of the degradation and rapid dilution (burst release) of these cytokines [93]. In addition, BMPs exhibit a dose-dependent efficacy [94]; however, their side effects are also dose-dependent [95], causing a dilemma in selecting an optimal dose. Therefore, enhancing the potency of BMPs and decreasing the use of high-dose BMPs would be clinically imperative.

5.4. Experimental Trials to Both Enhance the Anabolic Effect and Reduce the Side Effects of BMPs

The combined administration of PTH1-34 and BMP has been attempted to promote bone remodeling and lessen the amount of BMP dosage required and, thus, lowering the risk (and even preventing) the previously reported side effects of BMPs. Morimoto et al. [96] reported the positive effect of intermittent PTH1-34 administration on BMP induced bone formation in a rat model of spinal fusion. The fusion rate and bone volume density of newly formed bone in the group treated with BMP significantly increased with the concomitant administration of PTH1-34. Kaito et al. [97] also confirmed the modeling and remodeling effects of intermittent administration of PTH1-34 on BMP induced bone in a rat model of spinal fusion, and showed that PTH1-34 administration significantly decreased the tissue volume of the fusion mass at 12 weeks postoperatively, compared to 2 weeks postoperatively. According to an additional histomorphometric analysis of the cortical bone, periosteal bone resorption and endosteal bone formation were prominent.

In addition, several studies have reported that heterodimers, which are distinctive BMP family members are more potent than their constituent homodimers in inducing bone formation; in fact, BMP-2/6, -2/7 and -4/7 heterodimers have been shown to have a higher specific activity than their constituent homodimers [98–100]. Based on the sequence homology, BMPs are categorized into subfamilies. There are class I BMPs, comprising BMP2 and BMP4, and class II BMPs, comprising BMP5-8, and class I BMPs can form heterodimers with class II BMPs [101].

To date, although the underlying mechanism of the higher bone induction ability of BMP heterodimers remains partially understood, several clarifications have been suggested. First, heterodimers constitute a more stable receptor–ligand complex. Compared to BMP-2 or -6 homodimers [102], the BMP2/6 heterodimer exhibits a higher affinity to BMPRI and BMPRII, as well as a high SMAD1-dependent signaling activity. Second, heterodimers can better upregulate BMP receptor genes.

Reportedly, BMP2/6 induces the expression of the BMPRII gene more effectively than BMP-2 or -6 homodimers [100]. Third, hetero- and homo-dimeric BMPs vary in their ability to control the synthesis of BMP inhibitors or are differentially affected by these inhibitors. For example, BMP2/7 heterodimers are not antagonized by Noggin, one of the soluble BMP antagonists, compared to BMP homodimers [103]. Perhaps the weaker Noggin antagonism on BMP heterodimers might contribute to the enhanced osteogenic potency of heterodimers, compared to that of homodimers. Although these results suggest that BMP heterodimers could be an alternative to BMP homodimers, whether lower doses of BMP heterodimers result in bone formation to the same extent as BMP homodimers, while reducing the secondary inflammatory response, remains unclear [95].

5.5. Carrier Materials for Delivering BMPs

To date, various materials have also been assessed to enhance the delivery of BMPs. Carrier materials are classified into four main types: natural polymers, synthetic polymers, inorganic materials (mainly ceramics), and their composites [104]. Each class provides some advantages and disadvantages. Currently, the trend is to use composite carriers that provide the benefits of each class of materials. For example, semisynthetic polymers, which exhibit controlled release properties, were introduced due to their biocompatibility in combining with natural polymers, including polycaprolactone within collagen [105], PEGylated fibrinogen [106]. In another example, composites, that combined collagen to biphasic calcium phosphate, were superior to biphasic calcium phosphate alone for bone regeneration, while decreasing the incidence of burst release [107]. Therefore, developing an ideal carrier material for delivering BMPs that can localize the protein, prolong its retention time at the site of action and provide mechanical strength and a scaffold for bone ingrowth is essential.

6. Anti-Sclerostin Antibody

6.1. Mechanism of Action

Sclerostin, which is the product of the SOST gene, is a negative regulator of bone formation [108–110]. Sclerostin is considered to be mainly produced from osteocytes, although its messenger ribonucleic acid has also been detected in chondrocytes, the kidney, lung, liver, vascular tissue, and the heart [111–113]. Sclerostin works as an antagonist of BMP and Wnt signaling, with the main function of sclerostin on bone metabolism being the inhibition of the Wnt/β-catenin pathway in osteoblasts via binding to the low-density lipoprotein receptor-related protein 5/6 receptor on the membrane of osteoblasts [114–116]. Thus, the inhibition of sclerostin can induce the activation of osteoblasts and promote bone formation (Figures 1 and 2). For therapeutic use in humans, the anti-sclerostin antibody (romosozumab) has been developed for the treatment of osteoporosis, which decreases endogenous levels of sclerostin, allowing for osteogenesis through an improvement in osteoblast survival [117–119]. Several authors have reported on the anabolic effect of anti-sclerostin antibody in enhancing the bone formation and fracture healing in animal models [120–124]. In addition to the anabolic effect of anti-sclerostin antibodies, Suen et al. [122] suggested that anti-sclerostin antibodies could also induce an early increase in neovascularization around the fracture site, which would also contribute to enhanced fracture healing.

6.2. Experimental Studies in Animal Spinal Fusion Models and Clinical Trials for Human Spinal Fusion

There have been no studies on the use of anti-sclerostin antibodies for animal or human models of spinal fusion to date. However, taking into consideration the anabolic effect of anti-sclerostin on bone metabolisms and its efficacy in the treatment of osteoporosis, there is a promise that anti-sclerostin could enhance spinal fusion.

7. Prostaglandins Agonist

7.1. Mechanism of Action

Prostaglandins (PGs) have not only a stimulatory but also an inhibitory effect for bone metabolism depending on the physiological or pathological conditions. In particular, PGE2 produced by osteoblasts under cyclooxygenase (COX)-2 stimulation plays an important role in bone metabolism [125]. There are four subtypes of receptors for PGE2 (EP1, EP2, EP3, EP4), and studies have shown signaling, via EP2 and EP4, to play an important role in bone metabolism [126]. With regard to the anabolic aspect of bone metabolism, PGE2 induced the expression of the core-binding factor alpha1 (Runx2/Cbfa1) and enhanced the mineralized nodule formation. These phenomena could not occur in the culture of cells from EP4-deficient mice (Figures 1 and 2) [127]. In several animal and human studies of spinal fusion, non-specific non-steroidal anti-inflammatory drugs have been shown to exert a strong negative effect on the rate of spinal fusion, though there is no consensus about the effects of COX-2 inhibitors on spinal arthrodesis [126,128]. With regard to therapeutic trials, many studies have focused on EP4 receptor activation, demonstrating the effectiveness of EP4 agonist for fracture healing and osteoporosis in animal models [129–132].

7.2. Experimental Studies in Animal Models of Spinal Fusion and Issues for Clinical Use in Human Spinal Fusion

Namikawa et al. [131] revealed that the local administration of an EP4 receptor agonist promoted the osteoinductivity of BMP-2 in a rabbit posterolateral lumbar spinal fusion model. Recently, Kanayama et al. [133] showed that an IP (PGI2 receptor) agonist also promoted osteoblast differentiation and ectopic and orthotopic bone formation in vivo in a rat model of spinal fusion. PG receptor agonists may induce several specific side effects (such as local and/or systemic inflammation, hypotension, tachycardia, and diarrhea) and, thus, further research is required to elucidate these side effects for human clinical use. However, PG agonists may provide a therapeutic potential to enhance bone fusion in spinal arthrodesis.

8. Cell Therapies

8.1. Mechanism of Action and Cell Sources

Cell-based therapies, which aim to enhance osteogenesis, osteoconduction, and/or osteoinduction of bone graft, have been tried for spinal arthrodesis. Mesenchymal stem cells (MSCs) are key cells for these therapies and have been widely used to promote bone formation and regeneration in many animal and human trials [134,135]. Bone marrow-MSCs (BM-MSCs), isolated by bone marrow aspiration from the iliac crest or vertebral body, are considered to be suitable for spinal arthrodesis due to their intra-operative accessibility [136,137]. MSCs are multipotent stem cells that have the capability for self-renewal, plasticity, and multilineage potential, including osteogenic, chondrogenic, adipogenic, and myogenic lineages. Their differentiation relies on both intrinsic and extrinsic factors in their environments, where BMP signaling has an important role in the differentiation of MSCs to osteoblasts by activation of Runx2, via SMAD1/5/8 [14–16,138]. Adipose-derived stem cells (ASCs) have also been attracting attention as a source of MSCs. ASCs are attractive because they are easily accessible and adipose tissue has a high cellular content, but also, ASCs have a higher capacity for self-renewal and plasticity than BM-MSCs [134].

8.2. Experimental Studies in Animal Spinal Fusion Models, Clinical Trials for Human Spinal Fusion and Issues for Clinical Use

In an animal posterolateral spinal fusion model with rabbits, Nakajima et al. [139] reported that successful fusion observed in four of 5 rabbits with cultured osteogenic BM-MSCs in Type-1 collagen gel, compared to none of 6 rabbits with hydroxyapatite in Type-1 collagen gel. Yang et al. [140] also evaluated the effectiveness of osteogenic BM-MSCs in the rabbit anterior lumbar interbody fusion model. Four of 10 rabbits with porous collagen sponge with cultured osteogenic BM-MSCs and 7 of 10 rabbits with iliac crest bone graft achieved bony fusion, compared to none of 10 rabbits without bone graft or collagen sponge. Against these experiments from animal studies, several cellular bone matrices, which are allogenic bone grafts containing living MSCs, have been commercially available for human spinal arthrodesis. Though no randomized controlled trial has been conducted to evaluate the efficacy of cellular bone matrices in spinal arthrodesis and there is no evidence that MSCs can survive, differentiate, and regenerate after being transplanted into the human spinal fusion site, they can be a promising alternation for bone augmentation [141]. However, potential long-term drawbacks, such as mal-differentiation and tumorigenicity, are of concern and still need to be solved before MSCs can be used for clinical purposes in humans [142]. Instead of MSCs, bone marrow aspiration (BMA) combined with synthetic or allograft materials has been used to enhance bony fusion after spinal arthrodesis in clinical practice because they contain different cell populations including osteoprogenitors and hematoprogenitors [135,143]. One concern is that BMAs harvested from the iliac crest contains only one to five MSCs per 500,000 nucleated cells [141,144]. This could make the therapeutic effect of BMA uncertain. Moreover, there is no clear evidence that BMA combined with synthetic or allograft materials can be a substitute or supplementary graft to autologous bone [135,145]. Yousef et al. [145] reported that a collagen scaffold with BMA, using selective cell retention technology for the intraoperative concentration of MSCs, could lead to successful fusion and improved clinical outcomes after human posterolateral fusion [145]. Recently, it has been demonstrated that induced pluripotent stem (iPS) cells can be differentiated into osteoblasts and this technology may alter the strategy for bone regenerative cell therapies [146]. Several high-quality comparative studies aiming to reveal the efficacy of cell therapies are ongoing, and their evidence will be clarified in the future [134,135,141].

9. Gene Therapies

The main limitation of using osteogenic agents, such as BMPs, for inducing bone formation after spinal arthrodesis is the need for safe and effective drug delivery systems that will provide a sustained and biologically appropriate concentration of the osteogenic factor at the target sites [134]. Gene therapy approaches aim to deliver osteoinductive genes locally to induce bone formation and improve spinal fusion, with several approaches having been tried [134]. The vectors used for gene therapy approaches consist of an adenoviral vector, lentiviral vector, naked deoxyribonucleic acid, liposomes, and plasmids. Not only BMPs, but also Nell-like molecule, LIM mineralization protein, and SMAD1 have been tested as transduction genes to enhance the spinal fusion in animal models [98,134,147–149]. The main problems with genetic engineering are cell toxicity, immunization, insertional mutagenesis, and low cell selectivity. Thus, though further studies are still needed for the clinical application of gene therapies in spinal fusion, these therapies do hold the promise for eliminating the use of autograft and its associated morbidities.

10. Overview and Future Direction

In addition to anti-bone resorptive agents which have been widely used so far, the recent progress in bone pharmacophysiology provides us with newly developed bone anabolic agents. These agents certainly have an advantage over anti-bone-resorptive agents to enhance bone fusion after spinal fusion surgery. Furthermore, cell and gene engineering techniques have a great potential to make innovative changes in drug delivery systems or environment for bone formation. These attempts for biological enhancement of bone formation can offer a reliable fusion after spinal fusion or shorten the period for achieving bone fusion. The development of artificial bone grafts, using osteoinductivity and osteoconductivity, may reduce the necessity of harvesting autologous bone graft and the incidence of related complications. The limitation of previous experimental studies was that many studies about the biological enhancement for bone formation after spinal fusion were performed using small animals such as a rat, mouse, and rabbit. Pharmacokinetic and local environments around the fusion site can be different between such small animals and a human. The evaluation with large animals or establishment of experimental models closer to the human environment with small animals is desirable in the future. In particular, the establishment of the interbody fusion model in small animals is difficult because the vertebral endplates can be easily sacrificed and thus local environment in human interbody fusion cannot be reproduced. Recently, we have established a rat interbody fusion model without violating endplates and demonstrated the reproducibility of BMP-2 related dose-dependent complications such as soft tissue swelling and osteolysis (unpublished data). Furthermore, several issues remain to be solved particularly with regard to the safety and cost-effectiveness of such novel approaches for human clinical use. However, we believe that the development of the biological enhancement of spinal fusion would be of benefit to patients' health-related QOL outcomes, as well as being important for social health economics.

Author Contributions: T.M. provided overall direction, final editing, and contributed to original writing. H.T., Y.U. and D.T. contributed original writing and editing. H.Y. supervised this work. T.K. provided overall direction and final editing, and supervised this work.

Acknowledgments: The authors specially thanked Kunihiko Hashimoto (Department of Orthopedic Surgery, Osaka University Graduate School of Medicine, Suita, Osaka, Japan) for preparing figures.

Conflicts of Interest: The authors declare no conflict of interest.

Abbreviations

ACS	absorbable collagen sponge
ASC	adipose derived stem cell
BMA	bone marrow aspiration
BMD	bone mineral density
BM-MSC	bone marrow-mesenchymal stem cell
BMP	bone morphogenetic protein
BRONJ	bisphosphonate-related osteonecrosis of the jaw
Cbfa1	core-binding factor subunit alpha-1
COX	Cyclooxygenase
FDA	the US Food and Drug Administration
ICBG	iliac crest autologous bone grafting
OPG	Osteoprotegerin
PG	Prostaglandin
PKCδ	protein kinase Cδ
PTH	parathyroid hormone
QOL	quality of life
RANKL	receptor activator of nuclear factor κB ligand
rhBMP	recombinant human BMP
Runx2	Runt-related transcription factor 2

References

1. Rajaee, S.S.; Bae, H.W.; Kanim, L.E.; Delamarter, R.B. Spinal fusion in the United States: Analysis of trends from 1998 to 2008. *Spine* **2012**, *37*, 67–76. [CrossRef] [PubMed]
2. Cannada, L.K.; Scherping, S.C.; Yoo, J.U.; Jones, P.K.; Emery, S.E. Pseudoarthrosis of the cervical spine: A comparison of radiographic diagnostic measures. *Spine* **2003**, *28*, 46–51. [CrossRef] [PubMed]
3. Kornblum, M.B.; Fischgrund, J.S.; Herkowitz, H.N.; Abraham, D.A.; Berkower, D.L.; Ditkoff, J.S. Degenerative lumbar spondylolisthesis with spinal stenosis: A prospective long-term study comparing fusion and pseudarthrosis. *Spine* **2004**, *29*. [CrossRef]
4. Makino, T.; Kaito, T.; Fujiwara, H.; Honda, H.; Sakai, Y.; Takenaka, S.; Yoshikawa, H.; Yonenobu, K. Risk Factors for Poor Patient-Reported Quality of Life Outcomes After Posterior Lumbar Interbody Fusion: An Analysis of 2-Year Follow-up. *Spine* **2017**, *42*, 1502–1510. [CrossRef] [PubMed]

5. Makino, T.; Kaito, T.; Fujiwara, H.; Ishii, T.; Iwasaki, M.; Yoshikawa, H.; Yonenobu, K. Does fusion status after posterior lumbar interbody fusion affect patient-based QOL outcomes? An evaluation performed using a patient-based outcome measure. *J. Orthop. Sci.* **2014**, *19*, 707–712. [CrossRef] [PubMed]

6. Phillips, F.M.; Carlson, G.; Emery, S.E.; Bohlman, H.H. Anterior cervical pseudarthrosis. Natural history and treatment. *Spine* **1997**, *22*, 1585–1589. [CrossRef] [PubMed]

7. Lee, R. The outlook for population growth. *Science* **2011**, *333*, 569–573. [CrossRef] [PubMed]

8. Deyo, R.A.; Gray, D.T.; Kreuter, W.; Mirza, S.; Martin, B.I. United States trends in lumbar fusion surgery for degenerative conditions. *Spine* **2005**, *30*. [CrossRef]

9. Datta, H.K.; Ng, W.F.; Walker, J.A.; Tuck, S.P.; Varanasi, S.S. The cell biology of bone metabolism. *J. Clin. Pathol.* **2008**, *61*, 577–587. [CrossRef] [PubMed]

10. Hirsch, B.P.; Unnanuntana, A.; Cunningham, M.E.; Lane, J.M. The effect of therapies for osteoporosis on spine fusion: A systematic review. *Spine J.* **2013**, *13*, 190–199. [CrossRef] [PubMed]

11. Zipfel, G.J.; Guiot, B.H.; Fessler, R.G. Bone grafting. *Neurosurg. Focus* **2003**, *14*, e8. [CrossRef] [PubMed]

12. Boden, S.D.; Schimandle, J.H.; Hutton, W.C. An experimental lumbar intertransverse process spinal fusion model. Radiographic, histologic, and biomechanical healing characteristics. *Spine* **1995**, *20*, 412–420. [CrossRef] [PubMed]

13. Kalb, S.; Mahan, M.A.; Elhadi, A.M.; Dru, A.; Eales, J.; Lemos, M.; Theodore, N. Pharmacophysiology of bone and spinal fusion. *Spine J.* **2013**, *13*, 1359–1369. [CrossRef] [PubMed]

14. Lin, G.L.; Hankenson, K.D. Integration of BMP, Wnt, and notch signaling pathways in osteoblast differentiation. *J. Cell. Biochem.* **2011**, *112*, 3491–3501. [CrossRef] [PubMed]

15. Long, F. Building strong bones: Molecular regulation of the osteoblast lineage. *Nat. Rev. Mol. Cell Biol.* **2011**, *13*, 27–38. [CrossRef] [PubMed]

16. Rutkovskiy, A.; Stenslokken, K.O.; Vaage, I.J. Osteoblast Differentiation at a Glance. *Med. Sci. Monit. Basic Res.* **2016**, *22*, 95–106. [CrossRef] [PubMed]

17. Ikeda, K.; Takeshita, S. The role of osteoclast differentiation and function in skeletal homeostasis. *J. Biochem.* **2016**, *159*, 1–8. [CrossRef] [PubMed]

18. Boyle, W.J.; Simonet, W.S.; Lacey, D.L. Osteoclast differentiation and activation. *Nature* **2003**, *423*, 337–342. [CrossRef] [PubMed]

19. Walsh, M.C.; Choi, Y. Biology of the RANKL-RANK-OPG System in Immunity, Bone, and Beyond. *Front. Immunol.* **2014**, *5*, 511. [CrossRef] [PubMed]

20. Jung, A.; Bisaz, S.; Fleisch, H. The binding of pyrophosphate and two diphosphonates by hydroxyapatite crystals. *Calcif. Tissue Res.* **1973**, *11*, 269–280. [CrossRef] [PubMed]

21. Miller, P.D. Anti-resorptives in the management of osteoporosis. *Best Pract. Res. Clin. Endocrinol. Metab.* **2008**, *22*, 849–868. [CrossRef] [PubMed]

22. Rodan, G.A.; Fleisch, H.A. Bisphosphonates: Mechanisms of action. *J. Clin. Investig.* **1996**, *97*, 2692–2696. [CrossRef] [PubMed]

23. Lehenkari, P.P.; Kellinsalmi, M.; Napankangas, J.P.; Ylitalo, K.V.; Monkkonen, J.; Rogers, M.J.; Azhayev, A.; Vaananen, H.K.; Hassinen, I.E. Further insight into mechanism of action of clodronate: Inhibition of mitochondrial ADP/ATP translocase by a nonhydrolyzable, adenine-containing metabolite. *Mol. Pharmacol.* **2002**, *61*, 1255–1262. [CrossRef] [PubMed]

24. Hoppe, E.; Masson, C.; Laffitte, A.; Chappard, D.; Audran, M. Osteomalacia in a patient with Paget's bone disease treated with long-term etidronate. *Morphologie* **2012**, *96*, 40–43. [CrossRef] [PubMed]

25. Russell, R.G.; Croucher, P.I.; Rogers, M.J. Bisphosphonates: Pharmacology, mechanisms of action and clinical uses. *Osteoporos. Int.* **1999**, *9* (Suppl. 2), S66–S80. [CrossRef] [PubMed]

26. Stone, M.A.; Jakoi, A.M.; Iorio, J.A.; Pham, M.H.; Patel, N.N.; Hsieh, P.C.; Liu, J.C.; Acosta, F.L.; Hah, R.; Wang, J.C. Bisphosphonate's and Intermittent Parathyroid Hormone's Effect on Human Spinal Fusion: A Systematic Review of the Literature. *Asian Spine J.* **2017**, *11*, 484–493. [CrossRef] [PubMed]

27. Van Beek, E.R.; Lowik, C.W.; Papapoulos, S.E. Bisphosphonates suppress bone resorption by a direct effect on early osteoclast precursors without affecting the osteoclastogenic capacity of osteogenic cells: The role of protein geranylgeranylation in the action of nitrogen-containing bisphosphonates on osteoclast precursors. *Bone* **2002**, *30*, 64–70. [PubMed]

28. McDonald, M.M.; Dulai, S.; Godfrey, C.; Amanat, N.; Sztynda, T.; Little, D.G. Bolus or weekly zoledronic acid administration does not delay endochondral fracture repair but weekly dosing enhances delays in hard callus remodeling. *Bone* **2008**, *43*, 653–662. [CrossRef] [PubMed]
29. Huang, R.C.; Khan, S.N.; Sandhu, H.S.; Metzl, J.A.; Cammisa, F.P., Jr.; Zheng, F.; Sama, A.A.; Lane, J.M. Alendronate inhibits spine fusion in a rat model. *Spine* **2005**, *30*, 2516–2522. [CrossRef] [PubMed]
30. Lehman, R.A., Jr.; Kuklo, T.R.; Freedman, B.A.; Cowart, J.R.; Mense, M.G.; Riew, K.D. The effect of alendronate sodium on spinal fusion: A rabbit model. *Spine J.* **2004**, *4*, 36–43. [CrossRef]
31. Nakao, S.; Minamide, A.; Kawakami, M.; Boden, S.D.; Yoshida, M. The influence of alendronate on spine fusion in an osteoporotic animal model. *Spine* **2011**, *36*, 1446–1452. [CrossRef] [PubMed]
32. Yasen, M.; Li, X.; Jiang, L.; Yuan, W.; Che, W.; Dong, J. Effect of zoledronic acid on spinal fusion outcomes in an ovariectomized rat model of osteoporosis. *J. Orthop. Res.* **2015**, *33*, 1297–1304. [CrossRef] [PubMed]
33. Nagahama, K.; Kanayama, M.; Togawa, D.; Hashimoto, T.; Minami, A. Does alendronate disturb the healing process of posterior lumbar interbody fusion? A prospective randomized trial. *J. Neurosurg. Spine* **2011**, *14*, 500–507. [CrossRef] [PubMed]
34. Gasser, J.A.; Ingold, P.; Venturiere, A.; Shen, V.; Green, J.R. Long-term protective effects of zoledronic acid on cancellous and cortical bone in the ovariectomized rat. *J. Bone Miner. Res.* **2008**, *23*, 544–551. [CrossRef] [PubMed]
35. Chen, F.; Dai, Z.; Kang, Y.; Lv, G.; Keller, E.T.; Jiang, Y. Effects of zoledronic acid on bone fusion in osteoporotic patients after lumbar fusion. *Osteoporos. Int.* **2016**, *27*, 1469–1476. [CrossRef] [PubMed]
36. Tu, C.W.; Huang, K.F.; Hsu, H.T.; Li, H.Y.; Yang, S.S.; Chen, Y.C. Zoledronic acid infusion for lumbar interbody fusion in osteoporosis. *J. Surg. Res.* **2014**, *192*, 112–116. [CrossRef] [PubMed]
37. Buerba, R.A.; Sharma, A.; Ziino, C.; Arzeno, A.; Ajiboye, R.M. Bisphosphonate and Teriparatide Use in Thoracolumbar Spinal Fusion: A Systematic Review and Meta-Analysis of Comparative Studies. *Spine* **2018**. [CrossRef] [PubMed]
38. Marx, R.E. Pamidronate (Aredia) and zoledronate (Zometa) induced avascular necrosis of the jaws: A growing epidemic. *J. Oral Maxillofac. Surg.* **2003**, *61*, 1115–1117. [CrossRef]
39. Santini, D.; Vincenzi, B.; Avvisati, G.; Dicuonzo, G.; Battistoni, F.; Gavasci, M.; Salerno, A.; Denaro, V.; Tonini, G. Pamidronate induces modifications of circulating angiogenetic factors in cancer patients. *Clin. Cancer Res.* **2002**, *8*, 1080–1084. [CrossRef]
40. Rasmusson, L.; Abtahi, J. Bisphosphonate associated osteonecrosis of the jaw: An update on pathophysiology, risk factors, and treatment. *Int. J. Dent.* **2014**, *2014*, 471035. [CrossRef] [PubMed]
41. Adler, R.A.; El-Hajj Fuleihan, G.; Bauer, D.C.; Camacho, P.M.; Clarke, B.L.; Clines, G.A.; Compston, J.E.; Drake, M.T.; Edwards, B.J.; Favus, M.J.; et al. Managing Osteoporosis in Patients on Long-Term Bisphosphonate Treatment: Report of a Task Force of the American Society for Bone and Mineral Research. *J. Bone Miner. Res.* **2016**, *31*, 16–35. [CrossRef] [PubMed]
42. Takayanagi, H. Osteoimmunology: Shared mechanisms and crosstalk between the immune and bone systems. *Nat. Rev. Immunol.* **2007**, *7*, 292–304. [CrossRef] [PubMed]
43. Delmas, P.D. Clinical potential of RANKL inhibition for the management of postmenopausal osteoporosis and other metabolic bone diseases. *J. Clin. Densitom.* **2008**, *11*, 325–338. [CrossRef] [PubMed]
44. Cummings, S.R.; San Martin, J.; McClung, M.R.; Siris, E.S.; Eastell, R.; Reid, I.R.; Delmas, P.; Zoog, H.B.; Austin, M.; Wang, A.; et al. Denosumab for prevention of fractures in postmenopausal women with osteoporosis. *N. Engl. J. Med.* **2009**, *361*, 756–765. [CrossRef] [PubMed]
45. Miller, P.D.; Pannacciulli, N.; Brown, J.P.; Czerwinski, E.; Nedergaard, B.S.; Bolognese, M.A.; Malouf, J.; Bone, H.G.; Reginster, J.Y.; Singer, A.; et al. Denosumab or Zoledronic Acid in Postmenopausal Women with Osteoporosis Previously Treated with Oral Bisphosphonates. *J. Clin. Endocrinol. Metab.* **2016**, *101*, 3163–3170. [CrossRef] [PubMed]
46. Kostenuik, P.J.; Smith, S.Y.; Samadfam, R.; Jolette, J.; Zhou, L.; Ominsky, M.S. Effects of denosumab, alendronate, or denosumab following alendronate on bone turnover, calcium homeostasis, bone mass and bone strength in ovariectomized cynomolgus monkeys. *J. Bone Miner. Res.* **2015**, *30*, 657–669. [CrossRef] [PubMed]
47. Zebaze, R.M.; Libanati, C.; Austin, M.; Ghasem-Zadeh, A.; Hanley, D.A.; Zanchetta, J.R.; Thomas, T.; Boutroy, S.; Bogado, C.E.; Bilezikian, J.P.; et al. Differing effects of denosumab and alendronate on cortical and trabecular bone. *Bone* **2014**, *59*, 173–179. [CrossRef] [PubMed]

48. Cernes, R.; Barnea, Z.; Biro, A.; Zandman-Goddard, G.; Katzir, Z. Severe Hypocalcemia Following a Single Denosumab Injection. *IMAJ* **2017**, *19*, 719–721. [PubMed]

49. Tateiwa, D.; Outani, H.; Iwasa, S.; Imura, Y.; Tanaka, T.; Oshima, K.; Naka, N.; Araki, N. Atypical femoral fracture associated with bone-modifying agent for bone metastasis of breast cancer: A report of two cases. *J. Orthop. Surg.* **2017**, *25*, 2309499017727916. [CrossRef] [PubMed]

50. Yoshimura, H.; Ohba, S.; Yoshida, H.; Saito, K.; Inui, K.; Yasui, R.; Ichikawa, D.; Aiki, M.; Kobayashi, J.; Matsuda, S.; et al. Denosumab-related osteonecrosis of the jaw in a patient with bone metastases of prostate cancer: A case report and literature review. *Oncol. Lett.* **2017**, *14*, 127–136. [CrossRef] [PubMed]

51. Zhou, Z.; Chen, C.; Zhang, J.; Ji, X.; Liu, L.; Zhang, G.; Cao, X.; Wang, P. Safety of denosumab in postmenopausal women with osteoporosis or low bone mineral density: A meta-analysis. *Int. J. Clin. Exp. Pathol.* **2014**, *7*, 2113–2122. [PubMed]

52. Hock, J.M.; Gera, I. Effects of continuous and intermittent administration and inhibition of resorption on the anabolic response of bone to parathyroid hormone. *J. Bone Miner. Res.* **1992**, *7*, 65–72. [CrossRef] [PubMed]

53. Podbesek, R.D.; Mawer, E.B.; Zanelli, G.D.; Parsons, J.A.; Reeve, J. Intestinal absorption of calcium in greyhounds: The response to intermittent and continuous administration of human synthetic parathyroid hormone fragment 1–34 (hPTH 1–34). *Clin. Sci.* **1984**, *67*, 591–599. [CrossRef] [PubMed]

54. Tam, C.S.; Heersche, J.N.M.; Murray, T.M.; Parsons, J.A. Parathyroid-Hormone Stimulates the Bone Apposition Rate Independently of Its Resorptive Action—Differential-Effects of Intermittent and Continuous Administration. *Endocrinology* **1982**, *110*, 506–512. [CrossRef] [PubMed]

55. Canalis, E.; Giustina, A.; Bilezikian, J.P. Mechanisms of anabolic therapies for osteoporosis. *N. Engl. J. Med.* **2007**, *357*, 905–916. [CrossRef] [PubMed]

56. Rubin, M.R.; Bilezikian, J.P. The anabolic effects of parathyroid hormone therapy. *Clin. Geriatr. Med.* **2003**, *19*, 415–432. [CrossRef]

57. Horwitz, M.J.; Tedesco, M.B.; Sereika, S.M.; Prebehala, L.; Gundberg, C.M.; Hollis, B.W.; Bisello, A.; Garcia-Ocana, A.; Carneiro, R.M.; Stewart, A.F. A 7-day continuous infusion of PTH or PTHrP suppresses bone formation and uncouples bone turnover. *J. Bone Miner. Res.* **2011**, *26*, 2287–2297. [CrossRef] [PubMed]

58. Sato, M.; Zeng, G.Q.; Turner, C.H. Biosynthetic human parathyroid hormone (1–34) effects on bone quality in aged ovariectomized rats. *Endocrinology* **1997**, *138*, 4330–4337. [CrossRef] [PubMed]

59. Jerome, C.P.; Burr, D.B.; Van Bibber, T.; Hock, J.M.; Brommage, R. Treatment with human parathyroid hormone (1–34) for 18 months increases cancellous bone volume and improves trabecular architecture in ovariectomized cynomolgus monkeys (*Macaca fascicularis*). *Bone* **2001**, *28*, 150–159. [CrossRef]

60. Yamane, H.; Takakura, A.; Shimadzu, Y.; Kodama, T.; Lee, J.W.; Isogai, Y.; Ishizuya, T.; Takao-Kawabata, R.; Iimura, T. Acute development of cortical porosity and endosteal naive bone formation from the daily but not weekly short-term administration of PTH in rabbit. *PLoS ONE* **2017**, *12*, e0175329. [CrossRef] [PubMed]

61. Zebaze, R.; Takao-Kawabata, R.; Peng, Y.; Zadeh, A.G.; Hirano, K.; Yamane, H.; Takakura, A.; Isogai, Y.; Ishizuya, T.; Seeman, E. Increased cortical porosity is associated with daily, not weekly, administration of equivalent doses of teriparatide. *Bone* **2017**, *99*, 80–84. [CrossRef] [PubMed]

62. Graeff, C.; Timm, W.; Nickelsen, T.N.; Farrerons, J.; Marin, F.; Barker, C.; Gluer, C.C.; EUROFORS High Resolution Computed Tomography Substudy Group. Monitoring teriparatide-associated changes in vertebral microstructure by high-resolution CT in vivo: Results from the EUROFORS study. *J. Bone Miner. Res.* **2007**, *22*, 1426–1433. [CrossRef] [PubMed]

63. Neer, R.M.; Arnaud, C.D.; Zanchetta, J.R.; Prince, R.; Gaich, G.A.; Reginster, J.Y.; Hodsman, A.B.; Eriksen, E.F.; Ish-Shalom, S.; Genant, H.K.; et al. Effect of parathyroid hormone (1–34) on fractures and bone mineral density in postmenopausal women with osteoporosis. *N. Engl. J. Med.* **2001**, *344*, 1434–1441. [CrossRef] [PubMed]

64. Nakamura, T.; Sugimoto, T.; Nakano, T.; Kishimoto, H.; Ito, M.; Fukunaga, M.; Hagino, H.; Sone, T.; Yoshikawa, H.; Nishizawa, Y.; et al. Randomized Teriparatide [human parathyroid hormone (PTH) 1–34] Once-Weekly Efficacy Research (TOWER) trial for examining the reduction in new vertebral fractures in subjects with primary osteoporosis and high fracture risk. *J. Clin. Endocrinol. Metab.* **2012**, *97*, 3097–3106. [CrossRef] [PubMed]

65. Andreassen, T.T.; Ejersted, C.; Oxlund, H. Intermittent parathyroid hormone (1–34) treatment increases callus formation and mechanical strength of healing rat fractures. *J. Bone Miner. Res.* **1999**, *14*, 960–968. [CrossRef] [PubMed]

66. Kumabe, Y.; Lee, S.Y.; Waki, T.; Iwakura, T.; Takahara, S.; Arakura, M.; Kuroiwa, Y.; Fukui, T.; Matsumoto, T.; Matsushita, T.; et al. Triweekly administration of parathyroid hormone (1–34) accelerates bone healing in a rat refractory fracture model. *BMC Musculoskelet. Disord.* **2017**, *18*, 545. [CrossRef] [PubMed]

67. Zhang, W.; Zhu, J.; Ma, T.; Liu, C.; Hai, B.; Du, G.; Wang, H.; Li, N.; Leng, H.; Xu, Y.; et al. Comparison of the effects of once-weekly and once-daily rhPTH (1–34) injections on promoting fracture healing in rodents. *J. Orthop. Res.* **2017**. [CrossRef] [PubMed]

68. Andreassen, T.T.; Cacciafesta, V. Intermittent parathyroid hormone treatment enhances guided bone regeneration in rat calvarial bone defects. *J. Craniofac. Surg.* **2004**, *15*, 424–427. [CrossRef] [PubMed]

69. Aspenberg, P.; Genant, H.K.; Johansson, T.; Nino, A.J.; See, K.; Krohn, K.; Garcia-Hernandez, P.A.; Recknor, C.P.; Einhorn, T.A.; Dalsky, G.P.; et al. Teriparatide for acceleration of fracture repair in humans: A prospective, randomized, double-blind study of 102 postmenopausal women with distal radial fractures. *J. Bone Miner. Res.* **2010**, *25*, 404–414. [CrossRef] [PubMed]

70. Abe, Y.; Takahata, M.; Ito, M.; Irie, K.; Abumi, K.; Minami, A. Enhancement of graft bone healing by intermittent administration of human parathyroid hormone (1–34) in a rat spinal arthrodesis model. *Bone* **2007**, *41*, 775–785. [CrossRef] [PubMed]

71. O'Loughlin, P.F.; Cunningham, M.E.; Bukata, S.V.; Tomin, E.; Poynton, A.R.; Doty, S.B.; Sama, A.A.; Lane, J.M. Parathyroid hormone (1–34) augments spinal fusion, fusion mass volume, and fusion mass quality in a rabbit spinal fusion model. *Spine* **2009**, *34*, 121–130. [CrossRef] [PubMed]

72. Lehman, R.A., Jr.; Dmitriev, A.E.; Cardoso, M.J.; Helgeson, M.D.; Christensen, C.L.; Raymond, J.W.; Eckel, T.T.; Riew, K.D. Effect of teriparatide [rhPTH(1,34)] and calcitonin on intertransverse process fusion in a rabbit model. *Spine* **2010**, *35*, 146–152. [CrossRef] [PubMed]

73. Tokuyama, N.; Hirose, J.; Omata, Y.; Yasui, T.; Izawa, N.; Matsumoto, T.; Masuda, H.; Ohmiya, T.; Yasuda, H.; Saito, T.; et al. Individual and combining effects of anti-RANKL monoclonal antibody and teriparatide in ovariectomized mice. *Bone Rep.* **2015**, *2*, 1–7. [CrossRef] [PubMed]

74. Tsai, J.N.; Uihlein, A.V.; Lee, H.; Kumbhani, R.; Siwila-Sackman, E.; McKay, E.A.; Burnett-Bowie, S.A.; Neer, R.M.; Leder, B.Z. Teriparatide and denosumab, alone or combined, in women with postmenopausal osteoporosis: The DATA study randomised trial. *Lancet* **2013**, *382*, 50–56. [CrossRef]

75. Kitaguchi, K.; Kashii, M.; Ebina, K.; Kaito, T.; Okada, R.; Makino, T.; Noguchi, T.; Ishimoto, T.; Nakano, T.; Yoshikawa, H. Effects of single or combination therapy of teriparatide and anti-RANKL monoclonal antibody on bone defect regeneration in mice. *Bone* **2018**, *106*, 1–10. [CrossRef] [PubMed]

76. Ohtori, S.; Inoue, G.; Orita, S.; Yamauchi, K.; Eguchi, Y.; Ochiai, N.; Kishida, S.; Kuniyoshi, K.; Aoki, Y.; Nakamura, J.; et al. Teriparatide accelerates lumbar posterolateral fusion in women with postmenopausal osteoporosis: Prospective study. *Spine* **2012**, *37*, E1464–E1468. [CrossRef] [PubMed]

77. Ohtori, S.; Inoue, G.; Orita, S.; Yamauchi, K.; Eguchi, Y.; Ochiai, N.; Kishida, S.; Kuniyoshi, K.; Aoki, Y.; Nakamura, J.; et al. Comparison of teriparatide and bisphosphonate treatment to reduce pedicle screw loosening after lumbar spinal fusion surgery in postmenopausal women with osteoporosis from a bone quality perspective. *Spine* **2013**, *38*, E487–E492. [CrossRef] [PubMed]

78. Ohtori, S.; Orita, S.; Yamauchi, K.; Eguchi, Y.; Ochiai, N.; Kuniyoshi, K.; Aoki, Y.; Nakamura, J.; Miyagi, M.; Suzuki, M.; et al. More than 6 Months of Teriparatide Treatment Was More Effective for Bone Union than Shorter Treatment Following Lumbar Posterolateral Fusion Surgery. *Asian Spine J.* **2015**, *9*, 573–580. [CrossRef] [PubMed]

79. Cho, P.G.; Ji, G.Y.; Shin, D.A.; Ha, Y.; Yoon, D.H.; Kim, K.N. An effect comparison of teriparatide and bisphosphonate on posterior lumbar interbody fusion in patients with osteoporosis: A prospective cohort study and preliminary data. *Eur. Spine J.* **2017**, *26*, 691–697. [CrossRef] [PubMed]

80. Ebata, S.; Takahashi, J.; Hasegawa, T.; Mukaiyama, K.; Isogai, Y.; Ohba, T.; Shibata, Y.; Ojima, T.; Yamagata, Z.; Matsuyama, Y.; et al. Role of Weekly Teriparatide Administration in Osseous Union Enhancement within Six Months after Posterior or Transforaminal Lumbar Interbody Fusion for Osteoporosis-Associated Lumbar Degenerative Disorders: A Multicenter, Prospective Randomized Study. *J. Bone Joint Surg. Am. Vol.* **2017**, *99*, 365–372. [CrossRef] [PubMed]

81. Urist, M.R. Bone: Formation by autoinduction. *Science* **1965**, *150*, 893–899. [CrossRef] [PubMed]

82. Wozney, J.M.; Rosen, V.; Celeste, A.J.; Mitsock, L.M.; Whitters, M.J.; Kriz, R.W.; Hewick, R.M.; Wang, E.A. Novel regulators of bone formation: Molecular clones and activities. *Science* **1988**, *242*, 1528–1534. [CrossRef] [PubMed]

83. Lissenberg-Thunnissen, S.N.; de Gorter, D.J.; Sier, C.F.; Schipper, I.B. Use and efficacy of bone morphogenetic proteins in fracture healing. *Int. Orthop.* **2011**, *35*, 1271–1280. [CrossRef] [PubMed]

84. Bragdon, B.; Moseychuk, O.; Saldanha, S.; King, D.; Julian, J.; Nohe, A. Bone morphogenetic proteins: A critical review. *Cell. Signal.* **2011**, *23*, 609–620. [CrossRef] [PubMed]

85. Pneumaticos, S.G.; Triantafyllopoulos, G.K.; Basdra, E.K.; Papavassiliou, A.G. Segmental bone defects: From cellular and molecular pathways to the development of novel biological treatments. *J. Cell. Mol. Med.* **2010**, *14*, 2561–2569. [CrossRef] [PubMed]

86. Mahendra, A.; Maclean, A.D. Available biological treatments for complex non-unions. *Injury* **2007**, *38* (Suppl. 4), S7–S12. [CrossRef]

87. Burkus, J.K.; Heim, S.E.; Gornet, M.F.; Zdeblick, T.A. Is INFUSE bone graft superior to autograft bone? An integrated analysis of clinical trials using the LT-CAGE lumbar tapered fusion device. *J. Spinal Disord. Tech.* **2003**, *16*, 113–122. [CrossRef] [PubMed]

88. Burkus, J.K.; Sandhu, H.S.; Gornet, M.F.; Longley, M.C. Use of rhBMP-2 in combination with structural cortical allografts: Clinical and radiographic outcomes in anterior lumbar spinal surgery. *J. Bone Joint Surg. Am. Vol.* **2005**, *87*, 1205–1212. [CrossRef]

89. Simmonds, M.C.; Brown, J.V.; Heirs, M.K.; Higgins, J.P.; Mannion, R.J.; Rodgers, M.A.; Stewart, L.A. Safety and effectiveness of recombinant human bone morphogenetic protein-2 for spinal fusion: A meta-analysis of individual-participant data. *Ann. Intern. Med.* **2013**, *158*, 877–889. [CrossRef] [PubMed]

90. Martin, B.I.; Lurie, J.D.; Tosteson, A.N.; Deyo, R.A.; Farrokhi, F.R.; Mirza, S.K. Use of bone morphogenetic protein among patients undergoing fusion for degenerative diagnoses in the United States, 2002 to 2012. *Spine J.* **2015**, *15*, 692–699. [CrossRef] [PubMed]

91. McClellan, J.W.; Mulconrey, D.S.; Forbes, R.J.; Fullmer, N. Vertebral bone resorption after transforaminal lumbar interbody fusion with bone morphogenetic protein (rhBMP-2). *Clin. Spine Surg.* **2006**, *19*, 483–486. [CrossRef] [PubMed]

92. Shields, L.B.; Raque, G.H.; Glassman, S.D.; Campbell, M.; Vitaz, T.; Harpring, J.; Shields, C.B. Adverse effects associated with high-dose recombinant human bone morphogenetic protein-2 use in anterior cervical spine fusion. *Spine* **2006**, *31*, 542–547. [CrossRef] [PubMed]

93. Seeherman, H.; Wozney, J.M. Delivery of bone morphogenetic proteins for orthopedic tissue regeneration. *Cytokine Growth Factor Rev.* **2005**, *16*, 329–345. [CrossRef] [PubMed]

94. Boden, S.D.; Martin, G.J., Jr.; Morone, M.A.; Ugbo, J.L.; Moskovitz, P.A. Posterolateral lumbar intertransverse process spine arthrodesis with recombinant human bone morphogenetic protein 2/hydroxyapatite-tricalcium phosphate after laminectomy in the nonhuman primate. *Spine* **1999**, *24*, 1179–1185. [CrossRef] [PubMed]

95. Kaito, T.; Morimoto, T.; Mori, Y.; Kanayama, S.; Makino, T.; Takenaka, S.; Sakai, Y.; Otsuru, S.; Yoshioka, Y.; Yoshikawa, H. BMP-2/7 heterodimer strongly induces bone regeneration in the absence of increased soft tissue inflammation. *Spine J.* **2018**, *18*, 139–146. [CrossRef] [PubMed]

96. Morimoto, T.; Kaito, T.; Kashii, M.; Matsuo, Y.; Sugiura, T.; Iwasaki, M.; Yoshikawa, H. Effect of Intermittent Administration of Teriparatide (Parathyroid Hormone 1–34) on Bone Morphogenetic Protein-Induced Bone Formation in a Rat Model of Spinal Fusion. *J. Bone Joint Surg. Am. Vol.* **2014**, *96*, e107. [CrossRef] [PubMed]

97. Kaito, T.; Morimoto, T.; Kanayama, S.; Otsuru, S.; Kashii, M.; Makino, T.; Kitaguchi, K.; Furuya, M.; Chijimatsu, R.; Ebina, K.; et al. Modeling and remodeling effects of intermittent administration of teriparatide (parathyroid hormone 1–34) on bone morphogenetic protein-induced bone in a rat spinal fusion model. *Bone Rep.* **2016**, *5*, 173–180. [CrossRef] [PubMed]

98. Kaito, T.; Johnson, J.; Ellerman, J.; Tian, H.; Aydogan, M.; Chatsrinopkun, M.; Ngo, S.; Choi, C.; Wang, J.C. Synergistic effect of bone morphogenetic proteins 2 and 7 by ex vivo gene therapy in a rat spinal fusion model. *J. Bone Joint Surg. Am. Vol.* **2013**, *95*, 1612–1619. [CrossRef] [PubMed]

99. Suzuki, A.; Kaneko, E.; Maeda, J.; Ueno, N. Mesoderm induction by BMP-4 and -7 heterodimers. *Biochem. Biophys. Res. Commun.* **1997**, *232*, 153–156. [CrossRef] [PubMed]

100. Valera, E.; Isaacs, M.J.; Kawakami, Y.; Izpisua Belmonte, J.C.; Choe, S. BMP-2/6 heterodimer is more effective than BMP-2 or BMP-6 homodimers as inductor of differentiation of human embryonic stem cells. *PLoS ONE* **2010**, *5*, e11167. [CrossRef] [PubMed]

101. Guo, J.; Wu, G. The signaling and functions of heterodimeric bone morphogenetic proteins. *Cytokine Growth Factor Rev.* **2012**, *23*, 61–67. [CrossRef] [PubMed]

102. Isaacs, M.J.; Kawakami, Y.; Allendorph, G.P.; Yoon, B.H.; Izpisua Belmonte, J.C.; Choe, S. Bone morphogenetic protein-2 and -6 heterodimer illustrates the nature of ligand-receptor assembly. *Mol. Endocrinol.* **2010**, *24*, 1469–1477. [CrossRef] [PubMed]

103. Zhu, W.; Kim, J.; Cheng, C.; Rawlins, B.A.; Boachie-Adjei, O.; Crystal, R.G.; Hidaka, C. Noggin regulation of bone morphogenetic protein (BMP) 2/7 heterodimer activity in vitro. *Bone* **2006**, *39*, 61–71. [CrossRef] [PubMed]

104. El Bialy, I.; Jiskoot, W.; Reza Nejadnik, M. Formulation, Delivery and Stability of Bone Morphogenetic Proteins for Effective Bone Regeneration. *Pharm. Res.* **2017**, *34*, 1152–1170. [CrossRef] [PubMed]

105. Subramanian, G.; Bialorucki, C.; Yildirim-Ayan, E. Nanofibrous yet injectable polycaprolactone-collagen bone tissue scaffold with osteoprogenitor cells and controlled release of bone morphogenetic protein-2. *Mater. Sci. Eng. C Mater. Biol. Appl.* **2015**, *51*, 16–27. [CrossRef] [PubMed]

106. Ben-David, D.; Srouji, S.; Shapira-Schweitzer, K.; Kossover, O.; Ivanir, E.; Kuhn, G.; Muller, R.; Seliktar, D.; Livne, E. Low dose BMP-2 treatment for bone repair using a PEGylated fibrinogen hydrogel matrix. *Biomaterials* **2013**, *34*, 2902–2910. [CrossRef] [PubMed]

107. Lee, E.U.; Lim, H.C.; Hong, J.Y.; Lee, J.S.; Jung, U.W.; Choi, S.H. Bone regenerative efficacy of biphasic calcium phosphate collagen composite as a carrier of rhBMP-2. *Clin. Oral Implants Res.* **2016**, *27*, e91–e99. [CrossRef] [PubMed]

108. Compton, J.T.; Lee, F.Y. A review of osteocyte function and the emerging importance of sclerostin. *J. Bone Joint Surg. Am. Vol.* **2014**, *96*, 1659–1668. [CrossRef] [PubMed]

109. Poole, K.E.; van Bezooijen, R.L.; Loveridge, N.; Hamersma, H.; Papapoulos, S.E.; Lowik, C.W.; Reeve, J. Sclerostin is a delayed secreted product of osteocytes that inhibits bone formation. *FASEB J.* **2005**, *19*, 1842–1844. [CrossRef] [PubMed]

110. Weivoda, M.M.; Youssef, S.J.; Oursler, M.J. Sclerostin expression and functions beyond the osteocyte. *Bone* **2017**, *96*, 45–50. [CrossRef] [PubMed]

111. Balemans, W.; Ebeling, M.; Patel, N.; Van Hul, E.; Olson, P.; Dioszegi, M.; Lacza, C.; Wuyts, W.; Van Den Ende, J.; Willems, P.; et al. Increased bone density in sclerosteosis is due to the deficiency of a novel secreted protein (SOST). *Hum. Mol. Genet.* **2001**, *10*, 537–543. [CrossRef] [PubMed]

112. Brunkow, M.E.; Gardner, J.C.; Van Ness, J.; Paeper, B.W.; Kovacevich, B.R.; Proll, S.; Skonier, J.E.; Zhao, L.; Sabo, P.J.; Fu, Y.; et al. Bone dysplasia sclerosteosis results from loss of the SOST gene product, a novel cystine knot-containing protein. *Am. J. Hum. Genet.* **2001**, *68*, 577–589. [CrossRef] [PubMed]

113. Van Bezooijen, R.L.; Deruiter, M.C.; Vilain, N.; Monteiro, R.M.; Visser, A.; van der Wee-Pals, L.; van Munsteren, C.J.; Hogendoorn, P.C.; Aguet, M.; Mummery, C.L.; et al. SOST expression is restricted to the great arteries during embryonic and neonatal cardiovascular development. *Dev. Dyn.* **2007**, *236*, 606–612. [CrossRef] [PubMed]

114. Ott, S.M. Sclerostin and Wnt signaling—The pathway to bone strength. *J. Clin. Endocrinol. Metab.* **2005**, *90*, 6741–6743. [CrossRef] [PubMed]

115. Ten Dijke, P.; Krause, C.; de Gorter, D.J.; Lowik, C.W.; van Bezooijen, R.L. Osteocyte-derived sclerostin inhibits bone formation: Its role in bone morphogenetic protein and Wnt signaling. *J. Bone Joint Surg. Am. Vol.* **2008**, *90* (Suppl. 1), 31–35. [CrossRef] [PubMed]

116. Winkler, D.G.; Sutherland, M.K.; Geoghegan, J.C.; Yu, C.; Hayes, T.; Skonier, J.E.; Shpektor, D.; Jonas, M.; Kovacevich, B.R.; Staehling-Hampton, K.; et al. Osteocyte control of bone formation via sclerostin, a novel BMP antagonist. *EMBO J.* **2003**, *22*, 6267–6276. [CrossRef] [PubMed]

117. Cosman, F.; Crittenden, D.B.; Adachi, J.D.; Binkley, N.; Czerwinski, E.; Ferrari, S.; Hofbauer, L.C.; Lau, E.; Lewiecki, E.M.; Miyauchi, A.; et al. Romosozumab Treatment in Postmenopausal Women with Osteoporosis. *N. Engl. J. Med.* **2016**, *375*, 1532–1543. [CrossRef] [PubMed]

118. Liu, Y.; Cao, Y.; Zhang, S.; Zhang, W.; Zhang, B.; Tang, Q.; Li, Z.; Wu, J. Romosozumab treatment in postmenopausal women with osteoporosis: A meta-analysis of randomized controlled trials. *Climacteric* **2018**, *21*, 1–7. [CrossRef] [PubMed]

119. McClung, M.R. Sclerostin antibodies in osteoporosis: Latest evidence and therapeutic potential. *Ther. Adv. Musculoskelet. Dis.* **2017**, *9*, 263–270. [CrossRef] [PubMed]

120. Gao, F.; Zhang, C.-Q.; Chai, Y.-M.; Li, X.-L. Systemic administration of sclerostin monoclonal antibody accelerates fracture healing in the femoral osteotomy model of young rats. *Int. Immunopharmacol.* **2015**, *24*, 7–13.

121. Liu, Y.; Rui, Y.; Cheng, T.Y.; Huang, S.; Xu, L.; Meng, F.; Lee, W.Y.; Zhang, T.; Li, N.; Li, C.; et al. Effects of Sclerostin Antibody on the Healing of Femoral Fractures in Ovariectomised Rats. *Calcif. Tissue Int.* **2016**, *98*, 263–274. [CrossRef] [PubMed]

122. Suen, P.K.; He, Y.X.; Chow, D.H.; Huang, L.; Li, C.; Ke, H.Z.; Ominsky, M.S.; Qin, L. Sclerostin monoclonal antibody enhanced bone fracture healing in an open osteotomy model in rats. *J. Orthop. Res.* **2014**, *32*, 997–1005. [CrossRef] [PubMed]

123. Suen, P.K.; Zhu, T.Y.; Chow, D.H.; Huang, L.; Zheng, L.Z.; Qin, L. Sclerostin Antibody Treatment Increases Bone Formation, Bone Mass, and Bone Strength of Intact Bones in Adult Male Rats. *Sci. Rep.* **2015**, *5*, 15632. [CrossRef] [PubMed]

124. Virk, M.S.; Alaee, F.; Tang, H.; Ominsky, M.S.; Ke, H.Z.; Lieberman, J.R. Systemic administration of sclerostin antibody enhances bone repair in a critical-sized femoral defect in a rat model. *J. Bone Joint Surg. Am. Vol.* **2013**, *95*, 694–701. [CrossRef] [PubMed]

125. Fracon, R.N.; Teofilo, J.M.; Satin, R.B.; Lamano, T. Prostaglandins and bone: Potential risks and benefits related to the use of nonsteroidal anti-inflammatory drugs in clinical dentistry. *J. Oral Sci.* **2008**, *50*, 247–252. [CrossRef] [PubMed]

126. Abdul-Hadi, O.; Parvizi, J.; Austin, M.S.; Viscusi, E.; Einhorn, T. Nonsteroidal anti-inflammatory drugs in orthopaedics. *J. Bone Joint Surg. Am. Vol.* **2009**, *91*, 2020–2027.

127. Yoshida, K.; Oida, H.; Kobayashi, T.; Maruyama, T.; Tanaka, M.; Katayama, T.; Yamaguchi, K.; Segi, E.; Tsuboyama, T.; Matsushita, M.; et al. Stimulation of bone formation and prevention of bone loss by prostaglandin E EP4 receptor activation. *Proc. Natl. Acad. Sci. USA* **2002**, *99*, 4580–4585. [CrossRef] [PubMed]

128. Dumont, A.S.; Verma, S.; Dumont, R.J.; Hurlbert, R.J. Nonsteroidal anti-inflammatory drugs and bone metabolism in spinal fusion surgery: A pharmacological quandary. *J. Pharmacol. Toxicol. Methods* **2000**, *43*, 31–39. [CrossRef]

129. Graham, S.; Gamie, Z.; Polyzois, I.; Narvani, A.A.; Tzafetta, K.; Tsiridis, E.; Helioti, M.; Mantalaris, A.; Tsiridis, E. Prostaglandin EP2 and EP4 receptor agonists in bone formation and bone healing: In vivo and in vitro evidence. *Expert Opin. Investig. Drugs* **2009**, *18*, 746–766. [CrossRef] [PubMed]

130. Nakagawa, K.; Imai, Y.; Ohta, Y.; Takaoka, K. Prostaglandin E2 EP4 agonist (ONO-4819) accelerates BMP-induced osteoblastic differentiation. *Bone* **2007**, *41*, 543–548. [CrossRef] [PubMed]

131. Namikawa, T.; Terai, H.; Hoshino, M.; Kato, M.; Toyoda, H.; Yano, K.; Nakamura, H.; Takaoka, K. Enhancing effects of a prostaglandin EP4 receptor agonist on recombinant human bone morphogenetic protein-2 mediated spine fusion in a rabbit model. *Spine* **2007**, *32*, 2294–2299. [CrossRef] [PubMed]

132. Pagkalos, J.; Leonidou, A.; As-Sultany, M.; Heliotis, M.; Mantalaris, A.; Tsiridis, E. Prostaglandin E(2) receptors as potential bone anabolic targets—Selective EP4 receptor agonists. *Curr. Mol. Pharmacol.* **2012**, *5*, 174–181. [CrossRef] [PubMed]

133. Kanayama, S.; Kaito, T.; Kitaguchi, K.; Ishiguro, H.; Hashimoto, K.; Chijimatsu, R.; Otsuru, S.; Takenaka, S.; Makino, T.; Sakai, Y.; et al. ONO-1301 Enhances in vitro Osteoblast Differentiation and in vivo Bone Formation Induced by Bone Morphogenetic Protein. *Spine* **2017**, *43*, E616–E624. [CrossRef] [PubMed]

134. Barba, M.; Cicione, C.; Bernardini, C.; Campana, V.; Pagano, E.; Michetti, F.; Logroscino, G.; Lattanzi, W. Spinal fusion in the next generation: Gene and cell therapy approaches. *Sci. World J.* **2014**, *2014*, 406159. [CrossRef] [PubMed]

135. Khashan, M.; Inoue, S.; Berven, S.H. Cell based therapies as compared to autologous bone grafts for spinal arthrodesis. *Spine* **2013**, *38*, 1885–1891. [CrossRef] [PubMed]

136. Barbanti Brodano, G.; Terzi, S.; Trombi, L.; Griffoni, C.; Valtieri, M.; Boriani, S.; Magli, M.C. Mesenchymal stem cells derived from vertebrae (vMSCs) show best biological properties. *Eur. Spine J.* **2013**, *22* (Suppl. 6), S979–S984. [CrossRef] [PubMed]

137. Risbud, M.V.; Shapiro, I.M.; Guttapalli, A.; Di Martino, A.; Danielson, K.G.; Beiner, J.M.; Hillibrand, A.; Albert, T.J.; Anderson, D.G.; Vaccaro, A.R. Osteogenic potential of adult human stem cells of the lumbar vertebral body and the iliac crest. *Spine* **2006**, *31*, 83–89. [CrossRef] [PubMed]

138. Beederman, M.; Lamplot, J.D.; Nan, G.; Wang, J.; Liu, X.; Yin, L.; Li, R.; Shui, W.; Zhang, H.; Kim, S.H.; et al. BMP signaling in mesenchymal stem cell differentiation and bone formation. *J. Biomed. Sci. Eng.* **2013**, *6*, 32–52. [CrossRef] [PubMed]

139. Nakajima, T.; Iizuka, H.; Tsutsumi, S.; Kayakabe, M.; Takagishi, K. Evaluation of posterolateral spinal fusion using mesenchymal stem cells: Differences with or without osteogenic differentiation. *Spine* **2007**, *15*, 2432–2436. [CrossRef] [PubMed]

140. Yang, W.; Dong, Y.; Hong, Y.; Guang, Q.; Chen, X. Evaluation of Anterior Vertebral Interbody Fusion Using Osteogenic Mesenchymal Stem Cells Transplanted in Collagen Sponge. *Clin. Spine Surg.* **2016**, *29*, E201–E207. [CrossRef] [PubMed]

141. Skovrlj, B.; Guzman, J.Z.; Al Maaieh, M.; Cho, S.K.; Iatridis, J.C.; Qureshi, S.A. Cellular bone matrices: Viable stem cell-containing bone graft substitutes. *Spine J.* **2014**, *14*, 2763–2772. [CrossRef] [PubMed]

142. Parekkadan, B.; Milwid, J.M. Mesenchymal stem cells as therapeutics. *Annu. Rev. Biomed. Eng.* **2010**, *12*, 87–117. [CrossRef] [PubMed]

143. Muschler, G.F.; Midura, R.J. Connective tissue progenitors: Practical concepts for clinical applications. *Clin. Orthop. Relat. Res.* **2002**, *395*, 66–80. [CrossRef]

144. Livingston, T.L.; Gordon, S.; Archambault, M.; Kadiyala, S.; McIntosh, K.; Smith, A.; Peter, S.J. Mesenchymal stem cells combined with biphasic calcium phosphate ceramics promote bone regeneration. *J. Mater. Sci. Mater. Med.* **2003**, *14*, 211–218. [CrossRef] [PubMed]

145. Yousef, M.A.A.; La Maida, G.A.; Misaggi, B. Long-term Radiological and Clinical Outcomes after Using Bone Marrow Mesenchymal Stem Cells Concentrate Obtained with Selective Retention Cell Technology in Posterolateral Spinal Fusion. *Spine* **2017**, *42*, 1871–1879. [CrossRef] [PubMed]

146. Lou, X. Induced Pluripotent Stem Cells as a new Strategy for Osteogenesis and Bone Regeneration. *Stem Cell Rev.* **2015**, *11*, 645–651. [CrossRef] [PubMed]

147. Douglas, J.T.; Rivera, A.A.; Lyons, G.R.; Lott, P.F.; Wang, D.; Zayzafoon, M.; Siegal, G.P.; Cao, X.; Theiss, S.M. Ex vivo transfer of the Hoxc-8-interacting domain of Smad1 by a tropism-modified adenoviral vector results in efficient bone formation in a rabbit model of spinal fusion. *J. Spinal Disord. Tech.* **2010**, *23*, 63–73. [CrossRef] [PubMed]

148. Lu, S.S.; Zhang, X.; Soo, C.; Hsu, T.; Napoli, A.; Aghaloo, T.; Wu, B.M.; Tsou, P.; Ting, K.; Wang, J.C. The osteoinductive properties of Nell-1 in a rat spinal fusion model. *Spine J.* **2007**, *7*, 50–60. [CrossRef] [PubMed]

149. Viggeswarapu, M.; Boden, S.D.; Liu, Y.; Hair, G.A.; Louis-Ugbo, J.; Murakami, H.; Kim, H.S.; Mayr, M.T.; Hutton, W.C.; Titus, L. Adenoviral delivery of LIM mineralization protein-1 induces new-bone formation in vitro and in vivo. *J. Bone Joint Surg. Am. Vol.* **2001**, *83*, 364–376. [CrossRef]

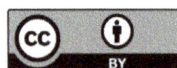

MDPI

St. Alban-Anlage 66

4052 Basel

Switzerland

Tel. +41 61 683 77 34

Fax +41 61 302 89 18

www.mdpi.com

International Journal of Molecular Sciences Editorial Office

E-mail: ijms@mdpi.com

www.mdpi.com/journal/ijms

www.ingramcontent.com/pod-product-compliance
Lightning Source LLC
Chambersburg PA
CBHW051710210326
41597CB00032B/5432